Information Retrieval in Biomedicine:
Natural Language Processing for Knowledge Integration

Violaine Prince
University Montpellier 2, France & LIRMM-CNRS, France

Mathieu Roche
University Montpellier 2, France & LIRMM-CNRS, France

MEDICAL INFORMATION SCIENCE REFERENCE

Hershey · New York

Director of Editorial Content: Kristin Klinger
Senior Managing Editor: Jamie Snavely
Managing Editor: Jeff Ash
Assistant Managing Editor: Carole Coulson
Typesetter: Amanda Appicello
Cover Design: Lisa Tosheff
Printed at: Yurchak Printing Inc.

Published in the United States of America by
Information Science Reference (an imprint of IGI Global)
701 E. Chocolate Avenue
Hershey PA 17033
Tel: 717-533-8845
Fax: 717-533-8661
E-mail: cust@igi-global.com
Web site: http://www.igi-global.com/reference

and in the United Kingdom by
Information Science Reference (an imprint of IGI Global)
3 Henrietta Street
Covent Garden
London WC2E 8LU
Tel: 44 20 7240 0856
Fax: 44 20 7379 0609
Web site: http://www.eurospanbookstore.com

Library of Congress Cataloging-in-Publication Data

Information retrieval in biomedicine : natural language processing for knowledge integration / Violaine Prince and Mathieu Roche, editors.
p. cm.
Includes bibliographical references and index.
Summary: "This book provides relevant theoretical frameworks and the latest empirical research findings in biomedicine information retrieval as it pertains to linguistic granularity"--Provided by publisher.
ISBN 978-1-60566-274-9 (hardcover) -- ISBN 978-1-60566-275-6 (ebook) 1. Medical informatics. 2. Biotechnology--Data processing. 3. Information storage and retrieval systems--Medical care. I. Prince, Violaine, 1958- II. Roche, Mathieu, 1975-
R858.I536 2009
651.5'04261--dc22

2008043763

British Cataloguing in Publication Data
A Cataloguing in Publication record for this book is available from the British Library.

Table of Contents

Detailed Table of Contents

Text mining provides the automated means to manage information overload and overlook. By adding meaning to text, text mining techniques produce a much more structured analysis of textual knowledge than do simple word searches, and can provide powerful tools for knowledge discovery in biomedicine. In this chapter, the authors focus on the text mining services for biomedicine offered by the United Kingdom National Centre for Text Mining.

The identification and mapping of terminology from large repositories of life science data onto concept hierarchies constitute an important initial step for a deeper semantic exploration of unstructured textual content. Accurate and efficient mapping of this kind is likely to provide better means of enhancing indexing and retrieval of text, uncovering subtle differences, similarities and useful patterns, and hopefully new knowledge, among complex surface realisations, overlooked by shallow techniques based on various forms of lexicon look-up approaches. However, a finer-grained level of mapping between terms as they occur in natural language and domain concepts is a cumbersome enterprise that requires various levels of processing in order to make explicit relevant linguistic structures. This chapter highlights some of the challenges encountered in the process of bridging free to controlled vocabularies and thesauri and vice versa. It investigates how the extensive variability of lexical terms in authentic data can be efficiently projected to hierarchically structured codes, while means to increase the coverage of the underlying lexical resources are also investigated.

This chapter argues for the integration of clinical knowledge extracted from medical ontologies in order to improve a Multi-Label Text Categorization (MLTC) system for medical domain. The approach is based on the concept of semantic enrichment by integrating knowledge in different biomedical collections. Specifically, the authors expand terms from these collections using the UMLS (Unified Medical Language System) metathesaurus. This resource includes several medical ontologies. The authors have managed two rather different medical collections: first, the CCHMC collection (Cincinnati Children's Hospital Medical Centre) from the Department of Radiology, and second, the widely used OHSUMED collection. The results obtained show that the use of the medical ontologies improves the system performance.

The present chapter discusses the use of terminological resources for Information Retrieval in the biomedical domain. It first introduces a number of example resources which can be used to compile terminologies for biomedical IR. The authors explain some of the common problems with such resources including redundancy, term ambiguity, insufficient coverage of concepts, and incomplete semantic organization of such resources for text mining purposes. They also discuss some techniques used to address each of these deficiencies, such as static polysemy detection as well as adding terms and linguistic annotation from the running text. In the second part of the chapter, the authors show how query expansion based on using synonyms of the original query terms derived from terminological resources potentially increases the recall of IR systems. Special care is needed to prevent a query drift produced by the usage of the added terms and high quality word sense disambiguation algorithms can be used to allow more conservative query expansion. In addition, the authors present solutions that help focus on the user's specific information need by navigating and rearranging the retrieved documents. Finally, they explain the advantages of applying terminological and semantic resources at indexing time. The authors argue that by creating a semantic index with terms disambiguated for the term's semantic types and larger chunks of text denoting entities and relations between them, they can facilitate query expansion, reduce the need for query refinement and increase the overall performance of Information Retrieval. Semantic indexing also provides support for generic queries for concept categories, such as genes or diseases, rather than singular keywords.

The automatic alignment between a specialized terminology used by librarians in order to index concepts and a general vocabulary employed by a neophyte user in order to retrieve medical information will certainly improve the performances of the search process, this being one of the purposes of the ANR VODEL project. The authors propose an original automatic alignment of definitions taken from different dictionaries that could be associated to the same concept although they may have different labels. The definitions are represented at different levels (lexical, semantic and syntactic), by using an original and shorter representation, which concatenates more similarities measures between definitions, instead of the classical one (as a vector of word occurrence, whose length equals the number of different words from all the dictionaries). The automatic alignment task is considered as a classification problem and three Machine Learning algorithms are utilised in order to solve it: a *k* Nearest Neighbour algorithm, an Evolutionary Algorithm and a Support Vector Machine algorithm. Numerical results indicate that the syntactic level of nouns seems to be the most important, determining the best performances of the SVM classifier.

This chapter presents a simple yet efficient approach to translate automatically unknown biomedical terms from one language into another. This approach relies on a machine learning process able to infer rewriting rules from examples, that is, from a list of paired terms in two studied languages. Any new term is then simply translated by applying the rewriting rules to it. When different translations are produced by conflicting rewriting rules, the authors use language modeling to single out the best candidate. The experiments reported here show that this technique yields very good results for different language pairs (including Czech, English, French, Italian, Portuguese, Spanish and even Russian). They also show how this translation technique could be used in a cross-language information retrieval task and thus complete the dictionary-based existing approaches.

This chapter is concerned with lexical enrichment of ontologies, that is, how to enrich a given ontology with lexical information derived from a semantic lexicon such as WordNet or other lexical resources. The authors present an approach towards the integration of both types of resources, in particular for the human anatomy domain as represented by the Foundational Model of Anatomy and for the molecular biology domain as represented by an ontology of biochemical substances. The chapter describes their approach on enriching these biomedical ontologies with information derived from WordNet and Wikipedia by matching ontology class labels to entries in WordNet and Wikipedia. In the first case, they acquire WordNet synonyms for the ontology class label, whereas in the second case they acquire multilingual translations as provided by Wikipedia. A particular point of emphasis here is on selecting the appropriate interpretation of ambiguous ontology class labels through sense disambiguation, which they address by use of a simple algorithm that selects the most likely sense for an ambiguous term by statistical significance of co-occurring words in a domain corpus. Acquired synonyms and translations are added to the ontology by use of the LingInfo model, which provides an ontology-based lexicon model for the annotation of ontology classes with (multilingual) terms and their linguistic properties.

Ambiguity is a common phenomenon in text, especially in the biomedical domain. For instance, it is frequently the case that a gene, a protein encoded by the gene, and a disease associated with the protein share the same name. Resolving this problem, that is assigning to an ambiguous word in a given context its correct meaning is called word sense disambiguation (WSD). It is a pre-requisite for associating entities in text to external identifiers and thus to put the results from text mining into a larger knowledge framework. In this chapter, the authors introduce the WSD problem and sketch general approaches for solving it. They then describe in detail the results of a study in WSD using classification. For each sense of an ambiguous term, they collected a large number of exemplary texts automatically and used them to train an SVM-based classifier. This method reaches a median success rate of 97%. They also provide an analysis of potential sources and methods to obtain training examples, which proved to be the most difficult part of this study.

Protein posttranslational modification (PTM) is a fundamental biological process, and currently few text mining systems focus on PTM information extraction. A rule-based text mining system, RLIMS-P (Rule-based LIterature Mining System for Protein Phosphorylation), was recently developed by our group to extract protein substrate, kinase and phosphorylated residue/sites from MEDLINE abstracts. This chapter covers the evaluation and benchmarking of RLIMS-P and highlights some novel and unique features of the system. The extraction patterns of RLIMS-P capture a range of lexical, syntactic and semantic constraints found in sentences expressing phosphorylation information. RLIMS-P also has a second phase that puts together information extracted from different sentences. This is an important feature since it is not common to find the kinase, substrate and site of phosphorylation to be mentioned in the same sentence. Small modifications to the rules for extraction of phosphorylation information have also allowed us to develop systems for extraction of two other PTMs, acetylation and methylation. A thorough evaluation of these two systems needs to be completed. Finally, an online version of RLIMS-P with enhanced functionalities, namely, phosphorylation annotation ranking, evidence tagging, and protein entity mapping, has been developed and is publicly accessible.

This chapter argues that in order to extract significant knowledge from masses of technical texts, it is necessary to provide the field specialists with programming tools with which they themselves may use to program their text analysis tools. These programming tools, besides helping the programming effort of the field specialists, must also help them to gather the field knowledge necessary for defining and retrieving what they define as significant knowledge. This necessary field knowledge must be included in a well-structured and easy to use part of the programming tool. The authors illustrate their argument by presenting a programming language, CorTag, which they have built in order to correct existing tags in a text, while trying to follow the informal specification given above.

The task of question answering (QA) is to find an accurate and precise answer to a natural language question in some predefined text. Most existing QA systems handle fact-based questions that usually take named entities as the answers. In this chapter, the authors take clinical QA as an example to deal with more complex information needs. They propose an approach using semantic class analysis as the organizing principle to answer clinical questions. They investigate three semantic classes that correspond to roles in the commonly accepted PICO format of describing clinical scenarios. The three semantic classes are: the description of the patient (or the problem), the intervention used to treat the problem, and the clinical outcome. They focus on automatic analysis of two important properties of the semantic classes.

Section III
Pragmatics, Discourse Structures and Segment Level as the Last Stage in the NLP Offer to Biomedicine

This chapter presents the challenge of integrating knowledge at higher levels of discourse than the sentence, to avoid "missing the forest for the trees". Characterisation tasks aimed at filtering collections are introduced, showing use of the whole set of layout constituents from sentence to text body. Few text descriptors encapsulating knowledge on text properties are used for each granularity level. Text processing differs according to tasks, whether individual document mining or tagging small or large collections prior to information extraction. Very shallow and domain independent techniques are used to tag collections to save costs on sentence parsing and semantic manual annotation. This approach achieves satisfactory characterisation of text types, for example, reviews versus clinical reports, or argumentation-type articles versus explanation-type. These collection filtering techniques are fit for a wider domain of biomedical literature than genomics.

In this chapter, a non-linear relevance feedback mechanism is proposed for increasing the performance and the reliability of information (medical content) retrieval systems. In greater detail, the user who searches for information is considered to be part of the retrieval process in an interactive framework, who evaluates the results provided by the system so that the user automatically updates its performance based on the users' feedback. In order to achieve the latter, the authors propose an adaptively trained neural network (NN) architecture that is able to implement the non-linear feedback. The term "adaptively" refers to the functionality of the neural network to update its weights based on the user's content selection and optimize its performance.

The fast growing content of online articles of clinical case studies provides a useful source for extracting domain-specific knowledge for improving healthcare systems. However, current studies are more focused on the abstract of a published case study which contains little information about the detailed case profiles of a patient, such as symptoms and signs, and important laboratory test results of the patient from the diagnostic and treatment procedures. This chapter proposes a novel category set to cover a wide variety of semantics in the description of clinical case studies which distinguishes each unique patient case. A manually annotated corpus consisting of over 5,000 sentences from 75 journal articles of clinical case studies has been created. A sentence classification system which identifies 13 classes of clinically relevant content has been developed. A golden standard for assessing the automatic classifications has been established by manual annotation. A maximum entropy (MaxEnt) classifier is shown to produce better results than a Support Vector Machine (SVM) classifier on the corpus.

Section IV
NLP Software for IR in Biomedicine

SNPs constitute key elements in genetic epidemiology and pharmacogenomics. While data about genetic variation is found at sequence databases, functional and phenotypic information on consequences of the variations resides in literature. Literature mining is mainly hampered by the terminology problem. Thus, automatic systems for the identification of citations of allelic variants of genes in biomedical texts are required. The authors have reported the development of OSIRIS, aimed at retrieving literature about allelic variants of genes, a system that evolved towards a new version incorporating a new entity recognition module. The new version is based on a terminology of variations and a pattern-based search algorithm for the identification of variation terms and their disambiguation to dbSNP identifiers. OSIRISv1.2 can be used to link literature references to dbSNP database entries with high accuracy, and is suitable for collecting current knowledge on gene sequence variations for supporting the functional annotation of variation databases.

Molecular Biology research projects produced vast amounts of data, part of which has been preserved in a variety of public databases. However, a large portion of the data contains a significant number of errors and therefore requires careful verification by curators, a painful and costly task, before being reliable enough to derive valid conclusions from it. On the other hand, research in biomedical information retrieval and information extraction are nowadays delivering Text Mining solutions that can support curators to improve the efficiency of their work to deliver better data resources. Over the past decades, automatic text processing systems have successfully exploited biomedical scientific literature to reduce the researchers' efforts to keep up to date, but many of these systems still rely on domain knowledge that is integrated manually leading to unnecessary overheads and restrictions in its use. A more efficient approach would acquire the domain knowledge automatically from publicly available biological sources, such as BioOntologies, rather than using manually inserted domain knowledge. An example of this approach is GOAnnotator, a tool that assists the verification of uncurated protein annotations. It provided correct evidence text at 93% precision to the curators and thus achieved promising results. GOAnnotator was implemented as a web tool that is freely available at http://xldb.di.fc.ul.pt/rebil/tools/goa/.

ABNER (A Biomedical Named Entity Recognizer) is an open-source software tool for text mining in the molecular biology literature. It processes unstructured biomedical documents in order to discover and annotate mentions of genes, proteins, cell types, and other entities of interest. This task, known as *named entity recognition* (NER), is an important first step for many larger information management goals in biomedicine, namely extraction of biochemical relationships, document classification, information retrieval, and the like. To accomplish this task, ABNER uses state-of-the-art machine learning models for sequence labeling called *conditional random fields* (CRFs). The software distribution comes bundled with two models that are pre-trained on standard evaluation corpora. ABNER can run as a stand-alone application with a graphical user interface, or be accessed as a Java API allowing it to be re-trained with new labeled corpora and incorporated into other, higher-level applications. This chapter describes the software and its features, presents an overview of the underlying technology, and provides a discussion of some of the more advanced natural language processing systems for which ABNER has been used as a component. ABNER is open-source and freely available from http://pages.cs.wisc.edu/~bsettles/abner/

Valuable knowledge has been distributed in heterogeneous formats on many different Web sites and other sources over the Internet. However, finding the needed information is a complex task since there is a lack of semantic relations and organization between them. This chapter presents a problem-solving map framework for extracting and integrating knowledge from unstructured documents on the Inter-

computational linguists but need to be revisited for this entirely new genre of materials. In returning to the past and studying the contents of these materials in retrospective studies the authors can plan to go forward to a future that provides technologies that better support clinicians. They need to produce both lexically and grammatically higher quality texts that can then be leveraged successfully for advanced translational research thereby bolstering its momentum.

Preface

NEEDS AND REQUIREMENTS IN INFORMATION RETRIEVAL AND KNOWLEDGE MANAGEMENT FOR BIOLOGY AND MEDICINE

Natural language processing (NLP) is a sub-field of computational sciences which addresses the operation and management of texts, as inputs or outputs of computational devices. As such, this domain includes a large amount of distinct topics, depending which particular service is considered. Nowadays, with the Internet spreading as a worldwide tremendous reservoir of knowledge, NLP is highly solicited by various scientific communities as a worthwhile help for the following tasks:

1. Information Retrieval, Knowledge Extraction

Human produced texts are seen as a valuable input, to be processed and transformed into representations and structures directly operable by computational systems. This type of service is highly required when human need is about a set of texts relevant for a given query (information retrieval), or when the need is to built up a machine readable structure (knowledge extraction) for further computer assisted developments. In both medicine and biology, these two aspects are crucial. Scientific literature is so abundant that only a computational setup is able to browse and filter so huge amounts of information. A plain search engine is too limited to undertake queries as complex as those which meet the researchers' requirements. From the knowledge extraction point of view, manually constructed ontologies seldom reach more than a few concepts and relationships, because of the tremendous effort necessary to achieve such a task.

For the past decades, artificial intelligence (AI) has undertaken an important endeavor in favor of knowledge management. Its result, a set of taxonomies, i.e. knowledge classifications formalized according to a graph-based representation (sometimes simplified into a tree-based representation when hierarchical ties between knowledge items are dominant) also commonly called ontologies, are obtained at a very high cost in manpower, and human involvement. As soon as statistical techniques and new programming skills have appeared through machine learning, the AI community has attempted to automate this task as much as possible, feeding systems with texts and producing, at the other end, an ontology or something similar to it. Naturally, human intervention, for validation, or re-orientation, was still needed. But the learning techniques were operated on the front filtering task, the one seen as the most tedious and the most risky. Results looked promising and a few ontologies were initiated with such processes. However, they were incomplete: Wrong interpretations were numerous (noisy aspect), structures were scarce (silent aspect), and most of all, the linguistic-conceptual relationship was totally ignored. When the community acknowledged that, it turned toward NLP works and tools to reorganize its processes, and NLP skills in separating between the linguistic and conceptual properties of words were of a great help. This conjunction shyly began a few years ago, but is going stronger now, since NLP tools have improved with time.

2. Knowledge Integration to Existing Devices

Knowledge integration is a logical sequel to knowledge extraction. Rejecting existing ontologies and terminological classifications is not affordable, even if they do not meet expectation, since their building is definitely expensive. A new trend has emerged from such a situation: Available digital data (but not machine operable), mostly texts and figures, is regularly mined in order to complete or correct existing knowledge structures. This explains the present success of data and text mining in AI, as well as in information systems (IS) and NLP communities. Several works have been devoted to ontologies enhancement or enrichment by adding concepts or terminology related to concepts. One has to know that in natural language, unlike mathematical originated formalisms, a given item (concept) could be addressed through several different symbols (i.e. words or phrases), these symbols not being exactly identical to each other in the way that they do not stress out exactly the same concept properties. This feature is called synonymy or mostly near-synonymy, since natural language elements are not mathematically equivalent. This has been for a long time one of the most important obstacles in building and completing ontologies for knowledge management. On the other hand, not only natural language symbols are prone to synonymy. At the same time, a given symbol (again, a word or a phrase) could address different items, illustrating polysemy, or multiple meanings phenomenon. Both aspects could be seen as terminological expansion (synonymy) or contraction (polysemy) processes. They have largely impeded automated procedures that mined texts in order to find concepts and relations. Therefore, new knowledge is as complicated to integrate to existing devices as to built a classification from scratch, if NLP techniques, that have been tackling the expansion-contraction phenomenon for long, are not solicited for such a task. As it is the case for the documents coming from the general field, the main classical linguistic phenomena can be observed when considering the biomedical corpora. Among these phenomena, polysemy (e.g., "RNA" which can mean "ribonucleic acid" or "renal nerve activity") appears, as well as synonymy (e.g., "tRNA" and "transfer RNA"). However, it should be noted that the biomedical texts contain linguistic specificities: Massive presence of acronyms (contracted forms of multiword expressions), scientific style of documents, and so forth.

3. Using and Applying Existing Knowledge Structures for Services in Information Retrieval

Ontologies are built and extended because they are needed as basic structures for further applications, otherwise, the effort would be vain. In a kind of loop process, information retrieval appears as one of the goals of such an effort, while in previous paragraphs, it seemed to be a launching procedure for knowledge extraction. Retrieving the relevant set of texts to a complex query cannot only rely on words, it has to grasp ideas, expressed by several distinct strings of words, either phrases, or sentences. Retrieving the appropriate portion in a relevant text needs going further: It requires topical classification. Browsing a given literature in a given domain often relies on multilingual abilities: Translation has its role to play. Even if science is nowadays focused on a major tongue (English) for its publications, nevertheless, depending on domains, more than half of worldwide publications is done in other languages. Terminological translation could be of a great help also in writing down articles for non-native English speakers. All these services, knowledgeable to an important target of users, are provided by AI, statistical and NLP techniques, altogether invoked to produce the most appropriate output.Considering the

BioNLP domain, there are a lot of resources such as the corpora (e.g., PubMed: http://www.ncbi.nlm.nih.gov/pubmed/), the Ontologies/Thesaurus (e.g., GeneOntolgy: http://www.geneontology.org/, Mesh Thesuarus: http://www.nlm.nih.gov/mesh/), etc. Many chapters of this book rely on these resources in order to achieve the various NLP tasks they address.

ORIGINALITY OF OUR APPROACH

This book topic meets the knowledge extraction, integration, and application triple goal expressed in the previous description, beginning with the information retrieval task. As explained before, the extraction process for either information retrieval or knowledge management is the same, the difference lying in the output shape: Raw in information retrieval or machine operable in knowledge extraction and integration.

Two properties define this book as both totally fitting in the ongoing research trend, and original in its presentation:

1. Emphasizing Natural Language Processing as the Main Methodological Issue

NLP has appeared to a majority of researchers in the fields of complex information retrieval, knowledge extraction and integration, as the most fitting type of approach going beyond obvious statistical highways. NLP tackles linguistic data and tries to extract from linguistic properties as much information as possible. If, very obviously, non specialists think about NLP as a 'word computing' science, this domain goes much beyond the level of words, since language productions, i.e. texts, are complex devices structured at least at two other levels:

- **The sentence level:** Words are not haphazardly thrown in texts as dice could be on a table, unlike what would some raw statistical models in text mining implicitly assume. Words contribution to sentences determines their role as meaning conveyors. A governance principle has been defined a long time ago by scholars (going back to Aristotle), but has been rejuvenated by the works of Noam Chomsky and Lucien Tesnière in the second half of the twentieth century. Words or phrases (groups of words) may govern others, and thus interact with them, and the sentence meaning results from words interactions as much as words meanings. One of the peculiarities of this book is to demonstrate the implication of NLP in information retrieval, knowledge extraction and integration, beyond the plain terminological involvement. In other words, beyond simple words.
- **The discourse, segment or text level:** As much as sentences are intended words structures, a text is also not randomly organized. It abides by discourse rules that convey the intentions of the writer about what is written and about the potential readers. Several phenomena appear at the text level, and could highly impact the importance of text segments relatively to each other. Paragraphs positions, paragraphs beginnings, lexical markers acting as particular position flags between sets of sentences, are among the several items used by human writers to organize their texts according to their goal. These 'clues' are generally ignored by most computational techniques. The few researchers that take them into account, do not hesitate to stress out the difficulties in identifying them automatically. Several NLP theories have provided a formal environment for these phenomena (e.g. DRT, discourse relations theory, DRST, discourse rhetorical structures theory, speech acts theory, etc.), but experiments have not succeeded in demonstrating their efficiency on important

volumes of data. Moreover, text organization, at this level, shows the dependence between language and its nonlinguistic environment. The underlying knowledge, beliefs, social rules and conventional implicatures are present, and strongly tie linguistic data to the outside world in organized macro-structures. This is why we have tried, in this book, not to neglect this part, or else our NLP grounding would have been lame, and certainly incomplete.

2. Studying the Interaction between NLP and its Application Domains: Biology and Medicine

We hope to have convinced the reader in the preceding paragraph that human language entails its outside world peculiarities, and is not a simple rewriting mechanism, with inner rules, that could be applied as a mask or a filter on reality. Language interacts with what it expresses, modifies and is modified by the type of knowledge, beliefs, expectations and intentions conveyed by a given theme, topic, domain or field. This point of view drives us to consider that NLP in Biomedicine is not plainly an NLP outfit set up on biological and medical data. BioNLP (the acknowledged acronym for NLP dedicated to biology and medicine) has recently appeared as a fashionable trend in research because of the dire need of biologists and medical scientists for a computational information retrieval and knowledge management framework, as explained in the earlier paragraphs. But BioNLP has developed its own idiosyncrasies, i.e. its particular way to process biological and medical language. A domain language is not a simple subset of the general language, unlike what a common belief tends to claim. It develops its own semantics, lexical organization, lexical choice, sentence construction rules and text organization properties that translate the way of thinking of a homogeneous community. From our point of view, it was really necessary to present a set of works in BioNLP that were not plain transpositions of works done in other domain and transferred to medicine and biology without adaptation. Also, it is as important to investigate the tremendous potential of this domain, because of the following reasons:

- Biology and medicine are multifaceted, and specialists tend to specialize too narrowly. This prevents the ability to discover, or recognize common topics among them. The most obvious and cited example is the cancer issue. Oncologists, chemists, pathologists, surgeons, radiologists, molecular biologists, researchers in genetics are all concerned by this domain. But they do not publish at all in the same journals, do not read what each other write, and very often do not even communicate with each other, although they are invited to do so. Hyper-specialization prevents scientific multidisciplinary exchange. Lack of time, huge volumes of data are the most usually invoked reasons. Also, the inability to read what the neighboring community has written, because its words appear a bit foreign, its way of writing is different, etc. How much useful information is lost like this, and how precious it would be to gather it, process it and re-present it to those who need it!
- Biology and medicine are far from being the only domains suffering such a dispersion, but they are those which have the greatest impact on human public opinion. Health is nowadays the most preoccupying issue. Life sustenance and maintenance is the prime goal of every living being. Sciences that deal with this issue have naturally a priority in people minds.
- The particular linguistic features of biological and medical languages are very interesting challenges from an NLP point of view, and tackling them is an efficient way of testing the techniques robustness.
- Last, bioinformatics has been widely spreading in these last years. Algorithmical and combinatorial approaches have been very much present in the field. Statistics and data mining have also enhanced the domain. It seems that NLP had also to provide its contribution, and tackle the bioinformatics

issue from the textual side, which was either neglected or only superficially processed by the other domains.

TARGET AUDIENCE

The audience of this book could be approached from several points of views. First, the reader's function or position: Researchers, teachers preparing graduate courses, PhD or masters students are the natural potential audience to such a work. Second, from the domain or community point of view: NLP researchers are naturally meant since they could discover through this book the particularities of the application domain language, and thus understand their fellow researchers' work from the NLP problem solving side. AI researchers dealing with building and enhancing ontologies are also concerned when they have to deal with biological and/or medical data. Terminologists, and more generally linguists could benefit from this book since some interesting experiments are related here, and could be seen as sets of data in which they could plough to illustrate phenomena there are interested in. The health information systems community could also see this book as a set of works at their more 'theoretical' side. Since this book also enumerate some existing and working NLP software, medical or biological teams could be interested into browsing some of the chapters addressing more practical issues. Last but not least, the BioNLP community is itself the most concerned by this book.

A BRIEF OVERVIEW OF THE CHAPTERS AND THEIR ORGANIZATION

The book is divided into six sections.

The chapter title "*Text Mining in Biomedicine*", is an introduction written by Sophia Ananiadou. She is one of the most renowned leaders in BioNLP, has edited a very interesting book about NLP, presenting the domain and its different aspects to the community of researchers in information retrieval, knowledge extraction and management, dedicated to biology and medicine. Sophia's book has stated the grounding principles of NLP. This book complements her work by showing a progressive interaction between NLP and its target domain through text mining as a task. Her introduction emphasizes the needs, the requirements, the nature of the issues and their stakes, and the achievements of the state of the art.

Sophia Ananiadou is the most appropriate writer for this chapter because of her extensive knowledge about the domain and the ongoing research.

The core sections of the book are four: Three that follow the NLP granularity scope, ranging from the lexical level to the discourse level as explained in an earlier paragraph, and one devoted to selected existing software. Chapters belonging to these sections are numbered from II to XIX.

Section I, named "*Works at a Lexical Level, Crossroads Between NLP and Ontological Knowledge Management*", is the most abundant, since research has reached here a recognized maturity. It is composed of nine chapters. The order in which chapters have been organized is set up by the following pattern:

1. **Using existing resources to perform document processing tasks:** Indexation(Chapter II), categorization (Chapter III) and information retrieval (Chapter IV). Indexation and categorization could be seen as previous tasks to an intelligent information retrieval, since they pre-structure textual data, according to topics, domain, keywords or centers of interest.
2. **Dealing with the cross-linguistic terminological problem:** From a specialists language to general language within one tongue (Chapter V), or across different tongues (Chapter VI).

3. **Enriching terminology: The beginning of a strong lexical NLP involvement** (Chapter VII).
4. **Increasing lexical NLP involvement in biomedical application** (Chapter VIII).

In a more detailed version, these chapters are very representative of the state-of-the art. Most works are devoted to words, word-concepts relations, word-to-word relations.

Chapter II titled, "*Lexical Granularity for Automatic Indexing and Means to Achieve It: The Case of Swedish MEsH®*", by Dimitri Kokkinakis from the University of Gothenburg, Sweden, is one of the three articles in this section involving MEsH, the Medical terminological classification that is currently one of the backbone of research and applications in BioNLP. Kokkinakis's paper emphasizes the indexing function, and clearly demonstrates the impact of lexical variability within a dedicated technical language (medical language). The authors explain the challenges met by researchers when they go beyond indexation with broad concepts (introducing vagueness, and thus noise), and try to tackle the fine grained level where the complex term-concept relationship creates mismatches, thus jeopardizing precision.

Chapter III named, "*Expanding Terms with Medical Ontologies to Improve a Multi-Label Text Categorization Systems*", by M. Teresa Martín-Valdivia, Arturo Montejo-Ràez, M.C. Diaz-Galiano, José Perea Ortega and L. Alfonso Ureña-Lopez from the University of Jaén, in Spain, tackles the categorization issue, which is in spirit, very close to indexation. An index highlights the importance of the word and its possible equivalents. A category is more adapted to needs, and conveys pragmatic knowledge. The chapter focuses on terminological expansion, that facet of the expansion-contraction linguistic phenomenon that troubles the ontological world so much. By trying to resolve multiple labels in different medical classification sets, the authors fruitfully complement Kokkinakis' approach.

A third representative of this type of work is Chapter IV, "*Using Biomedical Terminological Resources for Information Retrieval*", by Piotr Pezik, Antonio Jimeno Yepes and Dietrich Rebholz-Schuhmann, from the European Bioinformatics Institute at Cambridge, UK. It could be seen as the third volume of a trilogy: Previous chapters deal with introductory (as well as highly recommended) tasks to information retrieval, this one directly tackle the task in itself. Chapter II clearly states the complexity of the word-concept relationship and its variety, Chapter III focuses on expansion, Chapter IV focuses on contraction (ambiguity). Chapter II was centered on MesH, Chapter III enlarged this focus to other medical thesauri, Chapter IV provides an extensive account of biomedical resources, highlighting their linguistic properties. One of the added values of this chapter is that it largely describes queries properties and reformulation, thus shedding the light on the specific issues of information retrieval processes. This chapter is of a great help to understand why general search engines could not be efficient in biomedical literature.

Chapter V, "*Automatic Alignment of Medical Terminologies with General Dictionaries for an Efficient Information Retrieval*", by Laura Dioşan, Alexandra Rogozan, and Jean-Pierre Pecuchet (a collaboration between the Institut National des Sciences Appliquées, France, and the Babeş-Bolyai University, Romania), tackles the delicate issue of the neophyte-specialist linguistic differences. This aspect is crucial and often remains in the shadow, because the attention of researchers in information retrieval mostly focuses on the specialists' language, and addresses specialists. Mapping general language and technical language is a necessity since all technical texts contain general words. Moreover, meanings variations may introduce misinterpretations. The authors offer an automatic alignment system which classifies specialized and general terminology according to their similarity.

After stressing out the need of translating words within one language, depending on its specialization, Chapter VI named, "*Translation of Biomedical Terms by Inferring Rewriting Rules*", by Vincent Claveau (IRISA-CNRS, France), addresses the cross-linguistic aspect. The author ambitiously deals with several languages: Czech, English, French, Italian, Portuguese, Spanish, Russian. The idea is to provide an automatic translation between a pair of languages for unknown medical words (i.e. not existing in the available bilingual dictionaries), and to use this not only for terminological resources enhancement (which is its natural recipient) but also for a cross-linguistic information retrieval tasks. Results achieved look highly promising.

After the translation issue, two other chapters go deeper within the NLP classical issue of lexical functions, variety and ambiguity. Here the reader dives into the genuine 'NLP culture'.

Chapter VII, "*Lexical Enrichment of Biomedical Ontology*", by Nils Reiter and Paul Buitelaar, respectively from the universities of Heidelberg and Saarbrücken in Germany, is one of the most representative of what NLP research could offer to knowledge enrichment. Enhancing domain ontologies with semantic information derived from sophisticated lexica such as WordNet, using Wikipedia as another source of information (very fashionable in lexical NLP nowadays), and mostly selecting the most appropriate interpretations for ambiguous terms (the case of those broad concepts evoked beforehand), are but a few of the several contributions of this chapter to knowledge integration.

Chapter VIII, "*Word Sense Disambiguation in Biomedical Application: A Machine Learning Approach*", by Torsten Schiemann, Ulf Leser (both from the Humboldt-Universität zu Berlin, Germany) and Jörg Hackenberg (Arizona State University, USA) is the ideal complement to Chapter VII. Going deep in the ambiguity phenomenon, not only as it might appear in ontologies, but also as it happens in the existing texts (specialized texts have proven to convey ambiguity almost as much as non specialized literature, despite the common belief that specialization is logically assorted with disambiguation!)

Section II titled, "*Going Beyond Words: NLP Approaches Involving the Sentence Level*", groups three chapters. If the lexical level has been explored to a certain extent, broader linguistic granularities are yet to be investigated. A such, those three chapters could be considered as representative attempts to go beyond the lexical horizon. The need is certain: Chapters VII and VIII have shown the effects of ambiguity: Intrinsic ambiguity (localized in ontologies themselves) and induced ambiguities, detected in texts. A too fine-grained division might introduce such an effect, therefore, some researchers have turned their attention to the next complete linguistic unit, the sentence. The sentence context might erase lexical ambiguities effects in some cases. Sentences and not words might be queries or answers to queries.

Chapter IX named, "*Information Extraction of Protein Phosphorylation from Biomedical Literature*", by M. Narayanaswamy , K. E. Ravikumar (both from Anna University in India), Z. Z. Hu (Georgetown University Medical Center, USA) , K. Vijay-Shanker (Universitt of Delaware, USA) , and C. H. Wu (Georgetown University Medical Center, USA), describes a system that captures "the lexical, syntactic and semantic constraints found in sentences expressing phosphorylation information" from MEDLINE abstracts. The rule-based system has been designed as such because isolated words or phrases could possibly be thematic clues, but can by no means account for the different stages of a process. This means that event-type or procedure-type information cannot be encapsulated in a linguistic shape smaller than the significant text unit, the sentence. And according to the authors, a fair amount of the biomedical literature contains such information, which lexical approaches sometimes fail to capture.

Chapter X, "*CorTag: A Language for a Contextual Tagging of the Words Within Their Sentence*", by Yves Kodratoff, Jérôme Azé (both from the University Paris-Sud (Paris XI), France) and Lise Fontaine (Cardiff University, UK) complements the preceding one, which presented an application and a need, by offering a design to extract contextual knowledge from sentences. Knowledge extraction from text is generally done with part-of-speech taggers, mostly with lexical categories. Higher level tags such as noun or verb phrases, adjectival groups, and beyond, syntactic dependencies, are generally either neglected, or wrongly assigned by taggers in technical texts. CorTag corrects wrong assignments, and a few examples have been given by the authors, among other examples, about the same protein phosphorylation process tackled by Chapter IX. If Chapter IX has amply focused on knowledge extraction, Chapter X also deals with knowledge discovery, and how to induce relations between concepts recognized in texts, thanks to the services of syntactic and semantic information provided by sentences. In fact, sentences are the linguistic units that stage concepts and their relationships. Words or phrases capture concepts, but grammar expresses their respective roles.

Chapter XI titled, "*Analyzing the Text of Clinical Literature for Question Answering*", by Yun Niu and Graeme Hirst from the University of Toronto, Canada, is an ideal example of the usefulness of the sentence level information in a question-answer task, one of the most representative tasks in information retrieval. Focusing on clinical questions, and the need to retrieve evidences from corpora as automatically as possible, the authors propose here a method, a design and a system that not only deal with complex information at the sentence level, but also inchoate a possible argumentative articulation between fragments of sentences. As such, this chapter is the most adapted one to the intersection between the sentence level and the discourse level investigations. The use of semantic classes introduces a thematic, and thus a pragmatic approach to meaning (the authors are not frightened to use the word 'frame') completing lexical and sentence semantics. This attitude finds an echo in Chapter XIV, ending next section, but the latter mostly emphasizes the 'script' approach (isn't it bold to reuse frames and scripts in the late two thousands?) with a considerable highlight on situation pragmatics, whereas Chapter XI is closer to the heart of NLP literature in terms of linguistic material analysis. This chapter is also highly recommended to readers who need an accurate survey of question answering systems state-of-the art.

As a natural sequel to Section III titled, "*Pragmatics, Discourse Structures and Segment Level as the Last Stage in the NLP Offer to Biomedicine*" . It also groups three chapters.

Chapter XII, "*Discourse Processing for Text Mining*", by Nadine Lucas (GREYC CNRS, Université de Caen Basse-Normandie Campus 2, France), has to be considered as an educational chapter about discourse, the nature and effects of text structures, as well as the broad panel of inter-sentences relations available to readers and writers in order to organize information and knowledge in texts. The author is a linguist, and has deeply studied biomedical corpora from the linguistics point of view. This chapter is an 'opinion chapter': We have taken the risk to integrate such a text because it was important for us to offer a book which is not only a patchwork of present trends. We felt committed to research in NLP, IR, knowledge management, as well as to our target domain, biomedicine. Our commitment has been to give voice to criticism to approaches representatives of which been described in the same book. This chapter plays this role. It reveals the complexity of language that cannot be circumscribed by statistics, it shows that text mining scientific claims and trends still need to be improved, linguistically speaking. It emphasizes the fact that academic genre is not subsumed by its own abstracts features, and if texts are not 'bags of words', they are not 'bags of sentences' either. The longer the text, the more organized and the more conventional it is. The corpora analysis in this chapter is an interesting counter-argument to our gross computational attitudes toward text mining.

Chapter XIII titled, "*A Neural Network Approach Implementing Non-linear Relevance Feedback to Improve the Performance of Medical Information Retrieval Systems*", by Dimosthenis Kyriazis, Anastasios Doulamis and Theodora Varvarigou from the National Technical University of Athens, Greece, acknowledges the content reliability issue. In other words, whatever the technique is, the main stake is either not to loose information, or not to provide false tracks. Sole lexical approaches discard information, retrieved as much as possible by sentence level approaches. But both might provide wrong answers to users' needs. Including the user in the IR loop is a mandatory attitude. The authors attempt here to mathematically ground their information reliability hypothesis. Their contribution is in this section in the sense that they make room for pragmatics, if not for discourse structuration.

The increasing pragmatics involvment is clear in Chapter XIV, "*Extracting Patient Case Profiles with Domain-Specific Semantic Categories*", by Yifao Zhang and Jon Patrick, from The University of Sydney, Australia. Here the retrieved part is a complex structure and entails domain pragmatics. Authors tackle a particular issue, the role of fragments of patients medical records as diagnosis or symptoms clues. This naturally involve a discourse-type relationship. But if discourse relationships are difficult to retrieve with most means, according to the authors, the medical domain provides the researchers with 'sentences types' representing patterns to a given role. Acknowledging the existence of a conventional script for texts describing individual patients, authors have annotated a corpus and by acting at both the lexical and sentence level, have obtained most linguistic information from the linguistic material itself. The sentences types they present provide a kind of a text writing protocol in the particular application they investigate. Therefore the textual organization could be implicitely retrieved and used to complete information about patients, and thus help users in their queries. Chapter XIV is a mirror to Chapter XI. The latter focuses on the task (question answering) whereas Chapter XIV focuses on the need. Both are important pragmatic aspects. They could have been in the same section since sentence to text organization appears as a continuum in which the user is more and more concerned. Here we drop out of knowledge management, out of linguistics, to enter the outside world.

Section IV named, "*NLP Software for IR in Biomedicine*", is dedicated to software dealing with information or knowledge extraction or verification (Chapters XV to XIX). It is a good thing for readers to know the software state of the art and compare it with more theoretical and methodological studies, in order to assess the gap between semi-automatic and automatic productions.

Chapter XV called, "*Identification of Sequence Variants of Genes from Biomedical Literature: The OSIRIS Approach*", by Laura I. Furlong and Ferran Sanz from the Research Unit on Biomedical Informatics at Barcelona, Spain, deals with the problem of retrieving variants of genes described by literature. Their system, OSIRIS, integrates a cognitive module in its new version. This tries to relate more knowledge, NLP and algorithmics as a whole. Osiris can be used to link literature reference to biomedical databases entries, thus reducing the terminological variation.

Chapter XVI, "*Verification of Uncurated Protein Annotations*", by Francisco M. Couto, Mário J. Sylva (both from the Universidade de Lisboa, Portugal) and Vivian Lee, Emily Dimmer, Evelyn Camon, Rolf Apweiler, Harald Kirsch, and Dietrich Rebholz-Schuhmann (Euopean Bioinformatics Institute, Cambridge, UK) describes a tool that annotates literature with an available ontological description, GOAnnotator. Its aim is to assist the verification of uncurated protein annotations. In a way, it is a kind of a symmetrical tool to Osiris as a task (verification versus identification). GoAnnotator is a free tool, available on the Web, and is of a precious help to domain researchers.

Chapter XVII titled, "*A Software Tool for Biomedical Information Extraction (And Beyond)*", by Burr Settles, from the University of Wisconsin-Madison, USA, is dedicated to the description of ABNER, a biomedical named entity recognizer, which is an open-source software tool for mining in the molecular biology literature. Like its fellow tools, ABNER deals with molecular biology where literature is abundant, knowledge is volatile and research interest definitely keen. The 'named entity issue' is one of the most typical of the difficulties encountered in literature, since it is related to the 'unknown word or phrase' basic NLP issue. As the author describes it, entity recognition is the natural first step in information management. Unlike Osiris and GOAnnotator, ABNER does not necessarily relate to database or ontology labels. The strings it deals with could be real words, acronyms, abbreviated words, and so forth. This chapter is particularly interesting from an evaluation point of view. The author provides a very educational insight on techniques in named entities recognition and their comparison. So, beyond ABNER, there is the crucial issue of the accurate model for a given task, and this chapter is definitely informative.

Chapter XVIII, "*Problems-Solving Map Extraction with Collective Intelligence Analysis and Language Engineering*", by Asanee Kawkatrul (Kasetsart University and Ministry of Technology in Thailand), Chaveevari Petchsirim (University of Bangkok, Thailand), Sachit Rajbhandari (Food and Agriculture

Organization of the United Nations, Rome, Italy), and Frederic Andres (National Institute of Informatics Tokyo, Japan), is dedicated to the engineering of a framework aiming at reducing format heterogeneity in biological data. Their framework considers a collective action in knowledge management (extraction, enhancement, operation), and the issues they address are partly related to some of the other tools: Annotation (like Chapter XVI) but here for collaborative answers in question answering systems, named entity recognition (as in Chapter XVII), but also elements that could be related to our higher levels in NLP, discourse relations. This chapter is another bridge between AI and NLP. Ontologies and terminology are in the knowledge representation field of AI and the lexical level in NLP. Collective intelligence is at the social network, multi-agent level in AI and at the discourse and pragmatics level in NLP. Symmetry is preserved at every stage between language and intelligence.

Chapter XIX titled, "*Seekbio: Retrieval of Spatial Relations for System Biology*", by Christophe Jouis, Magali Roux-Rouquié , both from University Paris 3, Sorbonne Nouvelle and Jean-Gabriel Ganascia (University Paris 6) describes a software that retrieves spatial relations, i.e. topological relations between concepts (and their identifying terms), directly interesting system biology. The latter is an emerging field in which living organisms are considered as complex systemic devices, and it mainly focuses on dynamic interactions between the biological components of these organisms. If most terminological software retrieves static relations, Seek*bio* originality is its dedication to the dynamic aspect of knowledge relations system. The tool can be plugged at Pubmed, an important database in the medical field and provides the researcher in system biology with a promising insight for discovering new interactions.

Chapter II to XIX have described, through four main sections, the ongoing research, theoretical advances, and existing tools, produced by BioNLP, this crossroads field in which AI, NLP, statistics and application domains, biology and medicine, all interact.

Our last section, "*Conclusion and Perspectives*", with its sole chapter, the twentieth titled, "*Analysing Clincal Notes for Translation Research: Back to the Future*", by Jon Patrick and Pooyan Asgari from The University of Sydney, Australia, is meant not to be an end, but a window open on the future, already pending for most of the BioNLP community. The paper summarizes in its description several achievements that have been deeply investigated in this book through different applications. It has chosen, as a data field to plough, a type of text which is highly operational: No academic style, but something very heterogeneous, mixing images, sound, text, and in text, introducing abbreviations, acronyms, a particular grammar, a highly pragmatics-based way of organizing knowledge. This type of text is the patient folder (in health care institutions) and contains several units of clinical notes. Shifting from biology to medicine in this conclusion is also a way to shift from academic genre to a practitioner type of writing, in which general language is disturbed, noisy, because it is dedicated to a task in which time and goal are overwhelming: Caring of the sick and the dying. In this conclusion, we have tried, as editor to put a momentary final note to this volume (we could not go on for ever), but our baseline was to assess NLP presence and help as much in an intellectual research as in a day-to-day practice. Chapter XX could be a conclusion, or another chapter, but here we have chosen to show it as an opening to another world in which NLP is needed, with time and practice constraints.

HOW WE THINK THE BOOK IMPACTS THE FIELD

We emphasized the need for such a work and the originality of our collection of chapters in the first two sections of this preface. We described the different contributions in the light of our approach to NLP interaction with the application domains. The various authors of this volume chapters are very representative of the ongoing research in the field. They are spread all around the world, they belong to multidisciplinary areas, some of them are famous and renowned in BioNLP, some other are less known but present original theories and outcomes. We believe that this book is a most appropriate gathering of what is to be said about the field (an exhaustive approach would have needed an encyclopedia format). It is also a door open to discussion, opinion debates, scientific confrontation and other healthy attitudes that science nowadays is in a bad need for. As editors, we chose not to contribute ourselves, although we are running research in NLP, and apply it to BioNLP. But we believe that editors should be the gatherers of variety, not the speakers of a given trend, and certainly not advertisers of their own work. Under the magnifying lens of several of these contributions, we feel that all new work in BioNLP, whether dedicated to biology and academic production, or to medicine and its multiplicity of genres, has to integrate the idea that it is not a simple application of a given technique to a given domain, but a lively interaction between two scientific fields, giving birth to a hybrid with its specific properties. Theories or techniques have to be adapted, and 'dogmas' need to be discarded. On the other hand, rough statistical approximations have to be refined, in order not to produce noise and wrong directions. Language multiple layers must not be forgotten, but their integration has to be as customized as possible. We hope that, after reading this book, the scientific community will get a picture as accurate as possible of the enthusiastic challenges of our domain, as well as of its limitations and drawbacks. But let that not hinder our eagerness to continue in improving BioNLP achievements for the best of all.

Violaine Prince and Mathieu Roche
University Montpellier 2, France & LIRMM-CNRS, France

Chapter I
Text Mining for Biomedicine

Sophia Ananiadou
University of Manchester, National Centre for Text Mining, UK

ABSTRACT

Text mining provides the automated means to manage information overload and overlook. By adding meaning to text, text mining techniques produce a much more structured analysis of textual knowledge than do simple word searches, and can provide powerful tools for knowledge discovery in biomedicine. In this chapter, the author focus on the text mining services for biomedicine offered by the United Kingdom National Centre for Text Mining.

INTRODUCTION

Text mining covers a broad spectrum of activities and a battery of processes, but essentially the goal is to help users deal with information overload and information overlook (Ananiadou and McNaught, 2006). Key aspects are to discover unsuspected, new knowledge hidden in the vast scientific literature, to support data driven hypothesis discovery and to derive meaning from the rich language of specialists as expressed in the plethora of textual reports, articles, etc. With the overwhelming amount of information (~80%) in textual unstructured form and the growing number of publications, an estimate of about 2.5 million articles published per year (Harnad, Brody, Vallieres, Carr, Hitchcock, Gingras, Oppenheim, Stamerjohanns, and Hilf, 2004) it is not surprising that valuable new sources of research data typically remain underexploited and nuggets of insight or new knowledge are often never discovered in the sea of literature. Scientists are unable to keep abreast of developments in their fields and to make connections between seemingly unrelated facts to generate new ideas and hypotheses. Fortunately, text mining offers a solution to this problem by replacing or supplementing the human with automated means to turn unstructured text and implicit knowledge into structured data and thus explicit knowledge (Cohen, and Hunter,

2008; Hirschman, Park, Tsujii, and Wong, 2002; (McNaught and Black, 2006)(Jensen, Saric, and Bork, 2006; Hearst, 1999).

Text mining includes the following processes: information retrieval, information extraction and data mining.

Information Retrieval (IR) finds documents that answer an information need, with the aid of indexes. IR or 'search engines' such as Google™ and PubMed© typically classify a document as relevant or non relevant to a user's query. To successfully find an item relevant to a search implies that this item has been sufficiently well characterised, indexed and classified such that relevance to a search query can be ascertained. Unfortunately, conventional information retrieval technology, while very good at handling large scale collections, remains at a rough granular level. Moreover, such technology typically focuses on finding sets of individual items, leaving it up to the user to somehow integrate and synthesise the knowledge contained in and across individual items. Thus, the content of documents is largely lost in conventional indexing approaches. To address this problem, we have improved the search strategy by placing more emphasis on terms in a collection of documents. In Biomedicine new terms are constantly created creating a severe obstacle to text mining and other natural language processing applications. In addition, term variation and ambiguity exacerbate the problem. We extract the most significant words in a collection of documents by using NaCTeM's TerMine service.[a] TerMine extracts and automatically ranks technical terms based on our hybrid term extraction technique, C-value (Frantzi, Ananiadou, and Mima, 2000). The C-value scores are combined with the indexing capabilities of Lucene 2.2 for full text indexing and searching.

Based on the assumption that documents sharing similar words mention similar topics, the extracted terms can be used for subsequent associative search. The output of associative searching is a ranked list of documents similar to the original document. This allows us to link similar documents based on their content. Another enhancement of the search strategy is query expansion. One of the major criticisms with current search engines is that queries are effective only when well crafted. A desirable feature is automatic query expansion according to the users' interests, but most search engines do not support this beyond mapping selective query terms to ontology headings (e.g. PubMed[b]). Therefore, there are inevitable limitations of coverage. To address this, we have used term-based automatic query expansion drawing upon weights given to terms discovered across different sized document sets. Query expansion embedded in searching allows the user to explore the wider collection, focusing on documents with similar significance and to discover potentially unknown documents

Information Extraction (IE) is characterized as the process of taking a natural language text from a document source, and extracting the essential facts about one or more predefined fact types. We then represent each fact as a template whose slots are filled on the basis of what is found from the text.

A template is a "form" which, when filled, conveys a fact. Each form has a label which characterises the type of fact it represents, whilst the slots identify the attributes that make up the fact. An example of a simple fact is:

James Smith, Chief Research Scientist of XYZ Co.

Examples of events are:

XYZ Co. announced the appointment of James Smith as Chief Research Scientist on 4th August 2005.

We hypothesized that retinoic acid receptor (RAR) would activate this gene.

Tasks that IE systems can perform include:

- Named-entity recognition, which identifies the names in a document, such as the names of people, protein, gene, disease, organizations, etc.
- Fact extraction, which identifies and extracts complex facts from documents. Such facts could be relationships between entities or events.

A very simplified example of the form of a template and how it might be filled from a sentence is shown in Figure 1. Here, the IE system must be able to identify that *bind* is a kind of interaction, and that *myosin* and *actin* are the names of proteins (named entities). This kind of information might be stored in a dictionary or an ontology, which defines the terms in a particular field and their relationship to each other. The data generated during IE are normally stored in a database ready for analysis by the data mining component.

Data Mining (DM) is the process of identifying patterns in large sets of data. The aim is to uncover previously unknown associations. When used in text mining, DM is applied to the facts generated by the information extraction phase. Continuing with our protein interaction example, we may have extracted a large number of protein interactions from a document collection and stored these interactions as facts in a database. By applying DM to this database, we may be able to identify patterns in the facts. This may lead to new discoveries about the types of interactions that can or cannot occur, or the relationship between types of interactions and particular diseases and so on (Swanson and Smalheiser, 1994; Weeber, Vos, Klein, De Jong-Van Den Berg, Aronson, and Molema, 2003).

SEMANTIC METADATA FOR KNOWLEDGE DISCOVERY

Metadata are critical to discovery of new knowledge. The richer the metadata, and the more they are linked to other resources of different types, the better placed we are to support new knowledge discovery. By "richer" here is meant *semantic* metadata. However, our notion of semantic metadata has greater scope than its current restricted use in the context of the Semantic Web and ontologies (Spasic, Ananiadou, McNaught, and Kumar, 2005), where it essentially means a list of ontological labels attached to a document. Using text mining, the notion of semantic metadata is extended to include semantic representations of document content down to e.g. concepts and relationships among concepts (facts). Semantic layers of annotation obtained through text mining in the domain of biology can be seen in Figure 2 (adapted from Ananiadou, Kell, and Tsujii, 2006).

Such semantically enriched documents improve information access by freeing the user from the restrictions of keyword querying, enabling focused semantic querying. Thus, the users are able to carry out an easily expressed semantic query which delivers *facts* matching that semantic

Figure 1. An example of IE template filling

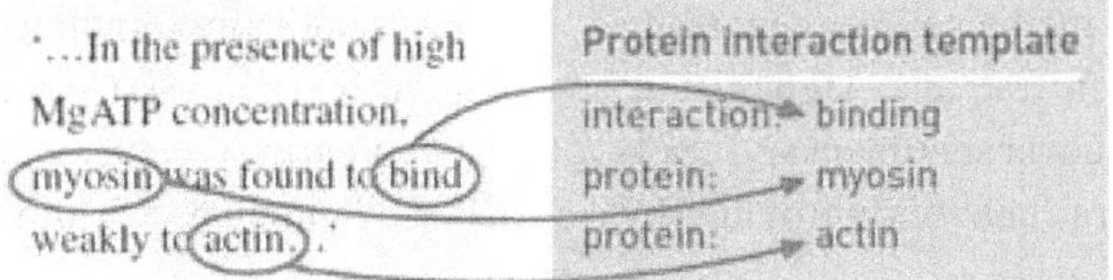

Figure 2. Layers of semantic annotation using text mining

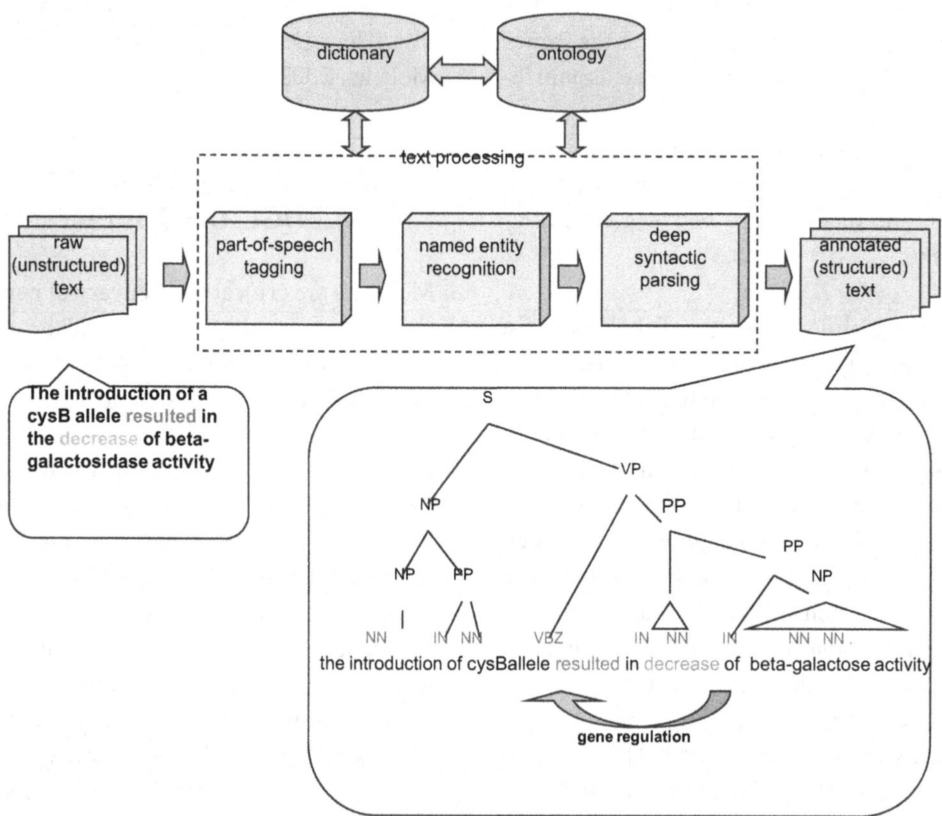

query rather than *just* sets of documents they have to read. For example, a biologist interested in protein-protein interactions might ask using a simple interface the semantic equivalent of "What does p53 activate?"; an emergency medicine specialist seeking to reduce unnecessary stays in hospital might ask "What complications may arise in patients with sternal fracture?", a social scientist interested in frame analysis in the media might want a visualisation of opinions and attitudes expressed by different media sources regarding the UK's involvement in Iraq and Afghanistan: semantic metadata can cover sentiment and opinion. An example of such an analysis is provided by NaCTeM's BBC project[c], where the results of text mining are also visualized (Ananiadou, Procter, Rea, Sasaki, and Thomas, 2007). An example of this visualization is shown in Figure 3.

MEDIE (Miyao, Ohta, Masuda, Tsuruoka, Yoshida, Ninomiya, and Tsujii, 2006) (http://www-tsujii.is.s.u-tokyo.ac.jp/medie/) is an example of an advanced search engine for the Life Sciences, which retrieves biomedical events. The service runs over the whole of MEDLINE and is based on semantically annotated texts using deep semantic text analysis (Miyao and Tsujii, 2008) and named entity recognition (Tsuruoka and Tsujii, 2004). Sentences are annotated in advance with

Figure 3. Visualisation of the results of document clustering and classification

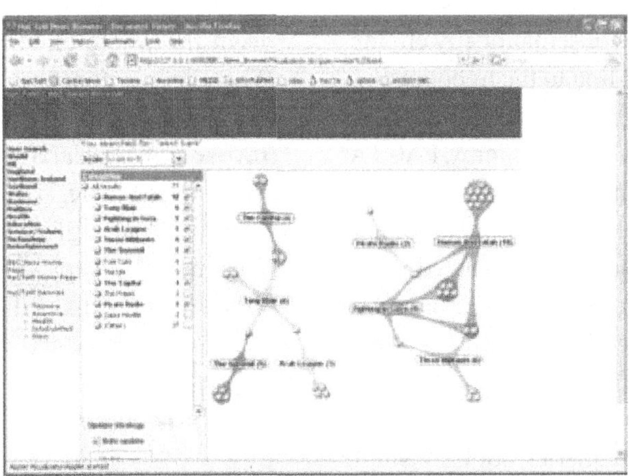

Figure 4. The user interface to MEDIE

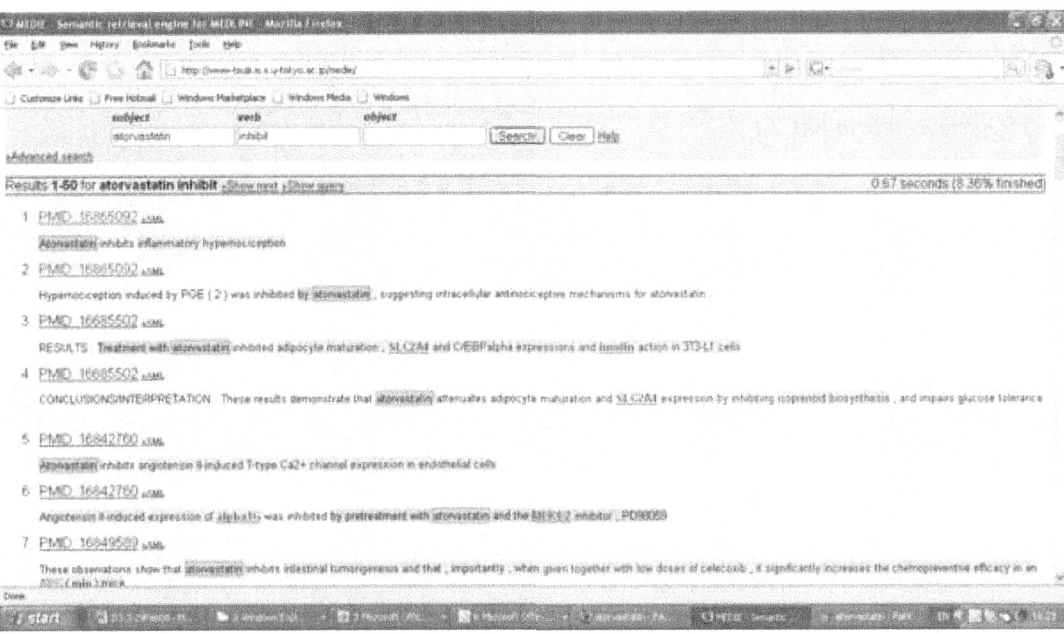

rich semantic metadata and stored in a structured database. User requests are converted on the fly into patterns of these semantic annotations, and texts are retrieved by matching these patterns with the pre-computed semantic annotations.

The user interface to MEDIE is shown in Figure 4. It allows the user to ask natural language questions such as *What does atorvastatin inhibit?* The system retrieves all relevant sentences to this query, in addition to pointing the user to the PMID and to relevant databases.

Furthermore, such rich semantic metadata can be automatically mined to discover associations among individual pieces of semantically characterized information, leading to the hypothesis of totally new knowledge. This strongly supports innovation and the knowledge economy. FACTA[d] is a system which automatically finds such associations between genes, diseases, drugs, compounds, enzymes, symptoms and their associated documents from the whole of MEDLINE, based on semantically annotated entities (Tsuruoka, Tsujii, and Ananiadou, 2008). FACTA is an interactive system—it responds to the user's query on the spot. FACTA accepts as queries not only single word concepts, but also arbitrary combinations of keywords, thus enabling the user to express a concept that cannot be captured by a single keyword. Figure 6 shows the user interface to FACTA. In the figure, the input query "nicotine" has been submitted. FACTA retrieved 15,988 documents from the whole of MEDLINE in 0.03 seconds. The relevant concepts from different categories are displayed in a tabular format. The user can invoke another search by clicking another concept name in the table.

FACTA also gives the user easy access to the documents by displaying snippets that are relevant to the query. This is illustrated in Figure 6.

TEXT MINING

An example of recent activities is engaging in extraction of rich metadata to add value to specialized repositories with a view to improving user search and supporting hypothesis genera-

Figure 5. Query results in FACTA

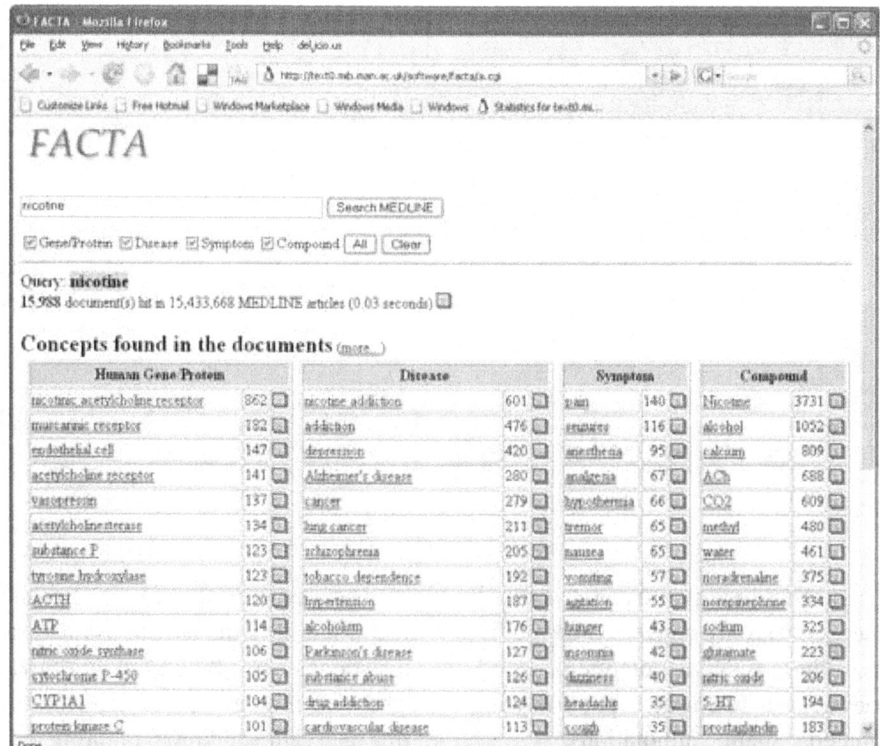

tion for discovery of new knowledge. In 2004, the National Centre for Text Mining (NaCTeM) (www.nactem.ac.uk) has been established with a remit to provide text mining services to academia focusing on biomedicine and, acting as a centre of expertise, to develop customised text mining solutions within collaborative funded projects to meet the individual needs of those projects, where text mining expertise would otherwise be unavailable. The extraction and exploitation of semantic metadata are prime applications of text mining technology. As an example, within the repository sphere, NaCTeM is working with Intute (http://www.intute.ac.uk/) to provide semantic search capabilities using concept-based document classification and personalised query expansion, thus going beyond traditional information retrieval techniques. Another recent development is UK PubMed Central (UKPMC, http://ukpmc.ac.uk/), funded by the Wellcome Trust. The aim is to turn PMC from a repository of publications into a premier resource and research tool for both the biomedical research community and for UK research funders..

The National Centre for Text Mining (www.nactem.ac.uk) has developed a suite of text mining tools and services which offer numerous benefits to a wide range of users. These range from considerable reductions in time and effort in finding and linking pertinent information from large scale textual resources, to customised solutions for semantic data analysis and knowledge management. Text mining is being used for subject classification, creation of taxonomies, information extraction, network building, controlled vocabularies, ontology building and Semantic Web

Figure 6. Sample of extracted snippets of information from text

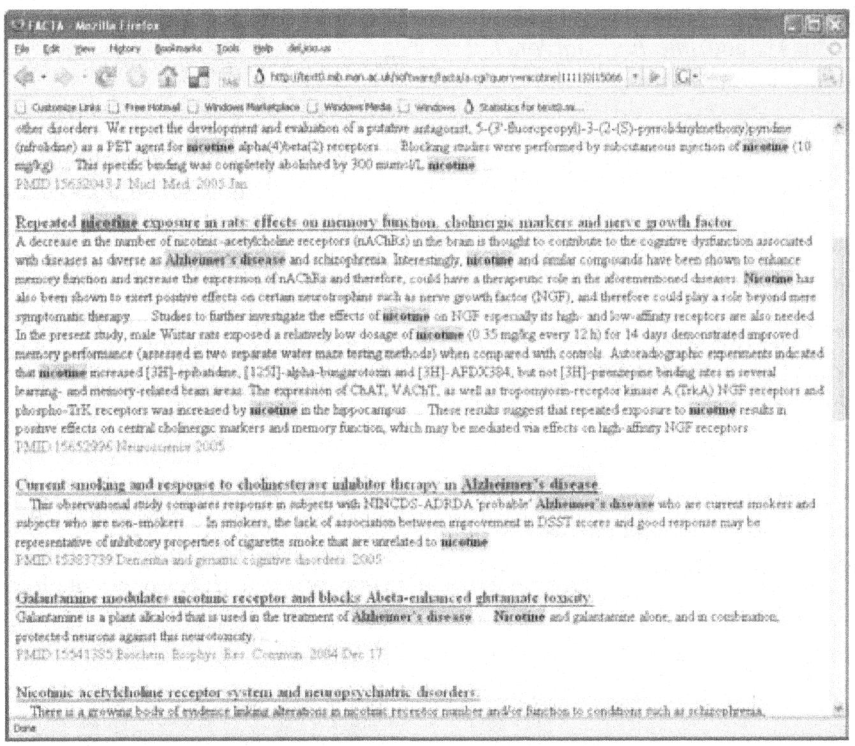

activities. Our goal is to bridge the gap between subject domains through an improved facility for constructing metadata descriptions from textual descriptions via text mining.

REFERENCES

Ananiadou, S., Kell, D. B., & Tsujii, J. (2006). Text mining and its potential applications in systems biology. *Trends Biotechnol, 24*, 571-579.

Ananiadou, S., & McNaught, J. (Eds.) (2006). *Text Mining for Biology and Biomedicine.* Boston / London: Artech House.

Ananiadou, S., Procter, R., Rea, B., Sasaki, Y., & Thomas, J. (2007). Supporting Systematic Reviews using Text Mining. *3rd International Conference on e-Social Science,* Ann Arbor.

Cohen, K. B., & Hunter, L. (2008). Getting started in text mining. *PLoS Comput Biol, 4*, e20.

Frantzi, K., Ananiadou, S., & Mima, H. (2000). Automatic Recognition of Multi-Word Terms: the C-value/NC-value Method. *International Journal on Digital Libraries, 3,* 115-130.

Harnad, S., Brody, T., Vallieres, F., Carr, L., Hitchcock, S., Gingras, Y., Oppenheim, C., Stamerjohanns, H., & Hilf, E. (2004). The Access/Impact Problem and the Green and Gold Roads to Open Access. *Serials review, 30.*

Hearst, M. (1999). Untangling Text Data Mining. *Proceedings of the 37th Annual Meeting of the Association for Computational Linguistics (ACL 1999)* (pp. 3-10).

Hirschman, L., Park, J. C., Tsujii, J., & Wong, L. (2002). Accomplishments and challenges in literature data mining for biology. *Bioinformatics, 18,* 1553-1561.

Jensen, L., Saric, J., & Bork, P. (2006). Literature mining for the biologist: From information retrieval to biological discovery. *Nature Reviews, Genetics, 7,*119-129.

McNaught, J., & Black, W. (2006). Information Extraction. In S.Ananiadou & J. McNaught (Eds.), *Text Mining for Biology and Biomedicine.* Artech house.

Miyao, Y., Ohta, T., Masuda, K., Tsuruoka, Y., Yoshida, K., Ninomiya, T., & Tsujii, J. (2006). Semantic Retrieval for the Accurate Identification of Relational Concepts in Massive Textbases. *Annual Meeting- Association for Computational Linguistics, 2,* 1017-1024.

Miyao, Y., & Tsujii, J. (2008). Feature Forest Models for Probabilistic HPSG Parsing. *Computational Linguistics, 34,* 35-80.

Spasic, I., Ananiadou, S., McNaught, J., & Kumar, A. (2005). Text mining and ontologies in biomedicine: making sense of raw text. *Brief Bioinform, 6,* 239-251.

Swanson, D., & Smalheiser, N. (1994). Assessing a gap in the biomedical literature: magnesium deficiency and neurologic disease. *Neuro-science Research Communications, 15,* 1-9.

Tsuruoka, Y., & Tsujii, J. (2004). Improving the performance of dictionary-based approaches in protein name recognition. *Journal of Biomedical Informatics, 37,* 461-470.

Tsuruoka, Y., Tsujii, J., & Ananiadou, S. (2008). FACTA: A text search engine for finding biomedical concepts. *Bioinformatics 2008*; doi: 10.1093/bioinformatics/btn46.

Weeber, M., Vos, R., Klein, H., De Jong-Van Den Berg, L. T., Aronson, A. R., & Molema, G. (2003). Generating hypotheses by discovering implicit associations in the literature: A case report of a search for new potential therapeutic uses for thalidomide. *J Am Med Inform Assoc, 10,* 252-259.

ENDNOTES

[a] http://www.nactem.ac.uk/software/termine/
[b] http://www.pubmed.gov
[c] http://www.nactem.ac.uk/bbc/
[d] http://text0.mib.man.ac.uk/software/facta/

Section I

Works at a Lexical Level:

Crossroads Between NLP and Ontological Knowledge Management

Chapter II
Lexical Granularity for Automatic Indexing and Means to Achieve It:
The Case of Swedish MeSH®

Dimitrios Kokkinakis
University of Gothenburg, Sweden

ABSTRACT

The identification and mapping of terminology from large repositories of life science data onto concept hierarchies constitute an important initial step for a deeper semantic exploration of unstructured textual content. Accurate and efficient mapping of this kind is likely to provide better means of enhancing indexing and retrieval of text, uncovering subtle differences, similarities and useful patterns, and hopefully new knowledge, among complex surface realisations, overlooked by shallow techniques based on various forms of lexicon look-up approaches. However, a finer-grained level of mapping between terms as they occur in natural language and domain concepts is a cumbersome enterprise that requires various levels of processing in order to make explicit relevant linguistic structures. This chapter highlights some of the challenges encountered in the process of bridging free text to controlled vocabularies and thesauri and vice versa. The author investigates how the extensive variability of lexical terms in authentic data can be efficiently projected to hierarchically structured codes, while means to increase the coverage of the underlying lexical resources are also investigated.

INTRODUCTION

Large repositories of life science data in the form of domain-specific literature, textual databases and other large specialised textual collections (corpora) in electronic form increase on a daily basis to a level beyond what the human mind can grasp and interpret. As the volume of data continues to increase, substantial support from new information technologies and computational techniques grounded in the form of the ever increasing applications of the *mining paradigm* is becoming apparent. In the biomedical domain, for instance, curators are struggling to effectively process tens of thousands of scientific references that are added monthly to the MEDLINE/ PubMed database. While, in the clinical setting vast amounts of health-related data are collected on a daily basis. They constitute a valuable research resource particularly if they by effective automated processing could be better integrated and linked, and thus help scientists to locate and make better use of the knowledge encoded in the electronic repositories. One example would be the construction of hypotheses based upon associations between extracted information possibly overlooked by human readers. *Web, Text* and *Data mining* are therefore recognised as the key technologies for advanced, exploratory and quantitative data-analysis of large and often complex data in unstructured or semi-structured form in document collections. Text mining is the technology that tries to solve the problem of information overload by combining techniques from natural language processing (NLP), information retrieval, machine learning, visualization and knowledge management, by the analysis of large volumes of *unstructured data* and the development of new tools and/or integration/adaptation of state of the art processing components. "Text mining aims at extracting interesting non-trivial patterns of knowledge by discovering, extracting and linking sparse evidence from various sources" (Hearst, 1999) and is considered a variation of *data mining,* which tries to find interesting patterns in *structured data*, while in the same analogy, *web mining* is the analysis of useful information directly from web documents (Markellos *et al.*, 2004). These emerging technologies play an increasingly critical role in aiding research productivity, and they provide the means for reducing the workload for information access and decision support and for speeding up and enhancing the knowledge discovery process (Kao & Poteet, 2007; Feldman& Sanger, 2007; Sirmakessis, 2004).

However, in order to accomplish these higher level goals and support the mining approach, a fundamental and unavoidable starting point is the identification, classification and mapping of terminology from the textual, unstructured data onto biomedical knowledge sources and concept hierarchies, such as domain-dependent thesauri, nomenclatures and ontologies. This first, but crucial step, constitutes the necessary starting point for a deeper semantic analysis and exploration of the unstructured textual content (Ananiadou & McNaught, 2006; Crammer *et al.*, 2007; Krauthammer & Nenadic, 2004; Névéol *et al.*, 2007; Vintar *et al.*, 2003). The task is considered as one of the most challenging research topics within the *biomedical natural language processing* community (bio-NLP), the field of research that seeks to create tools and methodologies for sequence and textual analysis that combine bioinformatics and NLP technologies in a synergistic fashion (Yandell & Majoros, 2002). Ananiadou & Nenadic (2006, pp. 67) point out that processing and management of terminology is one of the key factors for accessing the information stored in literature, since information across scientific articles is conveyed through terms and their relationships. Indexing, which is one of the main target activities of this mapping, is an indispensible step for efficient information retrieval engines and applications. A step that is realized as *the* most time consuming activity for librarians, *cf.* Névéol *et al.* (2005). Moreover, thesauri and ontologies are considered the backbone for various data and knowledge management systems. In our work, we take the position that such resources *do* exist in a digital form. We will use MeSH, Medical Subject Headings (edition 2006), as it is a free resource, which makes it potentially attractive as a component to build on and explore and therefore there is no need to create a thesaurus from scratch. Ontology learning and fully automatic, corpus-based thesaurus construction, as alternative methodologies for knowledge management application design, are beyond the scope of this chapter. For a description of such approaches the interested reader is referred to Buitelaar *et al.* (2005); Gómez-Pérez & Manzano-Macho (2003) and Navigli *et al.* (2003). However, a number of techniques for *thesaurus enrichment*, and how newly acquired terminology can be related to the original MeSH hierarchy are envisaged and will be explored in the following sections. This has the implication of drastically reducing the cost of updating resources such as MeSH, and improving human productivity using domain corpora.

The success of efficient terminology management for applications such as semantic relation acquisition/mining is dependant on the structure, quality and coverage of the underlying lexical resource (ontology or thesaurus) and the linguistic processing adopted (*cf.* Aronson, 2001). This chapter provides a description of the whole life-cycle of our work regarding terminology management on Swedish medical textual data including applications based on the results of this effort. For this purpose, we use one of the very few comprehensive biomedical terminological resources for Swedish, namely the Swedish MeSH thesaurus, and, for reasons explained in Section 2, we also work with its corresponding English original source. We are interested in exploring the thesaurus at its fullest and for this reason we are aiming at applying various techniques and paying particular attention to a number of processing and refinement steps in order to transform the original database tables into a fully-fledged processing oriented annotating resource, including means to increase its coverage. In parallel with this development, we will investigate how the extensive variability of lexical terms in authentic data can be efficiently and automatically projected to hierarchically structured MeSH codes with the highest possible accuracy and coverage. It is mutually important and beneficiary to work from both the resource perspective and the text perspective, since a large number of term forms, as they appear in text, are often not registered in official resources such as MeSH, which causes practical difficulties in sharing and disseminating knowledge in text (Tsujii & Ananiadou, 2005). In the following sections some of the challenges encountered in the process of bridging natural language text with the lexical content of the thesaurus and vice versa, will be exemplified. Although the various processing steps are the main focus of this chapter, the result of this synergy between text processing and thesaurus transformation, refinement and enhancement, will form the basis for applying it to different tasks, particularly relation mining and visualization of medical content.

This chapter is structured in the following six sections. Background information, particularly an overview of studies using MeSH, is given in Section 2. This section contains also a short presentation of a Swedish medical corpus used for acquiring terminological variants and testing various hypotheses. Section 3 provides the description of the transformation and normalization process of the original MeSH database tables into a processing resource for automatic indexing. Enhancements of MeSH by incorporating *external* and *corpus-based* terminology are also presented. Section 4 discusses the pre and post-processing of a text to be annotated by MeSH, including a number of complementary techniques to thesaurus enhancement, such as recognizing acronyms, approximate string matching and resolving elliptical coordination. In Section 5 experimental annotation of Swedish medical corpora is exemplified. This section also discusses evaluation issues, particularly the coverage of MeSH on Swedish data, and discusses a number of problematic cases. In Section 6 we present a number of applications and studies based on the automatic indexing. These include a system for relation mining based on binary solid compounds and visualization of medical content by the application of the vector space representation of document content. Finally, Section 6 summarizes the chapter and presents some thoughts and prospects for future research.

BACKGROUND

MeSH and MeSH Concepts

MeSH is the controlled vocabulary thesaurus of the U.S. National Library of Medicine (NLM). The work described in this chapter and the implementation of the terminology labelling system (henceforth MeSHLAB) we have developed are based on both the English and the Swedish translation of the year 2006 MeSH thesauri, approx. 24,000 descriptors. The motivation for integrating the English hierarchy in our work was the fact that it is fairly common that Swedish texts, intended both for professional and lay audience, contain portions of shorter or longer English segments. MeSH is a subset of the Unified Medical Language System Metathesaurus (UMLS, 2006), the world's largest domain-specific thesaurus and it is used for subject analysis of biomedical literature, particularly for indexing the MEDLINE/PubMed, the premier bibliography of NLM, a large repository of research papers from the medical domain. MEDLINE/PubMed contains bibliographic citations and abstracts from over 4,000 journals.

MeSH has been used for different purposes in a variety of applications and settings. Cooper & Miller (1998) developed and evaluated three different methods for mapping terms in clinical text to MeSH terms by suggesting a list of relevant MeSH terms to physicians to help them improve access to the literature. The best method reported was a hybrid system that achieved a recall of 66% and a precision of 20%. The results are rather poor for use in modern scientific research, but substantial achievements have been accomplished by the research community since that time, for instance Shin *et al.* (2004) have proposed various approaches to balance the manual and automatic indexing. Rosario *et al.* (2002) used MeSH for the analysis of compound nouns, by placing words from a noun compound into categories, and then using the category membership to determine the relation that holds between the nouns. Rechtsteiner & Rocha (2004) report on validation of gene expression clusters using MeSH; while Djebbari *et al.* (2005) applied the thesaurus to the identification of biological concepts that are significantly over-represented within the identified gene set relative to those associated with the overall collection of genes on the underlying DNA microarray platform. Moreover, Douyere *et al.*, (2004) enhance MeSH in order to adapt the terminology to a wider field of health internet resources instead of scientific articles, by introducing two new concepts, namely *resource types* and *metaterms*. Struble & Dharmanolla (2004) investigate the use of MeSH for discovering groupings within a collection of medical literature in MEDLINE/PubMED, in their study the authors conclude that MeSH is useful for document clustering but point out that yearly revisions of MeSH imply that systems must often adapt to these changes. In Sweden, documents in the Swedish database SveMed+ (<http://micr.kib.ki.se/>) are manually annotated using MeSH by human indexers at the Karolinska Institute in Stockholm.

Structure of MeSH Terms

In MeSH each atomic or composite concept has two kinds of "numbers" associated with it:

1. The identifier of the descriptor starting with a 'D' (e.g. [D000377] for *Agnosia*), a unique number for each descriptor and is the equivalent of the Gene Ontology (GO, <http://www.geneontology.org/>) accession number for GO terms or the Concept Unique Identifier (CUI) for UMLS concepts.
2. One or more alphanumeric semantic descriptor codes corresponding to particular positions in the hierarchy. The tree numbers have periods in them (except for the root)

and denote the position(s) of a descriptor in the polyhierarchical organization of MeSH - the place in the tree.

Thus, the codes have a "transparent" structure and each place in the hierarchy is unique, from which both the semantic class of a concept and its depth in the hierarchy can be inferred. The same MeSH descriptor often exists at several places within the same tree and may even belong to several trees. A tree number represents the path between a descriptor and the root of the tree to which it belongs. Still, using *Agnosia* as an example, there are three tree numbers, two from the *Diseases* [C] tree and one from the *Psychiatry and Psychology* [F]. What this means is that *Agnosia* can be seen from the perspective of both diseases and psychological disorders. But in both cases, this is the same "concept" *Agnosia.* Within diseases, there are two paths between *Neurologic manifestations* and the root of the C tree, leading to two paths between *Agnosia* (a descendant of Neurologic manifestations) and the root of the C tree, which are reflected in the two tree numbers starting with C. Thus, there are not three descriptors for *Agnosia* in MeSH, but only one, present in three different places in the MeSH organization (i.e., reachable through three different paths from the root of MeSH). Since there is only one descriptor, there is no need for disambiguation. MeSH indicates that *Agnosia* can be more or less indifferently a *Disease* (including symptoms) [C] or a *Psychological manifestation* [F]. Within C, the fact that *Agnosia* belongs to both *Neurologic Manifestations* [C10.597] and *Signs and Symptoms* [C23.888] can be understood as indicating that *Agnosia* is a neurologic symptom, inheriting from both ancestors; Bodenreider (2007), (Figure 1).

MeSHLAB uses all subtree hierarchies and all levels in MeSH. The higher level categorization (top level) of the hierarchy consists of 16 different semantic groups, or sub-hierarchies, and *nearly* each corresponds to a major branch of medical terminology. Nearly, since some of the hierarchies are more homogeneous and more strongly associated with medicine than others, e.g. *Anatomy* compared to *Information Science.* Depending of the annotation task and application needs, it might be beneficiary to filter out unnecessary levels of the tree hierarchy, and thus reduce the negative

Figure 1. The three MeSH paths of Agnosia (Retrieved March 01, 2008, from http://mesh.kib.ki.se/swemesh/show.swemeshtree.cfm?Mesh_No=C10.597.606.762.100)

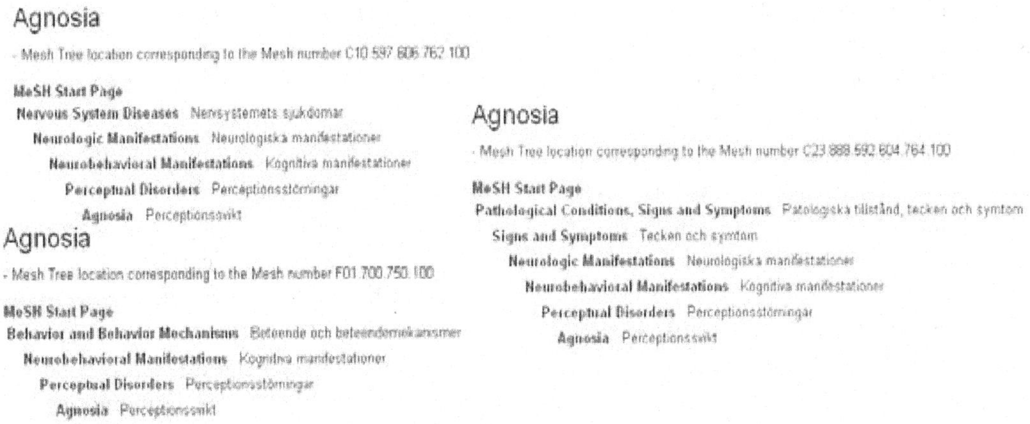

Agnosia

- Mesh Tree location corresponding to the Mesh number C10.597.606.762.100

MeSH Start Page
Nervous System Diseases Nervsystemets sjukdomar
Neurologic Manifestations Neurologiska manifestationer
Neurobehavioral Manifestations Kognitiva manifestationer
Perceptual Disorders Perceptionsstörningar
Agnosia Perceptionssvikt

Agnosia

- Mesh Tree location corresponding to the Mesh number F01.700.750.100

MeSH Start Page
Behavior and Behavior Mechanisms Beteende och beteendemekanismer
Neurobehavioral Manifestations Kognitiva manifestationer
Perceptual Disorders Perceptionsstörningar
Agnosia Perceptionssvikt

Agnosia

- Mesh Tree location corresponding to the Mesh number C23.888.592.604.764.100

MeSH Start Page
Pathological Conditions, Signs and Symptoms Patologiska tillstånd, tecken och symtom
Signs and Symptoms Tecken och symtom
Neurologic Manifestations Neurologiska manifestationer
Neurobehavioral Manifestations Kognitiva manifestationer
Perceptual Disorders Perceptionsstörningar
Agnosia Perceptionssvikt

Table 1. The 16 main descriptors in MeSH. Each category is further divided into subcategories, e.g. [A] in: Body regions [A01]; Musculoskeletal system [A02] and so on

Category	Description	Category	Description
A	Anatomy	I	Anthropology, Education, Sociology and Social Phenomena
B	Organisms	J	Technology and Food/Beverages
C	Diseases	K	Humanities
D	Chemicals and Drugs	L	Information Science
E	Analytical, Diagnostic and Therap. Techniques/Equipment	M	Persons
F	Psychiatry and Psychology	N	Health Care
G	Biological Sciences	V	Publication Characteristics
H	Physical Sciences	Z	Geographic Locations

effect that data sparseness may cause in various applications (*cf.* Rosario *et al.*, 2002; Vintar *et al.*, 2003). So for instance, the term *beta-Lactamases, Betalaktamaser* [D08.811.277.087.180] can be reduced to its main heading [D08] *Enzymes and Coenzymes*, if an application wishes to explore such simplified format. By this reduction, we assume that terms having multiple labels under the same level are similar. Table (1) shows an overview of the main headings, descriptors, in MeSH.

Swedish and English MeSH

The terms from both the English and Swedish MeSH editions of 2006 have been used in our work. The motivation for integrating the English hierarchy in MeSHLAB was the fact that it is fairly common that Swedish texts, intended both for professional (e.g. scientific texts, clinical notes) and lay audience (e.g. consumer health care texts), contain portions of shorter or longer English segments, usually in the form of citations. This phenomenon is illustrated by the following short example:

"Atenolol var effektivast, medan kalciumantagonisten nitrendipin (en dihydropyridin, som felodipin) stod för störst antal utsättningar på grund av biverkningar. Författarna konkluderade: »There is no evidence of superiority for antihypertensive effectiveness or tolerability of the new classes of antihypertensives (calcium channel blockers and angiotensin converting enzyme inhibitors).« Redovisningen av biverkningar i ALLHAT är bristfällig [...]."

Läkartidningen, vol. 100:6 (2003)

Moreover, the use of English simplex or compound terms in Swedish texts is also very common. This is probably due to the authors' unfamiliarity with the appropriate Swedish translation; by the influence from the English language, particularly in orthographic variation, e.g. use of 'ph' instead of 'f' (e.g. *lymfo-lympho*); use of 'th' instead of 't' (e.g. *hypothyreos-hypotyreos*; *thorax-torax*) and use of 'c' instead of 'k' (e.g. *bradycardi-bradykardi*); by spelling errors that might have a direct correspondence to English terms, the overuse of hyphen (e.g. *tetra-cyklin* instead of *tetracyklin*), or possibly because of an author finding the English spelling more appropriate or "correct". Moreover, in certain cases, we have observed the opposite phenomenon, that is the use of non-standard spelling variants instead of the pre-dominant nomenclature (e.g. *kancer* instead of *cancer*). Therefore, the integration of both languages opens up for greater coverage, more accurate results and more reliable statistics.

The MEDLEX Corpus

With the information overload in the life sciences there is an increasing need for annotated corpora (particularly with biological entities) which is the driving force for data-driven language processing applications and the empirical approach to language study. The GENIA corpus (Jin-Dong *et al.*, 2003) is one such corpus, extensively used in biomedical research. GENIA is a manually curated corpus of 2000 MEDLINE/PubMED abstracts with over 100,000 annotations for biological terms. Cohen *et al.* (2005) present a survey of biomedical corpora and the authors discuss the importance of format and annotation standards for usability and usefulness in research activities. In order to fulfil the needs of our research we have collected a Swedish medical corpus, MEDLEX, the first large structurally and linguistically annotated Swedish medical corpus (*cf.* Kokkinakis, 2006). The MEDLEX Corpus consists of a variety of text-documents related to various medical text subfields, and does not focus at a particular medical genre, primarily due to the lack of very large Swedish resources within a particular specialized area. All text samples (25 mil. tokens, 50,000 documents) are fetched from heterogeneous web pages during the past couple of years, and include: teaching material, guidelines, official documents, scientific articles from medical journals, conference abstracts, consumer health care documents, descriptions of diseases, definitions from on-line dictionaries, editorial articles, patient's FAQs and blogs etc. All texts have been converted to text files, and have been both structurally and linguistically annotated. All experiments described in this chapter use data from this collection.

MESH: CONVERSION, NORMALIZATION AND ENHANCEMENT

MeSHLAB is an *automatic indexing system*. Automatic indexing is an activity that exploits terms as means for assigning descriptors to documents in order to facilitate information access In this context two interrelated issues need to be taken under consideration in order to successfully map free text to control vocabularies and hierarchies such as MeSH. The first issue, further exemplified in this section, has to do with the necessary adaptations of the resource content to a format suitable for text processing. This is necessary, since it has been claimed by a number of researchers that many term occurrences cannot be identified in text if straightforward dictionary/database lookup is applied (*cf.* Hirschman *et al.*, 2003). Therefore a number of conversion and normalization steps have to be applied to the original material. Secondly, we have to efficiently deal with language variability by using, or even better, combining various techniques such as stemming (Jacquemin & Tzoukermann, 1999) and approximate string matching (Tsuruoka & Tsujii, 2003), see Section 4. Normalization is thus necessary before the actual application of the MeSH content due to the nature of the original data, in which the head word usually precedes its modifiers, e.g. *Lung Diseases, Obstructive* with the Swedish translation *Lungsjukdomar, obstruktiva.* Thus, a great effort has been put into the normalization of MeSH, since, compared to English and UMLS, for which a number of supporting software tools are available as part of the SPECIALIST lexicon, the situation for Swedish is diametrically different and there are no similar tools available. The SPECIALIST lexicon contains for each term, variants such as acronyms, abbreviations, synonyms, derivational variants, spelling errors, inflectional variants and meaningful combinations of all these.

Table 2. Head-modifier normalization

Original Swedish MeSH	Step-1 Tranformation	Glossing
Vacciner, orala	orala Vacciner	*Vaccines, Edible*
Astma, ansträngningsutlöst	ansträngningsutlöst Astma	*Asthma, Exercise-Induced*
Hepatit, viral, djur	viral Hepatit hos djur viral Hepatit , djur	*Hepatitis, Viral, Animal*
Lymfom, T-cell , kutant	kutant T-cellslymfom kutant t-cell Lymfom	*Lymphoma, T-Cell, Cutaneous*

Term Conversion and Normalization of the Head and Modifiers

The first step applied to the MeSH database was to change the order of the head and modifier complements, usually variants with commas, in the original material (Table 2) to the word order one would expect in free text. There are several hundreds of such cases in the database because of obvious terminological and lexicographic purposes, e.g. easier means of sorting based on head words. They had to be changed in order to be able to apply the lexical content to text data.

Term Conversion and Normalization of Inflected Variants

The second step was to normalize all inflected entries into a neutral *non-inflected* variant by applying a number of morphology stripping patterns. This was necessary since there is a combination of both inflected and uninflected terms in the database (Table 3). Although Swedish is morphologically more complex than English there was still a manageable number of inflectional patterns that covered the vast majority of inflected variants in the MeSH database, e.g. adjectives are usually inflected with the addition of *–t* (depending on the gender) and *–a* (depending on the number). Special patterns were constructed for a small number of noun terms with irregular inflection patterns, e.g. *öra* (ear) and *öron* (ears).

Case folding was applied to all terms at this stage, except those consisting of uppercase letters, acronyms. This was necessary in order not to introduce new forms of ambiguity, since the complete elimination of case information could introduce new ambiguities between homographs uppercase/ low case words, for instance, *kol* [D01.268.150] (carbon) and *KOL* [C08.381.495.389] (Chronic Obstructive Pulmonary Disease).

Addition of Inflectional Morphology and Variant Numeric Forms

At this stage, each entry is either of the form: $term_x$ => *mesh.tag(s)* or $term_x$' '$term_z$ => *mesh.tag(s)* in case of multiword terms. Depending on the

Table 3. Inflection normalization

Original Swedish MeSH	Step-2 Tranformation
Vaccin*er*, oral*a*	oral vaccin
Astma, ansträngningsutlös*t*	ansträngningsutlös astma
Hepatit, viral, djur	viral hepatit hos djur *and* viral hepatit, djur
Lymfom , T-cell , kutan*t*	kutan t-cellslymfom *and* kutan t-cell lymfom

suffixes of the adjectives and/or nouns in MeSH, we heuristically added inflectional morphological features and variants using regular expressions patterns to all entries, and in the case of multiword terms to both head and modifier(s). Thus, each term has actually been encoded as: $term_x(m_1|...|m_n)?$ => *mesh.tag(s)* or $term_x(m_1|...|m_n)?$' '$term_z(m_1|...|m_n)?$ => *mesh.tag(s)*, where m_1 to m_n are different optional inflectional suffixes. Here optionality is denoted by '?' and disjunction by '|'. This is a necessary step since MeSHLAB is meant to be applied on raw, unstemmed, texts and therefore we did not want to pose any particular restrictions to the nature of the input, which can be both ungrammatical and contain spelling errors, particularly at the declination level (Table 4). Therefore, apart from the *grammatically correct* inflectional patterns we also added wrong gender inflection patterns since we have noticed that particularly for the category [C] terms, grammatical gender (*–et* or *–en*) usually occurs in either forms, e.g. *adrenalin**et*** and *adrenalin**en***.

We also added variants to the Roman numbers e.g. for the use of "III" the addition of "3" (e.g. for *kollagen typ III* we added *kollagen typ 3*), and also to the Arabic numbers e.g. for the use of "2" the addition of "II" (e.g. for *Typ 2-diabetes* we added *Typ II-diabetes*).

Addition of Derivational Variants and Empty Suffixes

A small number of derivational patterns are also considered in order to add new entries through this affixation process. Particular emphasis was put on productive forms of making noun-to-adjective or noun-to-participle derivations with the suffixes *–sk* and *–nde*, as well as forms of making noun-to-noun derivations with the suffixes *–ik*, *–ing* and *–ion* (Table 5a).

In parallel, we developed a component utilizing a set of "empty" suffixation patterns to various MeSH groups (Table 5b). During the development cycle of the MeSHLAB we identified a number of such group-dependent markers that do not substantially change the meaning of a term, but simply act either as placeholders, or sometime add a slightly more detailed nuance to the term in question.

Addition of Variant Forms Based on Empirical Observations

Although a number of vocabularies, taxonomies and thesauri have been developed for the healthcare and biomedical domain, no single vocabulary can ever provide complete coverage of the information that can be found in free text. Therefore support from empirical studies provides an indispensable way to enhance existing taxonomies Almeida *et al.* (2003) argue that existing vocabularies may serve as content starting points to avoid duplication of work. During the development cycle of the MeSHLAB we observed a number of typographical variant cases of existing terms that we successively added to the database in an automatic fashion. Thus, apart from the cases discussed in the previous sections, we also added

Table 4. Morphological normalization

Original Swedish MeSH	Step-3 Tranformation
Vacciner, orala	oral*(t|a)?* vaccin*(en|et|er|erna)?*
Astma, ansträngningsutlöst	ansträngningsutlös*(t|a)?* astma*(n)?*
Hepatit, viral, djur	viral*(t|a)?* hepatit*(en|er|erna)?* hos djur*(et|en)?* viral*(t|a)?* hepatit*(en|er|erna)?* , djur*(et|en)?*
Lymfom , T-cell , kutant	kutan*(t|a)?* t-cellslymfom*(et|en)?* kutan*(t|a)?* t-cell lymfom*(et|en)?*

Table 5a-b. Common derivational patterns and "empty" suffixes

Original Swedish MeSH	Step-4 Derivations	Glossing
(a) farmakologi	farmakologi*sk*	*pharmacology, pharmacologic*
diagnos	diagnos*tik*	*diagnosis, diagnostic*
strålbehandling	strål*nings*behandling	*radiotherapy*
institut	insitut*ion*	*institute, institution*
(b) ögonlock [A]	ögonlocks*kanten*	*eyelids (edge)*
bakterie [B]	bakterie*typ*	*bacteria (type)*
Alzheimer [C]	alzheimer*typ*	*alzheimer disease (type)*
tetracyklin [D]	tetracyklin*tablett*	*tetracycline (tablet)*
gastrostomi [E]	gastrostomi*metod*	*gastrostomy (method)*

a large number of variants of multiword terms using pattern matching. Some of the most common text patterns had to do with various organisms as well as anatomical terms of Latin origin for which the text realization is usually found in an abbreviated form, particularly terms describing *muscles*, *nerves* and *arteries* (Table 6).

Automatically extracted paraphrase variant forms of solid MeSH compounds were also added after manual inspection (Table 7a). Compounds usually correspond to multiword phrases in other languages, such as English. A large number of such forms (roughly 500) were extracted from the MEDLEX Corpus, sometimes referred to as permutations (Jacquemin, 2001, pp. 162), and added to MeSH. Moreover, orthographic variant forms of compounds, compounds with acronyms and elisions were also added (Table 7b).

Errors in the Swedish MeSH

Some errors in the original material were also identified and added to the database (Figure 2), while other discrepancies were also minimized and normalized. For instance, there are both singular and plural forms for some head terms, such as *aortapulmonal* ***septumdefekt*** (aortopulmonary Septal Defect) in singular and *ventrikel****septum-defekter*** (Heart Septal Defects, Ventricular) in plural. Similarly, there were cases of both definite and indefinite forms, such as *bakterier i* ***urinen*** (bacteriuria) and *blod i* ***urin*** (hematuria), which were also normalised according the morphological normalization process described earlier.

Table 6. Abbreviated variations based on multiword terms

Original Swedish MeSH	Step-6 Tranformation
Nervus abducens	n. abducens
Vena cava inferior	v. cava inferior and v. cava inf.
Arteria iliaca	a. iliaca and art iliaca
Staphylococcus aureus	staph aureus and s. aureus
Helicobacter pylori	h pylori and h. pylori
Chlamydia pneumoniae	c. pneumoniae

Tables 7a-b. Lexical variations based on paraphrases

Original Swedish MeSH	Step-7 Tranformation	Glossing
(a) Bukspottkörtelcancer	cancer i bukspottkörtel	*Pancreatic Neoplasms*
Njurcancer	cancer i njuren	*Kidney Neoplasms*
Livmoderhalscancer	cancer i/på livmoderhalsen	*Uterine Cervical Neoplasms*
(b) Skivepitelcancer	skivepitelca	*Neoplasms, Squamous Cell*
Viral RNA	viral-rna	*Viral RNA*
Vitamin D3	d3-vitamin	*Vitamin D 3*
Parkinsons sjukdom	parkinsons	*Parkinsons Disease*
Restless Legs Syndrome	restless legs	*Restless Legs Syndrome*

Updating MeSH with Medical Brand Names

Apart from the work described in the previous section, particularly *"Addition of variant forms based on empirical observations"*, we have also explored other means for enhancing the content of MeSH. One such technique is to look up names of medicines, i.e. the trade name given by the manufacturers, and automatically map these names to their generic ones, if such a name is present in MeSH. This was accomplished using a handful handcrafted pattern matching rules.

For instance, *Cipramil®*, a medicine used for treatment of depression and anxiety disorders, contains the active ingredient *citalopram. Citalopram* can be found in MeSH under the nodes *D02.092.831.170, D02.626.320* and *D03.438.127.187*, but not *Cipramil®* which has been added by this matching process with the same alphanumeric coding as its generic name. In the MEDLEX Corpus there were 940 unique brand name contexts of the form shown in Table 8a. For a small number of these candidates (9%) only a part of the generic compound substance name was annotated by MeSH (Table 8b) and we chose not to add the brand name in the database. There were also cases in which neither the generic name or the trade name could be associated with a MeSH term (Table 8c).

External Lexical Resources

Although MeSH and its enhancements, as described previously, are a good starting point for mapping free text to structured codes, texts contain a lot of other types of medical terminology that need to be considered. MesH lacks for

Figure 2. Example of a MeSH spelling error; Trypsininhibiotor should be Trypsininhibitor (Retrieved March 01, 2008, from http://mesh.kib.ki.se/swemesh/show.swemeshtree.cfm?Mesh_No=D12.776.765.741.750)

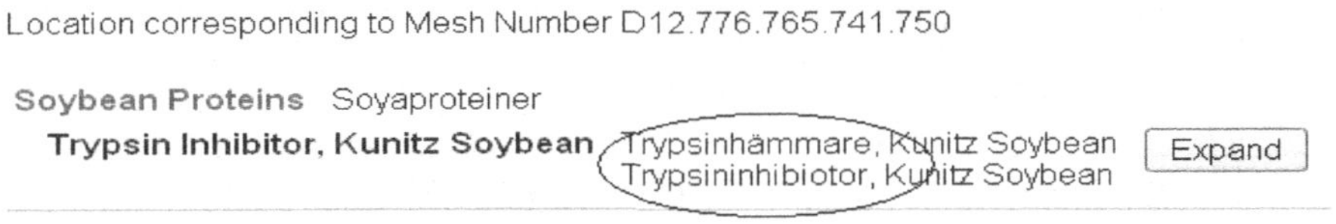

Location corresponding to Mesh Number D12.776.765.741.750

Soybean Proteins	Soyaproteiner	
Trypsin Inhibitor, Kunitz Soybean	Trypsinhämmare, Kunitz Soybean Trypsininhibiotor, Kunitz Soybean	Expand

instance information on (at least) two types of important terminology frequently occurring in free text: names of pharmaceutical products (drugs) and anatomical Greek and Latin terms. For that purpose, we have added several thousand names of pharmaceutical products, particularly names of drugs, by applying a generic annotation with simply the code [*D*] which in MeSH stands for *Chemicals and Drugs*, unless the generic name of the drug could be mapped to a structured MeSH code, in line with the previous discussion. The pharmaceutical names have been obtained from a reference book of all medicines that are approved and used in Sweden (<http://www.fass.se>), while terminology of Greek/Latin origin, particularly anatomical terms have been obtained from the Karolinska institutet (<http://www.karolinska.se>). In this case the generic annotation with code [*A*], which in MeSH stands for *Anatomy*, has been used.

TEXT PROCESSING

Even within the same text, a term can take many different forms. Tsujii & Ananiadou (2005, pp. 7) discuss that "a term may be expressed via various mechanisms including orthographic variation, usage of hyphens and slashes [...], lower and upper cases [...], spelling variations [...], various Latin/Greek transcriptions [...] and abbreviations [...]." This rich variety for a large number of term-forms is a stumbling block especially for Text Mining, as these forms have to be recognised, linked and mapped to terminological and ontological resources; for a review on normalization strategies see Krauthammer & Nenadic (2004). Consider the following examples for some terms extracted from the MEDLEX Corpus which clearly illustrate the term variability in authentic corpora (Table 9).

In order to capture cases as the ones shown in Table 9, we have generated permutation of the multiword terms in MeSH, supported by corpus evidence, and added the new forms to the database. However, even greater problems and challenges are posed by solid compound terms not included in MeSH, and the next two sections discuss how MeSHLAB effectively deals with these cases.

Compound Segmentation

Compounds pose a serious problem for many tasks in computerised processing of Swedish, particularly in applications that require morphological segmentation, such as Information Retrieval. In Swedish, compounds are written almost exclusively as one orthographic word (solid compounds) and are very productive. Therefore, for potential compound terms where there are no entries in

Table 8a-c. Brand names as MeSH candidates

Corpus Sample (before and after MeSH annotation)	New Entries
(a) *Ofta använda läkemedel är cisplatin (Platinol®) , vincristin (Oncovin®) , och metotrexat (Trexall®)*	Platinol® Oncovin® Trexall®
Ofta använda läkemedel är <mesh id="D01.210...">cisplatin</mesh> (Platinol®) , <mesh id="D03.132...">vincristin</mesh> (Oncovin®) , och <mesh id="D03.438...">metotrexat</mesh> (Trexall®) .	
(b) *...oxybutyninklorid (Ditropan XL®) och zoledronsyra (Zometa)*	--
...oxybutynin<mesh id="D01.210....">klorid</mesh> (Ditropan XL®) och zoledron<mesh id="D01.029...">syra</mesh> (Zometa)	
(c) *...sildenafil (Viagra) , tadalafil (Cialis) och vardenafil (Levitra)*	--

MeSH covering these forms, compound analysis is necessary. Inspired by the work of Brodda (1979) we have implemented a domain-independent, finite-state based analyser that builds on the idea of identifying "unusual" grapheme clusters (usually consonants) as means of denoting potential compound limits. The segmentation algorithm we have developed is a non-lexical, quantitative one and it is based on the distributional properties of graphemes, trying to recognize grapheme combinations, indicating possible boundaries. It proceeds by scanning word forms from left to right, trying to identify clusters of character combinations (n-grams) that are non-allowable when considering non-compound forms, and which carry information on potential token boundaries. The grapheme combinations have been arranged into groups of 2 to 8 characters. For instance, an example of a two-character cluster is the combination *sg* which segments compounds such as *virus||genom* (virus genome) and *fibrinolys||grupp* (fibrinolysis group); a three-character cluster is the combination *psd* which segments compounds such as *lewykropps||demens* (Lewy Body Dementia); a four-character cluster is *ngss* and *gssp* which segment compounds such as *sväljnings||svårighet* (swallowing difficulty) and *mässlings||specifik* (measles specific), and so forth. Special attention has been given to compounds where the head or modifier is a very short word (2-3 characters long), such as *lår* (thigh), *sår* (wound), *hår* (hair), *tå* (toe), *yt* (surface), *syn* (sight), *tum* (thumb), *hud* (skin) and *gen* (gene). For such cases we have manually added clusters of short characteristic contexts taken from the MEDLEX Corpus, usually 4-6 characters, before or after such short words. Compound splitting into its parts enables partial or whole annotation with MeSH codes, enhancing technologies such as relation mining (Section 6).

Elliptic Coordinations

The only requirement we pose prior to annotation with MeSHLAB is that the texts are tokenized (some basic form of separation between graphic words and punctuation). However, for maximum performance, the input texts can be optionally pre-processed in various ways (see previous section) in order to resolve certain frequent types of coordinated constructions with ellipsis. These can be of three types (Table 10).

Here, *binder* refers almost exclusively to a conjunction such as *och/and* or *eller/or*, while a few cases with the adverb *som* (as/like) as a binder were also found in the corpus. When such patterns are identified, the solid compound is

Table 9. Examples of lexical variants in the MEDLEX Corpus

Lexical Variants in the Swedish Corpus	Swedish MeSH
IBS/Inflammatory Bowel Syndrome, Infl Bowel Dis, Inflamm Bowel Dis, Inflammatory Bowel Diseases, Inflammatory Bowel Syndrome, Irritabile Bowel Syndrome, irritable bowel, Irritable Bowel Disease, irritable bowel syndrom, irritable bowel syndrome, Irritable Bowel Syndrome, Irritated Bowel Syndrome,...	Inflammatoriska tarmsjukdomar
diabetes typ 2, diabetes typ II, typ 2-diabetes, Typ 2-diabetes, typ II diabetes, typ II-diabetes, typ2 diabetes, typ-2 diabetes, typ2-diabetes, typ-2-diabetes, 'diabetes mellitus, rimligen typ 2',...	Typ 2-diabetes
Cox 2, cox-II hämmare, Cox II, COX-2 hämmare, COX-2-hämmare, cox 2-hämmare, COX2-hämmare, cox 2-hämmare,...	COX-2-hämmare
diarr, diarre, diarre´, diarré, diarrè, diarree, diarrée, diarrhea, diarrhoea, diarrhorea, diarrree,...	Diarre

automatically segmented and the elliptic, partial compound gets the head of the complete compound. This means that in the example *rygg- och nackvärk*, the compound *nackvärk* is segmented as *nack||värk* and *värk*, the head of the compound, is added as the head for *rygg*, and thus the whole phrase becomes *ryggvärk och nackvärk*. Here '||' denotes the border between the head and the modifier of the compound. In order to achieve this type of labelling, compound segmentation, as described previously, is applied and then the text is processed with a module that recognizes and restores candidate discontinuous structures. As soon as the segmentation is performed, the restoration of such structures becomes a trivial task using simple pattern matching. Note, that in case of more than one segmentation point, the rightmost segmentation is considered for the restoration. For instance, *stroke- och hjärtinfarktregister* (stroke registry and infarction registry) becomes *stroke- och hjärt||infarkt||register* after compound segmentation, with two segmentation points. But since the rightmost segmentation point is considered, the coordination will take the form *stroke||register och hjärt||infarkt||register*. Moreover this resolution approach is not limited to binary coordinations but to *n-ary*. For instance *alfa-, beta- och gammaglobulin* (alpha, beta and gamma globulin) becomes after compound segmentation *alfa-, beta- och gamma||globulin* and finally *alfa||globulin, beta||globulin och gamma||globulin*. By applying the process to the MEDLEX Corpus, 25,000 coordinations could be detected, 6,000 of those didn't receive a MeSH label at all and approx. 2,000 either consisted of simplex words or the compounds were not segmented by our segmenter. A random sample of 300 of those showed that 12 (4%) were restored erroneously due to complex non-elliptic compounds with multiple segmentation points, for which our method chose the rightmost one which appeared to be (partially) wrong, e.g. *fyra||stadiet eller åtta||cells||stadiet* (four-cell stage or eight-cell stage) instead of *fyra||cells||stadiet eller åtta||cells||stadiet*.

Approximate String Matching

We can safely assume that official, edited vocabularies will not be able to identify all possible terms in a text. There are a lot of cases that could be considered MeSH-term candidates but are left unmarked, particularly in the case of misspellings. Approximate string matching is fundamental to text processing for identifying the closest match for any text string not found in the thesaurus. Since we are interested in identifying as many terms as possible and with high accuracy, this technique seems very practical for achieving this goal. String matching is an important operation in information systems because misspelling is common in texts found on various web pages, particularly blogs. Therefore, we also calculate the orthographic similarity between potential candidates (≥ 7 characters long) and the MeSH content. We have empirically observed that the

Table 10. Patterns for elliptic coordination recovery

Pattern	Example	Glossing
solidCompound binder –partialCompound	binjurebarken och –märgen	*adrenal cortex and adrenal medulla*
partialCompound– binder solidCompound	rygg– och nackvärk	*back pain and neck pain*
multiW1 multiW2– binder multiW1 multiW3–Term	typ 1– och typ 2–diabetes	*type 1 diabetes and type 2 diabetes*

length of 7 characters is a reliable threshold, unlikely to exclude many misspellings.

As measure of orthographic similarity (or rather, difference) we used the Levenshtein distance (LD; also known as *edit distance*) between two strings. The LD is the number of deletions, insertions or substitutions required to transform a string into another string. The greater the distance, the more different the strings are. We chose to regard 1 as a trustworthy value and disregarded the rest (misspelled terms and MeSH terms usually differ in one character) although there were a few cases for which the value of 2 or 3 could provide compatible results. For instance, the misspelled *accneärr* (*Acne Keloid*) could be matched to *akneärr* with LD=2. By this approach and after manual inspection we actually chose to add the very frequent spelling errors in the thesaurus itself. The method is also applied on the fly while indexing arbitrary texts. Table 11 illustrates various cases and the obtained results. The number of occurrences is taken from the MEDLEX Corpus.

Integration of Acronyms

Long full names in (bio-) medical literature are almost always abbreviated, most frequently by the use of acronyms, which implies the creation of new sets of synonyms. Such abbreviated forms can introduce ambiguity since they might overlap with other abbreviations, acronyms or general Swedish or English vocabulary, as in *hemolytiskt uremiskt syndrome (HUS)*, where *HUS* also stands for the Swedish common noun *house*. Acronym identification is the task of processing text to extract pairs consisting of an acronym (a short form) and its definition or expansion. Discovering acronyms and relating them to their expanded forms is an essential aspect of text mining and terminology management. Shultz (2006) claims that online interfaces do not always map medical acronyms and initialisms to their corresponding MeSH phrases. If acronyms and initialisms are not used in search strategies it may lead to inaccurate results and missed information. Acronyms are rather rare in MeSH and freely available acronym dictionaries in Swedish are currently non existent. Still, acronyms are rather frequent in biomedical texts. Therefore, we applied a simple, yet effective, pattern matching approach to acronym identification, using a set of hand-coded patterns. The pattern matching approach is applied *after* the annotation of a text with MeSH labels. Appropriate annotations in conjunction with orthographic markers in the near vicinity of MeSH-annotations drive the recognition of acronyms throughout a document. Note that it is generally perceived that acronyms are usually introduced once in a text and then frequently used in the *same* document instead of the expanded form; this means that it is *not* safe to simply use an identified acronym in one document for the annotation of a seemingly similar acronym in another document. However, it is rather safe to consistently use the same *meaning*

Table 11. LD between potential terms and MeSH

Term candidate	#	Original MeSH	Accept?	Glossing
adrenaline	7	adrenalin	yes	*epinephrine*
bukspottskörtel	133	bukspottkörtel	yes	*pancreas*
adheranser	3	adherenser	yes	*adhesion*
abduktion	73	obduktion	no	*autopsy*
glucokortikoid	21	glucocorticoid	yes	*glucocorticoids*
aerophagi	10	aerophagy	yes	*aerophagy*

of an acronym throughout a single document. The applied approach has certain similarities with the work by Pustejovsky *et al.* (2001) and Schwartz & Hearst (2003), but here we apply more patterns with more variation and not merely the *Aaa Bbb Ccc (ABC)* where *Aaa*, *Bbb* and *Ccc* are words in a multiword term.

A handful of simple heuristic pattern matching rules (Table 12) can capture a large number of acronyms unknown to the resource and thus assign appropriate MeSH labels. In previous studies based on Swedish data the most frequent acronym patterns found were of the form 'D (A)' 66,2%, 'D, A,' 14,2% and 'A (D)' 5,7%; here *D* stands for the expanded form of an acronym *A* (*cf.* Kokkinakis & Dannélls, 2006).

ANNOTATION AND COVERAGE

Each identified MeSH term is annotated using a simple metadata scheme, based on eXtensible Markup Language (XML) technology with three attributes. The first attribute designates the alphanumeric MeSH code (id), the second the origin of the tag (src) and the third whether the term occurrence is negated or not (neg, with values *yes* or *no*), this attribute is currently not used but is planned for use in the near future. The origin's attribute of a MeSH-tag can take one of the following values:

swe for a term originating from the Swedish MeSH
e.g. *<meshid="C08..."src="swe">astma</mesh>*

eng for a term originating from the English MeSH
e.g. *<meshid="D11..."src="eng">ephrins</mesh>*

acr for a newly identified acronym
e.g. *<mesh id="C10..." src="acr">GBS</mesh>*, for *Guillain-Barres syndrome*

mdf a modified MeSH term, such as derivations and "empty" suffixes
e.g. *<mesh id="C23..." src="mdf">syndrom**typ**</mesh>*

new which stands for terms added to MeSH, e.g. brand names of medicines and misspelled terms
e.g. *<meshid="C14..."src="new">ischmi</mesh>*

In order to empirically investigate the coverage of the resources, by applying the previously discussed transformations and text processing, 50 random articles published by *Läkartidningen*, the

*Table 12. Examples of acronym identification patterns (u: upper case character; x: low case character, n: number; * after compound analysis)*

Pattern	Example	Glossing
<MeSH-term> (uuuu)	Posttraumatiskt stressyndrom (PTSD)	*Stress Disorders, Post-Traumatic*
<MeSH-term> (uuu)	Svår akut luftvägsinfektion (SAL)	*Severe Acute Respiratory Syndrome*
<MeSH-term>, uu-n,	Casein Kinase I, CK-1,	*Casein Kinase I*
<MeSH-term> (uuux)	RNA-interferens (RNAi)	*RNA Interference*
uuu (<MeSH-term>)	ALL (Akut Lymfatisk Leukemi)	*Leukemia, Lymphoid*
<MeSH-term> (uuu)	*låg|molekylärt heparin (LMH)	*Heparin, Low-Molecular-Weight*

Swedish Medical Association's official magazine (<http://www.lakartidningen.se>) during 2006-07 under section "Nya Rön" (New Findings), which usually contain a large portion of terminology, were automatically extracted and annotated. These documents are part of a manually inspected annotated corpus we are currently building (*cf.* Kokkinakis, 2008). In this sample we discovered some cases that had a negative effect on the evaluation results and we had not dealt with during the previous steps. For instance, the use of multiword compounds instead of solid compounds, e.g. in MeSH there is the solid compound *socialfobi* (*Phobic disorder*) but in the texts we could find a multiword variant *social fobi*. Also other forms of elisions were observed, e.g. in MeSH there is the term *chikungunya virus* but in the texts we could only find *chikungunya*.

A manual inspection of the obtained results showed a coverage of 74,7% considering a possible total of 2,516 terms, out of which 1,688 were completely covered, true positives (including new acronyms and terms as described earlier), and 391 were partially covered by MeSH. These were scored as half correct (0.5) if half of the term was covered by MeSH, e.g. *kronisk <trötthet>* (chronic fatigue); 0.3 if one third or less was covered, e.g. *lindrig <tyreoidea>rubbning* and 0.7 if more than two thirds were covered, e.g. *<color> duplex <sonography>*. A total of 437 terms (17.3%) were false negatives, left unannotated, e.g. *kalcipotriol*, *rimonabant*, which hints at the limitations of MeSH in terms of its coverage. The number of false positives, spuriously identified concepts, was low, 46. The majority of these cases are due to homography with non-medical words and are highly context dependent, such as *huvuddelen* (part of the head), which is more frequently used in an adverbial position, i.e. 'mainly'; *leder* (joints), which was used as the homograph verb 'to lead' and *tunga* (tongue), which was used as the homograph adjective 'heavy'. Note, that for homography between verbs and nouns or adjectives and nouns, part-of-speech tagging can be of great help for distinguishing the two forms from each other. The number of acronyms (36), the new terms (67) and the large number of terms originating from the English MeSH (265) in the sample indicates that the effort put into the pre-processing stages pays off both quantitatively and qualitatively. Some other, but less frequent cases had to do with the problem of multiple occurrences of acronyms with the same surface form within the same document but with different semantics. For instance the case of *BNP* in the fragment shown below:

Uppgiften om beslutsgränsvärdet för BNP (»brain natriuretic peptide« eller »B-type natriuretic peptide«) torde härröra från Maiselgruppens undersökning av patienter som söker akut för dyspné (breathing not properly , »BNP«) ."

Läkartidningen, vol. 103:19, (2006)

Which BNP is intended in the sentence *[...] metoden jämförts med andra, mer beprövade metoder för BNP-mätning [...]* following the previous fragment in the same document? The answer is fairly difficult for an automatic process.

Another, more frequent problem has to do with compound segmentation. Specifically in cases where the modifier ends in double consonant and the head starts with the same consonant as well, for instance, *galläckage* (bile leaking) and *skabbehandling* (treatment for scabies). Here, the first example actually stands for *gall+läckage* and the second for *skabb+behandling*. Our compound analyser did not segmented the first compound while the second was segmented as *skab||behandling* and *skab* could not be matched to the actual MeSH entry *skabb* since the approximate string matching approach ignores string less than 7 characters long. Another difficult problem arises when near synonyms of MeSH terms are used in text. For instance, *viktökning* (Weight Gain) is a MeSH term but the near synonym *viktuppgång* is not. In these cases a general thesaurus such as WordNet (Fellbaum, 1998) can be helpful, and once again compound analysis can play an important role for aiding the matching process between *ökning* and *uppgång*. Another important issue has to do with simplex head words that exist in MeSH only as heads of solid compounds. For instance, *retinopati* (retinopathy) exists in MeSH only in compound forms such as *prematuritetsretinopati* (retinopathy of prematurity) but not as a simplex term that can be found in corpora. Finally, it is noticeable that there are a number of rather frequent (lay) words that for reasons we are not aware of, are not covered by MeSH, such as *mage* (stomach) and *kropp* (body). However, such words do not contribute to the evaluation previously presented.

APPLICATIONS

Semantic Relation Mining

In the context of scientific and technical texts, meaning is usually embedded in noun compounds (NC) and the semantic interpretation of these compounds deals with the detection and semantic classification of the relation that holds between the compounds' constituents. *Semantic relation mining*, the technology applied for marking up, interpreting, extracting and classifying relations that hold between pairs of words, is an important enterprise that contribute to deeper means of enhancing document understanding technologies and applications. These range from the interaction of genes and gene products (Sekimizu *et al.*, 1998) to enhanced access to outbreak reports (Grishman *et al.*, 2002) and literature-based discovery by hypotheses generation for scientific research (Hristovski *et al.*, 2006). We explore the application of assigning semantic descriptors taken from MeSH to a large sample of solid compounds taken from MEDLEX, and determining the relation(s) that may hold between the compound constituents. This experiment is inspired by previous research in the area of using lexical hierarchies for identifying relations between binary NCs in the medical domain. In contrast to previous research, Swedish require further means of analysis, since NCs are written as one sequence with no space between the words. Our work replicates the methodology proposed by (Rosario *et al.*, 2002) who used the juxtaposition of category membership within the lexical hierarchy to determine the relation that holds between pairs of nouns (in English). We also apply predicate paraphrasing, inspired by (Nakov & Hearst, 2006), in order to propose a list of verbal predicates as designators of the relationship, without at this stage explicitly naming it.

We automatically annotated the MEDLEX Corpus with MeSH, the compound analysis determined whether the head and modifier parts of solid compounds could be annotated. From the annotated sample we selected all *binary* compounds, in which *both* constituents have been assigned a MeSH annotation, e.g.*<mesh id="B06..."> kakao</mesh><mesh id="D03... ">flavonoler</mesh>* (cacao flavonols). If a head and/or modifier fell under more than one MeSH IDs, we made multiple versions of this categorization. For instance, in the case of *andningsmuskler* (respiratory muscles), MeSHLAB produces *<mesh id="G09...">andning</mesh>s<mesh id= "A02.633;A10.690">muskler</mesh>* in which *A02.633* stands for *Musculoskeletal System* and *A10.690* stands for *Tissue*. In this case we made two versions of the annotated compounds, namely: *<mesh id="G09...">andning</mesh>s<mesh id="A02.633">muskler</mesh>* and *<mesh id="G09...">andning</mesh>s<mesh id="A10.690">muskler</mesh>*.

There were a total of 85,000 compounds having two annotations, of which 15,000 were unique and 46,000 were the final number after making the multiple versions. Having identified and extracted the MeSH labelled NCs the next step was to recognize binary relation(s) that can exist between these semantically labelled NCs. It should be noted however, that there is currently no consensus as to which set of relations should hold between nouns in a noun compound, but most existing approaches make use of a set of a small number of abstract relations, typically between 10 to 50. To constrain the scope of the task, we have chosen only to examine a set of relations involving the MeSH category 'A', *Anatomy* (Figure 3). The number of compounds with an 'A' descriptor, in either the head and/or modifier position, was 11,423. The number of groups in which 'A' was at the modifier position was 10,452 (e.g. A+A 1505, A+B 158, A+C 3171, A+D 1404 etc.), while the number of groups in which 'A' was in the head position was 2,476 (e.g. B+A 91, C+A 262, D+A 282, E+A 83 etc.). One way to characterize the semantic relationships that occur between the noun constituents is to discover the set of verbal predicates that paraphrase a NC. It has been shown (Nakov & Hearst, 2006) that this a promising approach, at least for English, compared to other forms of shallow semantic representations, such as preposition paraphrasing (i.e. N_2 preposition N_1, as a paraphrase of N_1N_2; Lapata & Keller, 2005). By applying paraphrases guided by a verbal predicate more finer-grained semantic representations can be compiled and captured. In order to achieve this goal the N_1 is paraphrased as a post-modifying relative clause, e.g. *bleedings disease* as: *disease that can-cause bleeding* or *disease that involves bleeding*. Following the methodology proposed by Nakov & Hearst we extracted sentences from the MEDLEX Corpus containing both N_1 and N_2 annotated them with part-of-speech information and filtered out relevant contexts based on the pattern:

N_2 REL-CLAUSE-INDICATOR AUX VERB PARTICLE? PREP? ARTICLE? ADJECTIVE(S)* N_1.*

Figure 3. Visualization of 1,427 unique binary compound combinations (descriptor level-1) and their occurrences (size of the dots). The x-axis presents the label of the head (N2) and the y-axis of the modifier (N1). A high concentration of NCs with heads having Body Regions [A01] and Signs and Symptoms [C23] can be easily detected in the left corner and middle part of the pane.

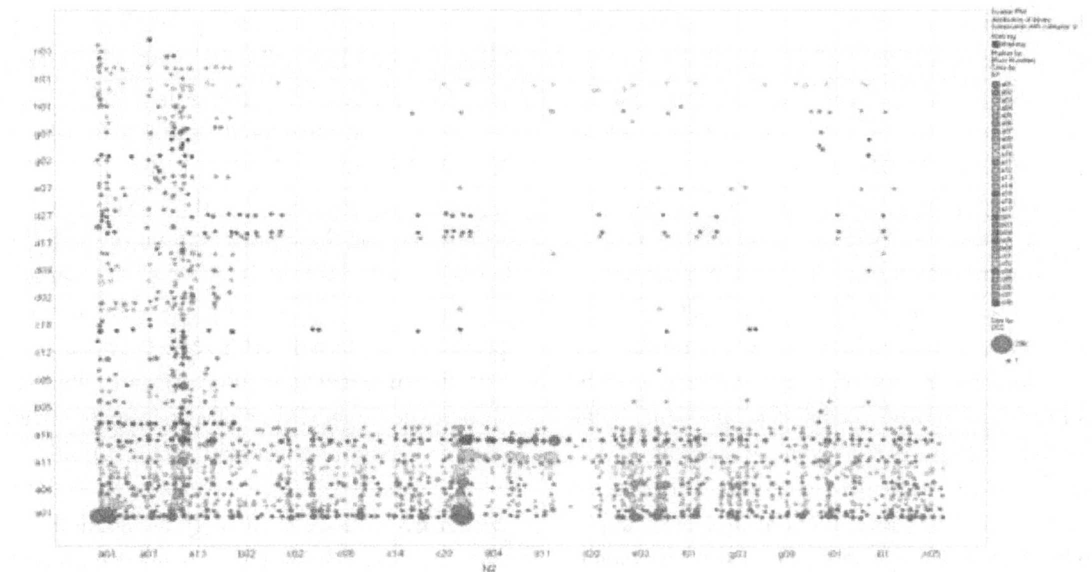

In which '?' denotes 0 or 1 occurrences and '*' denotes ≥0 occurrences. Predicates occurring more frequently with for instance Anatomy+infection, e.g. *hudinfektion* (skin infection) were: *drabba* (affect), *ta sig in* (get into) and a large number of locative verb constructions such as *ligga på* (is/lies on), *sitta på* (be on) and *sitta i* (is/lies in), while predicates occurring more frequently with for instance Anatomy+bakteria e.g. *hudbakterie* (skin bacteria) were *finns på* (occurs/exists), *infektera* (infect), *förekomma* (appear), *infiltrera* (infiltrate), *tillhöra* (belong), *befolka* (inhabit). A preliminary analysis showed that predicates that appear in combinations across the various semantic descriptors (e.g. A+C, B+E, D+M etc.) do not usually have any substantial overlap between their members. For instance the set of predicates for B+infection, e.g. *bakterieinfektion* (bacterial infection) were *för/orsakas av* (caused by), *bero på* (depend on); *infektera med* (infect with) and *spridda via* (spreading with).

In lack of suitable evaluation material, we manually determined if the identified verbs characterised the relationships between the descriptors at level-1 (A01, A02, A03 etc.) or there was a need to descent at lower levels, e.g. level-2 (A01.176, A01.236, A02.378 etc.). We found that this was necessary for very few categories in the examined set of NCs, such as *M* (Persons) where the *descending* of one level was necessary. For instance, *njurläkare* (kidney physician), *<mesh id="A05...">njur</mesh><mesh id="M01.526...">läkare</mesh>*, *vs. njurpatient* (kidney patient), *<mesh id="A05...">njur</mesh><mesh id="M01.643"> patient</mesh>*. There were many cases in which a paraphrase, as previously described, could not identify any relevant predicates between the paraphrased constituent even for NCs that this was clearly thinkable, e.g. *spädbarnsinfektioner* (neonatal infections). This is a drawback for the approach and in the future we plan to use the Web directly as a source for more material and even apply other paraphrasing models. There were also some problematic cases of NCs in which the head and/or modifier were referring to non-medical senses. This was particularly frequent with the noun *huvud* (head/main) as modifier e.g. *huvuddiagnos* (main diagnosis) annotated as *A01.456+E01*. The majority of the category pairs in hierarchy *A* could fit into discrete semantic relations with overlapping predicate sets. For instance, *A01+A02*, *ryggmuskel* (back muscle), *armled* (arm joint) with predicates *ligga* (lying), *sitta* (sitt), *finns* (be), *stabilisera* (stabilize); *A01+C17*, *ansiktspsoriasis* (face psoriasis), *handeksem* (hand eczema) with predicates *förekomma* (appear), *drabba* (affects), *finns* (be); *D12/D14+A11*, *insulincell* (insulin cell), *dopamincell* (dopamine cell) with predicates *bilda* (build), *tillverka/producera* (produce), *insöndra* (secrete) and *A02+C23*, *muskelvärk* (muscle pain), *skelettsmärta* (skeletal pain) with predicates *sitter* (sitt), *uppkomma* (arise/originate) and *bero på* (depends on).

Medical Content Visualization

With semantically annotated data we can easily apply more powerful information visualization and visual analytic software that supports ambitious exploration of the medical content. "Well-designed visual presentations make behavioral patterns, temporal trends, correlations, clusters, gaps, and outliers visible in seconds"; Shneiderman (2006). This way an end-user does not have to scan large-dimensional tabular data, which is time-consuming and difficult, but instead use a graphical view of selected concepts and their importance on the representation. In the following application we explore two such techniques which are based on the mining of the metadata produced by MeSHLAB. The first application is a time dependent visualization of the distribution of diseases per month in published newspaper articles and the second is a treemap visualization.

For these experiments we use a subset of the MEDLEX collection, namely a selection of all documents originating from Swedish daily newspapers (2,589 documents) published in 2006 and 2007. Each document in the sample was annotated with MeSHLAB as described in the previous sections. For each application we used the vector space model (Salton *et al.*, 1975) for representing the text documents as vectors of identifiers, which in our case are indexed MeSH terms, normalised by the *tf*idf* function. Here, *tf* is the frequency of a term in a document and *idf* is the inverse document frequency, defined as the log of the total number of documents in a collection and the number of documents containing the term. Each dimension corresponds to a separate MeSH descriptor (level 1). If a descriptor is not present in a document its value in the vector is 0. Figure 4 shows a sample of the distribution of diseases in the sub-corpora for two descriptors, namely *C01, Bacterial Infections* which are evenly distributed over the months (July having the highest value) and *C22, Animal Diseases* which are predominant in *February and March.*

Treemap Visualization of Medical Documents

Treemaps are a space-filling approach to showing hierarchies in which the rectangular screen space is divided into regions, and then each region is divided again for each level in the hierarchy (Shneiderman, 2006a; 2006b). Treemaps are very effective in showing attributes of leaf nodes using size and color coding and the technology has recently started to attract attention by practitioners within the biomedical domain (Arvelakis *et al.*, 2005; Chazard *et al.*, 2006). Treemaps enable users to compare nodes and sub-trees even at varying depth in the tree, and help them spot patterns and exceptions. Traditional means for representing medical data, such as pie charts and bar diagrams, have limitation with respect to the features they can represent. Chazard *et al.* (2006) mention at least four such problems, namely scale, data overlap, colour meaning and data labelling. The weak points associated with treemaps are the fact that they require certain training in order to get a thorough grasp of the advantages and that they are not suitable for representing chronological data.

Our experiments are based on the Treemap version 4.1 from the University of Maryland <http://www.cs.umd.edu/hcil/treemap>. Figure 5 illustrates the 2,589 documents, shown as nested rectangles (one document for each rectangle) for which the size and coloring are proportional features chosen by the user, here *C23 Symptoms* and *A01 Body Regions.*

CONCLUSIONS AND DISCUSSION

In this chapter we have discussed the transformation of a medical controlled thesaurus for Swedish and English as a resource that can be applied to indexing free text in the (bio-) medical domain with high quality results. Extensive effort has been put into various aspects of the normalization process in order to cover for a large range of phenomena that have implications on coverage. Our experiments revealed some incompleteness of the Swedish MeSH with respect to applying it to real data, since a number of potential medical terms are left unrecognized. This can partly be explained by the well-known distinction between the dynamic, constantly evolving nature of language and the static nature of lexical resources, which cannot adapt as rapidly to the stimuli from the text and the new discoveries continuously taking place in the biomedical domain. At the same time, simple steps (normalization and transformation) have the ability to considerably increase coverage and thus aid the enhancement of the current gaps. Swedish is a compounding language and compound analysis is a crucial step for fast access to partially annotated segments and it aids the enhancement of the results. In the near future we intend to utilize new means of enhancing MeSH and look deeper into the false negatives which might be a bit higher depending on who and how the judg-

Figure 4. Data from 2,589 news articles published in 2006-07. The top pie-chart shows that Bacterial Infections [C01] are evenly distributed over the months the bottom pie-chart shows that Animal Diseases [C22] were predominant in February and March.

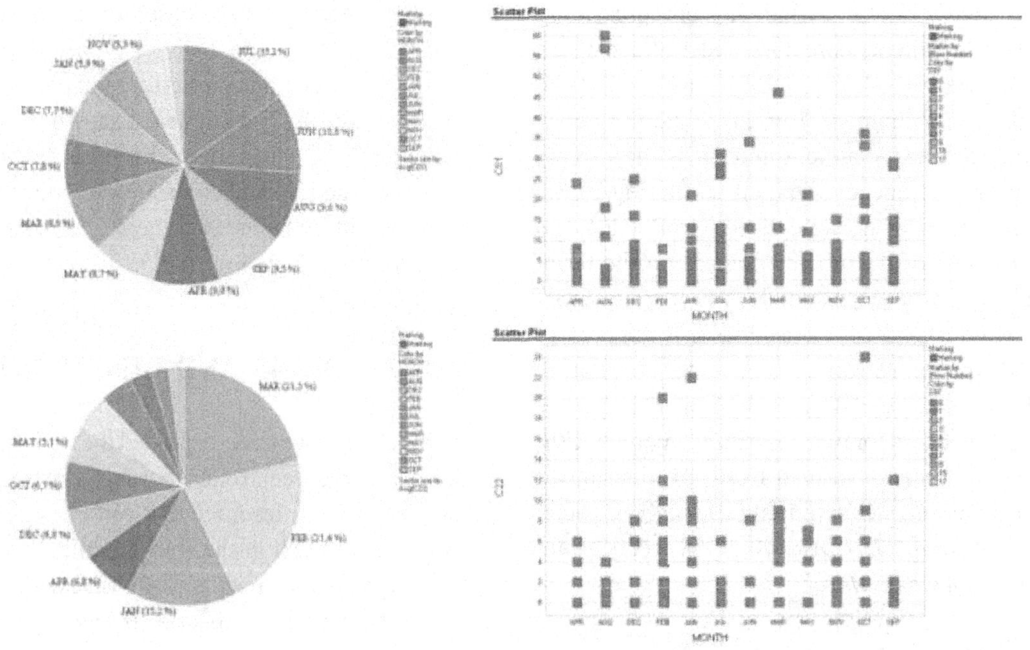

ment is performed since not all MeSH categories are homogeneous (*cf.* Rosario *et al.*, 2002) and therefore there is a risk that arbitrary decisions might be made. Compared to English, Swedish medical content on the Internet is quantitatively less, but nevertheless in the near future we intend to explore that option, for supporting the thesaurus enhancement process rather than merely using a sampled corpus despite its content.

Another important issue that we haven't addressed yet is the issue of anaphoric references, (including coreferential expressions, when two or more referring expressions refer to the same entity). In order to increase coverage for applications such as relation mining or information retrieval/extraction it is necessary to identify at least pronominal and sortal anaphors (e.g. various types of definite noun phrases). In its simplest form, anaphora resolution consists of tracking of mentions of named entities (e.g. terminology), usually pronouns, throughout a text and link them appropriately together with the entity they refer to (*cf.* Mitkov, 2002). A related issue we would like to explore in this domain is the use of lexico-syntactic patterns and templates for automatic lexical acquisition, which is a cost effective approach for overcoming the knowledge acquisition bottleneck, i.e. the difficulty of encoding knowledge into a system in a declarative fashion. Initially applied by Hearst (1992), in her pioneering work on the design and application of such patterns for extracting semantic relationships, e.g. *NP such as {NP, NP ..., (and/or)} NP*, such patterns have proven to be applicable to a whole range of domains, (*cf.* Bodenreider *et al.*, 2001; Oakes, 2005; Roberts, 2005) and recently

Figure 5. Treemap visualization of 2,589 newspaper articles according to the MeSH descriptors Body regions [A01] (size) and Pathological conditions, signs and symptoms [C23] (coloring)

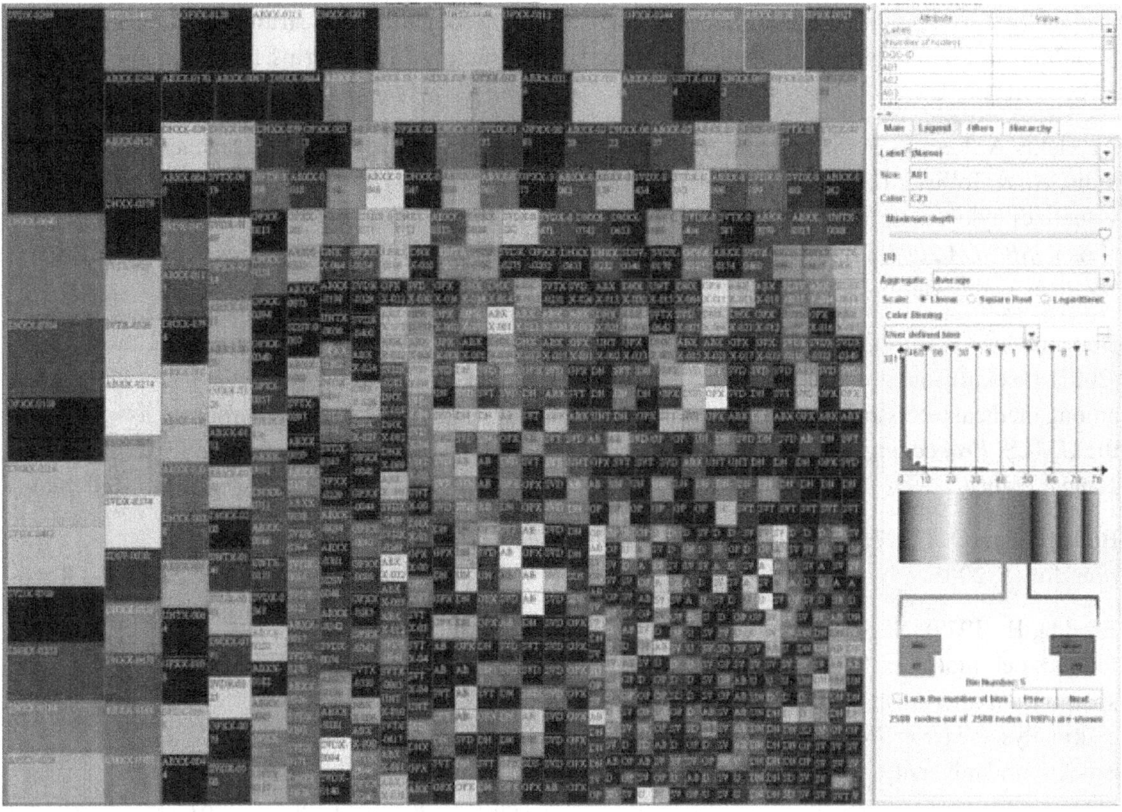

it was applied on the world wide web (Cimiano & Staab, 2004). The use of various types of similar patterns for Swedish (general corpora) have been reported by Kokkinakis *et al.* (2000), who applied techniques based on the productive compounding characteristic for Swedish and the semantic similarity in the enumerative noun phrases, by accessing corpora both in raw and parsed form for extending the lexical inventory of Swedish general semantic lexicons. Manual annotation and coding of scientific litterature is prone to omissions and errors and it is both expensive and inefficient, MeSHLAB operates automatically which guarantees consistency and completeness compared to manual efforts and can contribute to the annotation and curation process by increasing the productivity of human indexers.

REFERENCES

Almeida, F., Bell, M., & Chavez, E. (2003). Controlled health thesaurus for the CDC web redesign project. *AMIA Annu Symp Proc.* (p. 777).

Ananiadou, S., & McNaught, J. (2006). *Text mining for biology and biomedicine.* Artech House Books.

Ananiadou, S., & Nenadic, G. (2006). Automatic terminology management in biomedicine. In S.

Ananiadou & G. McNaught (Eds.), *Text mining for biology and biomedicine*. Artech House Books.

Aronson, A. R. (2001). Effective mapping of biomedical text to the UMLS Metathesaurus: The MetaMap program. *AMIA Annu Symp Proc.* (pp. 17-21). Oregon, USA.

Arvelakis, A., Reczko, M., Stamatakis, A., Symeonidis, A., & Tollis, I. (2005). Using Treemaps to visualize phylogenetic trees. In J. L. Oliveira *et al.* (Eds.), *ISBMDA 2005, LNBI 3745* (pp. 283–293). Springer-Verlag Berlin Heidelber.

Bodenreider, O., Burgun, A., & Rindflesch, T.C. (2001). Lexically-suggested hyponymic relations among medical terms and their representation in the UMLS. *Proceedings of the TIA Conference.* Nancy, France.

Bodenreider, O. (2007). *Personal Communication.* July 5, 2005.

Brodda, B. (1979). Något om de svenska ordens fonotax och morfotax: Iakttagelse med utgångspunkt från experiment med automatisk morfologisk analys. *PILUS nr 38.* Department of Swedish, Stockholm University. (In Swedish).

Buitelaar, P., Cimiano, P., & Magnini, B. (2005). Ontology learning from text: An overview. In P. Buitelaar, P. Cimiano & B. Magnini (Eds.), *Ontology learning from text: Methods, applications and evaluation* (pp. 3-12). IOS Press.

Chazard, E., Puech, P., Gregoire, M., & Beuscart, R. (2006). Using Treemaps to represent medical data. *Ubiquity: Technologies for Better Health in Aging Societies - Proceedings of MIE2006*, (pp. 522-527). Maastricht, Holland.

Cimiano, P. & Staab, S. (2004). Learning by Googling. *SIGKDD Explorations, 6*(2): 24-34.

Cohen, K. B., Ogren, P. V., Fox, L., & Hunter, L. (2005). Empirical Data on Corpus Design and Usage in Biomedical Natural Language Processing. *AMIA Annu Symp Proc.* (pp. 156–160). Washington, USA.

Cooper, G. F., & Miller, R. A. (1998). An experiment comparing lexical and statistical method for extracting MeSH terms from clinical free text. *Journal of Am Med Inform Assoc., 5*, 62–75.

Crammer, K., Dredze, M., Ganchev, K., Talukdar, P. P., & Caroll, S. (2007). Automatic code assignment to medical text. *Biological, Translational and Clinical Language processing (BioNLP 2007)* (pp. 129-136). Prague.

Djebbari, A., Karamycheva, S., Howe, E., & Quackenbush, J. (2005). MeSHer: identifying biological concepts in microarray assays based on PubMed references and MeSH terms. *Bioinformatics, 21*(15), 3324-3326. doi:10.1093/bioinformatics/bti503.

Douyere, M., Soualmia, L. F., Neveol, A., Rogozan, A., Dahamna, B., Leroy, J. P., Thirion, B., & Darmoni, S. J. (2004). Enhancing the MeSH thesaurus to retrieve French online health resources in a quality-controlled gateway. *Health Info Libr J., 21*(4), 253-61.

Feldman, R., & Sanger, J. (2006). *The Text Mining handbook: Advanced approaches in analyzing unstructured data.* Cambridge University.

Fellbaum, C. (1998). *WordNet: an Electronic Lexical Database.* Cambridge, Mass. MIT Press.

Gómez-Pérez, A., & Manzano-Macho, D. (2003). *OntoWeb D.1.5 A survey of ontology learning methods and techniques.* The OntoWeb Consortium. Retrieved March 07, 2008, from http://ontoweb.aifb.uni-karlsruhe.de/Members/ruben/Deliverable1.5.

Grishman, R., Huttunen, S., & Yangarber, R. (2002). Information extraction for enhanced access to disease outbreak reports. *Journal of Biomedical Informatics. Special Issue Sublanguage - Zellig Harris Memorial, 35*(4), 236-246.

Hearst, M. A. (1992). Automatic acquisition of hyponyms from large text corpora. *Proc. of the 14th International Conf. on Computational Linguistics*, (pp 539-545). Nantes, France.

Hirschman, L., Morgan, A. A., & Yeh, A. S. (2003). Rutabaga by any other name: extracting biological names. *Journal of Biomedical Informatics, 35*, 247-259. Elsevier.

Hristovski, D., Friedman, C., Rindflesch, T. C., & Peterlin, B. (2006). Exploiting semantic relations for literature-based discovery. *AMIA Annu Symp Proc.* (pp. 349-353). Washington, DC.

Jacquemin, C., & Tzoukermann, E. (1999). NLP for term variant extraction: A synergy of morphology, lexicon and syntax. In T. Strzalkowski (Ed.), *Natural Language Information Retrieval* (pp. 25-74). Kluwer: Boston.

Jacquemin, C. (2001). *Spotting and discovering terms through natural language processing.* Cambridge, MA, USA: MIT Press.

Jin-Dong, K., Ohta, T., Teteisi, Y., & Tsujii, J. (2003). GENIA corpus - a semantically annotated corpus for bio-textmining. *Bioinformatics, 19*(1), i180-i182. OUP.

Hearst, M. (1999). Untangling text data mining. *Proceedings of ACL'99: the 37th Annual Meeting of the Association for Computational Linguistics*, (pp. 20-26). Maryland, USA.

Kokkinakis, D., Toporowska Gronostaj, M., & Warmenius, K. (2000). Annotating, disambiguating & automatically extending the coverage of the Swedish SIMPLE lexicon. *Proceedings of the 2nd Language Resources and Evaluation Conference (LREC)*, Athens, Greece.

Kokkinakis, D., & Dannélls, D. (2006). Recognizing acronyms and their definitions in Swedish medical texts. *Proceedings of the 5th Conference on Language Resources and Evalutaion (LREC).* Genoa, Italy.

Kokkinakis, D. (2006). Collection, encoding and linguistic processing of a Swedish medical corpus – The MEDLEX experience. *Proceedings of the 5th Conference on Language Resources and Evalutaion (LREC).* Genoa, Italy.

Kokkinakis, D. (2008). A semantically annotated Swedish medical corpus. *Proceedings of the 6th Conference on Language Resources and Evalutaion (LREC).* Marrakech, Morocco.

Krauthammer, M., & Nenadic, G. (2004). Term identification in the biomedical literature. *Journal of Biomedical Informatics. Special issue: Named entity recognition in biomedicine, 37*(6), 512-526.

Lapata, M., & Keller, F. (2005). Web-based models for natural language processing. *ACM Transactions on Speech and Language Processing, 2*(1), 1-31.

MEDLINE/PubMed database. Accessed March XX, 2008: http://www.nlm.nih.gov/pubs/factsheets/medline.html.

Markellos, K., Markellou, P., Rigou, M., & Sirmakessis, S. (2004). Web mining: Past, present and future. In S. Sirmakessis (Ed), *Text Mining and Its Applications* (pp. 25-35). Springer.

Mitkov, R. (2002). *Anaphora resolution (Studies in Language & Linguistics).* Longman.

Nakov, P., & Hearst, M. (2006). Using verbs to characterize noun-noun relations. *Proc. of the 12th International Conference on AI: Methodology, Systems, Applications.* Bulgaria.

Navigli, R., Velardi, P., & Gangemi, A. (2003). Ontology learning and its application to automated terminology translation. *Intelligent Systems, IEEE, 18*(1), 22–31.

Névéol, A., Mary V., Gaudinat, A., Boyer, C., Rogozan, A., & Darmoni, S. (2005). *A benchmark evaluation of the French MeSH indexing systems.*

In S. Miksh, J. Hunter, & E. Keravnou (Eds.), *Springer's Lecture Notes in Computer Science, Artificial Intelligence in Medicine. Proc. AIME.* (pp. 251-255).

Névéol, A., Mork, J. G., & Aronson, A. R. (2007). Automatic indexing of specialized documents: Using generic vs. domain-specific document representations. *Biological, Translational and Clinical Language processing (BioNLP 2007).* (pp. 183-190). Prague.

Oakes, M. P. (2005). Using Hearst's rules for the automatic acquisition of hyponyms for mining a Pharmaceutical corpus. *Proc. of the RANLP 2005 Workshop* (pp 63-67). Bulgaria.

Pustejovsky, J. *et al.* (2001). Automation Extraction of Acronym-Meaning Pairs from MEDLINE Databases. *Medinfo 2001, 10*(Pt 1), 371-375.

Rechtsteiner, A., & Rocha, L. M. (2004). MeSH key terms for validation and annotation of gene expression clusters. In A. Gramada & E. Bourne (Eds), *Currents in Computational Molecular Biology. Proceedings of the Eight Annual International Conference on Research in Computational Molecular Biology (RECOMB 2004).* (pp 212-213).

Roberts, A. (2005). Learning meronyms from biomedical text. In C. Callison-Burch & S. Wan (Eds). *Proceedings of the Student Research Workshop of ACL,* (pp. 49-54). Ann Arbor, Michigan.

Rosario, B., Hearst, M. A., & Fillmore, C. (2002). The descent of hierarchy, and selection in relational semantics. *Proceedings of the ACL-02.* Pennsylvania USA.

Salton, G., Wong, A., & Yang, C. S. (1975). A vector space model for automatic indexing. *Communications of the ACM, 18*(11), 613–620.

Schwartz, A., & Hearst, M. (2003). A simple algorithm for identifying abbreviation definitions in biomedical texts. *Proceedings of the Pacific Symposium on Biocomputing (PSB).* Hawaii, USA.

Sekimizu, T., Park, H. S., & Tsujii, T. (1998). Identifying the interaction between genes and gene products based on frequently seen verbs in Medline abstracts. *Genome Inform Ser Workshop Genome Inform., 9,* 62-71 11072322.

Shin, K., Han, S-Y., & Gelbukh, A. (2004). Balancing manual and automatic indexing for retrieval of paper abstracts. *TSD 2004: Text, Speech and Dialogue. Lecture Notes in Computer Science.* (pp. 203-210) Brno.

Shneiderman, B. (2006a). Discovering business intelligence using treemap visualizations. *b-eye. HCIL-2007-20.* Retrieved February 29, from http://www.b-eye-network.com/view/2673.

Shneiderman, B. (2006b). Treemaps for space-constrained visualization of hierarchies. Retrieved March 10, 2008, from http://www.cs.umd.edu/hcil/treemap-history/.

Shultz, M. (2006). Mapping of medical acronyms and initialisms to Medical Subject Headings (MeSH) across selected systems. *Journal Med Libr Assoc., 94*(4), 410–414.

Sirmakessis, S. (2004). *Text Mining and Its Applications: Results of the Nemis Launch.* Springer.

Struble, C. A., & Dharmanolla, C. (2004). Clustering MeSH representations of biomedical literature. *ACL Workshop: Linking Biological Literature, Ontologies, and Databases, BioLINK.* (pp. 41-48). Boston USA.

Tsujii, J., & Ananiadou, S. (2005). Thesaurus or logical ontology, which one do we need for text mining? *Language Resources and Evaluation, Springer Science and Business Media B.V. 39*(1), 77-90. Springer Netherlands.

Tsuruoka, Y., & Tsujii, J. (2003). Probabilistic term variant generator for biomedical terms, *Pro-*

ceedings of the 26th annual international ACM SIGIR conference on Research and development in informaion retrieval. Toronto, Canada.

UMLS (2006). The Unified Medical Language System®. Accessed March 1st, 2008, from http://0-www.nlm.nih.gov.catalog.llu.edu/pubs/factsheets/umls.html.

Vintar, S., Buitelaar, P., & Volk, M. (2003). Semantic relations in concept-based cross-language medical information retrieval. *Proceedings of the Workshop on Adaptive Text Extraction and Mining.* Cavtat-Dubrovnik, Croatia.

Yandell, M. D., & Majoros, W.H. (2002). Genomics and natural language processing. *Nature Reviews Genetics*, *3*, 601-610. doi:10.1038/nrg861.

Chapter III
Expanding Terms with Medical Ontologies to Improve a Multi-Label Text Categorization System

M. Teresa Martín-Valdivia
University of Jaén, Spain

Arturo Montejo-Ráez
University of Jaén, Spain

M. C. Díaz-Galiano
University of Jaén, Spain

José M. Perea Ortega
University of Jaén, Spain

L. Alfonso Ureña-López
University of Jaén, Spain

ABSTRACT

This chapter argues for the integration of clinical knowledge extracted from medical ontologies in order to improve a Multi-Label Text Categorization (MLTC) system for medical domain. The approach is based on the concept of semantic enrichment by integrating knowledge in different biomedical collections. Specifically, the authors expand terms from these collections using the UMLS (Unified Medical Language System) metathesaurus. This resource includes several medical ontologies. They have managed two rather different medical collections: first, the CCHMC collection (Cincinnati Children's Hospital Medical Centre) from the Department of Radiology, and second, the widely used OHSUMED collection. The results obtained show that the use of the medical ontologies improves the system performance.

INTRODUCTION

This paper presents a method based on the use of medical ontologies in order to improve a Multi-Label Text Categorization (MLTC) system. Text Categorization (TC) is a very interesting task in Natural Language Processing (NLP) which consists in the assignment of one or more pre-existing categories to a text document and, more concisely, in text mining (Sebastiani, 2002). The simplest case includes only one class and the categorization problem is a decision problem or binary categorization problem (given a document, the goal is to determine whether the document is related to that class or not). The single-label categorization problem consists in assigning exactly one category to each document, while in multi-label assignment a document can be ascribed several categories.

Technological progress has greatly influenced all aspects of medical practice, education and research. In recent years, large biomedical databases (structured and non-structured) have been developed through the application of these technologies, but efficient access to this information is very difficult. For this reason, it is necessary to develop search strategies for easier retrieval of useful information. One of these strategies includes the use of linguistic resources in order to improve the access and management of information by expanding queries in information retrieval systems, enriching the databases semantically or extracting unknown data from collections.

These resources include training corpora and knowledge-based systems (e.g. ontologies). Training corpora, such as Reuters-21,578, OHSUMED or TREC collections are manually labelled document collections. Ontologies are repositories of structured knowledge (e.g. WordNet, EuroWordNet, MeSH, UMLS…).

Recent research shows that the use and integration of several knowledge sources improves the quality and efficiency of information systems. This is especially so in specific domains as, for example, medicine. Several studies show improvement in health information systems when a query is expanded using some ontology (Nelson et al., 2001). According to Gruber (1995), an ontology is a specification of a conceptualization that defines (specifies) the concepts, relationships, and other distinctions that are relevant for modelling a domain. The specification takes the form of the definitions of representational vocabulary (classes, relations, and so on), which provide meanings to the vocabulary and formal constraints on its coherent use.

Ontologies range from general to domain-specific. WordNeta, EuroWordNetb and Cycc are examples of general ontologies. Domain-specific ontologies have been constructed in many different application areas such as law, medicine, archaeology, agriculture, geography, business, economics, history, physics…

In this work, we have used the medical UMLSd (Unified Medical Language System) metathesaurus to expand terms automatically in the medical domain. We have trained, adjusted and tested a Multi-Label Text Categorization (MLTC) system using two different collections. Firstly, we have trained a MLTC system with the CCHMC collectione (Cincinnati Children's Hospital Medical Center) from the Department of Radiology. This collection includes short records of free text about children radiology reports. An MLTC system has also been trained using the widely used OHSUMEDf collection. This relied on more documents and on larger ones too. The OHSUMED corpus includes documents from several medical journals published in MEDLINEg and labelled with one or more categories from MeSHh (Medical Subject Headings).

This chapter is thus intended to show the improvement obtained over an MLTC system when we use the available data automatically extracted from the UMLS resource, and this information is integrated into a biomedical collection as external knowledge.

The rest of the chapter is organised as follows: first, a background section comments on some relevant works in the field; section 3 briefly introduces the UMLS resource; section 4 describes the two collections used for training and testing our system, and includes the method used for expanding the document with UMLS; section 5 presents a description of the multi-label text categorization system; section 6 explains our experiments and shows the results obtained. The conclusions are presented in the last section.

BACKGROUND

Our main objective is to improve a MLTC system by automatically integrating external knowledge from ontologies. Ontologies have been used for several natural language processing tasks such as automatic summarisation (Chiang et al., 2006), text annotation (Carr et al., 2001) and word sense disambiguation (Martín-Valdivia et al., 2007, among others.

One of the main applications of ontologies expands terms found in free textual documents/queries. Several works point out the advantage of using ontologies for query expansion in order to improve information retrieval systems. For example, Bhogal et al. (2007) present a review of various query expansion approaches including relevance feedback, corpus-dependent knowledge models and corpus-independent knowledge models. The work also analyzes the query expansion using domain-specific and domain-independent ontologies.

WordNet (Miller, 1995) is a large electronic lexical database of English language and was conceived as a full-scale model of human semantic organization, where words and their meanings are related to one another via semantic and lexical relations. WordNet has been used for query expansion in several works. Voorhees (1994) expand query nouns using WordNet synsets and the is-a relation. An early and relevant study by de Buenaga Rodríguez et al. (1997) showed that the expansion of document text by adding terms from synsets where the categories are included in enhance system performance.Gonzalo et al. (1998) use WordNet synset for index manually disambiguated test collection of documents and queries derived from the SemCor semantic concordance. Navigli and Velardi (2003) suggest that query expansion is suitable for short queries. They use WordNet 1.6 and Googlei for their experiments. Martín-Valdivia et al. (2007) integrate the WordNet concepts (synsets) of several semantic relationships to improve two different NLP tasks: a word sense disambiguation system and a text categorization system. The results obtained show that the expansion is a very promising approach.

The problem with domain-independent ontologies such as WordNet is that they have a broad coverage. Thus, ambiguous terms within the ontology can be problematic and the researchers prefer to use domain-specific ontologies because the terminology is less ambiguous. For narrower search tasks, domain-specific ontologies are the preferred choice. A domain-specific ontology models terms and concepts which are proper to a given domain. For example, Aronson and Rindflesch (1997) use the MetaMap program for associating UMLS Metathesaurus concepts with the original query. They conclude that the optimal strategy would be to combine the query expansion with the retrieval feedback. Hersh et al. (2000) observe that the UMLS Metathesaurus can provide benefit for Information Retreival tasks such as automated indexing and query expansion in a substantial minority of queries, therefore must be studied what queries are better for expansion. Nilsson et al. (2005) use synonyms and hyponyms, from domain specific ontology based on Stockholm University Information System (SUiS) to carry out query expansion. The experiments have shown a precision increase. Fu et al. (2005) present query expansion techniques based on both a domain and a geographical ontology. In their work, a query is expanded by derivation of its geographical footprint. Spatial terms such as place names are modelled in the geographical ontology and non-spatial terms such as 'near' are encoded in tourism domain ontology. The experiments show that this method can improve searches.

As to the biomedical domain, some recent works such as (Yu, 2006) review current methods in the construction, maintenance, alignment and evaluation of medical ontologies. Krallinger & Valencia (2005) make a very good review of text mining and information retrieval in molecular biology including a large amount of interesting references.

Many thesaurii and ontologies designed to maintain and classify medical knowledge are also available: GOj(Stevens, 2000), UniProt[1] (Apweiler et al., 2004), Swiss-Prot[2] (Bairoch et al., 2004), MeSH (Nelson et al., 2001) or UMLS (Bodenreider, 2004). These resources have been successfully applied to a wide range of applications in biomedicine from information retrieval (Ide et al., 2007) to integration and development of ontologies (Simon et al., 2006). For example, the Gene Ontology (GO) is a collaborative project to address the need for consistent descriptions of gene products in different databases including several of the world's major repositories for plant, animal and microbial genomes. The GO project has developed three structured controlled vocabularies (ontologies) that describe gene products in terms of their associated biological processes, cellular components and molecular functions in a species-independent manner. The controlled vocabularies are structured so that they can be queried at different levels. GO has been used in a number of research projects mainly aimed at identifying biomolecular entities or extracting particular relationships among entities. For example, Verspoor et al. (2005) propose a method for expanding terms associated with GO nodes, and an annotation methodology which treats annotation as categorization of terms to select GO nodes as cluster heads for the terms in the input set based on the structure of the GO. The evaluation results indicate that the method for expanding words associated with GO nodes is quite powerful.

Another harnessed medical resource is MeSH. This ontology, published by the United States National Library of Medicinek in 1954, mainly consists in the controlled vocabulary and a MeSH Tree. The controlled vocabulary contains several types of terms, such as descriptors, qualifiers, publication types, and entry terms. Díaz-Galiano et al. (2007) use two of these terms: descriptors and entry. Descriptor terms are main concepts or main headings. Entry terms are the synonyms or the related terms of the descriptors. The query terms are expanded using this biomedical information. In order to test the results, the approach uses the ImageCLEFmed collections supplied by the Cross Language Evaluation Forum (CLEF)[l] organization for the ImageCLEFmedm task (Müller et al., 2007). The ImageCLEFmed task includes a multi-modal and multilingual collection based on medical cases. The experiments show that the integration of MeSH information by expanding the query terms improves the biomedical multimodal information system greatly.

Finally, the UMLS metathesaurus has been widely used in biomedical environment. This is a repository of biomedical vocabularies developed by the United States National Library of Medicine. The UMLS integrates over 2 million names for some 900,000 concepts from more than 60 families of biomedical vocabularies, as well as 12 million relations among these concepts. In the same framework of the ImageCLEFmed competition, Lacoste et al. (2006) use the UMLS concepts over a multimodal information retrieval system in order to achieve a higher semantic level and improve the communication between visual and textual retrieval. In (Zou et al., 2003) the UMLS is used for extraction of key concepts from clinical text for indexing in order to improve a medical digital library. Meystre & Haug (2006) study the performance of the NLP to extract medical problems using the UMLS metathesaurus. The experiments are accomplished over a corpus that includes records of patients with free text. The results show a faster and significant improvement in recall without any less precision.

UMLS: A MEDICAL RESOURCE TO KNOWLEDGE INTEGRATION

An ontology is a formal, explicit specification of a shared conceptualization for a domain of interest (Gruber, 1995). Usually, an ontology is organized by concepts and identifies all the possible relationships among them. Ontologies are used to facilitate communication among domain experts and between domain experts and knowledge-based systems. This is done to reflect the expert view of a specific domain.

The UMLS project was born as a way to overcome two major barriers to efficient retrieval of machine-readable information (Humphreys et al., 1998; Lindberg et al., 1993): first, the different expression of the same concepts in different machine-readable sources and by different people; second, the distribution of useful information between databases and systems. The UMLS metathesaurus is a repository of biomedical ontologies and associated software tools developed by the US National Library of Medicine (NLM). The purpose of UMLS is to facilitate

Figure 1. UMLS elements and the interaction among them

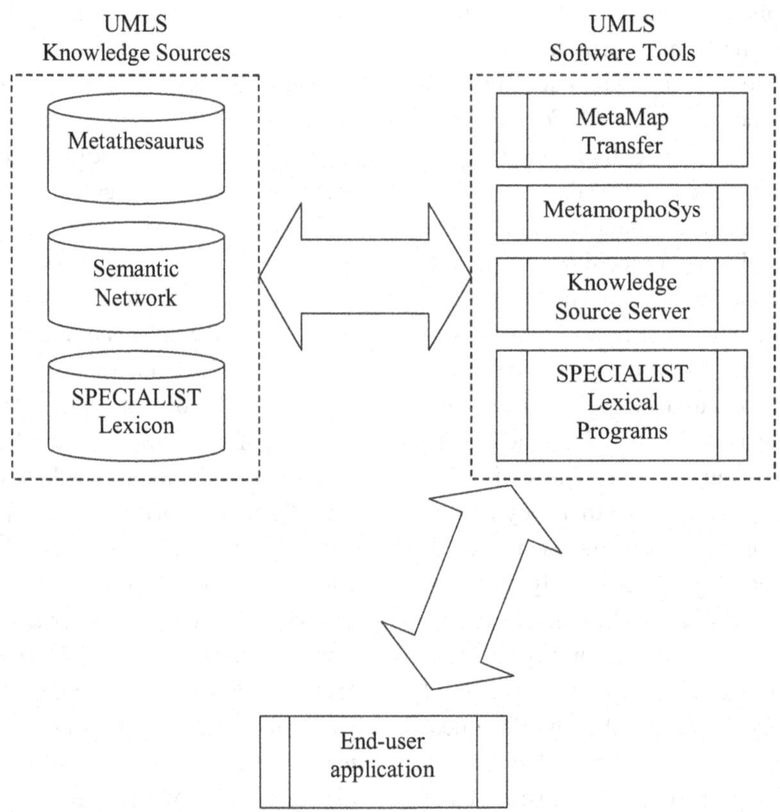

the development of computer systems that use the biomedical knowledge to understand biomedicine and health data and information. To that end, the NLM distributes two types of resources for use by system developers and computing researchers (Figure 1):

1. The UMLS Knowledge Sources (databases), which integrates over 2 million names for some 900,000 concepts from over 60 families of biomedical vocabularies, as well as 12 million relations between these concepts used in patient records, administrative data, full-text databases and expert systems (Bodenreider, 2004). There are three UMLS Knowledge Sources: the Metathesaurus, the Semantic Network and the SPECIALIST Lexicon.
2. Associated software tools (programs) to assist developers in customizing or using the UMLS Knowledge Sources for particular purposes. Some of the tools included in UMLS are, for example, MetamorphoSys (a tool for customization of the Metathesaurus), LVG (for generation of lexical variants of concept names) or MetaMap (for extraction of UMLS concepts from text).

The Metathesaurus is a very large multi-lingual vocabulary database that contains concepts, concept names and other attributes from over 100 terminologies, classifications, and thesaurii, some in multiple editions. The Metathesaurus also includes relationships between concepts.

The Metathesaurus is built from the electronic versions of many different thesaurii, classifications, code sets and lists of controlled terms used in patient care, health services billing, public health statistics, indexing and cataloguing biomedical literature, and /or basic, clinical, and health services research. It is organized by concept or meaning. Many of the words and multi-word

Figure 2. Example of a cluster for the term "Addison's disease" (CUI: C0001403)

Addison's disease (C0001403)			
Addison's disease	Metathesaurus	PN	
Addison's disease	SNOMED	CT	PT363732003
Addison's Disease	MedlinePlus	PT	T1233
Addison Disease	MeSH	PT	D000224
Bronzed disease	SNOMED Intl 1998	SY	DB-70620
Deficiency; corticorenal, primary	ICPC2-ICD10P Thesaurus	TM	THU021575
Primary Adrenal Insufficiency	MeSH	EN	D000224
Primary hypoadreanlism syndrome, Addison	MedDRA	LT	10036696

terms that appear in concept names or strings in the Metathesaurus also appear in the SPECIALIST Lexicon. The terms in the Metathesaurus are clustered by meaning. In every cluster a preferred term represents this cluster. Yet, a unique identifier (CUI) is assigned to each cluster (Figure 2).

The purpose of the Semantic Network is to provide a set of useful relationships between concepts represented in the UMLS Metathesaurus and to provide a consistent categorization of all these concepts. All the information about specific concepts is found in the Metathesaurus. The current release of the Semantic Network contains 135 semantic types and 54 relationships. There is a wide range of terminology in multiple domains that can be categorized by the UMLS semantic types.

The SPECIALIST Lexicon provides the lexical information of many biomedical terms. The information available for each word or term records includes syntactic, morphological, and orthographic information. This lexical information is very useful for natural language processing systems, specifically for the SPECIALIST NLP System.

Multi-word terms in the Metathesaurus and other controlled vocabularies may have word order variants in addition to their inflectional and alphabetic case variants. The lexical tools allow the user to abstract away from this sort of variation.

DATA COLLECTIONS

The empirical evaluation relies on two test collections. On the one hand, the CCHMC collection includes slightly under one thousand documents, with brief (usually one line) textual content. The OHSUMED collection provides documents with larger text, but its size is considerably large. For our experiments we have taken a subset of it (exactly, 6,000 samples). These two collections are detailed below.

CCHMC

The first collection expanded using UMLS is a corpus of clinical free text developed by "The Computational Medicine Center". The corpus includes anonymous medical records collected from the Cincinnati Children's Hospital Medical Center's Department of Radiology (CCHMC)n. The collection consists in a sample of radiology reports about outpatient chest X-ray and renal procedures for a one-year period. . It was released with 978 training documents and 976 test documents, with a total number of 150 different topics (appearing in an average of 1,9 topics per document).The collection was labelled with ICD-9-CM codes. The ICD-9-CM (International Classification of Diseases, Ninth Revision, Clinical Modification) is based on the World Health Organization's Ninth Revision, International Classification of Diseases (ICD-9). ICD-9-CM is the official system of assigning codes to diagnoses and procedures associated with hospital utilization in the United States.

An ICD-9-CM code is a 3 to 5 digit number with a decimal point after the third digit. ICD-9-CM codes are organized in a hierarchy, with the highest levels of the hierarchy simply concatenating some codes together by assigning consecutive numbers (Figure 3).

A radiology report has many components and two parts are fundamental for assigning ICD-9-CM codes:

1. **A clinical history:** Provided by an ordering physician before a radiological procedure.
2. **An impression**: Reported by a radiologist after the procedure.

The collection was annotated manually by three human annotators. Thus, there are three sets of annotations for each document. The majority annotation is calculated with only those codes which were assigned to the document by two or more of the annotators. All the data were

Figure 3. Example of an ICD-9-CM hierarchy

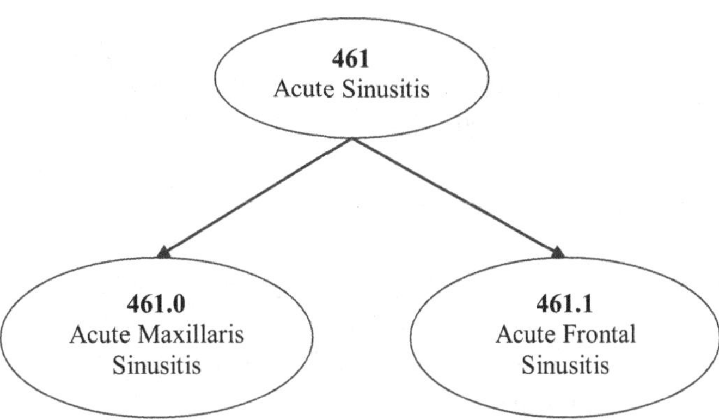

Figure 4. Example of a radiology report with annotations in XML format

```
<doc id="97635942" type="RADIOLOGY_REPORT">
   <codes>
     <code origin="CMC_MAJORITY" type="ICD-9-CM">780.6</code>
     <code origin="CMC_MAJORITY" type="ICD-9-CM">786.2</code>
     <code origin="COMPANY3" type="ICD-9-CM">780.6</code>
     <code origin="COMPANY3" type="ICD-9-CM">786.2</code>
     <code origin="COMPANY1" type="ICD-9-CM">780.6</code>
     <code origin="COMPANY1" type="ICD-9-CM">786.2</code>
     <code origin="COMPANY2" type="ICD-9-CM">780.6</code>
     <code origin="COMPANY2" type="ICD-9-CM">786.2</code>
   </codes>
   <texts>
     <text origin="CCHMC_RADIOLOGY" type="CLINICAL_HISTORY">Three - year-
old female with cough and fever.</text>
     <text origin="CCHMC_RADIOLOGY" type="IMPRESSION">Normal chest
radiograph.</text>
   </texts>
```

converted to an XML format that has two top-level subdivisions:

1. **Texts:** With the clinical history and the impression.
2. **Codes:** With human ICD-9-CM annotations and the majority annotation.

Figure 4 shows the structure of a document.

OHSUMED

The second test collection is taken from the OHSUMED corpus consisting of 348,566 medical documents excerpted from 270 medical journals published between 1987 and 1991 through the MEDLINE database, which was originally compiled by Hersh et al. (1994). For each of the MEDLINE document, title, publication type, abstract, author, and source information are provided. The OHSUMED corpus is available by anonymous ftpo and is divided across five very large files, one for each year between 1987 and 1991. Out of 50,216 original documents for the year 1991, the first 20,000 documents are classified into the 23 MeSH "disease" categories and labelled with one or multiple categories by Joachims (1998). This partition has not been considered in our work, as a higher number of classes is preferred for a more accurate evaluation of our MLTC system. Original topics in OHSUMED documents have been processed to discard non-main headers. In our subset, this results in 6,464 different classes, which is clearly higher than those selected by Joachims. The average number of topics per document is 18, which is much higher than that found in the collection previously introduced. These major differences has to be considered when analyzing and comparing results obtained on both data sets.

OHSUMED is a subset of the MEDLINE database, which is a bibliographic database of important, peer-reviewed medical literature maintained by the NLM. In MEDLINE most references allude to journal articles, but there is also a small number of references to letters to the editor, conference proceedings, and other reports. About 75% of the references contain abstracts, while the remainder (including all letters to the editor) has only titles. Each reference also contains human-assigned subject headings from the MeSH vocabulary. The NLM has agreed to make the MEDLINE references available for experimentation under certain conditions.The format for each MEDLINE document file follows the conventions of the SMART retrieval system. Each field is defined as detailed below (the NLM designator in brackets):

1. I: sequential identifier.
2. U: MEDLINE identifier (UI).
3. M: human-assigned MeSH terms (MH).
4. T: title (TI).
5. P: publication type (PT).
6. W: abstract (AB).
7. A: author (AU).
8. S: source (SO).

In some references of MEDLINE document files, the abstract field (W) has been truncated at 250 words, while some have no abstracts at all, only the titles.

Expanding Terms with UMLS

Term expansion using UMLS here relies on a tool widely used by many users of UMLS: MetaMap Transferp (MMTx). MMTx matches the text from documents or queries into concepts from the UMLS metathesaurus. MMTx offers a configurable programming environment available to researchers in general. Its main function is to discover metathesaurus concepts.

With MMTx, the text is processed through a series of modules. First, it is parsed into components including sentences, paragraphs, phrases, lexical elements and tokens. Variants are generated from the resulting phrases. Candidate concepts from the UMLS metathesaurus are retrieved and evaluated against the phrases. The best candidates are organized into a final mapping in such a way as to best cover the text. This final mapping is used in our system to carry out the term expansion. Figure 5 shows the processing of a document through the MetaMap modules.

The expansion terms sometimes consist of more than one word or token. This has been dealt with using two different strategies in the expansion process:

1. **Joint strategy**. For this case, we have considered the expansion terms consisting of more than one word as a single token. Thus, the spaces between the words of the expanded term have been replaced with the underlined symbol. Using this expansion strategy we manage to introduce more dif-

ferent expansion terms for the subsequent classification process. For example, if the UMLS string obtained from the expansion process is "reactive airways disease", the expansion term added to the document would be "reactive_airways_disease".

2. **Non-joint strategy**. In this case, we split the tokens of the expansion terms consisting of more than one word. In the expansion process for this strategy, each token is added to the document separately (if it had not already been added). Unlike the previous strategy, the total number of different expanded terms added to the documents is considerably lower.

An example of such expansion strategies applied to a document is shown in Figure 6.

On the other hand, the number of expanded terms for the OHSUMED collection has been 1,270,881 and 91,956 for the CCHMC collection. For the OHSUMED collection, the percentage of expanded terms belonging to ontologies which have supplied more terms in the expansion process for the joint strategy is shown in Table 1.

For the CCHMC collection, the percentage of expanded terms belonging to each ontology is shown in Table 2. In both cases, the number of ontologies or resources that have contributed some term to the expansions, was 80 for the OHSUMED collection and 70 for the CCHMC collection. This is because expanded terms come from different ontologies in an unbalanced way. Table 1 and Table 2 show only 6 resources which provide more terms because almost 70% of the expansions are provided from 6 resources out of 80 used ones within UMLS.

MULTI-LABEL TEXT CATEGORIZATION

With expansion we enlarge document content by adding terms from the UMLS metathesaurus. Once documents have been expanded according to the strategies described above, text categorization is accomplished.

Text categorization is a discipline which applies both to natural language processing and Machine Learning (ML) techniques. The former allows to turn documents into feature based representations that can be handled by the ML algorithms. In this way, a text, i.e. a list of words forming phrases, is transformed into a list of weighted features. Features are usually deeply mapped from words (known as the bag of words representation) and

Figure 5. Processing a document through the MetaMap modules

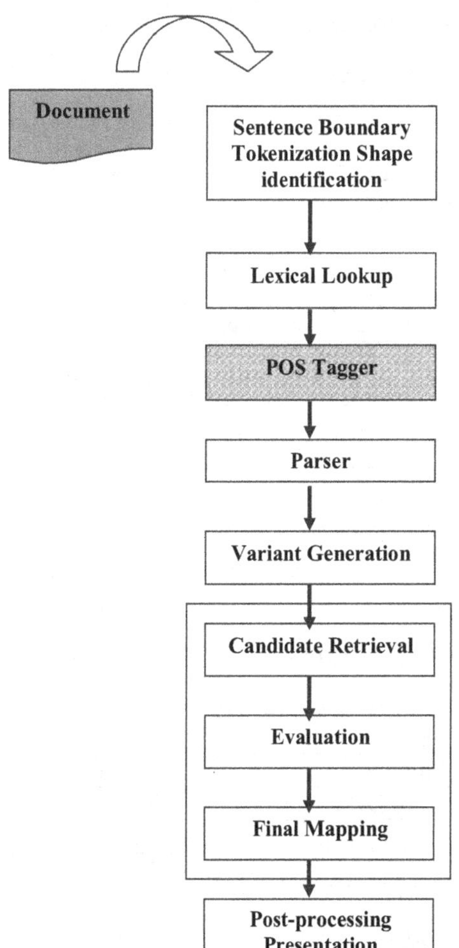

Figure 6. Examples of the expansion strategies using UMLS

Document

```
Seven month old with wheezing, congestion.
Findings consistent with viral or reactive
airway disease.
```

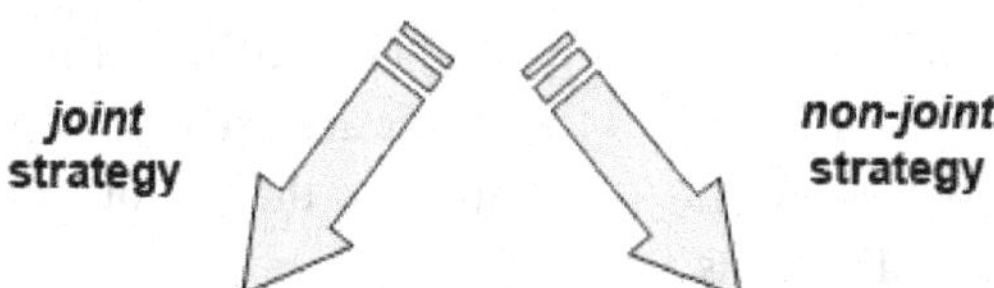


```
seven month old with wheezing,
congestion
old_episode wheeze
precision_month wheezings
wheezy
congestions precision_-_month
months wheezes
findings consistent with viral
or reactive airway disease
reactive_airways_disease
airway_equipment
hyperactive_airway_disease
airways_disease dz diseases
disorders
airway_disease_reactive
airway_device airways
airway_structure
breathing_passages disorder
respiratory_airway aw_airway
viruses
```

```
seven month old with wheezing,
congestion
wheeze episode precision
wheezings wheezy - congestions
months wheezes
findings consistent with viral
or reactive airway disease
structure dz hyperactive
airways breathing equipment
disorders diseases aw passages
respiratory disorder device
viruses
```

Table 1. Terms per ontology using the OHSUMED collection

Ontology	% of Expanded Terms
SNOMEDCT	39.87
NCI	24.00
MSH	23.44
MTH	21.53
RCD	20.48
SNMI	13.79

Table 2. Terms per ontology using the CCHMC collection

Ontology	% of Expanded Terms
SNOMEDCT	47.19
RCD	29.01
NCI	25.33
MSH	20.94
MTH	19.61
SNMI	17.24

weights computed with adjustments over word frequencies. Additional processing in the aim of capture content and meaning from the original text is, however, usually more complex (Sebastiani, 2002). The representations of documents obtained are then suitable for ML algorithms, which are intended to produce models from training data to predict classes for new incoming samples.

We have applied the Adaptive Selection of Base Classifiers (ASBC) algorithm as a classification strategy for multi-label text categorization (Montejo-Ráez et al., 2007). It is trained by selecting, for each class independently, a binary classifier algorithm from a given set according to a given evaluation measure. Thus, each class selects the most suitable classifier algorithm on the predefined evaluation measure from a set of candidate learning algorithms. In this way, we reduce a multi-label classification problem into several binary ones (Allwein et al., 2000). The process is described in Algorithm 1.

It learns from a training set of already labelled samples. These texts are processed so that stemmer and stop words removal is performed. Also, classes and terms (stemmed words) are discarded as follows:

1. A term or a class is discarded if it does not appear in more than two documents.
2. Information gain is computed on every single term. The set of 50,000 terms with highest information gain value is kept.
3. Classes not appearing in a training folder and also in a testing folder are also discarded.

For every final term, the well known TF.IDF weight is computed (Salton & Buckley, 1987). Then, a binary classification model (i.e. a classifier) is learned from every associated class (also known as category, topic or descriptor) found in the labelled collection. A set of candidate learning approaches are passed to the algorithm, and they all are trained on every class. These binary classifiers can be chosen from a wide range of available approaches: Support Vector Machines (Joachims, 1998), PLAUM (Li et al., 2002), Widrow-Hoff, Rocchio and many others (Lewis et al., 1996). Only one binary classifier will be related to each class by selecting the one with the best performance on a given evaluation measure. The classifier must also reach a minimum value on that measure (the α threshold in Algorithm 1), otherwise it is discarded.This measure can be any of the metrics used commonly in TC and in Information Retrieval (Baeza-Yates & Ribeiro-Neto,1999) like precision, recall, F1, accuracy and so on. How these measures are computed is detailed in the following subsection.

At the end of the training process, a list of binary classifiers (one or none per class) is obtained. It is important to underline that in many cases not every class gets an associated classifier. This is due to the lack of samples (we can have one sample with that class but no one else in order to evaluate it) or because none of the trained classifiers produced an acceptable performance (i.e. none of them was over the threshold). In our experiments, the first case of class discarding leads to disregard the class in the evaluation process (simply because there are not enough data), although in the second case, even when the class has no related classifier, it is taken into account for computing the system's performance.

Evaluating Text Categorization

The evaluation of a text categorization system is based on test samples that have been already labelled by human experts. For text categorization systems, the evaluation strategy used is inherited from traditional Information Retrieval experience. Lewis (1991) has an interesting review of how evaluation is carried out in TC systems. The starting point is to compare the matches between human- and computer-assigned key words. We can

Algorithm 1.Adaptive selection of base classifiers

```
Input:
- A set Dt of multi-labelled training documents
- A set Dv of validation documents
- A threshold ? over a given evaluation meassure
- A set L of possible labels (categories)
- A set C of candidate binary classifiers
Output:
- A set C' = {c1, ..., ck, ..., c|L|} of trained
  binary classifiers
Algorithm:
C' ← Ø
For each li in L:
  T ← Ø
  For each cj in C:
    train (cj, li, Dt)
    T ← T ∪ {cj}
   End For
  $cbest ← best(T, Dv)
   If evaluate(cbest) > ?
          C' ← C' ∪ {cbest}
   End if
End For
```

summarize four possible situations in the following contingency table when assigning class c_i:

		Assigned by expert	
	Class c_i	YES	NO
Assigned by system	YES	TP_i	FP_i
	NO	FN_i	TN_i

where

1. TP_i True positive. Assessments where the system and the human expert agree in label assignment.
2. FP_i False positive. Labels assigned by the system that do not agree with expert assignment.
3. FN_i False negative. Labels which the system assigned differently from the human expert.
4. TN_i True negative. Non-assigned labels that were also discarded by the expert.

By combining these measurements, some well-known performance values can be calculated (Baeza-Yates & Ribeiro-Neto,1999):

Precision: $$P = \frac{TP}{TP + FP}$$

Recall: $$R = \frac{TP}{TP + FN}$$

F1 measure: $$F1 = \frac{2PR}{P + R}$$

As can be seen, this is computed for every class. For an overall evaluation of the system, we can compute subtotals for TP, FP, TN and FN values. Computing measures above from these subtotals is named Micro-averaging, and these final measures provide values for precision, recall, F1 or any similar statistical value on the system as a whole. If we first compute these P, R and F1 on every class and then we average, we obtain the so-called Macro-averaging metrics. In multi-label categorization we could also obtain the macro-averaging measure in a document basis, as discussed in the following subsection.

Regardless of the averaging approach chosen, ten-fold cross validation (Witten & Frank, 2000) is a good practice to generate testing sets in self-promoted experiments. This technique splits the collection into ten different and disjoint partitions, and the process of training and evaluating is performed ten times, each one using one of the subsets for testing and the rest for training. Then, the ten measurements obtained are averaged for final results. In this way, we avoid results to be dependent on a given predefined testing set. Thus, our conclusions are led by more robust statistics.

Some Issues about Micro and Macro-Averaging on MLTC

When evaluating text categorization, micro-averaging measures have been traditionally chosen as indicators of the goodness of a system. In multi-label text categorization we could, nevertheless, consider the possibility of evaluating following two additional bases: macro-averaging measures by document and macro-averaging measures by class. These are totally different. Depending on how we want to apply our system, the choice may be crucial to really understand the performance of a proposed solution. In this way, macro-averaging precision by document, for instance, will tell about how valid the labels assigned to every single document are. On the other hand, macro-averaging precision by class will tell how precise we are in assigning classes to documents in general. Significant differences arise since it is only rarely that most of the classes are assigned to most of the documents (there are many rare classes in real classification systems). Therefore, macro-averaging by document is an interesting indicator when the system is intended for individual document labelling. Of course, the counterpoint here is that, if the system is good with most frequent classes, then macro-averaging measurements by document will report good results, hiding bad behaviour in rare classes. This is so even when rare classes may be of higher relevance, because they are better discriminators when labels are used for practical matters. In order to avoid this discussion, only micro-averaging values have been computed here.

EXPERIMENTS

At this point, the collections used along with the expansion and learning phases have been described. We have conducted our experiments according to the variety of combinations of configurations detailed. We have used two binary base classifiers to ensure that term expansion is robust against the selected learning model. Also, the experiments have been carried out using the collections described in Section 4: the CCHMC collection and a partition of 6,000 documents of the OHSUMED collection. The multi-label text categorization system has been trained, adjusted and tested using these collections. We have also used the medical knowledge resource UMLS for the terms expansion of these collections. In order to integrate the clinical knowledge from UMLS metathesaurus, we have used two different approaches: the joint strategy and the non-joint strategy.

In our experiments, topics have been considered to exist at the same level, i.e. no hierarchical relations have been taken into account. For instance, 518 and 518.3 in the CCHMC corpus are considered two distinct topics.

Finally, another parameter used in the experiments has been the machine learning algorithm employed for training the MLTC system. We have tried two ML algorithms as base classifiers within the ASBC strategy. The α threshold used was based on the F1 metric, set to a minimum value of 0.5 (i.e. classifiers below 0.5 or above F1 measure on the validation set are not considered as valid base classifiers):

1. The Support Vector Machine (SVM). It was first used in text categorization by Joachims (1999). The goal of this algorithm is to find the optimal level that maximizes the distance between the positive and the negative cases.
2. The Perceptron Learning Algorithm with Uneven Margins (PLAUM). The algorithm is an extension of the Perceptron algorithm adapted to problems of linear separation of data over a plane (Li et al., 2002).

Since the goal was to know the behaviour of the MLCT system when we integrate the UMLS resource, we have simply considered the default configurations for the two ML algorithms without changing any parameter. The TECAT[q] toolkit has been used as implementation of the ASBC approach. PLAUM algorithm is originally implemented within TECAT, although SVM-Light[r] has been called from this tool as an external binary classifier for the SVM learning algorithm.

Combining all these factors, we present the following experiments carried out for this work. They are summarized in Table 3. For each base classifier and each collection, a base case (without expansion) was run. In addition, join and non-joint strategy was accomplished with each configuration. A total of 12 runs were analyzed (2 collections x 2 ML algorithms x 3 expansion strategies).

Results

In order to evaluate the quality of our system, we have used the usual measures for text categorization: precision, recall and F1. The results obtained for the experiments carried out are shown in Table 4.

As regards the term expansion method, it is worth mentioning that the use of term expansion with UMLS improves the baseline (experiments without expansion, i.e. documents are not

Table 3. Configurations for the experiments

Experiment	Collection	ML Algorithm	Expansion Strategy
Exp_CSNN	CCHMC	SVM	None
Exp_CPNN	CCHMC	PLAUM	None
Exp_CSUJ	CCHMC	SVM	Joint
Exp_CPUJ	CCHMC	PLAUM	Joint
Exp_CSUN	CCHMC	SVM	Non-joint
Exp_CPUN	CCHMC	PLAUM	Non-joint
Exp_OSNN	OHSUMED	SVM	None
Exp_OPNN	OHSUMED	PLAUM	None
Exp_OSUJ	OHSUMED	SVM	Joint
Exp_OPUJ	OHSUMED	PLAUM	Joint
Exp_OSUN	OHSUMED	SVM	Non-joint
Exp_OPUN	OHSUMED	PLAUM	Non-joint

Table 4. Results

Experiment	Precision	Recall	F1
Exp_CSNN	90.48 %	61.79 %	73.43 %
Exp_CPNN	80.91 %	64.08 %	71.52 %
Exp_CSUJ	92.98 %	64.80 %	76.37 %
Exp_CPUJ	84.97 %	71.13 %	77.44 %
Exp_CSUN	92.04 %	62.92 %	74.74 %
Exp_CPUN	85.17 %	69.49 %	76.53 %
Exp_OSNN	77.16 %	26.50 %	39.45 %
Exp_OPNN	64.84 %	31.36 %	42.28 %
Exp_OSUJ	77.89 %	27.30 %	40.43 %
Exp_OPUJ	63.86 %	34.07 %	44.44 %
Exp_OSUN	78.69 %	27.66 %	40.93 %
Exp_OPUN	67.35 %	33.03 %	44.33 %

enriched with terms coming from UMLS) in some cases. Actually, if we analyze the results focusing on expansion benefits, we can state that the integration of UMLS greatly improves the results without expansion. Specifically, for the PLAUM algorithm and the CCHMC collection, the F1 measure improves by 5.01 points if we use the non-joint strategy in the expansion process, and by 5.92 points if we use the joint strategy. The same applies to the SVM algorithm, only a smaller difference than for PLAUM (1.75 points with non-joint expansion strategy and 3.84 with joint expansion strategy, for the CCHMC collection). We can see that the same happens when we use the OHSUMED collection. With PLAUM the improvement of using UMLS exceeds by 2 points (for joint and non-joint strategy) while with SVM it does by about 1 point. Otherwise, the differences between the two types of expansion (joint and non-joint) are not very significant. All in all, the integration of the knowledge from the UMLS methatesaurus is a very promising approach.

As to the learning algorithms used, the expansion works for PLAUM and SVM, but it should be noted that PLAUM works better than SVM (if we focus on F1 measurements). Only one experiment with SVM gives better results than the PLAUM experiment (2.6 points better when we do not apply term expansion over the CCHMC collection). Otherwise, we have obtained better results using PLAUM for the rest of the experiments. Specifically, for the CCHMC collection PLAUM is better than SVM by 2.33 points with the non-joint expansion strategy and by 1.38 points with the joint strategy. With the OHSUMED collection, PLAUM is better than SVM for none, joint and non-joint expansion (byy 2.83 points, 4.01 points and 3.9 points, respectively).

Differences according to the use of joint or non-joint strategies are rather small. It may indicates that the specificity of the terms introduced as joint terms do not add more information than using terms separatedly. This is maybe due to the specialization of the UMLS metathesaurus, so deeper levels of detail could be worthless. The differences between the two collections are also clear. The results show that the improvement is higher when we use the CCHMC collection. We believe that this is because very short texts profit from expansion more than those in OHSUMED.

CONCLUSION

This paper presents a term expansion method based on the UMLS metathesaurus in order to improve a multi-label text categorization system based on machine learning methods. We have tested our approach using two biomedical corpora. On the one hand, we have trained a MLTC system with the CCHMC collection from the Department of Radiology. This corpus includes short records of free text about children radiology reports. On the other hand, another MLTC system has been trained using the widely used OHSUMED collection. In the latter case, the documents are much larger and there are many more of them too..

We propose the integration of clinical knowledge extracted from several medical ontologies in order to improve the MLTC system for medical domain. The approach is based on the idea of semantic enrichment by integrating knowledge in different biomedical collections. For the integration of this clinical knowledge we have used the UMLS metathesaurus. This resource has been applied using two expansion approaches: joint and non-joint. The joint strategy adds more UMLS terms to the final expansion than the non-joint strategy. Another parameter used in our experiments has been the machine learning algorithm employed for the training of the MLTC system. We have tried two ML algorithms: The SVM and the PLAUM.

The accomplished experiments show that the integration of medical knowledge from a resource such as the UMLS metathesaurus is a very promising approach. Independently of the document features (shorter or larger texts) and the expansion type (joint or non-joint), the use of UMLS improves the performance of the MLTC system.

Some new issues have also arisen during the development of our research: The MetaMap tool provides a score value on the terms expanded that could be used to filter them, and terms come from different resources in an unbalanced way. Actually, almost 70% of the expansions are provided from 6 resources out of 80 used ones within UMLS, so some noise may have been brought in by such a wide range of resources. Finally, as working on a supervised paradigm, expanded terms could be ranked according to the information provided regarding the classes they are related through documents. In this way, values like gain ratio could be determined for every expanded term on the training set, that value being useful for additional filtering of expansions.

ACKNOWLEDGMENT

This research has been partially funded by a grant from the Spanish Government, project TIMOM (TIN2006-15265-C06-03).

REFERENCES

Allwein, E. L., Schapire, R. E., & Singer, Y. (2000): Reducing Multiclass to Binary: A Unifying Approach for Margin Classifiers. *In Proceedings of the 17th International Conf. on Machine Learning* (pp. 9-16). San Francisco, CA.: Morgan Kaufmann.

Apweiler, R., Bairoch, A., & Wu, et al. (2004). UniProt: the Universal Protein knowledgebase. *Nucleic Acids Res,* (32), 115-119.

Aronson, A. R., & Rindflesch, T. C. (1997). Query Expansion Using the UMLS Metathesaurus. *Proceedings of the 1997 AMIA Annual Fall Symposium*, (pp. 485-489).

Baeza-Yates, R., & Ribeiro-Neto, B. (1999). *Modern Information Retrieval.* Addison Wesley.

Bairoch, A., Boeckmann, B., Ferro, S., & Gasteiger E. (2004). Swiss-Prot: Juggling between evolution and stability Brief. *Bioinform,* (5), 39-55.

Bhogal, J., Macfarlane, A., & Smith, P. (2007). A review of ontology based query expansion. *Information Processing & Management, 43*(4), July 2007, 866-886.

Bodenreider, O. (2004). The Unified Medical Language System (UMLS): integrating biomedical terminology. *Nucleic Acids Research, 32*, 267-270.

Carr, L., Hall, W., Bechhofer, S., & Goble, C. (2001). Conceptual linking: ontology-based open hypermedia. *In Proceedings of the 10th international Conference on World Wide Web* (Hong Kong, Hong Kong, May 01 - 05, 2001). WWW '01. ACM, New York, NY, (pp. 334-342).

Chiang, J. H., Shin, J. W., Liu, H. H., & Chin, C. L. (2006). GeneLibrarian: an effective gene-information summarization and visualization system. *Bioinformatics, 7*, 392.

De Buenaga Rodríguez, M., Gómez Hidalgo, J. M., & Díaz Agudo, B. (1997). Using WordNet to Complement Training Information in Text Categorization. *Proceedings of RANLP-97. 2nd International Conference on Recent Advances in Natural Language Processing*. Tzigov Chark, Bulgary. 11-13 September 1997.

Díaz-Galiano, M. C., García-Cumbreras, M. A., Martín-Valdivia, M. T., Montejo-Ráez, A., & Urea-López, L. A. (2007). SINAI at ImageCLEF 2007. *Workshop of the Cross-Language Evaluation Forum.*

Fu, G., Jones, C. B., & Abdelmoty, A. I. (2005). *Ontology-Based Spatial Query Expansion in Information Retrieval ODBASE: OTM Confederated International Conferences.*

Gonzalo, J., Verdejo, F., Chugur, I., & Cigarrán, J (1998). Indexing with WordNet synsets can improve text retrieval. *Coling-ACL 98*, (pp. 38-44).

Gruber, T. (1993). A translation approach to portable ontologies. *Knowledge Acquisition, 5*(2), 199–220.

Gruber, T. (1995). Towards Principles for the Design of Ontologies used for Knowledge Sharing. *International Journal of Human-Computer Studies, 43*, 907-928.

Hersh, W., Buckley, C., Leone, T. J., & Hickam, D. (1994). OHSUMED: an interactive retrieval evaluation and new large test collection for research. In Springer-Verlag New York, Inc. *SIGIR '94: Proceedings of the 17th annual international ACM SIGIR conference on Research and development in information retrieval* (pp. 192-201).

Hersh, W., Price, S., & Donohoe, L. (2000). Assessing Thesaurus-Based Query Expansion Using the UMLS Metathesaurus. *In Proceedings of the AMIA Symposium* (pp. 344-348).

Humphreys, B. L., Lindberg, D. A. B., Schoolman, H. M., & Barnett, G. O. (1998). The Unified Medical Language System: An Informatics Research Collaboration. *Journal of the American Medical Informatics Association (JAMIA), 5*, 1-11.

Ide, N. C., Loane, R. F., & Demner-Fushman, D. (2007). Essie: A Concept Based Search Engine for Structured Biomedical Text. *Journal of the American Medical Informatics Association, 14*(3), 253-263.

Joachims, T. (1998). Text categorization with support vector machines: learning with many relevant features. *In Proceedings of ECML-98, 10th European Conference on Machine Learning*, 1398 (pp. 137-142). Berlin, Germany: Springer Verlag, Heidelberg.

Krallinger, M., & Valencia, A. (2005). Text mining and information retrieval services for Molecular Biology. *Genome Biology, 6*, 224.

Lacoste, C. Chevallet, J. P., Lim, J. H., Wei, X. Raccoceanu, D., Thi Hoang, D. L., Teodorescu, R., & Vuillenemot, N. (2006). IPAL Knowledge-based Medical Image Retrieval in ImageCLE-Fmed 2006. *Workshop of the Cross-Language Evaluation Forum.*

Lewis, D. D. (1991). *Evaluating Text Categorization. In Proceedings of Speech and Natural Language Workshop* (pp. 312-318). Morgan Kaufmann (publisher).

Lewis, D. D., Schapire, R. E., Callan, J. P., & Papka, R. (1996). Training algorithms for linear text classifiers. *In Proceedings of SIGIR-96, 19th ACM International Conference on Research and Development in Information Retrieval* (pp. 298-306). New York, US: ACM Press.

Li, Y., Zaragoza, H., Herbrich, R., Shawe-Taylor, J., & Kandola, J. (2002) The Perceptron Algorithm with Uneven Margins. *In Proceedings of the International Conference of Machine Learning (ICML'2002)* (pp. 379-386).

Lindberg, D. A. B., Humphreys, B. L., & McCray, A. T. (1993). The Unified Medical Language System. *Methods of Information in Medicine, 32*, 281-291.

Martín-Valdivia, M. T., Ureña López, L. A., & García Vega, M. (2007). The learning vector quantization algorithm applied to automatic text classification tasks. *Neural Networks, 20*(6), 748-756.

Meystre, S., & Haug, P. J. (2006). Natural language processing to extract medical problems from electronic clinical documents: Performance evaluation. *Journal of Biomedical Informatics, 39*, 589-599.

Miller, G. A. (1995). Introduction to WordNet: A lexical database for English. *Communication ACM, 38*, 39-41.

Montejo-Ráez, A., Martín-Valdivia, M. T., & Ureña-López, L. A. (2007). Experiences with the LVQ algorithm in multilabel text categorization. *In Proceedings of the 4th International Workshop on Natural Language Processing and Cognitive Science* (pp. 213-221.), Funchal, Madeira - Portugal.

Müller, H., Deselaers, T., Lehmann, T., Clough, P., & Hersh, W. (2007). Overview of the Image-CLEFmed 2006 medical retrieval and annotation tasks. Evaluation of Multilingual and Multi-modal Information Retrieval. *Workshop of the Cross-Language Evaluation Forum 2006, Springer Lecture Notes in Computer Science* (2007).

Navigli, R., & Velardi, P. (2003). An Analysis of Ontology-based Query Expansion Strategies. *Workshop on Adaptive Text Extraction and Mining (ATEM 2003), in the 14th European Conference on Machine Learning (ECML 2003),* (pp. 42-49).

Nelson, S. J., Johnston, D., & Humphreys, B. L. (2001). Relationships in medical subject headings. In C. A. Bean & R. Green (Eds.), *Relationships in the Organization of Knowledge.* New York: Kluwer Academic Publishers (pp. 171-184).

Nilsson, K., Hjelm, H., & Oxhammar, H. (2005). SUiS – cross-language ontology-driven information retrieval in a restricted domain. *In Proceedings of the 15th NODALIDA conference,* (pp. 139-145).

Salton, G., & Buckley, C. (1987). *Term Weighting Approaches in Automatic Text Retrieval.* Technical Report, Cornell University. Ithaca, NY, USA.

Sebastiani, F. (2002). Machine learning in automated text categorization. *ACM Comput. Surv., 34*(1), 1–47.

Simon, J., Dos Santos, M., Fielding, J., & Smith, B. (2006). Formal ontology for natural language processing and the integration of biomedical databases. *International Journal of Medical Information, 75*(3-4), 224-231.

Stevens, R., Goble, C. A., & Bechhofer, S. (2000). Ontology-based knowledge representation for bioinformatics. *Brief Bioinformatics 2000, 1,* 398-414.

Verspoor, K., Cohn, J., Joslyn, C., Mniszewski, S., Rechtsteiner, A., Rocha, L. M., & Simas, T. (2005). Protein Annotation as Term Categorization in the Gene Ontology using Word Proximity Networks. *BMC Bioinformatics, 6*(Suppl 1), S20.

Voorhees, E. (1994). Query expansion using lexical-semantic relations. *In Proceedings of the 17th annual international ACM SIGIR conference,* (pp. 61-69).

Witten, I. H., & Frank, E. (2000). *Data Mining.* Morgan Kaufmann.

Yu, A. C. (2006). Methods in biomedical ontology. *Journal of Biomedical Informatics, 39,* 252-266.

Zou, Q., Chu, W. W., Morioka, C., Leazer, G. H., & Kangarloo, H. (2003). IndexFinder: A Method of Extracting Key Concepts from Clinical Texts for Indexing. *AMIA Annual Symposium Proceeding,* (pp. 763-767).

ENDNOTES

[a] http://wordnet.princeton.edu/
[b] http://www.illc.uva.nl/EuroWordNet/
[c] http://www.cycfoundation.org/
[d] http://www.nlm.nih.gov/research/umls/
[e] http://www.computationalmedicine.org/challenge/index.php
[f] ftp://medir.ohsu.edu/pub/ohsumed/
[g] http://medlineplus.gov/
[h] http://www.nlm.nih.gov/mesh/meshhome.html
[i] http://www.google.com
[j] http://www.geneontology.org/
[k] http://www.nlm.nih.gov/
[l] http://www.clef-campaign.org/
[m] http://ir.ohsu.edu/image/
[n] http://www.computationalmedicine.org/challenge/cmcChallengeDetails.pdf
[o] ftp://medir.ohsu.edu/pub/ohsumed
[p] http://mmtx.nlm.nih.gov
[q] http://sinai.ujaen.es/wiki/index.php/TeCat
[r] http://svmlight.joachims.org
[1] http://www.ebi.uniprot.org/index.shtml
[2] http://www.expasy.org/sprot/

Chapter IV
Using Biomedical Terminological Resources for Information Retrieval

Piotr Pezik
European Bioinformatics Institute, Wellcome Trust Genome Campus, UK

Antonio Jimeno Yepes
European Bioinformatics Institute, Wellcome Trust Genome Campus, UK

Dietrich Rebholz-Schuhmann
European Bioinformatics Institute, Wellcome Trust Genome Campus, UK

ABSTRACT

The present chapter discusses the use of terminological resources for Information Retrieval in the biomedical domain. The authors first introduce a number of example resources which can be used to compile terminologies for biomedical IR and explain some of the common problems with such resources including redundancy, term ambiguity, and insufficient coverage of concepts and incomplete Semantic organization of such resources for text mining purposes. They also discuss some techniques used to address each of these deficiencies, such as static polysemy detection as well as adding terms and linguistic annotation from the running text. In the second part of the chapter, the authors show how query expansion based on using synonyms of the original query terms derived from terminological resources potentially increases the recall of IR systems. Special care is needed to prevent a query drift produced by the usage of the added terms and high quality word sense disambiguation algorithms can be used to allow more conservative query expansion. In addition, they present solutions that help focus on the user's specific information need by navigating and rearranging the retrieved documents. Finally, they explain the advantages of applying terminological and Semantic resources at indexing time. The authors argue that by creating a Semantic index with terms disambiguated for their Semantic types and larger chunks of text denoting entities and relations between them, they can facilitate query expansion, reduce the need for query refinement and increase the overall performance of Information Retrieval. Semantic indexing also provides support for generic queries for concept categories, such as genes or diseases, rather than singular keywords.

INTRODUCTION

Researchers in the life science domain have high hopes for the automatic processing of scientific literature. Consequently, there has been a growing interest in developing systems retrieving domain-specific information without making users read every document. (Rebholz-Schuhmann et al., 2005). Over the recent years, Text Mining and Information Retrieval in the life science domain have evolved into a specialized research topic, as the exploitation of biomedical data resources becomes more and more important (Hirschman et al., 2005/2008).

The genomics era has lead to the generation of large-scale data resources containing sequence information about genes and proteins (EMBL database, UniProtKb), and keep track of experimental findings such as gene expression profiles measured in MicroArray experiments (GEO, ArrayExpress). All of these types of data require specialized databases that represent scientific findings with the highest level of detail possible. To address this need, standardization efforts have been launched to develop well-defined database schemas and controlled vocabularies that represent named concepts and entities, for example genes, proteins, parts of genes, functions of proteins and the biological processes that proteins and chemicals are involved in.

In principle, text mining solutions (both information retrieval as well as information extraction oriented ones) benefit from the availability of terminological resources. In the case of information retrieval such resources improve a number of tasks, such as the expansion of user queries, and recognition of concepts in texts, linking them to existing databases and conducting a first order analysis of textual data. Terminological resources are essential in tackling the problem of synonymy, where a single concept has multiple orthographic representations as well as that of polysemy, where a single term may refer to multiple concepts. Lexical metadata encoding hypernymic relations between terms may also come in handy when implementing search engines supporting queries for a generic Semantic type rather than for a specific keyword.

In this chapter we first focus on the availability of terminological resources for the biomedical domain, and discuss different aspects of adopting them for Information Retrieval tasks (section 2 and 3). Then we introduce query refinement as one use scenario of lexicons for improved Information Retrieval (section 4). Finally, we present Semantic indexing as an alternative and complementary approach to integrating the use of terminological resources into the early stages of text processing of biomedical literature (section 5).

COMPILATION OF LEXICAL RESOURCES

A number of life science data resources lending support to text mining solutions are available, although they differ in quality, coverage and suitability for IR solutions. In the following section we provide an outline of the databases commonly used to aid Information Retrieval and Information Extraction.

Public Resources for Biomedical and Chemical Terminologies

The **Unified Medical Language System** (UMLS)[a]: is a commonly used terminological resource provided by the National Library of Medicine. UMLS is a compilation of several terminologies and it contains terms denoting diseases, syndromes and gene ontology terms among others. The UMLS is characterized by a wide coverage and a high degree of concept type heterogeneity, which may make it difficult to use when a specific subset of terms is required. The ***UMLS Metathesaurus*** forms the main part of UMLS and it organizes over 1 million concepts denoted by 5 million term variants. The Metathesaurus has been used for the task of named entity recognition e.g. (Aronson et al., 2001). Also, more specialized subsets have been compiled out of this resource and used for the identification of disease names, e.g. (Jimeno et al., 2008). An assessment of UMLS's suitability for language processing purposes was carried out by (McCray et al., 2001).

Medical Subject Headings (MeSH) (included in UMLS). An organized controlled vocabulary encompassing a set of terminological descriptors developed with a view to supporting the retrieval of Medline abstracts. MeSH annotations have been used for query expansion and text categorization, e.g. (Ruch, 2006).

SNOMED-CT (Systematized Nomenclature of Medicine - Clinical Terms) is a comprehensive taxonomy of medical terms. It is used in commercial IT solutions to achieve consistent representations of medical concepts and it has recently gained some importance in public IT solutions. It is included in UMLS, although license agreements have to be checked by the potential users of the resource. SNOMED-CT has been integrated into a decision support solutions that links patient data to genomics information (Lussier et al., 2002).

The **NCBI taxonomy**[b] "database is a curated set of names and classifications for all organisms represented in GenBank" (quote from Website). It is used to offer cross-linking between the different data resources at the NCBI.

The **Gene Ontology** (GO) is a taxonomy of concepts for molecular functions, cellular components and biological processes (GO-Consortium, 2004). It is used as a controlled vocabulary for the annotation of database entries, for the categorization of genes in microarray experiments and for the extraction of terms representing the concepts from the scientific literature (Couto et al., 2005). GO is now part of UMLS.

Medline Plus[c] provides information on disease and drugs that can be used to compile controlled vocabularies.

BioThesaurus is a collection of protein and gene names extracted from a number of different data resources, e.g. UniProtKb, EntrezGene, Hugo, InterPro, Pfam and others (Liu et al., 2006). The database contains several million entries and is difficult to integrate into an information extraction solution due to its huge size. We discuss some ways of adapting this resource for IR tasks in the sections below.

GPSDB[d] is a thesaurus of gene and protein names that have been collected from 14 different resources (Pillet et al., 2005). It serves as a controlled vocabulary for named gene and protein entities and is thus similar to the BioThesaurus.

DrugBank[e] is a database that collects information for bioinformatics and cheminformatics use. The resource contains information on drug brand names, chemical IUPAC names, chemical formula, generic names, InCHI identifiers, chemical structure representations and relevant links to other data bases, e.g. ChEBI, PharmGKB and others. A comprehensive list of names representing drugs has been used to identify and categorize mentions of drugs in the scientific literature (Rebholz-Schuhmann et al., 2008; Kolárik et al., 2007).

ChEBI[f] is a taxonomy of chemical entities of biological interest developed at the European Bioinformatics Institute.

The **PubChem**[g] database contains information on small chemical entities (currently 17 million chemical entities are represented). This public resource is meant to keep track of information relating small chemical entities to biological experiments. Similarly to DrugBank, it gives access to the names, structures and kinetic parameters of small chemical entities.

Both CHEBI and PubChem have been used as terminological resources for the identification of chemical names (Corbett et. al. 2007).

Other biomedical data resources that can be exploited for terminology include **EntrezGene**[h], the **EMBL Nucleotide Sequence Database**[i] and **GenBank Database**[j]. These are large databases containing sequence information and annotations for proteins and genes. Apart form names, they also provide definitions and other annotations which can be used to compile and enrich a terminological resource.

The **Specialist lexicon**[k] is a lexical resource covering some 20,000 terms relevant to the biomedical domain. This core part was populated in a bottom-up fashion from a corpus of Medline abstracts, and it has been complemented with some 12,000 additional words from existing dictionaries of general English. The Specialist Lexicon contains words of different part of speech categories annotated with basic morphological information on inflectional variants.

Even this short overview shows that databases which can be potentially used as terminological resources by the text mining community in the biomedical domain come in many different shapes and sizes. Generally, they may be said to fall roughly under the following three major categories with respect to their suitability for IR and IE applications:

databases which were not originally designed as terminological resources in the first place, but can still to some degree be used as such (e.g., the NCBI Taxonomy), multi-purpose top-down resources which were not designed to be used for information retrieval or text mining exclusively but can well be taken advantage of for such purposes (e.g., controlled vocabularies and ontologies such as GO and ChEBI), and finally terminological resources which were constructed with specific text mining applications in mind (e.g., Specialist lexicon).

Because of the importance of having access to terminological databases on the one hand, and the scarcity of text-mining oriented lexicons on the other, in practice resources of the first two types are often adopted for text mining purposes. In the following sections we discuss the most common issues arising in the compilation of terminological resources for the biological domain, which include:

redundancy (pseudo terms),
polysemous entries (ambiguous terms),
lack of explicit links between Semantically related terms and
incomplete coverage of terms used in naturally occurring language.

Next, we suggest some ways of alleviating these problems. In particular we focus on reducing ambiguity through the assignment of polysemy indicators, grouping sets of synonyms containing similar terms, and complementing a terminological resource through bottom-up population.

REDUNDANCY

Examples of resources of the first type include protein and gene databases which contain names, synonyms in addition to more specialized biological annotation of genes and proteins. Typical problems with such resources include artificial and erroneous names. For instance, the aforementioned *Biothesaurus*, which (depending on the version) is a compilation of more than 30 existing gene/protein databases, groups together protein and gene names (PGNs) by their unique Uniprot accession numbers. Due to the sheer number of the resources it covers, not all the terms contained can be regarded as equally valid. Different fields imported from different databases contain terms of varying quality. **Table 1** shows an example entry from the Biothesaurus, where different entries from the UniProt, ENTREZGENE and Rat Genome databases have been grouped together as synonymous through the shared accession number Q4KMB9. Interestingly, the entry lists the term *human* as a fully-fledged synonym of such unambiguous terms as *Ush1c* or *Usher syndrome 1C homolog.* Obviously, this pseudo-term originally appeared in a descriptor field of a rat homolog of the human *Usher syndrome 1C* (*Ush1c*) gene, since the accession number under which this term is listed in the UniProt database is annotated with the species identifier of *Rattus norvegicus.*

Redundant pseudo-terms have to be taken into consideration when compiling a terminological resource from existing databases which were not originally meant for text-processing purposes.

Genuine Polysempy

The example of *human* as a false gene name can be regarded as a case of artificial term polysemy resulting from noisy database fields. However, in many other cases, terminological resources contain terms which are genuinely ambiguous even within the same domain. As an example the UMLS Metathesaurus groups together the terms *cancer, tumour* and *neoplasm* as synonymous, although they are rather a case of vertical polysemy, where one term has a more general sense (i.e., *tumour*) than the others (*cancer* is even a subtype of *neoplasm*) (Jimeno et al. 2007). The problem of polysemy is particularly common in PGNs. (Pezik et al. 2008b) point out four major cases of PGN polysemy:

- A PGN has a common English word homograph. We call this a case of **domain-independent polysemy**, e.g. (but, WHO). Sometimes this type of polysemy is introduced by pseudo terms by resulting from the poor quality of a lexical resource, e.g. Biothesaurus contains partial PGN terms such as *human* or, due to the fact that they were gathered from less trustworthy database description fields.

Table 1. Example entry from Biothesaurus

NUM	TERM	SOURCE
Q4KMB9	Ush1c	UniProt:GENE:PRIMARY:Q4KMB9
Q4KMB9	harmonin a1	ENTREZGENE:SYNONYMS:308596
Q4KMB9	Human	ENTREZGENE:DESCRIPTION:308596
Q4KMB9	Usher syndrome 1C homolog (human)	RGD:NAME:1303329
Q4KMB9	MGC112571	ENTREZGENE:SYNONYMS:308596
Q4KMB9	Usher syndrome 1C homolog	UniProt:PROTEIN:PRIMARY:Q4KMB9
Q4KMB9	Human	UniProt:PROTEIN:OTHER:Q4KMB9

- A PGN has a number of hyponyms and it is sometimes used synonymously with them. Examples of this type of polysemy include generic enzyme names, such as *oxidoreductase*). Sometimes a more specified case of holonymy triggers similar ambiguity, e.g. an operon name can be interpreted to denote any of the genes it contains. We call this a case of **vertical polysemy**.
- A PGN is used for a number of **orthologous genes**. Thus the ambiguity in the gene name results from the fact that the same name is used for structurally identical gene found in different species. We ignore an even finer case of polysemy where a distinction is made between homologous genes.
- A PGN has a biomedical homograph, e.g. *retinoblastoma.* We refer to this as a case of domain-specific polysemy.

Many of these types of polysemy apply to other Semantic types as well. Taking terms from ad-hoc lexicons at face value and using them to expand queries as described below may lead to a rather devastating concept drift. In other words, polysemous terminological entries may result in expanding the query with irrelevant terms and thus lower the precision of the result set. Therefore it is important to consider different ways of reducing term polysemy when utilizing automatically compiled resources.

Implicit Semantic Relations

The opposite problem of having an incomplete number of synonyms for a given concept may occur, as well. When compiling lexical resources from biological databases, we may take simplified assumptions about the Semantic relations between terms suggested by the structure of such resources. In the example above 7 terms for the same gene were assigned the same accession number Q4KMB9 and assumed to be synonymous. Obviously, a term with a different accession number would be considered to belong to a different lexical entry. However, it would not always be reasonable to expect terms to be *equally* different from each other just because they happen to have different accession numbers in an automatically generated thesaurus. Sets of synonyms in human-crafted thesauri often overlap with each other, and they are characterized by different level of intra-cluster coherence, with some synonyms being more similar to each other than others. If, for example, we were to take all the PGNs assigned to the accession number P10274 and make a ranked list of sets of synonymous PGNs which are assigned to a different accession number according to the number of terms they share, we may end up with a list similar to the one illustrated in **Table 2**. A brief look at the list reveals that, for instance, the number of terms shared between different synsets seems to be inversely correlated with the distance in the species taxonomy nodes to which these terms are assigned[1] indicating that sets of synonymous protein and gene names happen to be more similar for closely related species. This in turn proves that sense distinctions based on UniProt accession numbers only are rather coarse-grained and that they conceal a variety of finer sense distinctions implicitly present in Biothesaurus as a lexical resource. In some contexts we might want to ignore the fine-grained distinction between two strains of the two gene identifiers *P10274* and *P14074* for the Human T-cell lymphotrophic virus type 1. The similarity between the two different sets of terms used to denote these genes can be inferred from external resources such as the NCBI species taxonomy (the two strains of the virus have an immediate common parent). Another way of detecting such latent sense relations shown below is based on comparing the number of terms shared by both synsets.

One conclusion that results from this example is that explicit sense distinctions derived directly from existing databases do not translate easily into a consistent lexical representation which can

Table 2. Synset similarity measured in terms of the number of shared terms

#	UniProt	Cosine	Synset	Species	Tax distance
0	P10274	1	| Protease | PRT | aspartic proteinase | HIV-1 retropepsin | Human immunodeficiency virus type 1 protease | prt	11926	0—0
1	P14074	0.89	| Protease | PRT | HIV-1 retropepsin | Human immunodeficiency virus type 1 protease | prt	11927	1—1
2	P04024	0.70	| Protease | PRT | prt	11942	4—3
3	P10271	0.68	| Protease| PRO | HIV-1 retropepsin | Human immunodeficiency virus type 1 protease | prt	11758	4—3
4	P03353	0.67	| Protease | HIV-1 retropepsin | Human immunodeficiency virus type 1 protease	11909	3—2
5	P21407	0.61	| proteinase | Protease | PRT | prt	11856	4—2
6	P51518	0.57	| Protease | PRT	39068	4—3
7	P05960	0.43	| POL| Pol polyprotein | HIV-1 retropepsin | Human immunodeficiency virus type 1 protease	11687	4—4
8	P12498	0.43	| POL| Pol polyprotein | HIV-1 retropepsin | Human immunodeficiency virus type 1 protease	11694	4—4
9	P11204	0.4	| POL| pol| Pol polyprotein | HIV-1 retropepsin | Human immunodeficiency virus type 1 protease	11670	8—34
10	P10394	0.32	| POL| FlyBase:412 | HIV-1 retropepsin | Human immunodeficiency virus type 1 protease| Retrovirus-related Pol polyprotein from transposon 412	7227	3—2

always be relied upon in Information Retrieval techniques such as query expansion.

Recall and Abstraction from Text

Databases used to compile terminological resources are often prepared in abstraction from the literature. This may mean that some concepts described in the literature are not represented in the databases used to compile a terminological resource. One reason for that situation is that curators find it difficult to keep their databases up to date with the research reported in the literature. In other cases, concepts may be present in both the database and the literature, but no obvious link is provided between the two due to the different wording used to name the same entities or relations. As an example, the aforementioned Gene Ontology (GO) is a database containing over 23,000 biological concepts annotated with a category label and a definition and integrated into a taxonomic structure. GO relates terms denoting molecular functions, cellular components and biological processes, thus offering potentially interesting possibilities of advanced Information Retrieval (e.g. Müller et al. 2004). However, GO controlled vocabulary is difficult to use directly as a terminology because of the different wording of GO concepts in naturally occurring language. In fact, identifying mentions of GO concepts in running text has been tackled as a separate text mining task (Gaudan et al. 2008; Blaschke 2005).

LEXICON REFINEMENT AND ENRICHMENT

In view of the problems typical of term repositories compiled from biomedical databases it is worthwhile to consider some ways of refining the quality of terminological resources. In the next three sections we discuss possible methods of identifying and filtering highly synonymous terms in a dictionary combining several Semantic types. Then we briefly focus on the types of linguistic and domain-specific metadata that can be added to a terminological resource to increase its coverage and general usefulness for IR tasks.

Reducing Polysemy

Term polysemy can be dealt with at two levels. On the one hand, Named Entity Recognition and Word Sense Disambiguation techniques can be applied in the context where a given term occurs in text. In the context of IR systems, however, such techniques would have to be applied either at indexing time or only at post-retrieval time, when refining the first set of results retrieved with polysemous query terms.

Interestingly, it is possible to statically assign features that can help to identify highly polysemous terms without having to analyze their context of occurrence. If we consider the four major types of PGN ambiguity sketched above, it is possible to design a set of features which can indicate possible ambiguity for each term in a lexicon. For instance, if a word form is highly frequent in a corpus of general English, such as the British National Corpus (BNC), then there is a high chance of the word being a frequent common English homograph (see Type 1 polysemy above). If the word happens to be a PGN, but it can be found with a high number of accession numbers or species identifiers, it may be a case of type 2 or type 3 polysemy. Also, if the word is highly frequent in Medline, or if it occurs under many different nodes of a biomedical taxonomy such as MESH, then it is quite likely to be a case of type 4 polysemy. (Pezik et al. 2008b) have examined the use of such features to predict highly polysemous terms. The set of static dictionary features examined is listed in **Table 3**, with the polysemy type addressed by each of the features indicated in the third column. The values for the features were computed and assigned to PGNs imported from Biothesaurus. Two corpora annotated for PGN mentions were used to implement and train a J48 decision-tree based classifier using the abovementioned feature set to recognize false protein names in biomedical texts.

The evaluation showed that it is possible predict highly polysemous terms with some of the

Table 3a. Set of potenial polysemy indicators

#	Feature	Polysemy type
1	BNC frequency	1
2	Number of acc. numbers	2,3
3	NCBI taxonomy ids	3
4	Generic enzyme	2
5	Medline frequency	4,1
6	MESH nodes	4

static dictionary features tested alone, and that the prediction and resolution of true PGNs can be further improved with contextual features. BNC and Medline frequencies have turned out to be the strongest predictors of PGN polysemy. Just using the Biothesaurus to recognize human PGNs through direct dictionary look-ups resulted in a relatively high recall rate of 0.83, but rather unacceptable precision of 0.03, which means that 97 per cent PGNs matching dictionary entries were resolved incorrectly, either because these terms were not PGNs in the context considered or because they were a case of Type 2 or Type 3 polysemy introduced above. Applying static dictionary features as predictors of polysemy increased the precision to 0.36 and combining static dictionary features with contextual clues resulted in a further increase of 0.79 precision (see Figure 1).

Clearly, the most polysemous terms can be predicted to a significant extent based on the static information about the terms which can be encoded in the terminological resource. This offers a polysemy-sensitive way of selecting the terms to expand or refine queries in Information Retrieval systems. The last sections of the performance improvement graphs also show that named entity resolution is further augmented by applying context-driven disambiguation clues. We return to this point when presenting the advantages of Semantic indexing in the final sections of this chapter.

Adding Linguistic Metadata

Typical linguistic metadata annotated in terminological resources includes morphological variants of terms such as inflectional endings, which provides a basic way of term normalization, thus ensuring a better rate of term recognition in texts. As we have shown, it is also possible to explicitly represent basic Semantic relations between terminological units such as synonymy or hypernymy. Some lexicons and text mining

Figure 1. Reducing the polysemy of terminological entries with static and contextual features

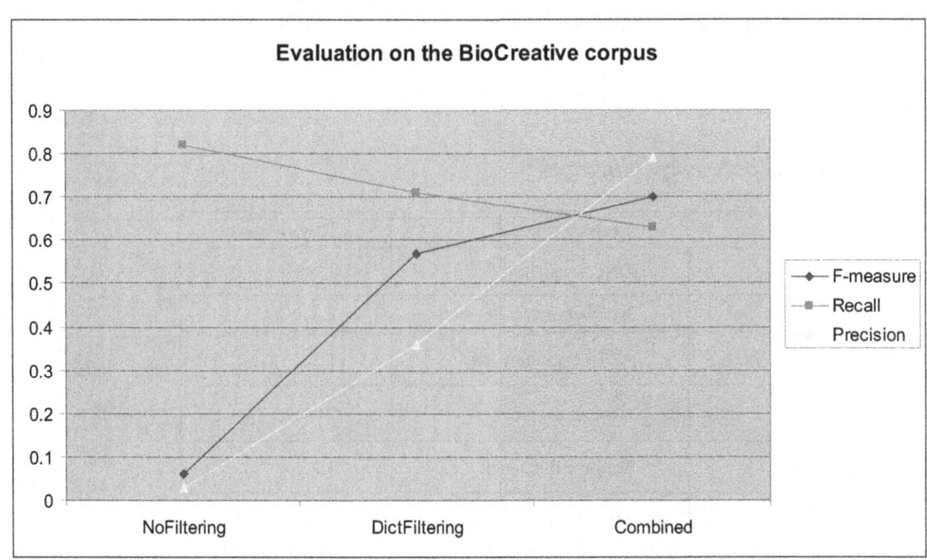

systems are also designed to represent syntactic information, such as the most frequent arguments of verbs, also known as subcategorization frames (e.g. Wattarujeekrit et al. 2004). Subcategorization frames roughly reflect the Semantic relations typically denoted by a given verb, thus enabling queries for terms which occur in a certain Semantic relation. For example, the typical arguments of the verb *inhibit* in a collection of texts on molecular biology could involve the participants of a gene regulation event. Having categorized similar verbs by their syntactic arguments, one can form generic queries about all possible gene regulation events between two named entities, e.g. *gene1 AND (activate OR inhibit) AND gene2*, where *activate* and *inhibit* are antonyms sharing a common subcategorization frame.

Bottom-Up Population

So far we have only discussed the possibilities of importing and refining existing resources which can be transformed into biomedical term repositories. Such approaches to lexicon population can be described as top-down in that they derive vocabularies from conceptual representations which are often abstracted from the naturally occurring language. A complementary bottom-up approach would involve extracting terms directly from the biomedical literature, normalizing and incorporating them into a terminological resource. Bottom-up population of a lexical resource can either result in completely new senses or new variants of existing senses being added to the lexicon. The aforementioned *Specialist* lexicon is an example of the former as it was partly populated with terms from a collection of Medline documents. The *BioLexicon* developed within the BootStrep project[m] contains variants of terms such as gene names which were found in relevant corpora. However, in the latter case it is not new concepts that are added to the lexicon, but rather new wording of the concepts already attested in the existing resources.

We have discussed some of the available biomedical databases which can be compiled into terminological resources. We have outlined the typical problems posed by such databases, such as redundancy (noisy entries), polysemy (ambiguous entries) insufficient coverage of concepts and term variants, as well as the incomplete representation of Semantic relations between terms (implicit similarity between terms with different sense identifiers). Assuming that we can deal with these problems and produce a relatively reliable terminological resource, we now focus on demonstrating how terminological resources can be used for the purposes of Information Retrieval.

TERMINOLOGICAL RESOURCES FOR QUERY REFORMULATION

Users of an ad-hoc information retrieval system have to translate their information demand into a representation of the system's query language under the additional constraint that the retrieval is efficient in terms of processing time. Users tend to query for concept representations, i.e. terms, and have to consider all different terms that may be used to express their information need in the collection as well as the specificity linked to the terms within the document collection in order to reduce the number of non-relevant documents.

Query Reformulation

Concepts in specialised domains can be expressed using different terms (synonymy). In the biomedical domain we can identify proteins and diseases that may be represented using several synonymous terms. A user may face the problem of missing documents simply because he or she is not aware of all the possible synonyms. Query reformulation (QR) is a well-known technique applied from the very beginning of information retrieval and it may rely on lexical resources and statistical techniques or a combination of both. QR comprises different operations that are applied to the original user query in order to improve its performance either in itself or in relation to the representation of ideas in the documents (Efthimiadis, 1996). Query reformulation is a relatively lightweight IR technique because it affects only the query side of the retrieval engine. QR can be applied using different lexicons and ontologies to select the reformulation terms without the need to rebuild existing indexes. QR can be categorized into query expansion and query refinement. Query expansion is intended to increase recall and query refinement is intended to increase the precision of the user query by specifying its possible meanings.

Query Expansion (QE)

We can distinguish between different QE techniques based on the resource used to provide expansion terms, which can be derived both from the document collection or a lexical resource. In this chapter we will focus more on information retrieval based on existing lexical resources after introducing both expansion types.

Document-Analysis for Query Expansion

Relevance feedback is the most popular QE technique used to expand the query by analyzing those retrieved documents which the user identified as relevant or irrelevant to the query. One of the most well known relevant feedback approaches is based on Rocchio's formula (Buckley, 1994). In this formula the vector of the original query is modified according to the vectors of the relevant documents (D_r) and the non-relevant documents (D_{nr}). The parameters (*α*, *β* and *γ*) are used to adjust the importance of the relevance of the original query, the vector of the relevant documents and the vector of the non-relevant queries respectively.

$$\vec{q}_m = \alpha \vec{q}_0 + \beta \frac{1}{|D_r|} \sum_{\vec{d}_j \in D_r} \vec{d}_j - \gamma \frac{1}{|D_{nr}|} \sum_{\vec{d}_j \in Dn_r} \vec{d}_j$$

This formula produces a smoothed vector that is placed in the region of the document space containing the relevant documents. Relevant documents are assumed to occur in complementary distribution to the irrelevant ones. One drawback of this method of relevance feedback is that it is intended to produce a coherent prototype vector of relevant documents (Joachims, 1997), based on the assumption that all the relevant documents are to be found in a single cluster. In reality, relevant documents may be distributed over different clusters (Sebastiani, 2002).

One advantage of this approach to finding expansion terms over terminology-based approaches is that the reformulation of the query is based on example relevant documents from the collection at hand. The generated context may contain collection-specific information which is unavailable from terminological resources. To complement the information on term similarity found in terminological resources, it has been suggested to use term co-occurrences in the entire collection as a measure of collection-specific term similarity. This approach is known as a *global analysis*, and it can be contrasted with the *local analysis strategy* where only co-occurrences of terms in the relevant documents from the initially retrieved result set are used to find terms similar to the original query terms. The global strategy has been proposed to improve existing resources like WordNet (Mandala et al., 1998). Methods combining global and local strategies have been proposed in (Xu and Croft, 1996).

Explicit feedback from the user is expensive and difficult to obtain. Therefore, in some systems the method of *blind relevance feedback* is used, where an arbitrary number of documents retrieved by the original query are assumed to be relevant. This set of initially retrieved document is then used to find terms for query expansion, without asking for the user's explicit feedback. These techniques have been only found useful in those retrieval systems which show a high precision rate at the top ranks of the retrieved set of documents. Modifications to existing systems to provide high precision at top ranks are proposed by (Mitra et al., 1998), to satisfy this condition. In the Genomic Track in TREC[n] different approaches for pseudo-relevance feedback have been used, but they did not provide interesting results, since it was not possible to obtain high precision at the top ranks.

Other techniques analyse the relation between the different terms in the collection and create mathematical models relating the different terms that in some cases can be considered as automatically extracted thesauri (Qiu and Frei,1993). To conclude, it is not always useful to do the expansion of the queries. Approaches that measure the appropriateness of the expansion have been proposed in the literature.

Using Terminological Resources for Query Expansion

The most basic approach to query expansion involving terminological resources is to expand the query terms with available synonyms from an existing lexicon, taxonomy or ontology. In the biomedical domain, systems like PubMed provide automatic query expansion by default. PubMed expands the original queries with synonyms of the query term and other more specific terms (hyponyms) from the MeSH taxonomy. As we can see in the following table the query "colon cancer" submitted to PubMed has been expanded with the synonym "colonic neoplasm" and hyponyms such as "colonic neoplasms". This example shows as well how the expansion can involve the use of Boolean operators, in order to relate synonymous terms with the OR operator.

Research in information retrieval (Voorhees, 1994) has shown that it is difficult to provide a general procedure for query expansion and the different problems are related to the specificities of each individual query. Another conclusion resulting from this study is that query expansion is effective when the queries are short, since longer queries already contain terms that identify better the context of the information need.

In the biomedical domain query expansion has shown to be useful in specific tasks and specific terminologies, and not so useful in others. For instance, (Sehgal et al. 2006, Aronson et al., 1997, Liu et al, 2005) worked with the Medline collection using UMLS and the LocusLink database to retrieve documents specific to genes showing successful results. On the other hand, fewer benefits of query expansion benefits have been demonstrated in the work of (Hersh et al., 2000) with the Oshumed collection and the UMLS. (Chu and Liu, 2004) have applied query expansion using the UMLS and the OSHUMED collection based on template specific queries in which the expanded terms are combined based on the relations in the UMLS and the document collection (similar to local context techniques). The Genomics Track in TREC provides a document collection in which different expansion techniques have shown to be

Table 4. Query expanded by PubMed with MeSH terms

Original query: Colon cancer
Expanded query:
("colonic neoplasms"[TIAB] NOT Medline[SB]) OR "colonic neoplasms"[MeSH Terms] OR colon cancer[Text Word]

useful based on LocusLink and the disease branch of the MeSH (Aronson, 2001).

The automatic expansion of user queries requires the mapping of the query terms to the corresponding entities or concepts in existing resources. In addition, very accurate word sense disambiguation needs to be applied on the concepts appearing in the query. High quality word sense disambiguation is a difficult task as we have already seen is section 2 for PGNs and GO terms or as in the case of the disambiguation of terms denoting diseases (Jimeno et al., 2008). The annotation of entities is useful as well in other retrieval tasks as cross-lingual information retrieval in combination with multilingual resources like the UMLS. In this case, the original query is mapped to concept identifiers and then to terms in the target language (Ruch, 2004). Furthermore word sense disambiguation is very difficult to achieve because the query lacks the contextual information needed for the disambiguation. The mistakes resulting from the sense disambiguation in query expansion induce a *query drift* changing the intention of the original user query.

Another source for *query drift* stems from the fact that biomedical lexicons may not provide a clean set of terms as the ones required by the information retrieval. The above-mentioned example of the vertical polysemy of the term *neoplasm* is a case in point. Because *neoplasm* is a hypernym of *cancer*, the set of documents retrieved for the query term *cancer* expanded with *neoplasm* is likely to lose focus of the user's possible original information need. Other cases of polysemy identified in section 2 may cause a similar depression in the precision rate.

But query drift may happen as well even if the query concepts are properly disambiguated. We have to remember that the exact mechanism of query expansion depends on the query language (i.e. Boolean operators or vector space model or language models). In the case of the Boolean operators, with the exception of the extended vector space model based on Boolean operators no weight is needed. Kekäläinen and Järvelin, 1998) have shown the impact of the usage of different Boolean operators for the same information need.

As a conclusion query expansion can provide an increase in the performance of biomedical information retrieval in specific cases. It seems to be especially useful in queries where the terms are not the one commonly used wording of the relevant concepts in the underlying collection. Expanding with synonyms has also been found useful in short queries which are difficult to map to all relevant documents.

Query Refinement

Search engines for document collections like Medline or the Web may easily retrieve a large quantity of documents due to term ambiguity. As a result, false positives may appear in the retrieved result set, where the original user query is not specific enough leading to several potential interpretations. Query refinement attempts to modify the query in order to improve the precision of the retrieved set of documents, by filtering out irrelevant documents.

As we have seen in the QR definition introduced above, the different techniques needed to find the appropriate interpretation of the user query may have to utilize not only available terminological resources, but also the documents found in the collection at hand. This is necessary in situations where a term is not explicitly marked as ambiguous in a term repository but it is used ambiguously in the document collection.

For instance, users interested in documents about *APC* in PubMed may obtain documents concerning *adenomatous polyposis coli* or documents dealing with *anaphase-promoting complex*. Although, the different techniques of disambiguation of the entities appearing in the query may provide the right interpretation of the term, as we have shown for QE a query drift might still occur. Solving this problem may require learning the specificities of a given document collection and may turn out to be collection-specific.

The essential problem is then one of discarding non-relevant documents which could possibly occur in the result set due to term ambiguity. We have to identify keywords that target the non-relevant documents and integrate them in the query language. In a Boolean model, negative keywords can be specified with the NOT operator. In a vector space model a negative weight can be added to an ambiguous term. Obviously, it is possible to require the user to manually identify such negative keywords while browsing through the set of originally retrieved documents. The selection of these terms may in fact require some feedback provided by the user. One way of automating this process is through the analysis of query logs of an information retrieval system. This means that the performance of an IR system is relative to its usage. In other cases it has proved useful to use explicit feedback information in template based queries (Ruch et al., 2006).

A more relaxed approach would involve grouping the retrieved document sets according to different criteria. The main idea of this approach is to show the different possible topical clusters identified in the set retrieved documents. Again, we may identify methods that rely on the retrieved set of documents or on existing terminological resources to achieve that goal. Some approaches propose the clustering of the retrieved documents, e.g. *scatter/gather*. This is the case of Vivisimo[o] an information retrieval engine, which processes documents and gathers terms from text to cluster and label sets of documents. The labels guide the user to the cluster of highest relevance.

Other approaches rely on existing knowledge sources like OntoRefiner (Safar et al., 2004) and GoPubMed[p]; which maps the retrieved document set to the GO and MeSH taxonomies, so that the user can target a more refined subset of documents.

As we have seen interpreting the intended focus of the query may be problematic. Both the information contained in terminological resources and the document collection itself can contribute to refining the intention of the user getting it closer to the right sense and the right group of documents. MedEvi (**Figure 2**) (Pezik et al. 2008a) implements a retrieval engine as a special concordancer which identifies marching query terms in the retrieved documents and shows the context in which they occur. Other applications provide structured results using domain-specific information extracted from the initial result set (e.g. EBIMed).

SEMANTIC INDEXING

In the previous sections of this chapter we have focused on compiling and adopting terminological resources for the purposes of Information Retrieval. Query expansion and query refinement have been identified as some of the most common use cases of terminological resources in IR. We have shown that query expansion is aimed at increasing the recall of IR systems and this goal is achieved by finding synonyms of the original query terms, while query refinement is a technique for boosting precision by eliminating irrelevant or highly ambiguous query terms.

In this section we present the concept of Semantic indexing. We argue that Semantic indexing has the potential of increasing the performance of IR systems in query expansion scenarios and that it reduces the need for query refinement by resolving ambiguity at indexing time.

Information Extraction for Semantic Indexing

The basic prerequisite for creating a Semantic index is the thorough analysis of the collection of documents at hand utilizing the different techniques of information extraction. Information Extraction solutions are applied to associate terms with named entities resolved to concept identifiers (thus resulting in the Semantic annotation of documents). Concept identifiers in the biomedical

Figure 2. Latent relations between diseases and genes linked to the centrosome as retrieved by MedEvi

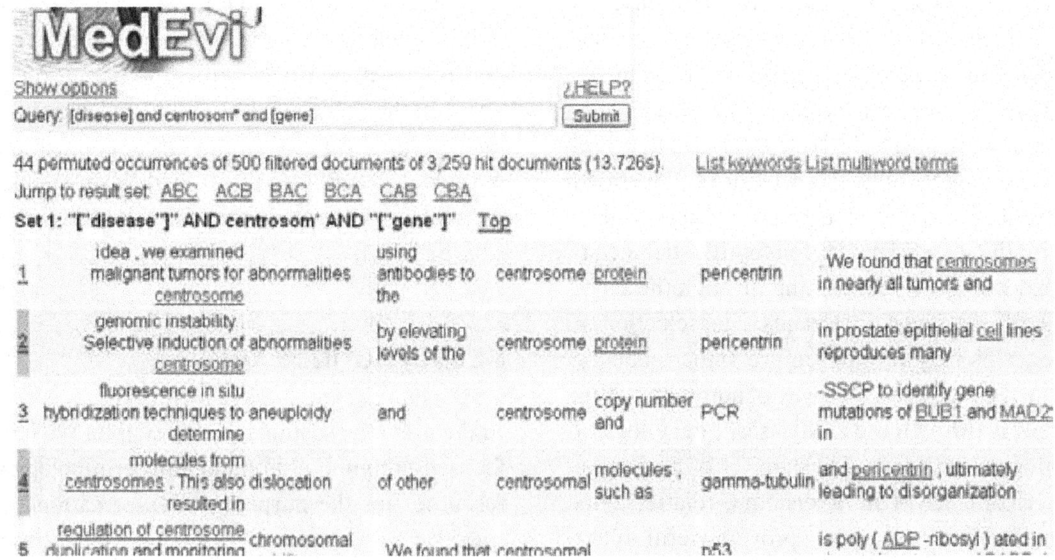

domain are available for terms denoting named entities such as gene or protein names, chemical entities, diseases or organism names (see section 2.1). Apart from single concepts, more complex spans of text reporting on relations such as protein-protein interactions or gene regulation events can also be annotated, with the participants of these events explicitly identified. Whenever possible, it is also useful to resolve the entities and events identified and map them to databases of reference (e.g. UniProtKb), so that a standard interpretation of these entities can be achieved across different text mining systems.

From the technical point of view such information can be added to the running text either as inline or stand-off annotation (Rebholz-Schuhmann et al., 2006). The typical Information Extraction techniques used to enrich the documents with a domain-specific Semantic interpretation of the text include Named Entity Recognition and Resolution, as well as relation extraction and event identification. Needles to say, domain specific terminological and ontological resources play an important role in the process of Semantic enrichment.

Indexing

Once the running text of a document collection is annotated with concept identifiers, a Semantic index can be created. One example technique of compiling such an index would involve storing the concept identifier of a recognized and resolved named entity together with the term or span of terms denoting it at the same position in the index, e.g. Whatizit and EBIMed (Rebholz-Schuhmann et al., 2007; Rebholz-Schuhmann et al., 2008). Other examples of retrieval systems based on Semantic indexing include (William and Greenes, 1990; Müller et al., 2004; Wright et al., 1998).

One of the benefits resulting from compiling a Semantic index is the optimization of query expansion. As we have demonstrated in the first part of this chapter, automatically compiled terminological resources may contain redundant synonyms. Since a Semantic index can be queried with concept identifiers, there is no need to expand the queries with synonyms which are never used in the indexed collection. Also, the need for query refinement is reduced, since term ambiguity is resolved at indexing time. As we have demonstrated when discussing the use of polysemy indicators, using contextual features for the resolution of named entities can improve the success rate of disambiguation techniques which rely only on static information derived from terminological resources.

One more advantage of having an index derived from a Semantic annotation is the possibility of using queries for generic entity types as opposed to querying with lists of keywords. To illustrate this capability, let us briefly consider the following query which can be submitted to the MedEvi retrieval engine (Pezik et al., 2008a):

The query specifies a UniProtKb accession number *P38398* which is resolved in the index to the *BRCA1* gene and its possible variant representation *BRCA-1*. The next query term is the generic Semantic type of diseases (indicated by the use of square brackets). The user does not have to enumerate a long list of diseases which may co-occur in the context of a number of term variants denoting the gene identified by the abstract accession number.

Figure 3. In order to create a Semantic index, all documents in a collection are processed. In addition to the positions of possibly normalized word tokens, the index also contains annotations of terms and spans of texts with the biological concept identifiers. Such an index enables retrieval with specific concept identifiers or even classes of concepts (e.g. any disease), as well as focusing retrieval with a specific criterion that can be derived from the databases linked to the concept (e.g. searching for proteins found in a given species).

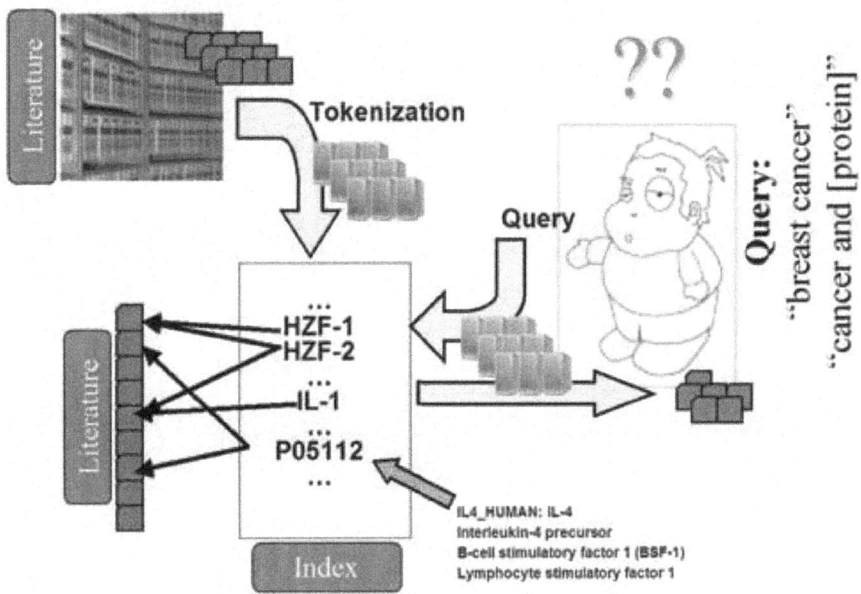

Obviously Semantic indexing comes with a few special requirements which do not have to be considered in traditional term-oriented indexes. First of all, the quality of the index and the resulting retrieval system is the function of the techniques, such as NER or relation extraction used to compile it. Secondly, the production and maintenance of the Semantic index is more problematic. The range of Semantic types to be indexed has to be defined in advance and possible changes in the external resources used to compile the index (such as biomedical ontologies or terminologies) necessitate regular updates of the index which are not triggered by the changes in the document collection itself. Finally, as demonstrated above, a special syntax has to be supported for an information retrieval engine to be able to translate user queries into the Semantic representation hard-coded in the underlying Semantic index.

SUMMARY

The present chapter has focused on the use of terminological resources for Information Retrieval in the biomedical domain. We first introduced a number of example resources which can be used to compile terminologies for biomedical IR. We explained some of the common problems with such resources including redundancy, term ambiguity, insufficient coverage of concepts and incomplete Semantic organization of such resources for text mining purposes. We also discussed some techniques used to address each of these deficiencies, such as static polysemy detection as well as adding terms and linguistic annotation from the running text.

In the second part of the chapter, we have shown that query expansion based on using synonyms of the original query terms derived from terminological resources potentially increases the recall of IR systems. Special care is needed

Figure 4. An example query for a gene concept identifier co-occurring with the Semantic type [disease]

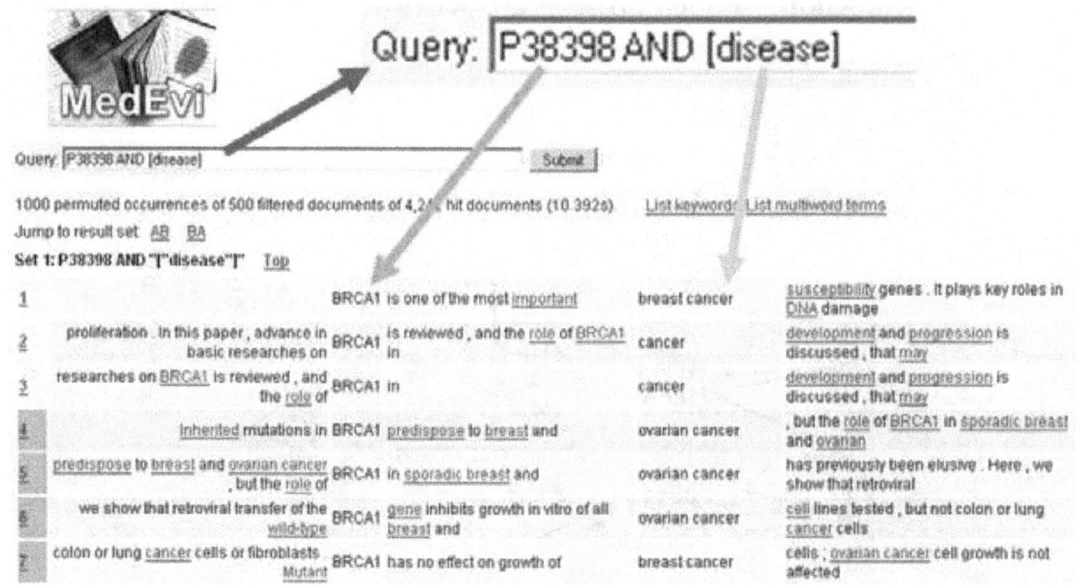

to prevent a query drift produced by the usage of the added terms and high quality word sense disambiguation algorithms can be used to allow more conservative query expansion. We explained that query refinement is used to define more precisely the intention of the user query, although it is still difficult to provide a generic approach that can automatically filter out irrelevant documents. In addition, we have presented several solutions which help focus on the user's specific information need by navigating and rearranging the initially retrieved result sets.

Finally, we explained the advantages of applying terminological and Semantic resources at a very early stage of IR – at indexing time. We argued that by creating a Semantic index with terms disambiguated for their Semantic types and larger chunks of text denoting entities and relations between them, we facilitate query expansion, reduce the need for query refinement and increase the overall performance of Information Retrieval. Semantic indexing also provides support for generic queries for concept categories, such as genes or diseases, rather than singular keywords.

REFERENCES

Aronson, A. (2001). *Effective mapping of biomedical text to the UMLS Metathesaurus: the MetaMap program.* Technical report.

Aronson, A., & Rindflesch T. (1997). Query expansion using the UMLS Metathesaurus. *In Proc. AMIA Annu. Fall Symp*, (pp. 485–489).

Blaschke, C., Leon, E., Krallinger, M., & Valencia, A. (2005). Evaluation of Biocreative assessment of task 2. *BMC Bioinformatics, 6*, S16.

McCray, A.T., Bodenreider, O., Malley J. D., & Browne (2001). Evaluating UMLS Strings for Natural Language Processing. *AC Proc AMIA Symp,* (pp. 448-52).

Buckley, C., Salton, G., Allan, J., & Singhal, A. (1994). Automatic query expansion using SMART: TREC 3. *In Text REtrieval Conference.*

Chu, W., & Liu, V. (2004). *A knowledge-based approach for scenario-specific content correlation in a medical digital library.*

Corbett P., Batchelor, C., & Teufel S. (2007). Annotation of Chemical Named Entities. *Biological, translational, and clinical language processing,* (pp. 57-64).

Couto, F., Silva, M., & Coutinho, P. (2005). Finding genomic ontology terms in text using evidence content. *BMC Bioinformatics, 6*(S1), S21.

Efthimiadis, E. (1996). Query expansion. Im M. E. Williams (Ed.), *Annual Review of Information Systems and Technologies (ARIST), v31*, 121-187.

Gaudan, S., Jimeno, A., Lee, V., & Rebholz-Schuhmann, D. (2008) Combining evidence, specificity and proximity towards the normalization of Gene Ontology terms in text. *EURASIP JBSB*, Hindawi Publishing Group.

GO-Consortium (2004). The Gene Ontology (GO) database and informatics resource. *Nucleic Acids Research, 32*(Database issue), D258–D261.

Hersh, W. R., Price, S., & Donohoe, L. (2000). Assessing thesaurus-based query expansion using the UMLS Metathesaurus. *Proceedings of the 2000 Annual AMIA Fall Symposium*, (pp. 344-348).

Hirschman, L., Yeh, A., Blaschke, C., & Valencia, A. (2005). Overview of BioCreAtIvE: critical assessment of information extraction for biology. *BMC Bioinformatics, 6*(Suppl 1), S1.

Jimeno, A., Jimenez-Ruiz, E., Lee, V., Gaudan, S., Berlanga-Llavori, R., & Rebholz-Schuhmann, D. (2008). Assessment of disease named entity recognition on a corpus of annotated sentences. *BMC Bioinformatics.*

Jimeno, A., Pezik, A., & Rebholz-Schuhmann, D. (2007). Information retrieval and information extraction in TREC Genomics 2007. *In Text REtrieval Conference.*

Joachims, T. (1997). A probabilistic analysis of the Rocchio algorithm with TFIDF for text categorization. In D. H. Fisher, (Ed.), *Proceedings of ICML-97, 14th International Conference on Machine Learning*, (pp. 143-151), Nashville, US, 1997. Morgan Kaufmann Publishers, San Francisco, US.

Kekäläinen, J., & Järvelin, K. (1998). The impact of query structure and query expansion on retrieval performance. *In Proceedings of the 21st annual international ACM SIGIR conference on Research and development in information retrieval*, (pp. 130-137). ACM Press.

Kolárik, C., Hofmann-Apitius, M., Zimmermann, M., & Fluck, J. (2007). Identification of new drug classification terms in textual resources. *Bioinformatics, 23*(13), i264-72.

Liu, H., Hu, Z., Zhang, J., & Wu, C. (2006). BioThesaurus: a Web-based thesaurus of protein and gene names. *Bioinformatics, 22*(1), 103-105.

Liu, Z., & Chu, W. (2005). Knowledge-based query expansion to support scenario-specific retrieval of medical free text. *In SAC '05: Proceedings of the 2005 ACM symposium on Applied computing*, (pp. 1076-1083), New York, NY, USA: ACM Press.

Lussier, Y. A., Sarkar, I. N., & Cantor, M. (2002). An integrative model for in-silico clinical-genomics discovery science. *Proc AMIA Symp.* (pp. 469-73).

Mandala, R., Tokunaga, T., & Tanaka, H. (1998). The use of WordNet in information retrieval. In S. Harabagiu, (Ed.), *Use of WordNet in Natural Language Processing Systems: Proceedings of the Conference*, (pp. 31-37). Association for Computational Linguistics, Somerset, New Jersey.

Mitra, M., Singhal, A., & Buckley, C. (1998). Improving automatic query expansion. *In Research and Development in Information Retrieval*, (pp. 206-214).

Müller, H., Kenny, E., & Sternberg, P. (2004). Textpresso: an ontology-based information retrieval and extraction system for biological literature. *PLOS Biology, 2*(11), E309.

Pezik, P, Jimeno, A., Lee, V., & Rebholz-Schuhmann, D. (2008b). *Static Dictionary Features for Term Polysemy Identification submitted to Workshop Proceedings of 5th International Conference on Language Resources and Evaluation (LREC 2008).*

Pezik, P., Kim, J., & Rebholz-Schuhmann, D. (2008a). MedEvi – a permuted concordancer for the biomedical domain. *In Proceedings of PALC 2008 Conference.*

Qiu, Y., & Frei, H. (1993). Concept-based query expansion. *In Proceedings of SIGIR-93, 16th ACM International Conference on Research and Development in Information Retrieval*, (pp. 160-169), Pittsburgh, US.

Rebholz-Schuhmann, D., Kirsch, H., & Couto, F. (2005). Facts from text - is text mining ready to deliver? *PLoS Biology, 3*(2), e65.

Rebholz-Schuhmann, D., Kirsch, H., & Nenadic, G. (2006). IeXML: towards a framework for interoperability of text processing modules to improve annotation of Semantic types in biomedical text. *Proc. of BioLINK, ISMB 2006*, Fortaleza, Brazil.

Rebholz-Schuhmann, D., Kirsch, H., Arregui, M., Gaudan, S., Rynbeek, M., & Stoehr, P. (2007). EBIMed: Text crunching to gather facts for proteins from Medline. *Bioinformatics, 23*(2), e237-44.

Rebholz-Schuhmann, D., Arregui, M., Gaudan, S., Kirsch, H., & Jimeno, A. (2008). Text processing through Web services: Calling Whatizit. *Bioinformatics 2008* (to appear).

Ruch, P., Jimeno, A., Gobeill, J., Tbarhriti, I., & Ehrler, F. (2006). Report on the TREC 2006 Experiment: Genomics Track. *TREC 2006.*

Ruch, P. (2004). Query Translation by Text Categorization. *COLING 2004.*

Ruch, P. (2006). Automatic assignment of biomedical categories: toward a generic approach. *Bioinformatics, 22,* 6(Mar. 2006), 658-664.

Safar, B., Kefi, H., & Reynaud, C. (2004). OntoRefiner, a user query refinement interface usable for Semantic Web Portals. *In Applications of Semantic Web technologies to Web communities, Workshop ECAI.*

Sebastiani, F. (2002) Machine learning in automated text categorization. *ACM Computing Surveys, 34*(1), 1-47.

Sehgal, A. K., & Srinivasan, P. (2006). Retrieval with Gene Queries. *BMC Bioinformatics* (Research Paper), 7, 220.

Voorhees, E. (1994). Query expansion using lexical-Semantic relations. *In Proceedings of the 17th annual international ACM SIGIR conference on Research and development in information retrieval,* (pp. 61-69). Springer-Verlag New York, Inc.

Wattarujeekrit, T., Shah, P., & Collier, N. (2004). PASBio: predicate-argument structures for event extraction in molecular biology. In *http://www.biomedcentral.com/bmcbioinformatics/, 5,* 155.

William, H., & Greenes, R. (1990). SAPHIRE-an information retrieval system featuring concept matching, automatic indexing, probabilistic retrieval, and hierarchical relationships. *Comput. Biomed. Res, 0010-4809, 23*(5), 410-425. I Academic Press Professional, Inc

Wright, L., Grossetta, H., Aronson, A., & Rindflesch, T. (1998). Hierarchical concept indexing of full-text documents in the UMLS information sources map. *Journal of the American Society for Information Science, 50*(6), 514-23.

Xu, J., & Croft, W. (1996). Query expansion using local and global document analysis. *In Proceedings of the Nineteenth Annual International ACM SIGIR Conference on Research and Development in Information Retrieval,* (pp. 4-11).

ENDNOTES

[a] http://www.nlm.nih.gov/pubs/factsheets/umls.html
[b] http://130.14.29.110/Taxonomy/
[c] http://medlineplus.gov/
[d] http://biomint.pharmadm.com/protop/bin/bmstaticpage.pl?userType=guest&p=gpsdb
[e] http://redpoll.pharmacy.ualberta.ca/drugbank/
[f] http://www.ebi.ac.uk/chebi/
[g] http://pubchem.ncbi.nlm.nih.gov/
[h] www.ncbi.nlm.nih.gov/projects/LocusLink/
[i] www.ebi.ac.uk/embl/
[j] www.ncbi.nlm.nih.gov/Genbank/
[k] http://lexsrv3.nlm.nih.gov/SPECIALIST/index.html
[l] The taxonomic distance is shown in the last column of the table (Tax distance) as the number of nodes from both sides between the two accession numbers and the nearest common parent node.
[m] http://www.bootstrep.org/
[n] http://ir.ohsu.edu/genomics
[o] http://vivisimo.com/
[p] http://www.gopubmed.org/

Chapter V
Automatic Alignment of Medical Terminologies with General Dictionaries for an Efficient Information Retrieval

Laura Dioşan
Institut National des Sciences Appliquées, France & Babeş-Bolyai University, Romania

Alexandrina Rogozan
Institut National des Sciences Appliquées, France

Jean-Pierre Pécuchet
Institut National des Sciences Appliquées, France

ABSTRACT

The automatic alignment between a specialized terminology used by librarians in order to index concepts and a general vocabulary employed by a neophyte user in order to retrieve medical information will certainly improve the performances of the search process, this being one of the purposes of the ANR VODEL project. The authors propose an original automatic alignment of definitions taken from different dictionaries that could be associated to the same concept although they may have different labels. The definitions are represented at different levels (lexical, semantic and syntactic), by using an original and shorter representation, which concatenates more similarities measures between definitions, instead of the classical one (as a vector of word occurrence, whose length equals the number of different words from all the dictionaries). The automatic alignment task is considered as a classification problem and three Machine Learning algorithms are utilised in order to solve it: a k Nearest Neighbour algorithm, an Evolutionary Algorithm and a Support Vector Machine algorithm. Numerical results indicate that the syntactic level of nouns seems to be the most important, determining the best performances of the SVM classifier.

INTRODUCTION

The need for terminology integration has been widely recognized in the medical world, leading to efforts to define standardized and complete terminologies. It is, however, also acknowledged in the literature that the creation of a single universal terminology for the medical domain is neither possible, nor beneficial because different tasks and viewpoints require different, often incompatible conceptual choices (Gangemi, Pisanelli & Steve, 1999). As a result, a number of communities of practice, differing in that they only commit to one of the proposed standards, have evolved. This situation demands for a weak notion of integration, also referred to as *alignment,* in order to be able to exchange information between different communities. In fact, the common points of two different terminologies have to be found in order to facilitate interoperability between computer systems that are based on these two terminologies. In this way, the gaps between general language and specialist language could be bridged.

Information retrieval systems are based on specific terminologies describing a particular domain. Only the domain experts share the knowledge encoded in those specific terminologies, but they are completely unknown to the neophytes. In fact, neophyte users formulate their queries by using naïve or general language. An information retrieval system has to be able to take into account the semantic relationships between concepts belonging to both general and specialised language, in order to answer the requests of naive users. The Information retrieval system has to map the user's query (expressed in general terms) into the specialised dictionary. The search task must be done by using both general and specialised terms and, maybe, their synonyms (or other semantic related concepts - hypernyms, hyponyms, and antonyms) from both terminologies.

The problem is how to automatically discover the connections between a specialised terminology and a general vocabulary shared by an average user for information retrieval on Internet (see Figure 1). This problem could be summarised as

Figure 1. VODEL and Information Retrieval. The elements designed by dot lines refer to the classic techniques of Information Retrieval domain, while those designed by solid lines relate to our models, developed during VODEL project.

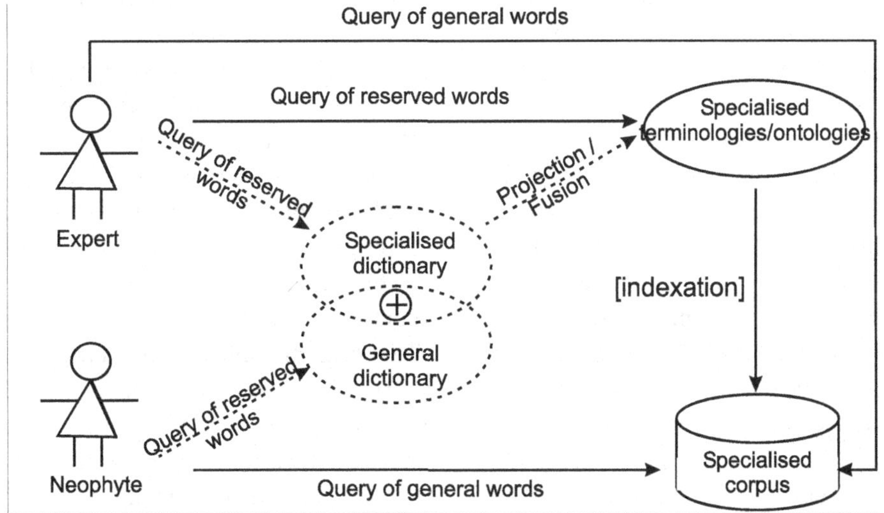

the automatic alignment of specialized terminologies and electronic dictionaries in order to take full advantage of their respective strengths.

The main objective of our work is to enrich the information retrieval system with a set of links, which allow for a better exploitation of specialised terminologies and electronic dictionaries. Several algorithms, well known in the community of Machine Learning, are utilised in order to realise an automatic alignment process. A non-expert user would therefore access documents indexed through the concepts of a professional dictionary if these notions are correlated by semantic links to a general dictionary. An important idea is to look for the terms of the non-expert query by using a specialized terminology and vice versa.

Therefore, one of the most important tasks is to achieve an automatic alignment of specialized *vs.* general terms that correspond to the same (or very similar) concepts. The main aim is to find a mapping between different formulations, but of the same meaning, in our case the sense of a concept being represented by its definition(s) from one or more dictionaries (i.e. to associate definitions from different dictionaries that correspond to the same/similar concept(s). This alignment of definitions, which is one of the goals of the French VODEL project[a] as well (Lortal et al. 2007, Dioşan et al. 2007, Dioşan et al. 2008a, Dioşan et al. 2008b), certainly needs to improve the fusion between the specialized terminology and the general vocabulary employed by a neophyte user in order to retrieve documents from Internet.

The main aim is to design a Machine Learning's algorithm that will decide whether two given definitions, expressed as text sentence(s), refer to the same concept or not. In order to perform this alignment, each definition (corresponding to a given concept and taken from a dictionary), is first turned into a bag of words (by using some NLP techniques), each word being than enriched with syntactic and semantic information.

The literature shows that a purely statistical approach on the plain text provides weak results for automatic text understanding. The text must be undergo several linguistic treatments, as the labelling at the syntactic level (POS – Parts of speech – tagging) and/or at the semantic level (extensions of terms to synonyms, hypernyms or hyponyms). Therefore, in order to achieve an efficient automatic classification ("aligned" *vs.* "not aligned" couples of definitions), the following (structural and semantic) linguistic processings have been performed: segmentation, lemmatisation and syntactic labelling.

Syntactic labelling led us to compare the automatic definition alignment performance at different syntactic levels (of nouns, adjectives, verbs or adverbs). Thus, a definition representation (based on a bag of "special" words) that is precise and meaningful is obtained. We thought it was proper to look at these levels in order to measure the contribution of each syntactic form to the performance of the alignment system. *A priori*, we do not know which are the most important: the nouns, adjectives, verbs and/or adverbs. We search to answer this question because, unlike text analysis, in the definition context, we deal with short, simple and concise phrases, where the figures of speech (metaphors, synecdoche, etc) are not present.

Each pair of "*special*" word bags corresponding to two definitions is transformed into a feature vector in a lower dimensional space by using several similarity measures. Instead of using the classical vectors of occurrences (whose lengths have to be equal the different word number from all the definitions), we propose a representation that concatenates five similarities measures and the length of the definitions. The similarity measures are generally based on the common words of two definitions, such that the word order is not taken into account in the models we propose. This original representation based on similarity measures avoids the problems associated with a classical representation TFIDF from bags of words, which involves very large sparse input vectors. The definitions are poorly represented because they can have only few common words and the semantic sensitivity is increased since definitions with a similar context, but denoted by a different term will not be associated, resulting in a "false negative match" (the proportion of positive instances – aligned definitions – that were erroneously reported as negative – not-aligned definitions). The vectors obtained are utilised as observations for a classifier trained to decide if two definitions are aligned or not (in other words if they refer to the same concept or not). The compact representation we propose allows for a fast and efficient learning of definition alignment.

The medical domain represents an area where the vocabulary of users (or the general terminology) is very different from the medical language (the specialist terminology). Thus, the need of an efficient information retrieval system is crucial. Therefore, we have chosen to represent the specialised terminology by several concepts taken from the French version of thesaurus MeSH[b] (provided by the CISMeF[c] team) and from the VIDAL dictionary[d], while the general medical vocabulary is represented by definitions from the encyclopaedia WIKIPEDIA and from the semantic network of LDI[e] provided by MEMODATA[f] - CISMeF and MEMODATA being members of VODEL project. A representative corpus has been created in order to determine the performances of our models for the automatic alignment of definitions[g].

As we have briefly mentioned, aligning two definitions actually means solving a binary classification problem. Several couples of definitions (which could be aligned or not aligned) are required, so that the classifier could learn to correctly discriminate between such relationships. In order to perform this alignment by such a classification approach, several couples of definitions from the above-mentioned dictionaries are considered. For each combination of two dictionaries, all the possible couples of definitions are considered. In this way, if a dictionary contains n definitions we will obtain n^2 couples of definitions for each combination of two dictionaries (n of them are aligned couples and $n^2 - n$ are not-aligned couples).

The alignment of terminologies is investigated by using three different models that involve well-known machine-learning approaches: a k-nearest neighbour (*kNN*) algorithm (Cover & Hart, 1967, Dasarathy, 1991), an evolutionary algorithm (EA) (Goldberg, 1989) and an SVM algorithm (Vapnik, 1995). One of them is based only on one similarity measure, while the *other* two models take into account several similarity measures simultaneously. Such multiple distance could determine a better alignment of definitions than a simple one measure done.

The alignment performances of these three models are analysed at the different syntactic levels already mentioned. Several performance measures, borrowed from the information retrieval domain, are used in order to evaluate the quality of the automatic alignments: the precision, the recall and the *F*-measure of alignments.

The chapter is structured as follows: Section II presents several text alignment models. Section III describes the problem of definition alignment, while Section IV details the characteristics of the corpora and of the linguistic treatments that have been performed. A brief theoretical review of the Machine Learning techniques involved in the alignment models we propose is given in Section V. Three original alignment models are described and analysed (through several numerical experiments) in the next section. Finally, Section VII concludes the chapter.

RELATED RESEARCH WORK

Bilingual Sentence Alignment

To our best knowledge, the problem of aligning sentences from parallel bilingual corpora has been intensively studied for automated translation. While much of the research has focused on unsupervised models (Brown, Pietra, Pietra &

Mercer, 1993, Gale & Church, 1991, Chen, 1993), a number of supervised discriminatory approaches have been recently proposed for automatic alignment (Taskar, Lacoste & Klein, 2005, Moore, 2002, Ceausu, Stefanescu & Tufis, 2006). One of the first algorithms utilised for the alignment of parallel corpora proposed by Brown (1993) and developed by Gale (1991) is solely based on the number of words/characters in each sentence. Chen (1993) has developed a simple statistical word-to-word translation model. Dynamic programming is utilised in order to search for the best alignment in these models.

Concerning the supervised methods, Taskar, Lacoste & Klein (2005) have cast the word alignment as a maximum weighted matching problem in which each pair of words in a sentence pair is associated with a score, which reflects the desirability of the alignment of that couple. The alignment for the sentence pair is then the highest scoring matching under some constraints, for example, the requirement that the matching should be one-to-one. Moore (2002) has proposed a hybrid and supervised approach that adapts and combines the sentence length-based methods with the word correspondence-based methods. Ceausu, Stefanescu & Tufis (2006) have proposed another supervised hybrid method that uses an SVM classifier in order to distinguish between aligned and non-aligned examples of sentence pairs, each pair being represented by a set of statistical characteristics (like translation equivalence, word sentence length-correlation, character sentence length-correlation, word rank-correlation, non-word sentence length – correlation).

Related to the utilisation of linguistic information, a more recent work (Moreau, Claveau & Sebillot, 2007) shows the benefits of combining multilevel linguistic representations (enriching query terms with their morphological variants). By coupling NLP and IR and by combining several levels of linguistic information through morphological (lemma, stem), syntactic (bigrams, trigrams) and semantic (terms and their morphological and/or semantic variants) analyses, the language is enriched. Moreover, data fusion has been exhaustively investigated in the literature, especially in the framework of IR (Moreau, Claveau & Sebillot, 2007, Croft, 2000). The difficulty is to find a way to combine the results of multiple searches conducted in paralel on a common data set for a given query, in order to obtain higher performances than for each individual search.

Ontology Alignment

Ontology Alignment, or ontology matching, is the process of determining correspondences between concepts of different ontologies. A set of correspondences is also called an alignment (Euzenat, 20007). For computer scientists, concepts are expressed as labels for data. Historically, the need for ontology alignment arose out of the need to integrate heterogeneous databases developed independently and thus each having their own data vocabulary. In the Semantic web context, where many actors providing their own ontologies are involved, the ontology matching plays a critical part in order to help heterogeneous resources to interoperate. Ontology alignment tools find classes of data that are "*semantically equivalent*". These tools have been generally developed in order to operate on database schemas, XML schemas, taxonomies, formal languages, entity-relationship models, dictionaries, and other label frameworks. They are usually converted into a graph representation before being matched. In this context, the ontology alignment is sometimes referred to as "*ontology matching*".

According to Shvaiko & Euzenat (2005), there are two major dimensions for similarity: the syntactic dimension and the semantic dimension. This classification refers to the manner in which matching elements are computed and the similarity relation is used.

In syntactic matching the key intuition is to map the labels (of nodes) and to look for the similarity using syntax driven techniques and syntactic similarity measures. As its name says, *in semantic matching* the main idea behind semantic matching is to map the meanings (of nodes). Thus, the similarity relation is specified in the form of a semantic relation between the extensions of concepts at the given nodes. Possible semantic relations between nodes are equality (=), overlapping (∩), mismatch (⊥) or more general/specific (⊆, ⊇).

At present, there is a line of semi-automated schema matching and ontology integration systems; see, for instance, Madhavan, Bernstein & Rahm (2001), Do & Rahm (2002), Li & Clifton (2000), Castano, Antonellis & Vimercati (2001), Arens, Hsu & Knoblock (1996), Mena, Kashyap & Sheth (2000), Doan, Madhavan, Domingos & Halevy (2002). Most of them implement syntactic matching.

The definition alignment is a different problem and quite a difficult one, too. The parallelism of corpora actually refers to the meaning of the content, which is expressed in the same language, but using different vocabularies.

PROBLEM STATEMENT

The alignment between the specialized terminology used by librarians to index concepts and a general vocabulary employed by a neophyte user in order to retrieve documents on the Internet will certainly improve the performances of the information retrieval process. Therefore, one of the most important tasks is to achieve an automatical alignment of the concepts. For this purpose, different methodologies could be considered. In our case, the meaning of a concept is represented by its definition(s) from one or more dictionaries and the terminology alignment is performed in terms of these definitions. This alignment is not a trivial task, since a concept could be represented by:

- different "*vedettes*" – the same notion can be expressed in different forms (e.g. *rhume* and *rhinite* are two terms semantically close, but graphically different). This fact excludes the alignment of concepts based only on their "*vedettes*".
- different definitions – the same concept could be explained by using different vocabularies: general and specialised.

In order to automatically perform this alignment, several definitions from four dictionaries (LDI, MeSH, VIDAL, WIKIPEDIA) have been considered. Pairs of definitions (that could define the same concept – and in this case we are dealing with two aligned definitions – or different concepts – the definitions being not aligned in this case) are formed. Thus, the alignment issue can be considered a binary classification problem: the inputs of the classifier are the pairs (of two definitions with different representations) and the outputs are the labels "*aligned*" or "*not aligned*" corresponding to each pair.

OUR CORPORA AND THE LINGUISTIC PROCESSING

The aim of the current research is to align the definitions from the electronic dictionaries in order to establish the correspondences between a specialised terminology and a general one. A representative corpus has been created from a user vocabulary and a medical one in order to allow the intermediation of the two terminologies in question. We describe the characteristics of each terminology and dictionary we have used in our experiments. These resources have been selected because all of them have an electronic version and some NLP tools (such as the Semiograph for LDI) that help us to enrich the definitions with syntactic and semantic information. In addition, the CISMeF team is one of the members of the VODEL project and it helps us to process the "raw" form of the definitions.

Dictionaries

In order to improve the search process *n* concepts and their definitions from four dictionaries have actually been utilised: the definitions from the French version of MeSH and VIDAL being considered specialised definitions, while those from LDI and WIKIPEDIA are non-specialised definitions. For each concept, four definitions are extracted, one from each dictionary. Six data sets of definition couples are formed by considering definitions from two different dictionaries: MeSH *vs.* MEMODATA, MeSH *vs.* VIDAL, MeSH *vs.* WIKIPEDIA, MEMODATA *vs.* VIDAL, MEMODATA *vs.* WIKIPEDIA, VIDAL *vs.* WIKIPEDIA. Therefore, each data set contains n^2 couples of definitions (all the possible combinations among the *n* definitions of two different dictionaries), each couple containing either two aligned definitions (referring to the same concept) or two not aligned definitions (referring to different concepts).

MeSH - The medical thesaurus MeSH[h] indexes health documents. It was proposed in 1960 by the United States National Library of Medicine - NLM. MeSH is a huge controlled vocabulary (or metadata system) which is used to index journal articles in the life sciences. Created and updated by NLM, it is used by the MEDLINE/PubMed article database and by NLM's catalog of book holdings. MeSH can be browsed and downloaded free of charge on the Internet. MeSH is the most frequently used terminology in order to index the medical articles by using a list of descriptors. The descriptors are arranged in a hierarchy that could be used to identify the context of a concept. Thus, the MeSH terminology provides a „controlled" or consistent way of retrieving information that may use different terminology for the same concept. The terms in the MeSH thesaurus are usually connected by relationships such as "is - a" or lexical relationships (synonyms), which bring together terms under a single theme. The 2005 version of MeSH contains 22,568 subject headings, also known as descriptors. Most of these are accompanied by a short definition, links to related descriptors, and a list of synonyms or very similar terms (known as entry terms). When browsing MeSH, the term being searched will be displayed within a hierarchy of broader (more general) headings above it, and narrower (more specific) headings below it.

The French keywords and qualifiers are those of MeSH bilingual directed by the Department of Scientific Information and Communication of INSERM. In addition to this, the types of resources and some meta terms are considered. Thus, CISMeF describes and indexes the most important resources of institutional health information in French (Darmoni et al., 2000).

Even if MeSH is enriched with this semantic information, no syntactic notes about the words or texts are provided. We have only selected the definitions of a concept from MeSH (and no other information) in order to facilitate the alignment with any other terminologies (structured or un-structured, enriched with other semantic information or not).

VIDAL - The VIDAL dictionary[i] is *destined* especially meant for the patients and their families. Written in clear and understandable language, the VIDAL family dictionary provides patients with reliable and detailed information on all the types of medicine available in pharmacies and other medical explanations. It also allows for better dialogue with the doctor or pharmacist. It contains 5000 types of medicine, advices, practical information for practical health, a table of generics and an on-line access.

In addition to this, the VIDAL dictionary contains a section called *Lexique médical* where different medical concepts are explained (and, certainly, indexed). This dictionary is renewed every year. On the other hand, the definitions of VIDAL explain to a non-specialist user the specialised vocabulary. This could be the main advantage (from the point of view of a neophyte user) of the VIDAL dictionary. Furthermore, this is the most important feature, which has determined us to use VIDAL in our experiments.

LDI - The semantic network LDI used by MEMODATA represents the knowledge shared by non-experts. LDI is a multilingual semantic network consisting of a heterogeneously directed graph and structured by the merger of three semantic models (Dutoit, 2003) that complement one other. LDI does not cover a specific domain, but it contains a large set of concepts used by a neophyte user in a natural language. It consists of several types of dictionaries (i.e. dictionary of synonyms, ontological dictionary, thesaurus WordNet) and approximately 1 million nodes and 3 million relations. A part of this organization records direct and oriented relationships between the meanings of two words based on the scheme of lexical functions. A second part of this organization manages several structures and indirect relationships between the word meanings. A third part of this organization manages concepts linked together by syntactic relationships, i.e. manages families of phrases.

The coverage of the French language in LDI is of about 185000 words; LDI has a greater number of relationships that WordNet. The relationships of LDI can connect word meanings, but also classes and concepts. More than 100 types of relationships have currently been defined. All these relations are typed and weighted in order to adapt the use of LDI to the task and area of application. Similarly, the comparison of two words is based on the structure of the graph and the calculation of proximity and activation on whether there are some common ancestors or not. Furthermore, LDI allows us to use a word in its general context (neighbourhood). The word and its environment can then be utilised as a conceptual beginning for the alignment of definitions.

Due to its structure, the semantic network LDI can provide semantic information about each term that it contains: synonyms, hyponyms and hypernyms. This functionality is similar to that of the MeSH thesaurus, but it is more complex because LDI is a general dictionary (for all the people and for all the domains), while MeSH only regards the medical domain. In addition to this, LDI is able to provide,, by using tools such as the Semiograph, some syntactic information about a word (for instance, its grammatical category or its derivations).

WIKIPEDIA - For the sake of completeness, we have considered a set of medical concepts with their definitions from the encyclopaedia WIKIPEDIA[J]. WIKIPEDIA is a multilingual on-line encyclopaedia highly controversial as it is written and maintained by Web users, more or less specialised in the domain described. Similarly to LDI, WIKIPEDIA contains definitions expressed in a general language, but Internet users propose these definitions (anyone can edit in the free encyclopedia WIKIPEDIA). The main criterion used for the choosing of the WIKIPEDIA dictionary instead of another general dictionary was to have definitions expressed in a general vocabulary.

A corpus of 51 concepts with 4 definitions for each concept have been created manually by several experts involved in the VODEL project. The size of the corpus is not very large; because its creation has required specialised knowledge, an automatic creation of such corpus could be extremely difficult. Still, our work is mainly focused on developing the aligner, which should be able to create a correspondence between the definitions referring to the same notion. Numerical experiments performed with the current corpus encourage us to continue our work and extending and enriching the definition data base.

These dictionaries have been selected for several reasons. Both the MeSH and the VIDAL dictionaries contain specialised medical information, being important references in the medical domain. The French version of MeSH is able to assist health professionals in their search for electronic information available on the Internet. In order to index the MeSH concepts, the „father" of its French version, CISMeF, respects the Net Scoring and the HON Code, criteria to assess the quality of health information on the Internet. VIDAL is a medical dictionary especially meant for the patients and their families. The information from VIDAL is not ranked.

The information provided by LDI and WIKIPEDIA refers to a general content, or, in other words, it addresses everyone/the general public. LDI is actually a reference dictionary containing an alphabetical list of words, with information given for each word, enriched with synonyms, analogies, rhymes and cross-words, anagrams, word derivatives (masculine and feminine forms, conjugation forms, singular and plural form). The purpose of WIKIPEDIA is to popularise various information. Like in the case of VIDAL, in both dictionaries the information is not ranked.

Linguistic Processing

French is the common language for all these dictionaries. Therefore, for each concept we have four different definitions, one from each dictionary. This provides us with six data sets, which represent pairs of definitions taken from two different dictionaries. In this way, a definition from a dictionary can be always aligned with a definition from another dictionary.

The definition corpus has been structured as an XML schema in order to facilitate the data parsing and as a consequence of the advantages of XML files (structured and easy to extend). It takes into account a higher level of each concept and its definitions (from the four dictionaries mentioned). The definition words are described by stating their form, lemma and grammatical category.

Each definition is split into phrases and the resulting phrases into words. Several types of linguistic processing are considered in order to improve the performances of the automatic alignment:

- *segmentation* – consists in cutting a sequence of characters so that various characters that form a single word can be brought together. Classic segmentation means cutting the sequences of characters depending on several separation characters such as "space", "tab" or „backspace".
- *stop-word filter* – stop words is the name given to words which are filtered out prior to, or after, the processing of natural language data (text). Hans Peter Luhn, one of the pioneers in information retrieval, is credited with coining the phrase and using the concept in his design. It is controlled by human input and not automated, which is sometimes seen as a negative approach to the natural articles of speech
- *lemmatisation* – is the process of reducing inflected (or sometimes derived) words to their stem, base or root form. The stem does not have to be identical to the morphological root of the word; it is usually sufficient that related words map the same stem, even if this stem is not a valid root in itself.
- *syntactic labelling* – is an important treatment that affixes a syntactic label, such as "noun", "adjective" or "verb" to each word. This treatment allows us to determine the empty words (such as the punctuation signs) and eliminate them, keeping only those that are considered important being meaningful.

Moreover, a set of synonyms has been extracted for each word. These pre-treatments have been performed[k] by using the Semiograph (Dutoit and Nugues, 2002, Dutoit et al., 2003), a specialised tool provided by MEMODATA. A tool can extract the contents of LDI and thus enable the analysis of a word, sentence or text. The Semiograph has two main functionalities: a syntagmatic one – used for labelling, computing the distance between words, comparing texts, resuming texts – and a paradigmatic one – used for expanding the words by their derivatives, synonyms, hypernyms and hyponyms and for lemmatisation.

The Semiograph prototype was designed to elimintate the semantic disambiguaty to compute the genericity, to index nomenclatures (e.g. as in the case of The Yellow Pages). The Semiographe manages all the LDI data: it represents thousands of pieces of information by word-meaning.

By its set of APIs that exploit the power of LDI, the Semiograph can be utilised in many applications (indexing of documents, comparing texts, routing e-mails, gaining access to nomenclatures, etc.).

The Semantic Description

In the Semiograph, most meanings linked to a specific area or a linguistic population - (be they common or rare) are incorporated into the basic dictionary. There are no restrictions on words and meanings *a priori*.

Thus, the word „*renard*" (fox) is understood *a priori* by the system as well as:

- a wild dog (*Le corbeau et le renard*),
- a leak in a hydraulic structure (*Jean a obturé le renard du barrage*) or
- a coat (*Justine a revêtu son magnifique renard*).

A 1-N relationship relating to the frequency of use (e.g. *frequent, rare*), the fields of employment (e.g. *hydrology*), where a phrase courses occurs (e.g. *Quebec*), and other pieces of similar information are used to distinguish between the current meaning of the concepts.

In the Semiograph, the semantic description is done with the help of links between lexical semantic units (word meaning) and concepts, on the one hand, and between some lexical semantic units and other lexical semantic units, on the other hand.

The first component of these semantic descriptions represents the ontological axis of the description. The second component is the linguistic acix of the description. The ontological description includes links between the lexical semantic units and concepts, and the relationships between concepts. The classification of these types of links can be done according to several points of view: the fortuity or necessary/required relationship, the meaning of ontological belonging and its utilisation of semantic features, with numerous differences such as the ontological nature of a component (a hunter is a person), its action (the hunter hunts), its field of interest (a florist sells flowers) and the description and utilization of all the syntactic links (any animal eats, reproduces or dies, a florist sells flowers), for fortuity or required knowledge. The graph contains approximately 280,000 ontological links, which reflects billions of associations that may be used by the system, since these links are between important sets of words. These ontological links are used in order to make the list of synonyms, hyponyms or hypernyms for each concept.

The Linguistic Description

The linguistic description concerns the relationships between words or expressions of the same language or the relationships (translation) between words or expressions of different languages. The linguistic description between words of the same language is designed to retain the use of the ontological axis by allowing the substitution of words between them on simple syntax criteria (paraphrases). At the simplest level, there is a variety of synonyms. For these levels, the substitutions are performed element/position by element/position, without changing the syntactic structure of the sentence. At higher levels, there are some phenomena of creating a change in the order of words in the sentence (*les negociations ont abouti* → *l'aboutissement des negociations*) or the number of words contained by a sentence (*la foret gabonaise* → *la foret du Gabon*). There are approximately 60,000 such relations in the graph.

For instance, the first part of an XML file of definitions is presented in Figure 1.

Figure 2. The XML structure of the corpus


```
<?xml version="1.0" encoding="ISO-8859-1" standalone="no" ?>
- <document>
- <vedette nom="abcès">
  - <definition type="MEMODATA">
      <texte>amas de pus formant une poche dans un tissu ou un organe.</texte>
    - <phrase num="1">
        <contenu>amas de pus formant une poche dans un tissu ou un organe.</contenu>
        <lemmePhrase>amas de pus formant un poche dans un tissu ou un organe .</lemmePhrase>
        <paraphrase />
      - <terme num="1">
          <forme>amas</forme>
          <lemme>amas</lemme>
        - <derive>
            <unDerive>amas</unDerive>
            <unDerive>amas</unDerive>
            <unDerive>amas</unDerive>
          </derive>
        - <categorieGrammaticale>
            <categorie>N</categorie>
            <type>c</type>
          </categorieGrammaticale>
```


It is very simple to observe that each definition is represented as a sequence of words. The order of the occurrence of the words in a phrase is retained (see the term *num* label) in order for the analysis that implies the word order to be carried out (for instance, by considering the bi-grams or tri-grams from a definition). In our experiments, we have not actually utilised the word order. In French, this order is not that important; the meaning of a phrase being preserved even if the (groups of) words change their order. Furthermore, several experiments with models considering the bi-grams or tri-grams from the definitions or a dynamic alignment model working with word sequences have been shown to be less efficient.

Each word of a definition is enriched with its lemma and its grammatical category (its category – noun, verb, adjective, pronoun, determinant, adverb, conjunction, interjection, etc. – and its type – e.g. *commun* (*c*), *propre* (*p*) or *cardinal* (*l*) for a noun). Lemmatisation consists in the recognition of the root of a word (the lemma or the canonical form) starting from a derived form (conjugated, feminine form, plural form). The derived form represents the result of the joining of an affix (suffix or prefix) to a root (affix derivation) or of the conversion (transformation) operation (improper derivation). Furthermore, for each word its synonyms, hyponyms and hypernyms are added. This semantic information is also extracted by using the Semiograph tool from MEMODATA too.

Levels of Definition Representation

The alignment of all these definitions could be performed at three relevant levels:

- lexical,
- semantic or
- syntactic.

A lexical analysis has to take into account each definition as a bag of word. In this case two words v and w are equal if and only if they are represented by the same strings of characters: $v = w \Leftrightarrow |v| = |w|^l \text{ and } v_i = w_i, i=1,|v|$. We have used a bag of words representation instead of a TFIDF one especially due the very high dimensionality and the sparseness of the vectors used to represent each definition. Unlike in the text analysis case (where many words are available for each example), in our case we are only dealing with several words for each definition (the number of words from a definition is much smaller than the number of words from a usual text). Moreover, the dimension of each vector is a fixed value (equal to the number of all the different words from all the definitions) that does not allow to consider new words (when new definitions are added *in* to the corpus).

On what concerns the semantic level, a bag of words representation is also used, but two words v and w are equal if and only if they have the same sense: $v = w \Leftrightarrow semantic(v) = semantic(w)$. For the semantic equality between two words (in other words, for „the same meaning") we have investigated several models:

- common synonyms (SYN) - two words have the same semantic if and only if they have at least one common synonym: $v = w \Leftrightarrow synonyms(v) \cap synonyms(w) \neq \varnothing$,
- common hyponyms (HYPO)- two words have the same semantic if and only if they have at least one common hyponym: $v = w \Leftrightarrow hyponyms(v) \cap hyponyms(w) \neq \varnothing$„
- common hypernyms (HYPE) - two words have the same semantic if and only if they have at least one common hypernym: $v = w \Leftrightarrow hypernyms(v) \cap hypernyms(w) \neq \varnothing$, and
- common synonyms and hyponym/hypernym inclusion (SHH) - two words have the same semantic if and only if one of them is found in the set of hyponyms of the other word or if they have at least one common synonym: $v = w \Leftrightarrow synonyms(v) \cap synonyms(w) \neq \varnothing$, *or* $v \subset hyponyms(w)$ *or* $w \subset hyponyms(v)$ *or* $v \subset hypernyms(w)$ *or* $w \subset hypernyms(v)$.

The syntactic analysis could be performed in three ways, namely by tacking into account only some of the syntactic form present in a definition or by weighting the importance of each syntactic form in the alignment process or by tacking into account the sequences of syntactic labels associated to each definition.

In the first case, the syntactic labelling led us to the comparison of the automatic definition alignment performance at different syntactic levels: one that retains only the nouns from each definition (the N level); one that retains only the nouns and the adjectives from each definition (the NA level); one that retains the nouns, the adjectives and the verbs from each definition (the NAV level); one that retains the nouns, the adjectives, the verbs and the adverbs from each definition (the NAVR level). The definitions have been considered at each of these syntactic levels, respectively. We have chosen to perform an analysis for each of these syntactic forms in order to measure the relative importance of each of them. This analysis could help us to achieve better alignment performances by considering only several forms or by eliminating some of them (during the alignment process).

The definitions could also be aligned by tacking into consideration the sequences of syntactic labels and by computing some dynamic distances (e.g. Levenshtein distance, Needleman-Wunsch distance, Smith-Waterman) based on these sequences. Following such an analysis it is possible to identify whether some nominal groups (nouns-adjectives-verbs or nouns-verbs-adverbs) are more relevant than others . The process is, however, difficult especially due to the concise form of a definition (a short description of a concept). Furthermore, the syntactic analysis of definitions strictly depends on the quality of the process of syntactic labelling.

Because each term of a definition has been enriched with synonyms, hyponyms and hypernyms, it could be possible to perform a semantic analysis of the definition corpus. This information has been obtained (extracted) by using the Semiograph tool (from MEMODATA) which has three important functions: *Synonymes* (that provides the synonyms and the antonyms of a word), *Spécifiques* (that provides the hyponyms of a word) and *Génériques* (that provides the hypernyms of a word). Because the Semiograph *was the only tool used* for this task and for all the dictionaries, some noise has been produced. Moreover, this semantic information has not been contextualised to the specific of the definitions (the medical domain). Further numerical experiments have been initiated in order to extract the synonyms, hyponyms and hypernyms from the same dictionary which has previously been used for the definition.

In order to perform the numerical experiments, several data sets have been constructed. Each data set contains couples of definitions taken from two dictionaries. The definitions from the dictionaries considered (MEMODATA, MeSH, VIDAL and WIKIPEDIA) have been actually organised in six datasets (C_4^2), each of them containing n^2 couples of definitions (*n* representing the number of definitions/concepts from each dictionary, in fact, 51 concepts). Each data set has been divided into a training part (2/3 of couples) and a testing part (1/3 of couples), in order to fulfil the requirements of an ML algorithm.

MACHINE-LEARNING TECHNIQUES ADAPTED TO TEXT MINING

The main goal of annotating and classifying texts is to allow efficient information retrieval and extraction. Although ontologies are quite good for representing text, the expense required in maintaining them and populating knowledge bases means that they are not usually sufficient on their own. Consequently, numerous word-based text-mining methods are being used to backup the cost and even improve the success in this area. Although pre-processing tasks are certainly important, the most useful text mining methods are the machine learning techniques. Some of these methods include the k Nearest Neighbour algorithm (*kNN*) (Cover & Hart, 1967, Dasarathy, 1991), Evolutionary algorithms (*EAs*) (Goldberg, 1989) and Support Vector Machine (*SVM*) (Vapnik, 1995).

kNN is a memory-based approach and it skips the learning phase, while *EAs* and *SVMs* are supervised model-based approaches that first build a model out of the available labelled items and than use the model to make recommendations. As a learning method *SVM* is regarded as one of the best classifiers with a strong mathematical foundation. On the other hand, evolutionary computational technique is characterized as a soft computing learning method with its roots in the theory of evolution. During the past decade, *SVM* has been commonly used as a classifier for various applications. The evolutionary computation has also attracted a lot of attention in pattern recognition and has shown significant performance improvement in a variety of applications.

k-Nearest Neighbour Classifier

In pattern recognition, the k-Nearest Neighbour algorithm (*kNN*) (Cover & Hart, 1967, Dasarathy, 1991), is a method for classifying objects based on the closest training examples in the feature space. *kNN* is a type of instance-based learning, or lazy learning where the function is only approximated locally and all computation is deferred until classification. The *kNN* algorithm is amongst the simplest of all machine-learning algorithms, while it is also remarkably fast. We have chosen to perform the alignment task by a *kNN* algorithm due to these two very useful characteristics. The main idea behind a *kNN* classifier is as follows: a majority of vote from its neighbours classifies an object, with the object being assigned to the *most common* class amongst its *k* nearest neighbours. *k* is a positive integer, typically small. If $k = 1$, then the object is simply assigned to the class of its nearest neighbour. In binary (two classes) classification problems, it is helpful to choose *k* to be an odd number as this avoids tied votes.

The training examples are vectors in a multidimensional feature space. The space is partitioned into regions by locations and labels of the training samples. A point in the space is assigned to the class *c* if it is the most frequent class label among the *k* nearest training samples. Euclidean distance is frequently used. The training phase of the algorithm consists only of storing the feature vectors and class labels of the training samples. In the actual classification phase, the test sample (whose class is not known) is represented as a vector in the feature space. Distances from the new vector to all the stored vectors are computed and *k* closest samples are selected. There are a number of ways to classify the new vector to a particular class; one of the most frequently used techniques is predicting the new vector to the most common class amongst the *k* nearest neighbours. A major drawback of using this technique in order to classify a new vector to a class is that the classes with the more frequent examples tend to dominate the prediction of the new vector, as they tend to come up in the k nearest neighbours when the neighbours are computed due to their large number. One of the ways to overcome this problem is to take into account the distance of each k nearest neighbours with the new vector that is to be classified and predict the class of the new vector based on these distances. The best choice of *k* depends upon the data; in general, larger values of k reduce the effect of noise on the classification, but make less distinct the boundaries between the classes.

In our case, an object corresponds to a definition (or to its representation as bag of "special" words at different syntactic levels). The distance between two objects (definitions) is computed by using a similarity measure. The smallest distance (or the largest similarity measure) between two definitions (from all the possible combinations) will indicate that the two definitions are aligned.

Evolutionary Algorithms

Evolutionary algorithms (*EAs*) form a subset of evolutionary computation, a generic population-based meta-heuristic optimization algorithm (Holland, 1975, Goldberg, 1989). An *EA* uses some mechanisms inspired by biological evolution: reproduction, mutation, recombination, and selection. Candidate solutions to the optimization problem play the part of individuals in a population, and the cost function determines the environment within which the solutions "live" (= the fitness function). The evolution of the population takes place after the repeated application of the above-mentioned operators. Evolutionary algorithms consistently perform well approximating solutions to all the types of optimisation problems because they do not make any assumption about the underlying fitness landscape; this generality is shown by the successes in various fields, as diverse as engineering, art, biology, economics, genetics, social sciences, or linguistics.

Evolutionary algorithms actually evolve a set of candidate solutions (individuals, chromosomes). The passage from one generation of individuals to another is performed by means of the genetically-inspired operators.

The selection operator chooses from the current population, the individuals which will act as parents for the next generation. Selection has to provide high reproductive chances to the fittest individuals but, at the same time, it has to preserve the exploration of the search space. The choice of the proper individuals for reproducing determines the choice of the regions in the search space to be visited next. Indeed, achieving equilibrium between the exploration and the exploitation of the search space is very important for the search process. The individuals selected will be the subject of recombination and mutation. Recombination (or crossover) creates new individuals by combining the genetic information of the parents. The way recombination between individuals takes place depends on their representation. Mutation is another genetic operator that acts different from a codification of the chromosomes to another codification. Mutation creates new individuals by small and stochastic perturbations of a single individual. The algorithm ends after a certain number of generations or when the solution is found (in the case when it is known). The best solution obtained in the last generation or in the whole search process is considered the solution of the given problem.

We have already seen that in order to align a set of definitions it is possible to compute the distances between a definition def_i and another definition def_j, $i \neq j$; if this distance is less than or equal to a threshold, then the definitions are aligned. This distance could be a simple similarity *measure* or a more generic distance that combines in a linear manner (by weighting) more similarity measures. The key problem is how to select, or even better, how to adapt these weights in order to obtain the best performance of a combined linear distance. The *EAs* could evolve these weights and the fitness of a chromosome could be estimated by the proportion of the correctly aligned definitions (by using the resulted combined measure).

Support Vector Machines

Support Vector Machines (*SVMs*) are a set of related supervised learning methods used for classification and regression. They belong to a family of generalized linear classifiers[m]. A special property of *SVMs* is that they simultaneously minimize the empirical classification error and maximize the geometric margin; hence, they are also known as maximum margin classifiers.

Basic Principles of SVMs

The *SVM* algorithm has initially been proposed in order to solve binary classification problems (Vapnik, 1995). These algorithms have later been generalized for multi-classes problems. Consequently, we will explain the theory behind *SVM* only on binary-labelled data. Suppose the training data has the following form: $D = (x_i, y_i)_{i=1,m}$, where $x_i \subset R^d$ represents input vectors (predictor variables) and each y_i, $y_i \subset \{-1, 1\}$, the output labels associated to the item x_i. A learning algorithm has to be able to generalize some unseen data points. In the case of a binary classification problem, given some new input $x \subset R_d$, we want to predict the corresponding label $y \subset \{-1, +1\}$. In other words, we want to choose y such that (x,y) is in some sense similar to the training examples.

The *SVM* algorithm tries to separate the two classes of points using a linear function of the form $f(x) = w^T x + b$, with $w \subset R^d$ and $b \in R$. Such a function assigns a label $+1$ to the points x with $f(x) \geq 0$, and a label -1 to the points x with $f(x) < 0$. The problem is therefore to learn such a function f from a data set of observations D. For a candidate function $f(x) = w^T x + b$, one can check for each observation (x_i, y_i) whether it is correctly classified by f, that is, whether $y_i f(x_i) \geq 0$ or not. A natural criterion to choose f might be to minimize the number of classification errors on D; the number of indices $i \in \{1, 2, ..., n\}$ so that $y_i f(x_i) \geq 0$. This general principle is called empirical risk minimization.

The *SVM* algorithm maps the input vectors to a higher dimensional space where a maximal separating hyper-plane is constructed (Vapnik, 1998). Learning the SVM implies to minimize the norm of the weight vector (w in Eq. (1)) under the constraint that the training items of different classes belong to opposite sides of the separating hyper-plane. Since $y_i \in \{-1, +1\}$ we can formulate this constraint as:

$$y_i (< w, x_i > + b) \geq 1, i = 1, 2, \ldots, m. \quad (1)$$

The items that satisfy Eq. (\ref{optim1}) with equality are called support vectors since they define the resulting maximum-margin hyper-planes. To account for the misclassification, e.g. items that do not satisfy Eq. (1), the soft margin formulation of *SVM* has introduced some slack variables $\xi_i \in R$ (Cristianini & Taylor, 2000).

Moreover, the separation surface has to be nonlinear in many classification problems. SVM can be extended to handle nonlinear separation surfaces by using a feature function $\varnothing(x)$. The SVM extension to nonlinear datasets is based on the mapping of the input variables into a feature space *F* of a higher dimension and then performing a linear classification in that higher dimensional space. The important property of this new space is that the data set mapped by $\varnothing$ might be linearly separable in it if an appropriate feature function is used, even when that data set is not linearly separable in the original space. Hence, in order to construct a maximal margin classifier, one has to solve the convex quadratic programming problem encoded by Eq. (2), which is its primal formulation *of it*:

$$\text{minimise}_{w,b,\xi}\ \tfrac{1}{2} w^T w + C\textstyle\sum_i \xi i$$
$$\text{subject to: } y_i(w^T\varnothing(x_i) + b) \geq 1 - \xi_{i,}\ \xi_i\varnothing \geq 0 \quad (2)$$

The coefficient *C* is a tuning parameter that controls the *trade off* between maximizing the margin and classifying without error. The primal decision variables *w* and *b* define the separating hyper plane.

Instead of solving Eq. (2) directly, it is a common practice to solve its dual problem described in Eq. (3):

$$\text{maximise } a\in R^m \textstyle\sum_i a_i - 1/2\sum_{i,j} a_i a_j\, y_i\, y_j\, \varnothing(x_i)\varnothing(x_j)$$
$$\text{subject to: } \textstyle\sum_i a_i y_i = 0,\ 0 \leq a_i \leq C \quad (3)$$

In Eq. (3), a_i denotes the Lagrange variable for the ith constraint of Eq. (2).

The optimal separating hyper plane $f(x) = w\varnothing(x)+b$, where *w* and *b* are determined by Eqs. (2) or (3) could be used to classify the un-labelled input data:

$$y_k = \text{sign}(\textstyle\sum_{x_i\in S} a_i\, \varnothing(x_i)\, \varnothing(x_k) + b) \quad (4)$$

where *S* represents the set on support vector items x_i. We will see in the next section that is more convenient to use a kernel function $K(x,z)$ instead of the dot product $\varnothing(x)\ \varnothing(z)$.

Kernel Formalism

The original optimal hyper-plane algorithm proposed by Vapnik in 1963 was a linear classifier (Vapnik, 1995). However, in 1992, Boser, Guyon and Vapnik (1992) have suggested a way to create non-linear classifiers by applying the kernel trick (originally proposed by Aizerman et al. (1964)) to maximum-margin hyper planes. Kernel methods work by mapping the data items into a high-dimensional vector space *F* called feature space where the separating hyper-plane has to be found. This mapping is implicitly defined by specifying an inner product for the feature space via a positive semi-definite kernel function: $K(x, z)=\varnothing(x)\varnothing(z)$, where $\varnothing(x)$ and $\varnothing(z)$ are the transformed data items *x* and *z*.

Note that all we have required are the results of such an inner product. Therefore we do not even need to have an explicit representation of the mapping $\varnothing$, or to know the nature of the feature space. The only requirement is to be able to evaluate the kernel function on all the pairs of data items, which is much easier than computing the coordinates of those items in the feature space. Evaluating the kernel yields a symmetric, positive semi definite matrix known as the kernel or Gram matrix (Cortes & Vapnik, 1995). In order to obtain an SVM classifier with kernels one has to solve the following optimization problem:

$$\text{maximise } a \in R^m \textstyle\sum_i a_i - 1/2\sum_{i,j} a_i\, a_j\, y_i\, y_j\, K(x_i, x_j)$$
$$\text{subject to: } \textstyle\sum_i a_i y_i = 0,\ 0 \leq a_i \leq C \quad (5)$$

In this case, Eq. (4) becomes:

$$y_k = \text{sign}(\textstyle\sum_{xi\in S} a_i\, K(x_i, x_k) + b) \quad (6)$$

One of the well-known and efficient kernel functions is the RBF kernel: $K(x_i, x) = \sigma |x_i - x_j|^2$.

Parameter Setting

In order to use a basic *SVM* for binary classification, two kinds of parameters have to be determined: the regularization parameter *C* of the SVM and the kernel and its parameters. A proper choice of these parameters is crucial for a good performance of the algorithm. A temptation to be avoided is to set the parameters based on the performance of the *SVM* on the training set, because this is likely to lead to over fitting: the performance increases on the training set used, but decreases on new samples. A standard way to fix parameters is to use cross-validation.

Regarding our problem of definition alignment, the single elements that must be provided to *SVM* algorithm are the inputs and the outputs of the classification problem. Therefore, we form couples (of two) definitions that can be labelled as aligned and not-aligned. All the five similarity measures and the length of each definition represent each couple. A kernel function will map these inputs in a higher dimensional space where the decision „aligned" or „not aligned" takes place easier than in the initial space. In fact, the definition alignment is considered as a binary classification problem.

THE PROPOSED ALIGNMENT MODELS

Performance Measures

Several performance measures, borrowed from the information retrieval domain, can be used in order to evaluate the quality of automatic alignments: the *precision of alignments* - the percent of relevant alignments among the proposed alignments; the *recall of alignments* - the percent of relevant alignments that are effectively retrieved and *F-measure* - the weighted harmonic mean of precision and recall. Grater F-measure (the maximal value being 1) signifies a correct and complete alignment.

These measures reflect the classification performance of the classification algorithm in a confidence interval. The confidence intervals associated to the performances of some systems must be computed in order to decide if a system outperforms another. If these intervals are disjoint, then one system outperforms the other one. A confidence interval of 95% is used in order to perform a statistical examination of the results. Therefore, the probability that the accuracy estimations are not in the confidence interval is 5% (see Equation (7)).

$$\Delta I = 1.96 \sqrt{(Acc(100 - Acc)/N)}\% \qquad (7)$$

Similarity Measures

Several or all of the following measures of similarity could be involved in our alignment models: *Matching* coefficient (Cormen, 1990), *Dice* coefficient (Dice, 1945), *Jaccard* coefficient (Jaccard, 1912), *Overlap* coefficient (Clemons, 2000) and *Cosine* measure (Salton, 1989}.

These statistics are generally used in order to compute the similarity and diversity of two sample sets, but they can be adapted to our definition couples and to their representation. In order to compute a similarity measure between two definitions, each of them is tokenized (segmented), lemmatised and syntactically labelled. In this way, a bag of labelled lemmas is obtained for each definition. Then, the similarity measure of two definitions is computed based on the elements of the corresponding bags. The considered definitions can be taken from the same dictionary or from different dictionaries (a general one and a specialised one). Based on the similarity measures obtained, the classifier will automatically decide if the two definitions are aligned or not.

In order to align the definitions by using these measures we have several possibilities:

1. to select (choose) one of these similarity measures: in fact the measure that works best;
2. to select (choose) some of them: in fact, to choose those that improve the alignment process;
3. to eliminate the similarity measures that do not "help" the target (objective) task;
4. to consider all the measures, since they could improve the classification performances due to their complementarity.

By working only with a representation based on these measures, instead of a classical one, the model we propose is able to map the initial vectors (based on a bag of word approach) into a space of reduce dimension. Thus, the computational effort is reduced and, at the same time, it does not allow for the loss of relevant information.

Therefore, in order to align the corpus of definitions three approaches are investigated:

- one based on a kNN classifier, taking into account only a similarity measure,
- one based on an evolutionary classifier, taking into account all the five similarity measures *simultaneously*
- one based on an SVM algorithm, taking into account all the five similarity measures and the length of each definition simultaneously.

The kNN-Based Alignment Model

The first investigated model (Lortal et al. 2007) considers each of the similarity measures in a separate frame. For instance, the *Matching* coefficient is computed for all the definition couples (which are taken from two different dictionaries). The largest similarity between two definitions indicates that the definitions are aligned (actually, the definitions represent the same concept).

For instance, we can consider three definitions: two for the concept *abcès* from two different dictionaries (MEMODATA and MeSH) and one for the concept *acne* from the MEMODATA dictionary.

Def_1: *amas de pus formant une poche dans un tissu ou un organe* (MEMODATA defintion for *abcès)*

Def_2: *Amas de pus formant une poche* (VIDAL defintion for *abcès)*

Def_3: *lésion de la peau au niveau des follicules pilo-sébacés.* (MEMODATA definiton for *acné*).

The couple *(Def_1, Def_2)* represents a couple of correctly aligned definitions (true positive), while the couples *(Def_1, Def_3)*, *(Def_2, Def_3)* correspond to not-aligned definitions (true negative).

The current model will be denoted in what follows as the *kNN*-based one similarity model (shortly, *kNN-S1* model). The *kNN-S1*model is actually based on the k-nearest neighbour algorithm (*kNN*) which is a method for classifying objects based on the closest training examples in the feature space.

In our case, *k=1*, which means that a definition is aligned to its nearest neighbour definition. The neighbours of a definition from the first dictionary are taken from the set of the definitions from the second dictionary. This can be thought of as the training set for the algorithm, though no explicit training step is required. Instead of using the Euclidean or Manhattan distance (like in the classic *kNN* algorithm), our alignment algorithm uses a similarity measure in order to compare two definitions.

Several numerical experiments are performed by using the kNN-S1 model for six different combinations of dictionaries: MEMODATA *vs.* MeSH, MEMODATA *vs.* VIDAL, MEMODATA *vs.* WIKIPEDIA, MeSH *vs.* VIDAL, MeSH *vs.* WIKIPEDIA and VIDAL *vs.* WIKIPEDIA, and to different levels:

- the lexical level - all the words in a definition are taken into account (ALL level);
- the semantic level - all the words in a definition are taken into account, with the difference that for each additional word additional semantic information are considered:
    - synonym - SYN level,
    - hyponyms - HYPO level,
    - hypernyms - HYPER level,
    - synonyms, hyponyms and hypernyms ➢ SHH level); and
- the syntactic level - only the nouns (N level), the nouns and the adjectives (NA level) or the nouns, the adjectives and the verbs (NAV level) are considered from each definition.

We present the results obtained only for these syntactic levels because the nominal groups N, NA and NAV are well known in computational linguistic. Moreover, because we deal with concise phrases for which a representation only based on adjectives or verbs could not determine a good alignment (several numerical experiments, using only this information have reached this conclusion). Note that for each level only the best similarity measure is retained and the F-measure (Rijsbergen, 1979), which combines the recall and precision of the alignment is computed. (see Table 1). This statistical performance measure is only computed for alignment examples (the definition couples referring the same concept) because the purpose in to create a parallelism between the explanations for the same notion. The results obtained by the kNN-based model are not so good because the aligner always tries to align a definition with another one. In addition, Table 1

Table 1. F measures of the aligned couples and their confidence intervals of kNN-S1 alignment model

Representation level	*MEMODATA vs. MeSH*	*MEMODATA vs. VIDAL*	*MEMODATA vs. WIKIPEDIA*	*MeSH vs. VIDAL*	*MeSH vs. WIKIPEDIA*	*VIDAL vs. WIKIPEDIA*
ALL	Matching	Cosine	Matching	Cosine	Matching	Matching
	40.38±13.34	40.38±13.34	48.08±13.58	36.54±13.09	38.46±13.22	40.38±13.34
SYN	Dice	Overlap	Overlap	Matching	Overlap	Overlap
	26.92±12.06	34.62±12.93	36.54±13.09	21.15±11.1	26.92±12.06	32.69±12.75
HYPO	Jaccard	Overlap	Matching	Jaccard	Dice	Jaccard
	23.08±11.45	28.85±12.31	30.77±12.54	15.38±9.81	19.23±10.71	19.23±10.71
HYPER	Overlap	Overlap	Overlap	Overlap	Overlap	Dice
	23.08±11.45	36.54±13.09	36.54±13.09	21.15±11.1	25.00±11.77	25.00±11.77
SHH	Dice	Overlap	Overlap	Matching	Overlap	Overlap
	25.00±11.77	36.54±13.09	34.62±12.93	19.23±10.71	25.00±11.77	26.92±12.06
N	Matching	Overlap	Cosine	Cosine	Cosine	Overlap
	40.00±13.34	48.00±13.58	50.00±13.59	46.00±13.55	52.00±13.58	63.00±13.12
NA	Matching	Overlap	Cosine	Cosine	Cosine	Overlap
	44.00±13.49	54.00±13.55	50.00±13.59	48.00±13.58	54.00±13.55	56.00±13.49
NAV	Matching	Overlap	Cosine	Cosine	Cosine	Matching
	44.00±13.49	52.00±13.58	52.00±13.58	46.00±13.55	42.00±13.42	48.00±13.58

displays the corresponding confidence intervals (estimated by using Eq. (7)).

Taking into account the dictionary combinations, the best performance[n] is obtained for the couples of definitions considered from the VIDAL and the WIKIPEDIA dictionaries.

By taking into account the representation level, the results indicate that the alignment to the syntactic level leads to the best performances. Furthermore, by introducing semantic information, the alignment performances are noised: each semantic level considered determines a degradation of the alignment performance of the lexical level. The Semiograph tool that does not extract "contextual" semantic information could induce this noise; for instance *amas* is synonym with *accumulation*, but also with *armes*.

If we compare the results obtained at the lexical level with those obtained by considering the definitions at a syntactic level, the latter ones are better, the best being obtained at the NA level. This fact could indicate that the nouns and adjectives contain the most important information in a definition. This is different from a text-processing task, because in our case we are only dealing with short and very concise phrases. Moreover, the adverbs or prepositional groups seem to be irrelevant to our task, since the performances obtained at NA level are better than those obtained at ALL level (where all the nouns, the adjectives, the verbs, the adverbs or the prepositional phrases are taken into account).

We can see that the adjectives bring more performance to the alignment model, since several improvements can be observed for the NA based model as compared to the N model. In addition to this, the verbs don't seem to to enrich the aligner with useful information. Therefore, the nouns and the adjectives seem to be the most important syntactic categories that have to be taken into account.

Regarding the similarity measures used in order to align two definitions, the best results are obtained in general by computing the Cosine and Overlap coefficients. These results prove that it is impossible to select only one similarity measure which performs best for any dictionary combination or for any lexical level and encourage the idea that the similarity measures could be complementary and their combination could improve the performance of an alignment system.

As a general conclusion, the best results are obtained for the VIDAL *vs.* WIKIPEDIA combination at the level of nouns by using the Overlap measure of similarity. However, even in this case, the F-measure reaches only 63% (which is below the expected performances). VIDAL and WIKIPEDIA are created for general users, so they share the same register. Furthermore, the purpose of both dictionaries could be associated to that of information dissemination or popularisation. This fact could explain, at least partially, the reason why the best alignment is obtained for the VIDAL - WIKIPEDIA combination.

However, the alignments provided by the kNN-S1 model are "biased" because the model considers that one definition must be aligned with one and only one second definition This model can be improved by determining an adaptive threshold (k) in order to align a definition not only with the closest definition, but also with a set of definitions. In this case it is possible to align a definition from a dictionary with any definition, with one definition or with several definitions from other dictionaries. In other words, the k-NN algorithm will use a dynamic strategy for the value of k: given a definition D, its definition neighbours DN_i will be those for which the similarity measure $SM(D, DN_i)$ is greater than the given threshold.

The Evolutionary Alignment Model

The performances achieved by each of the *kNN-S1* model have indicated that we cannot find a similarity measure that provides the best alignments for all the dictionary combinations. Therefore, we propose two new supervised models for the automatic alignment of definitions that take into account the complementarities between these similarity measures. This time all the five similarity measures are simultaneously considered, either in a linear combination or in a non-linear one. The new models are based on two well-known supervised machine-learning techniques: Evolutionary Algorithms and Support Vector Machines.

As regards the linear combination of the similarity measures, this could be a linear one, like that described in Eq. (8).

$$LCM = \sum \mu_q M_q, \text{ where } q = 1, NoSM \qquad (8)$$

where each M_q is a similarity measure, μ_q is its weight in the final combination ($\mu_q \in [0,1]$ and $\sum \mu_q = 1$) and *NoSM* is the number of individual similarity measures involved in the combination (in fact, 5 similarity measures are used). The weighting coefficients w_t could reflect the relative importance of an individual similarity measure in the linear combination. This linear combination of more similarity coefficients is able to provide a better classification of definition couples because the combined measure could be better adapted to the characteristics of the definition sets than a simple similarity measure.

In order to identify the optimal values of the weights w_t and to adapt them to the current definition alignment problem, an evolutionary approach, denoted *Ev-S5* (Lortal et al., 2007), is used. A Genetic Algorithm (GA) (Goldberg, 1989) evolves the weights of the linear combination. Each GA chromosome is a fixed length array of genes. The number of genes is equal to the number of individual measures involved in the combination. Each gene g_t is initialised with a real number in the *[0,1]* range. Because each gene must correspond to a weight, the following transformation has to be performed: $\mu_q = g_q / \sum g_q$, *where* $q \in \{1,2,..., NoSM\}$.

The quality of an evolved combined measure, which is encoded in the current GA chromosome, can be measured by the classification accuracy rate estimated by using this evolved distance. If the combined measure of a definition couple is less than or equal to a threshold, then the current couple is classified as aligned and otherwise (if the combined measure is greater than the threshold), the definitions are considered to be not aligned. The accuracy rate represents the number of correctly classified examples over the total number of examples (an example being represented by a couple of definitions). The quality is approximated on the validation set which is disjoint with the test set. In fact the best combination is searched for by using the training set and then it is validated on the test set.

The architecture of *Ev-S5* model is depicted in Figure 2.

We investigate the performance of the *Ev-S5* model for the definition alignment problem. All the five similarity measures computed for each definition couple are involved in the Linear Combined Similarity Measure. The steady-state evolutionary model (Syswerda, 1989) is involved as an underlying mechanism for the GA implementation: the new individual O^* (obtained after mutation) replaces the worst individual W in the current population if O^* is better than W. A population of 50 individuals is evolved during 50 generations. In order to obtain a new generation, binary tournament selection, convex crossover and Gaussian mutation are performed. The values for crossover and mutation probabilities ($p_c = 0.8$ and $p_m = 0.05$) were chosen so that a good diversity of the population and a stochastic search in the solution space could be ensured. The crossover and mutation operators are specific for real encoding and the values used for the population size and for the number of generation were empirically chosen based on the best results obtained during several tests performed with different values for these parameters.

The performances of the current model are not satisfactory (less acceptable), proving that a more complex combination of the similarity measures has to be considered in order to obtain a good alignment.

The syntactic levels of N, NA and NAV, respectively, are investigated for all the combinations of the MEMODATA dictionary with another dictionary (MEMODATA *vs.* MeSH, MEMODATA *vs.* *VIDAL*, MEMODATA *vs.* WIKIPEDIA)°. The numerical results are presented in Table 2.

By using this evolutionary approach in order to align the definitions from different dictionaries, the best results (43%) are obtained for the MEMODATA *vs.* MeSH combination at the syntactic level of nouns. We can observe that the results are worse than those obtained only with one similarity measure. A cause of this degradation could be the value of the threshold that influences the quality of the proposed model. Furthermore, the set of definition couples contains many not-aligned examples and only a few aligned ones. This distribution of examples could determine a good accuracy of the overall classification process; the precision of not-aligned examples is very large, while the precision corresponding to aligned examples is very poor. The linear form of the combined measure could also explain this degradation. It is possible to improve the performance of the aligner by using a non-linear form of the combined measure. We will see in the next section the manner in which a non-linear combination of the similarity measures improves the performance of the alignment model.

The SVM-Based Alignment Model

In order to learn a non-linear combination of similarity measures, we propose to also use a kernel-based SVM classifier, as well, because it is able to decide whether two definitions are to be considered as aligned or not aligned. In fact, the input of the SVM is a compact representation of two definitions, i.e. the concatenation of all the similarity measures considered to which we add the length of each definition. All this information will be used by the kernel function (actually an RBF kernel) of the *SVM* algorithm (Vapnik, 1995, Vapnik, 1998) in order to distinguish between aligned and non-aligned couples of definitions. Unlike the *kNN-S1* model and similarly to the *Ev-S5* model, the inputs of the SVM classifier are represented by all the five elements of the previous representation (all five-similarity measures which correspond to a couple of two definitions).

Figure 3. The architecture of Ev-S5 model

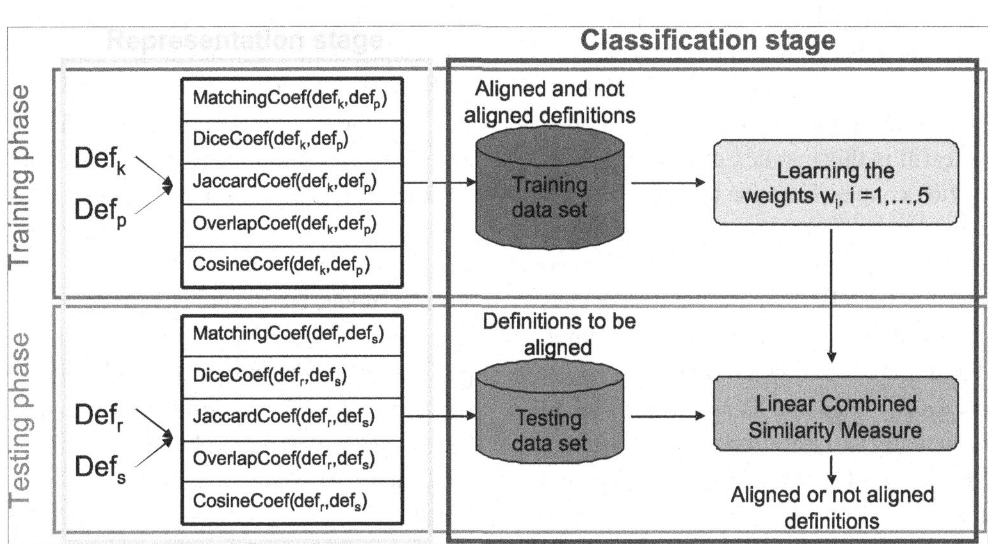

Table 2. F-measures corresponding to aligned couples and their confidence intervals of Ev-S5 alignment model

Representation level	*MEMODATA vs. MeSH*	*MEMODATA vs. VIDAL*	*MEMODATA vs. WIKIPEDIA*	*MeSH vs. VIDAL*	*MeSH vs. WIKIPEDIA*	*VIDAL vs. WIKIPEDIA*
N	43.32±3.98	42.34±3.97	36.23±3.86	38.01±3.90	32.39±3.76	31.44±3.73
NA	27.77±3.60	30.52±3.70	23.05±3.38	24.76±3.47	18.86±3.14	20.60±3.25
NAV	27.53±3.59	29.60±3.67	22.95±3.38	24.06±3.43	18.79±3.14	19.81±3.20

In addition to this, the length of each definition is taken into account by the non-linear measure[p]. Therefore, vectors of seven elements will represent the inputs and the resulted alignment approach will be denoted as the *SVM-S7* model. The output is represented by the class or label (aligned or not aligned) to be associated to each couple.

The classification process takes place in two phases that reflect the principles of the SVM algorithm: a training phase - the SVM model is learnt starting from the labelled examples and the hyper parameters are optimised - and a test phase - the unseen definition couples are labelled as aligned or not aligned. Therefore, each data set[q] has been divided into two parts: one for training and another one for testing. The training part has divided again into a learning sub-set – used by the SVM algorithm in order to find the hyper plane that makes the class separation – and a validation set – used in order to optimise the values of the hyper parameters C and σ. The SVM model, which is learnt in this manner, classifies (labels) the definition couples from the test set.

The parameter C of the SVM algorithm, representing the penalty error of the classification, as well as the RBF kernel parameter (σ) has been optimized by using the parallel grid search method and a cross-validation approach. Thus, we automatically adapt the SVM classifier to the problem, actually to the alignment of definitions. The architecture of *SVM-S7* model is depicted in Figure 3.

Several numerical experiments are performed for six different combinations of dictionaries and for the following syntactic levels: N, NA, NAV, NAVR with the supervised *SVM-S7* model – see Table 3.

The C-SVM algorithm, provided by LIBSVM[r], with an RBF kernel is used in the experiments. The optimisation of the hyper parameters is performed by a parallel grid search method in the following ranges: the tuning coefficient C is optimised in the $[2^{-10}, 2^{10}]$ range; the bandwidth σ of the RBF kernel is optimised in the interval $[2^{-4}, 2^{1}]$; a 10-fold cross validation is performed during the training phase.

The results on the test set disjoint from the training set show that the F-measure has reached 88%, thus demonstrating the relevance of the SVM-S7 approach. Moreover, these results are interesting since we do not have the bias from the *kNN-S1* model. Indeed, by using the SVM-model it is possible to align a definition from a dictionary with any definitions from another dictionary (either with one definition from another dictionary or with several definitions from other dictionaries, respectively).

The model based on learning from nominal groups NA (Nouns-Adjectives) leads to the best performances. The numerical results indicate that the verbs reduce the performance of the alignment, if we compare the results obtained at the NAV level with those obtained at the N level. However, an exception appears for the MeSH *vs.* WIKIPEDIA

Figure 4. The architecture of SVM-S7 model

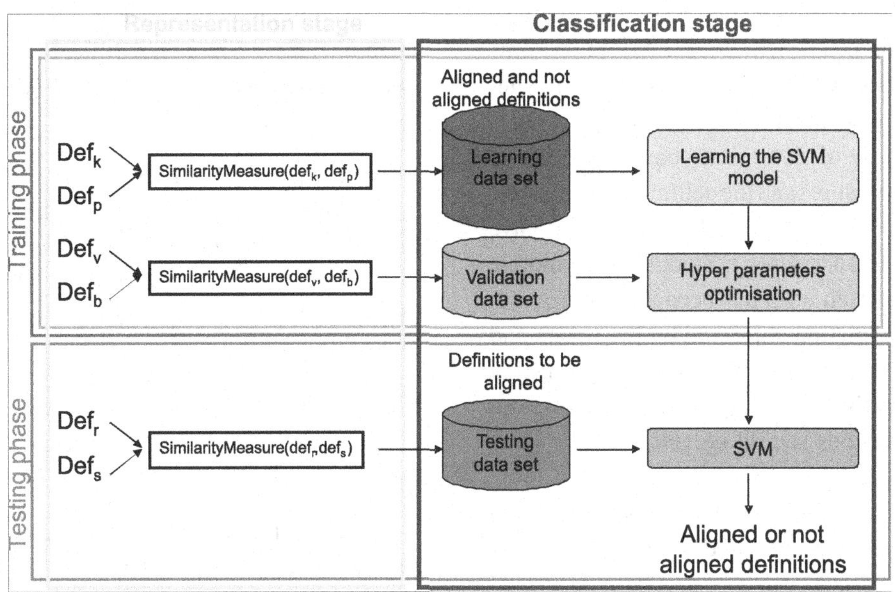

Table 3. F measures and their confidence intervals obtained with the SVM-S7 model

Representation level	*MEMODATA vs. MeSH*	*MEMODATA vs. VIDAL*	*MEMODATA vs. WIKIPEDIA*	*MeSH vs. VIDAL*	*MeSH vs. WIKIPEDIA*	*VIDAL vs. WIKIPEDIA*
N	80.95±3.16	81.54±3.12	84.27±2.93	81.39±3.13	79.6±3.24	87.35±2.67
NA	77.10±3.38	73.58±3.54	85.71±2.81	80.00±3.21	84.78±2.89	87.99±2.61
NAV	77.10±3.38	79.06±3.27	85.39±2.84	80.00±3.21	80.00±3.21	84.08±2.94
NAVR	78.05±3.33	82.76±3.04	68.42±3.74	76.54±3.41	68.42±3.74	71.79±3.62

and the MEMODATA *vs.* WIKIPEDIA combinations, where the F-measure computed by the NAV model is greater than the measure computed by the N model. Moreover, the NA model performs better than the NAV one. Reporting the results of the NAV model to those of the NA model, we reach the conclusion that better results are only obtained for the combination MEMODATA *vs.* WIKIPEDIA (both dictionaries using a general language).

In addition to this, the adverbs seem to bring a negative contribution to the performance of the aligner. Excepting the MEMODATA *vs.* VIDAL combination, the results obtained at the NAVR syntactic level are worse than the other results. This degradation could either be caused by the effective presence of the adverbs in the vicinity of nouns, adjectives and verbs, or by a not so good syntactic labelling performed during the pre-processing stage. However, these conclusions should be checked on a larger corpus.

CONCLUSIONS AND REMARKS

This chapter has presented three models for the automatic alignment of definitions taken from general and specialised dictionaries. The definition alignment has been considered as a binary classification problem and three ML algorithms have solved it: kNN, EAs and SVMs. In order to achieve this aim the classifiers have used a representation of definitions based on several similarity measures and the definition lengths that are compact and pertinent. The definitions have been considered at three syntactic levels and the influence of each level has been analysed.

The information conveyed by the nouns and adjectives seems to be more relevant than that conveyed by the verbs and adverbs are. However, these conclusions should be validated for some larger corpora.

Further work will be focused on developing a definition alignment based on a bag of morpho syntactic patterns.

A representation of definitions enriched by semantic and lexical extensions (synonyms, hyponyms, and antonyms) will also be considered.

REFERENCES

Arens, Y., Hsu, C. N., & Knoblock, C. A. (1996). Query processing in the SIMS information mediator. In A. Tate (Ed.), *Advanced Planning Technology* (pp. 61-69). Menlo Park, California, USA: AAAI Press.

Boser, B. E., Guyon, I., & Vapnik, V. (1992). A training algorithm for optimal margin classifiers. In H. Haussler (Ed.), *The 5th Annual ACM Workshop on Computational Learning Theory* (pp. 144-152). Pittsburgh, PA, USA: ACM.

Brown, P. F., Pietra, S. D., Pietra, V. J. D., & Mercer, R. L. (1994). The mathematic of statistical machine translation: Parameter estimation. *Computational Linguistics, 19(2),* 263-311.

Castano, S., Antonellis, V. D., & di Vimercati, S. D. C. (2001). Global viewing of heterogeneous data sources. *IEEE Transaction Knowl. Data Eng., 13(2),* 277-297.

Ceausu, A., Stefanescu, D., & Tufis, D. (2006). Acquis communautaire sentence alignment using Support Vector Machines. In L. Marconi (Ed.), *The 5th LREC Conference* (pp. 2134-2137). Paris, France: ELRA.

Chen, S. F. (1993). Aligning sentences in bilingual corpora using lexical information. In L. Schubert (Ed.), *The 31st Annual Meeting of the Association for Computational Linguistics* (pp.9-16). Morristown, NJ, USA: Association for Computational Linguistics.

Clemons, T. E., Edwin L., & Bradley, J. (2000). A nonparametric measure of the overlapping coefficient. *Comput. Stat. Data Anal., 34(1),* 51-61.

Cormen, T., Leiserson, C., & Rivest, R. (1990). *Introduction to Algorithms.* Cambridge, MA, USA: MIT Press.

Cortes, C., & Vapnik, V. (1995). Support-vector networks. *Machine Learning, 20(3),* 273-297.

Cover, T. M., & Hart, P. E. (1967). Nearest neighbor pattern classification. *IEEE Transactions on Information Theory, 13(1)*, 21-27.

Cristianini, N., & Shawe-Taylor, J. (2000). *An Introduction to Support Vector Machines.* Cambridge, UK: Cambridge Univ. Press.

Croft, W. B. (2000). Combining approaches to information retrieval. In W. B. Croft (Ed.), *Advances in Information Retrieval: Recent Research from the CIIR* (pp. 1-36). Norwell, MA, USA: Kluwer Academic Publishers.

Darmoni, S. J., Leroy, J. P., Baudic, F., Douyere, M., Piot, J., & Thirion, B. (2000) CISMeF: a structured health resource guide. *Methods of information in medicine, 39(1)*, 30-35.

Dasarathy, B. V. (1991). *Nearest Neighbor (NN) Norms: Nearest Neighbor Pattern Classification Techniques.* New York, USA: IEEE Press.

Dice, L. (1945). Measures of the amount of ecologic association between species. *Ecology 26*(3), 297-302.

Dioşan, L., Rogozan, A., & Pécuchet, J. P. (2007). Alignement des definitions par un apprentissage SVM avec optimisation des hyper-paramtres. In *Grand Colloque STIC 2007* (pp. 1-6). Paris, France.

Dioşan, L., Rogozan, A., & Pécuchet, J. P. (2008a). Apport des traitements morpho-syntaxiques pour l'alignement des dénitions par SVM. In F. Guillet & B. Trousse (Eds.), *Extraction et gestion des connaissances (EGC'2008), Actes des 8μemes journees Extraction et Gestion des Connaissances, Sophia-Antipolis, France,* (pp. 201-202). France: Cepadues-Editions.

Dioşan, L., Rogozan, A., & Pécuchet, J. P. (2008b). Automatic alignment of medical *vs.* general terminologies. In *11th European Symposium on Artificial Neural Networks, ESANN 2008,* Bruges, Belge.

Do, H. H., & Rahm, E. (2002). COMA - A system for flexible combination of schema matching approaches. In P. A. Bernstein et al. (Eds.), *International Conference on Very Large Data Bases* (pp. 610-621). Los Altos, CA, USA: Morgan Kaufmann.

Doan, A., Madhavan, J., Domingos, P., & Halevy, A. Y. (2002). Learning to map between Ontologies on the Semantic Web. In D. Lassner (Ed.), *The World-Wide Web Conference* (pp. 662-673). New York, NY, USA: ACM.

Dutoit, D, & Nugues P. (2002). A lexical network and an algorithm to find words from definitions. In F. van Harmelen (Ed.), *European Conference on Artificial Intelligence, ECAI 2002* (pp. 450-454). Amsterdam: IOS.

Dutoit, D., Nugues, P., & de Torcy, P. (2003). The integral dictionary: A lexical network based on componential semantics. In V. Kumar et al. (Eds.), *Computational Science and Its Applications - ICCSA 2003* (pp. 368-377). Berlin, DE: Springer.

Euzenat, J., & Shvaiko, P. (2007). *Ontology matching.* Berlin, DE: Springer.

Gangemi, A., Pisanelli, D. M., & Steve, G. (1999). An overview of the ONIONS project: Applying ontologies to the integration of medical terminologies. *Data Knowledge Engeneering., 31*(2), 183- 220.

Gale, W. A., & Church, K. W. (1991). A program for aligning sentences in bilingual corpora. *ACL, 19*(1), 177-184.

Goldberg, D. E. (1989). *Genetic Algorithms in Search, Optimization and Machine Learning.* Reading, MA, USA: Addison Wesley.

Holland, J. H. (1975). *Adaptation in Natural and Artificial Systems.* Michigan, USA: University of Michigan Press.

Jaccard, P. (1912). The distribution of the flora in the alpine zone. *New Phytologist, 11(2),* 37-50.

Li, W. S., & Clifton, C. (2000). SEMINT: A tool for identifying attribute correspondences in heterogeneous databases using neural networks. *Data Knowledge Engeneering, 33*(1), 49-84.

Lortal, G., Diosan, L., Pecuchet, J. P., & Rogozan, A. (2007). Du terme au mot: Utilisation de techniques de classification pour l'alignement de terminologies. In *Terminologie et Intelligence Artificielle, TIA2007, Sophia Antipolis, France.*

Madhavan, J., Bernstein, P. A., & Rahm, E. (2001). Generic schema matching with Cupid. In P. M. G. Apers et al. (Eds.), *The 27th International Conference on Very Large Data Bases VLDB '01* (pp. 49-58). Orlando, USA: Morgan Kaufmann.

Meadow, T. C. (1992). *Text Information Retrieval Systems.* San Diego, CA, USA: Academic Press.

Mena, E., Kashyap, V., Sheth, A., & Illarramendi, A. (2000). OBSERVER: An approach for query processing in global information systems based on interoperation across pre-existing ontologies. *Journal on Distributed and Parallel Databases, 8*(2), 223-272.

Moore, R. C. (2002). Fast and accurate sentence alignment of bilingual corpora. In S. D. Richardson (Ed.), *Machine Translation: From Research to Real Users, 5th Conference of the Association for Machine Translation in the Americas* (pp. 135-144). Berlin, DE: Springer-Verlag.

Moreau, F., Claveau, V., & Sebillot, P. (2007). Automatic morphological query expansion using analogy-based machine learning. In G. Amati et al. (Eds.), *Advances in Information Retrieval, 29th European Conference on IR Research, ECIR 2007, Vol. 4425* (pp. 222-233), Berlin, DE: Springer.

Salton, G. (1989). *Automatic text processing: the transformation, analysis, and retrieval of information by computer.* Reading, MA, USA: Addison Wesley.

Shvaiko, P., & Euzenat, J. (2005). A survey of schema-based matching approaches. *Journal on data semantics, 4*(1), 146-171.

van Rijsbergen, C. J. (1979). *Information Retireval.* Butterworths, London, UK: Butterworths.

Syswerda, G. (1989). Uniform crossover in Genetic Algorithms. In J. D. Schaffer (Ed.), *The Third International Conference on Genetic Algorithms* (pp. 2-9). San Mateo, California, USA: Morgan Kaufmann.

Taskar, B., Lacoste-Julien, S., & Klein, D. (2005). A discriminative matching approach to word alignment. In J. Chai (Ed.), *Human Language Technology Conference and Conference on Empirical Methods in Natural Language Processing* (pp. 73–80). Vancouver, USA: Association for Computational Linguistics.

Vapnik, V. (1995). *The Nature of Statistical Learning Theory.* Heidelberg, DE: Springer.

Vapnik, V. (1998). *Statistical Learning Theory.* New York, USA: Wiley.

ENDNOTES

a Valorisation Ontologique de Dictionnaires ELectroniques (Ontological Enrichment of Electronic Dictionaries) - http://vodel.insa-rouen.fr/

b http://ist.inserm.fr/basismesh/mesh.html

c Catalogue et Index des Sites Medicaux Francophones, founded in 1995 by CHU Rouen: http://www.cismef.org. It indexes the main French sites and documents from medical domain, while also adding some quality criteria based on Net Scoring.

d http://www.vidal.fr

e Le Dictionnaire Integral

f Mémodata is a small society specialising in electronic dictionaries and in Alexandria application in order to enrich a website by online access to definitions, translations or citations related to a designed term – http://www.memodata.com. Mémodata is the author of Alexandria (a *contextual multisource hypermedia enhancing dissemination) and* Semiograph (a program based on hypergraphs and heterogenous topologies and its task is to make a text make sense for a computer (at least partially)).

g The set of definitions with their morpho-syntactic and semantic relationships has been achieved by G. Lortal, I. Bou Salem and M. Wang throughout the VODEL project

h Medical Subject Headings http://www.nlm.nih.gov/mesh

i http://www.vidal.fr

j The free encyclopaedia http://www.wikipedia.org

[k] by Gaelle Lortal

[l] $|v|$ represents the number of characters of v

[m] In the field of Machine Learning, the goal of classification is to group items that have similar feature values, fara virg aici into groups. A linear classifier achieves this by making a classification decision based on the value of the linear combination of the features.

[n] in this case the Precision, the Recall and the F-measure are all equal

[o] The other levels (lexical or semantic) are not investigated due to the poor results previously obtained.

[p] The previous models did not take into account the length of each definition, since in both cases the alignment models work with a distance - a simple similarity measure or a linear combination of similarity measures. By including the length of the definitions, for instance in the linear combination, the *resulted* measure resulted will not be a distance as well. The SVM-based model works with a kernel that maps all the inputs (distance or not) in another space where the inputs can be linearly separated.

[q] that corresponds to all the couples formed by the definitions from two dictionaries

[r] http://www.csie.ntu.edu.tw/~cjlin/libsvm.

Chapter VI
Translation of Biomedical Terms by Inferring Rewriting Rules

Vincent Claveau
IRISA-CNRS, France

ABSTRACT

This chapter presents a simple yet efficient approach to translate automatically unknown biomedical terms from one language into another. This approach relies on a machine learning process able to infer rewriting rules from examples, that is, from a list of paired terms in two studied languages. Any new term is then simply translated by applying the rewriting rules to it. When different translations are produced by conflicting rewriting rules, we use language modeling to single out the best candidate. The experiments reported here show that this technique yields very good results for different language pairs (including Czech, English, French, Italian, Portuguese, Spanish and even Russian). The author also shows how this translation technique could be used in a cross-language information retrieval task and thus complete the dictionary-based existing approaches.

INTRODUCTION

In the biomedical domain, the international research framework makes knowledge resources such as multilingual terminologies and thesauri essential to carry out many researches. Such resources have indeed proved extremely useful for applications such as international collection of epidemiological data, machine translation (Langlais & Carl, 2004), and for cross-language access to medical publication. This last application has become an essential tool for the biomedical community. For instance, PubMed, the well-known biomedical document retrieval system gathers over 17 millions citations and processes about 3 millions queries a day (Herskovic et al., 2007)!

Unfortunately, up to now, little is offered to non-English speaking users. Most of the existing terminologies and document collections are in English, and the foreign or multilingual resources are far from being complete. For example, there are over 4 millions English entries in the 2006 UMLS Metathesaurus (Bodenreider, 2004), 1.2 million Spanish ones, 98 178 for German, 79 586 for French, 49 307 for Russian, and only 722 entries for Norwegian. Moreover, due to fast knowledge update, even well-developed multilingual resources need constant translation support. All these facts point up the need for automatic techniques to produce, manage and update these multilingual resources and to be able to offer cross-lingual access to existing document databases.

Within this context, we propose to present in this chapter an original method to translate biomedical terms from one language to another. This method aims at getting rid of the bottleneck caused by the incompleteness of multilingual resources in most real-world applications. As we show hereafter, this new translation approach has indeed proven useful in a cross-language information retrieval (CLIR) task.

The new word-to-word translation approach we propose makes it possible to translate automatically a large class of simple terms (i.e., composed of one word) in the biomedical domain from one language to another. It is tested and evaluated on translations within various language pairs (including Czech, English, French, German, Italian, Portuguese, Russian, Spanish).

Our approach relies on two major hypotheses concerning the biomedical domain:

- A large class of terms from one language to another are morphologically related;
- Differences between such terms are regular enough to be automatically learned.

These two hypotheses make the most of the fact that, most of the time, biomedical terms share a common Greek or Latin basis in many languages, and that their morphological derivations are very regular (Deléger et al., 2007). These regularities appear clearly in the following French-English examples: ophtalmorragie/ophthalmorrhagia, ophtalmoplastie/ophthalmoplasty, leucorragie/leukorrhagia...

The main idea of our work is that these regularities can be learnt automatically with well suited machine-learning techniques, and then can be used to translate new or unknown biomedical terms. We thus proposed a simple yet efficient machine learning approach allowing us to infer a set of rewriting rules from examples of paired terms that are translation of each other (different languages can be considered as source or target). These rules operate are the letter level; once they are learnt, they can be used to translate new and unseen terms into the target language. It is worth noting that neither external data nor knowledge is required besides the gathering of examples of paired terms for the languages under consideration. Moreover, these examples are simply taken from the multilingual terminologies that we aim at completing; thus, this is an entirely automatic process.

In the following sections, after the description of related studies, we present some highlights of our translation approach. The section entitled *Translation technique* is dedicated to the description of the method; Section *Translation experiments* gives some of its results for a pure translation task and the last section presents its performances when used in a simple CLIR application.

SCIENTIFIC CONTEXT

Few researches aim at translating terms directly from one language to another. One close work is the one of S. Schulz et al. (2004) about the translation of biomedical terms from Portuguese into Spanish with rewriting rules which are further used for biomedical information retrieval (Markó et al., 2005). Unfortunately, contrary to our work, these rules are hand-coded making this approach not portable.

In a previous work (Claveau & Zweigenbaum, 2005), an automatic technique relying on inference of transducers (finite-state machines allowing rewriting while analyzing a string) was proposed. The main drawback of this approach was that it could only handle language pairs sharing the same alphabet and produced less reliable results than the one presented in this paper (see the discussion in the section of translation experiments).

More recently, Langlais & Patry (2007) proposed a very interesting approach to translate unknown words based on analogical learning. This technique seems promising and its use to translate biomedical terms is under study (Langlais et al., 2007).

Apart from these studies, related problems are often addressed in the domain of automatic corpus translation. Indeed, the cognate detection task (cognates are pairs of words with close forms) relies on morphological operations (edit distance, longest common sub-string...) sometimes very close to the rewriting rules we infer (Flurh et al., 2000, inter alia). Other studies rely on corpus-based analysis using statistical techniques or lexical clues (punctuation marks, digits...) in order to discover alignments –thus, possible translation relations- between terms in aligned corpora (Ahrenberg et al., 2000; Gale & Church, 1991; Tiedemann, 2004) or comparable corpora (Fung & McKeow, 1997b, Fung & McKeow, 1997a). Besides the problem of the lack of such specialized corpora, these approaches differ from ours in that their goal is to exhibit the translation of a word in a text (relationship problem) whereas we are addressing the problem of producing the translation of a term without other information (generation problem). Moreover, most of the times, these alignment techniques actually need pairs of terms that are translation of each other as a starting point (Véronis, 2000, for a state-of-the-art).

More generally, statistical machine translation (Brown et al., 1990) addresses a close problem; of course, in our case, the sequence to translate is composed of letters and not words. Yet, the method we propose bears many similarities with the standard statistical approach that uses a translation model and a language model (Brown et al., 1993). Nonetheless, the kind of data we manipulate implies important differences. First, we are not concerned with the problem of reordering words, taken into account in the IBM models through the distortion parameter: indeed, the morpheme order (and thus the letter order) of our terms hardly varies from one language to another. Similarly, the fertility parameters or null words –used to tackle the word-to-word translation exceptions in these models— are not suited for our data. Such problems are indeed naturally handled by our inference technique which allows us to generate rewriting rules translating not only letter to letter but also from a string of letter to another string of letter of different length.

Studies on transliteration, for instance for Japanese (katakana) (Qu et al., 2003; Tsuji et al., 2002; Knight & Graehl, 1998, for example) or for Arabic (Al-Onaizan & Knight, 2002a; AbdulJaleel & Larkey, 2003) and their use to interlingual IR bears lots of similarities with our approach. Indeed, the techniques used in this domain are often close to the one we detail hereafter, but usually only concern the representation of foreign words (mainly named entities) in languages having a different alphabet than the source words. These techniques, which usually include a step aiming at transforming the term as a sequence of phonemes, are said *phonetic-based.* They must be set apart from *spelling-based* techniques such as the one we present in this chapter. *Phonetic-based* or hybrid techniques (Al-Onaizan & Knight, 2002a) thus require external knowledge (letters-to-phonemes table, source-language phonemes to target-language phonemes table...) which makes the approach efficient but not portable to other pairs of languages. Moreover, in the existing studies about named-entity transliteration, the two translation directions are not considered as equivalent: one speaks about *forward transliteration* (for example, transliteration of an Arabic name into the Latin alphabet) and the other of *backward transliteration* (retrieving the original Arabic name from its Latin transliteration). This distinction –that often implies differences in the techniques used— is not relevant to our approach. Our technique is fully symmetric even if the performances may vary from one translation direction to the other.

Finally, let us mention the studies on computational morphology in which machine learning approaches have been successfully used to lemmatize (Erjavec & Džeroski, 2004), to discover morphologic relations (Gaussier, 1999; Moreau et al., 2007) or to perform morphographemic analysis (Oflazer & Nirenburg, 1999). The technique of rewriting rule inference presented in the next section falls within the scope of such studies.

This lack of automatic methods to translate biomedical terms is reflected in the biomedical CLIR domain. Most of the studies on this subject adopt a dictionary-based approach (usually using the UMLS to translate queries (Eichmann et al., 1998; Fontelo et al., 2007); nonetheless, every author underscores the problem of the incompleteness of their multilingual resources, forcing them to use additional data such as (mono- or bilingual) specialized corpora (Tran et al., 2004). The work of K. Markó et al. (2005) also relies on a multilingual dictionary, but in this case their dictionary is partly generated with the hand-coded rewriting rules brought up above. Thus, the use of an automatic translation method in a CLIR system that we propose to describe in this chapter is new and original.

TRANSLATION TECHNIQUE

The translation technique we propose here works in two steps. First, rewriting rules (see below for examples) are learnt from examples of terms that are translations of each other in the considered language pair. This set of rules is then used to translate any new term, but conflicting rules may produce several rivaling translations. In order to choose only one translation, we use a language model, learnt on the training data, and keep the most probable translation.

Rewriting Rules

Our translation technique aims at learning rewriting rules (that can also be seen as transliteration rules). These rules, inferred from lists of bilingual term pairs (cf. next section), have the following form:

<input string> → *<output string>*

In the remaining of this chapter, we note *r* a rewriting rule; *R* is the list of every rule inferred during an experiment, *input(r)* and *output(r)* respectively refer to the input and output strings of the rule *r*.

Algorithm 1 gives an overview of our machine learning approach. The first step is performed by the software DPalign (http://www.cnts.ua.ac.be/~decadt/?section=dpalign). It is used to align two sequences by minimizing their edit distance with the dynamic programming approach proposed by Wagner & Fischer (1974); the necessary costs of substituting characters are computed on the whole set of pair to be aligned. Thus, this software does not rely on a formal similarity between characters; it makes it possible to align terms that do not share the same alphabet.

A list of paired terms is provided in input of DPalign; to each term, we add two characters # to represent the beginning and the end of the string of letters. The output list *L* then contains the paired terms aligned at a letter-level; Table 1 presents some examples for two language pairs ('_' means *no character*).

Algorithm 1. Inferring rewriting rules

```
align term pairs at the letter level, put the results in L
for all term pair W1 in L
        for all letter alignment of W1 in which the 2 letters differ
                find the best hypothesis of rule r in the search space E
                add r to the set of rules R
        end for
end for
```

Table 1. Examples of alignments produced for two language pairs

L Portuguese-English	*L* English-Russian
#cetosteróides# #ketosteroid_s#	#adenosinetriphosphatase# #аденозин_триф_осф_атаза#
#electroporação_# #electroporation#	#hydrox_ypregnenolone# #гидроксипрегненолон_#
#encef_alograf_ia# #encephalography_#	#keratoplasty__# #кератопластика#

Hereafter, the source term of pair p (respectively the target term of p) is written *input(p)* (resp. *output(p)*); moreover, *align(x,y)* means that the sub-string x is aligned with sub-string y in the considered term pair.

For each difference between two aligned letters, our algorithm has to generate the best rewriting rule. Many rules are eligible: consider for example the difference i/y in the French-English word pair #opht_almologie#/#ophthalmology_#; some of the rewriting rules our algorithm could generate in this context are i → y, gi → gy, ie → y (note that we do not write the _ character), ologie# → ology#, and so on.

The score of a rule is computed from the list L; it is defined as the ratio between the number of times the rule can actually be applied and the number of times the premise of the rule matches a source term from the example list. Thus, formally, it is defined as:

$$score(r) = \frac{\left|\{p \in L \mid input(r) \subseteq input(p) \wedge output(r) \subseteq align(input(r), p)\}\right|}{\left|\{s \in L_{input} \mid input(r) \subseteq s\}\right|}$$

where $\subseteq$ represents the inclusion of character string (for example, $abc \subseteq aabca$).

Lattice of Rules

In order to efficiently choose the best rule among these possibilities, we define a hierarchical relation between rules.

Definition 1 - Hierarchical Relation

Let r_1 and r_2 be two rules, then $r_1 \preccurlyeq r_2 \Leftrightarrow (input(r_1) \subseteq input(r_2) \wedge output(r_1) \subseteq output(r_2))$.

If $r_1 \preccurlyeq r_2$, then r_1 is said more general than r_2. This hierarchical relation defines a partial order in the search space *E*; thus, it makes it possible to order rules hierarchically in *E*, resulting in a lattice of rules.

Proof

Reflexivity

For any rule *r*, we obviously have $input(r) \subseteq input(r) \wedge output(r) \subseteq output(r)$, thus $r \preccurlyeq r$.

Transitivity

Let r_1, r_2 and r_3 be three rules such that $r_1 \preccurlyeq r_2$ and $r_2 \preccurlyeq r_3$. We have $input(r_1) \subseteq input(r_2)$, $input(r_2) \subseteq input(r_3)$, thus $input(r_1) \subseteq input(r_3)$, and similarly we have $output(r_1) \subseteq output(r_3)$. Finally, we have $r_1 \preccurlyeq r_3$.

Figure 1. Search lattice E from the example `i/y` *in* `#opht_almologie#/#ophthalmology_#`

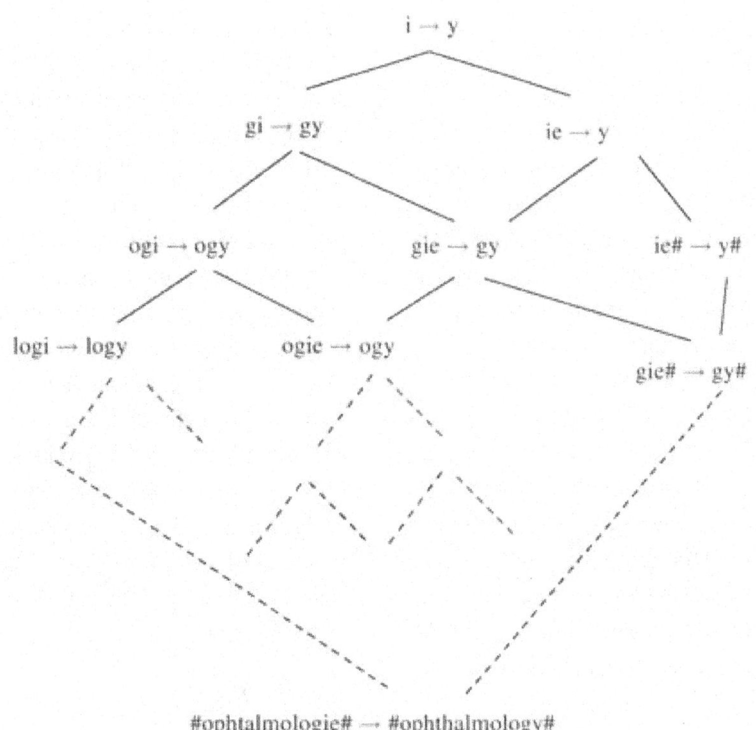

Anti-Symmetry

Let r_1 and r_2 be two rules such that $r_1 \preccurlyeq r_2$ and $r_2 \preccurlyeq r_1$. We have $input(r_1) \subseteq input(r_2)$, $input(r_2) \subseteq input(r_1)$, thus $input(r_1) = input(r_2)$, and similarly we have $output(r_1) = output(r_2)$. Finally, we have $r_1 = r_2$.

Thus, this relation defines a partial order. It is not a total order since we can have r_1 and r_2 such that we do not have $r_1 \preccurlyeq r_2$ or $r_2 \preccurlyeq r_1$.

One lattice is generated for each difference in the aligned pairs of terms. Figure 1 presents such a search space built from the difference i/y in the alignment #opht_almologie#/#ophthalmology_#.

In practice, these lattices of rules are explored top-down; the rules are generated on the fly with a very simple operator that generates more specialized rules from an existing one. Consider the rule r_1 = i → y in the previous example. This is the most general rule for the difference i/y in the alignment #opht_almologie#/#ophthalmology_#.

After the computing of its score the algorithm will generate and score every rule that is immediately more specific, that is:

$$\{ r_2 \mid r_1 \preccurlyeq r_2 \wedge \nexists\ r_3 \text{ s.t. } r_1 \succ r_3 \succ r_2 \}$$

The generation of these specific rules is simply done by adding the letter on the right (respectively on the left) from the input word of the paired term used as example to the input of r_1 and adding the corresponding aligned letter to the right (resp. to the left) of its output. Thus, by applying this to r_1 we have: g $input(r_1) \rightarrow$ g $output(r_1)$ and $input(r_1)$ e → output(r_1) _ , that is, gi → gy and ie → y.

The inheritance properties of the lattices and this specialization operator make it possible to choose quickly the best rewriting rules for each example according to the score function which is consistent with the specialization operator. Indeed, computing the score is the most time-consuming task of our algorithm because it necessitates analyzing every word in the training set L. However, by considering the hierarchical relation and the way hypothesis are generated, a big amount of time can be saved: for a term pair used as an example, consider two rules r_1 and r_2 such that $r_1 \preccurlyeq r_2$. When computing the score of r_2, we have for any word pair p:

$$input(r_1) \subseteq input(r_2) \subseteq input(p),$$

that is, if p is such that $input(r_2) \subseteq input(p)$ then necessarily p was analyzed when computing the score of r_1. Therefore, we do not need to examine every word of L to compute the score of r_2 but only those that were covered by the denominator of r_1.

Using the Rules and Language Modeling to Translate

Every difference between two aligned letters in every term pair thus ends up with one rewriting rule chosen in the corresponding lattice. All the rules are collected in R. Given a new term to translate, every rewriting rule of R that can be applied (i.e. rules inferred in the training set in which the input string corresponds to a sub-string of the term) is indeed applied. In case of conflicting rules (rules with the same or overlapping premise), all possibilities are generated. Thus, at this stage, a word can receive several concurrent translations. Therefore, the second step of our approach consists in a post-processing technique in order, on the one hand, to select only one of these proposed translations, and on the other hand, to give the user a confidence factor for the result.

These two tasks are conjointly performed by assigning a probability to each possible translation according to a language model (LM). That is, with standard notations, for a word w composed of the letters $l_1, l_2, \ldots, l_m$:

$$P(w) = \prod_{i=1}^{m} P(l_i \mid l_1, \ldots, l_{i-1})$$

In practice, the probabilities $P(l_i|...)$ are estimated from the list of output words used as examples in the first step (i.e. L_{output}), decomposed in n-grams of letters. As usual with language modeling, to prevent the problem of unseen sequences, the probabilities are actually computed with a limited history, that is, we only consider the n-1 previous letters:

$$P(w) = \prod_{i=1}^{m} P(l_i \mid l_{i-n+1}, \dots, l_{i-1})$$

In the experiments presented below, we use n = 7 letters. A simple smoothing technique is also used to provide more reliable estimations.

Intuitively, the LM aims at favoring translations that "look like" correct words of the output language. Thus, among all the proposed translations, we only keep the one with the better LM score. Moreover this language modeling approach also enables to avoid some problems. As it was underlined by Claveau & Zweigenbaum (2005b), some words have similar forms but different Part-of-Speech or Semantic role. If available, these additional pieces of information may avoid translation errors. For example, a word in -ique in French may be translated in English in -ic if it is an adjective (e.g. dynamique/dynamic) or in -ics if it is a noun (e.g. linguistique/linguistics). Similarly, a word in -logie in French may be translated in -logy if it concerns a science (biologie/biology) or in -logia if it concerns a language disorder (dyslogie/dyslogia). It is worth noting that this part-of-speech and Semantic information, if available in the data, can easily be used with the language model: the probabilities estimated from the training data are simply conditioned to the information we want to consider, that is:

$$P(w, PoS) = \prod_{i=1}^{m} P(l_i \mid l_{i-n+1}, \dots, l_{i-1}, PoS)$$

or

$$P(w, sem) = \prod_{i=1}^{m} P(l_i \mid l_{i-n+1}, \dots, l_{i-1}, sem)$$

where *PoS* and *sem* respectively denote the Part-of-Speech and Semantic information.

TRANSLATION EXPERIMENTS

This section presents some of the experiments we made with the translation technique previously described. We describe the data, the experimental framework we used and finally the results obtained for this translation task.

Data

Two different kinds of data are used for these experiments. First, in order to compare our translation approach with previous work, we use the same French-English pairs of terms used by Claveau & Zweigenbaum (2005a), that is a list of terms taken from the Masson medical dictionary (http://www.atmedica.com). The second set of data used in our experiments is the UMLS Metathesaurus (Tuttle et al., 1990; Bodenreider, 2004). This collection of thesauri brings together biomedical terms from 17 languages with a language-independent identifier allowing us to form the necessary bilingual pairs of terms. For these two sets, we only consider simple terms (i.e. one-word terms) in both studied languages, and we disregard acronyms.

Experimental Framework

In order to evaluate our results, we follow a standard protocol. The word pair list is split into two parts: the first one is used for the learning process as described above (rule inference and language modeling), and the second one, set to contain 1000 pairs, is used as a testing set. Once the rules have been inferred and language modeling has been done, we apply them to every input word of the testing set. We then compare the generated translation with the expected output word; if the two strings exactly match, the translation is considered as correct, in every other case, it is considered as wrong.

The results are evaluated in terms of precision (percentage of correct translations generated). Nonetheless, since the LM gives a confidence factor to each translation, we can decide to keep only those with a LM score greater than a certain threshold. If this threshold is set high the precision may be high, but the number of words actually translated may be low, and conversely. Thus, in order to represent all the possibilities, results below are presented as graphs where each point corresponds to the precision and the percentage of words translated for a certain LM score threshold.

Results

Translation Between French and English

As a first experiment, we focus our attention on the French-English language pair with the help of the Masson data in order to compare these results to those of Claveau & Zweigenbaum (2005a). Figure 2 and 3 respectively present the precision graph of the French into English and English into French translation experiments. In close languages such as French and English, many specialized words are exactly the same. Thus, as a simple baseline, we compute the precision that would be obtained by a system systematically proposing the input term as its own translation. We also indicate the best precision obtained by the transducer based technique exposed by Claveau & Zweigenbaum (2005a) within the same experimental framework and data.

Whatever the translation direction, the two graphs show that our approach performs very well: for French into English translations, it yields a precision of 85.4% when every word is translated, and 84.8% for English into French. In both cases, it represents a 10% improvement over the transducer-based approach (Claveau & Zweigenbaum, 2005a). Our technique clearly outperforms the baseline results, but it is also worth noting that about 25% of the biomedical terms are identical in French and English, which indicates that the two languages are close enough to make the learning task relatively easy.

Figure 2. Performances of translation from French into English

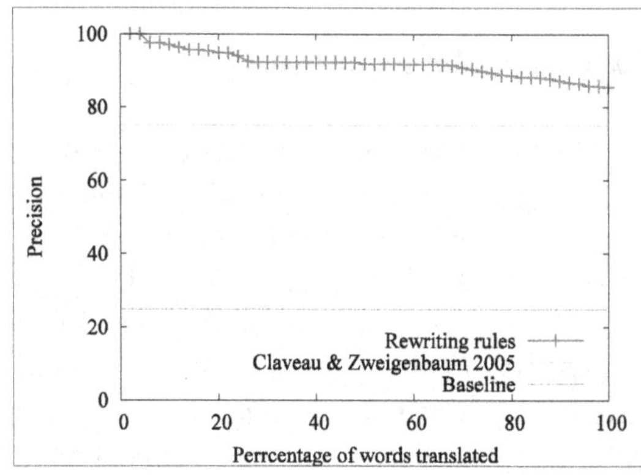

Figure 3. Performances of translation from English into French

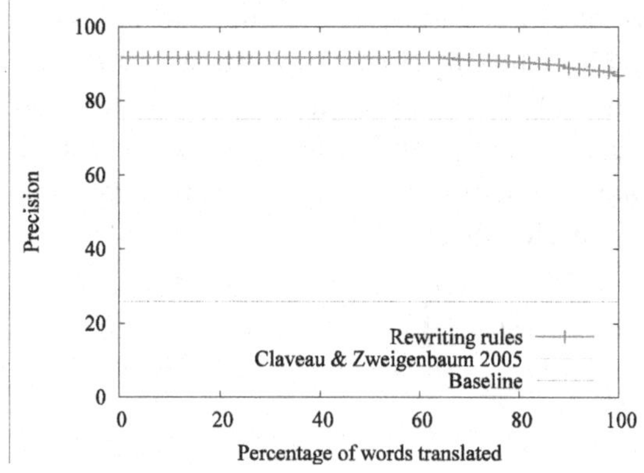

Concerning the use of the language modeling, several things are noteworthy. First, without including the Part-of-speech information, the precision rates are a bit lower (82.6% for French to English and 84.8% for English to French). Secondly, if we choose the translation at random among all the generated ones instead of choosing the one with the best LM score, the precision rate falls to about 50% for both translation directions. Lastly, if the good translations were always chosen (when it appears in the list of potential translations produced by the rewriting rules), the precision would reach 90%. It means that the language model makes very few mistakes at choosing the final translation among the different proposals. These facts clearly show the interest of using language modeling and, if available, to include the Part-of-Speech information in it.

Computation Time and Performances vs. Number of Examples

In the previous experiments all the available examples (i.e. all the paired terms but those kept for the test set) were used to infer the rewriting rules. Let us now examine the results and the computation time when this number varies. Table 2 displays the results we obtain when we keep different numbers of examples to infer the rewriting rules and to learn the language model probabilities. In this table, we indicate the precision rate in the worst case (i.e. every translation is kept), the number of rules that are inferred, as well as the computing time due to the alignment step and the total inference time (including the alignment time). The experiments were carried out on a 1.5GHz Centrino Laptop running Linux, and the algorithm presented in the previous section was entirely implemented in Perl.

One can notice that the precision rates remain very good, even with very few examples ending up with few rules. This is particularly interesting since gathering such paired terms could be difficult for certain language pairs due to the lack of multilingual resources. Concerning the computation time, the inference process is fast enough to process several language pairs in a minimal amount of time, thanks to our efficient search in the rewriting rule lattices. Yet, the whole process is slowed down by the alignment step for which the dynamic programming algorithm clearly constitutes a bottleneck.

Table 2. Computation time and precision as a function of the number of term pairs used as examples

Number of term pairs	Alignment time	Total execution time	Number of rules	Precision
5400	132s	146s	727	85.4%
3600	73s	84s	537	83.5%
2800	54s	62s	406	82.0%
1800	36s	42s	309	82.8%
1400	21s	28s	249	82.3%
660	10s	13s	164	80.4%
320	6s	9s	77	77.3%
130	3s	8s	39	76.3%

Other Language Pairs

The same experiment can be carried out with different language pairs from the UMLS Metathesaurus. We only exhibit some results from many possible combinations; contrary to the previous experiments, we do not include any part-of-speech information in the language modeling.

Figures 4 and 5 present the results obtained with two languages known to be close: Spanish and Portuguese. These results are very good: in the worst case (i.e. no LM threshold is set: every term is proposed a translation), 87.9% of Portuguese terms are correctly translated into Spanish and 85% for Spanish into Portuguese. This is not surprising given the closeness of the two languages, a closeness which further appears in the very high baseline precision.

We now focus on translation into English, as it is the way which is later used in our CLIR experiments. As shown in Figures 6 and 7, translation from Spanish into English provides 71.7% of terms correctly translated; translation from Portuguese into English gives 75.5% of precision. Here again, the results are quite good; they also are in accordance with the proximity of Spanish and Portuguese since both languages perform similarly when translated into English.

Italian or Czech to English yields almost similar results as illustrated in Figures 8 and 9, even if these languages are not reputed to be specially close: in the worst case, 70% of Italian terms and 75.5% of Czech terms are correctly translated.

A more surprising result is obtained for German; although these two languages share strong historical links, Figure 10 clearly shows that German and English biomedical terms do not exhibit enough regularities to achieve the same precision rates than the previous languages. Nonetheless, in the worst case, our technique still yields 68.8% of correctly translated terms.

Language Pairs with Different Alphabets

Let us now examine the translation performances of the Russian-English language pair. As we previously said, contrary to the technique of Claveau

Figure 4. Performances of translation from Portuguese into Spanish

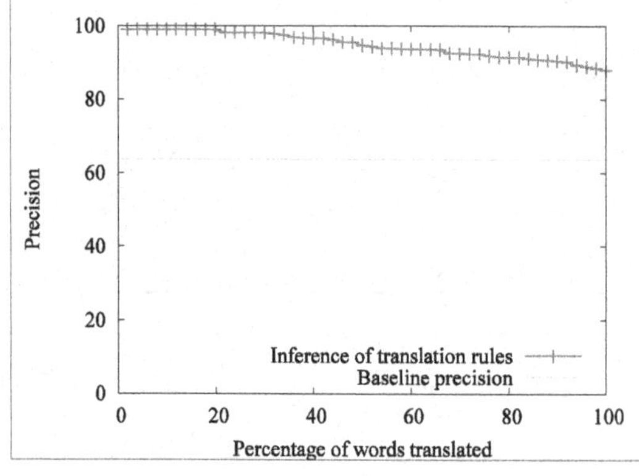

Figure 5. Performances of translation from Spanish into Portuguese

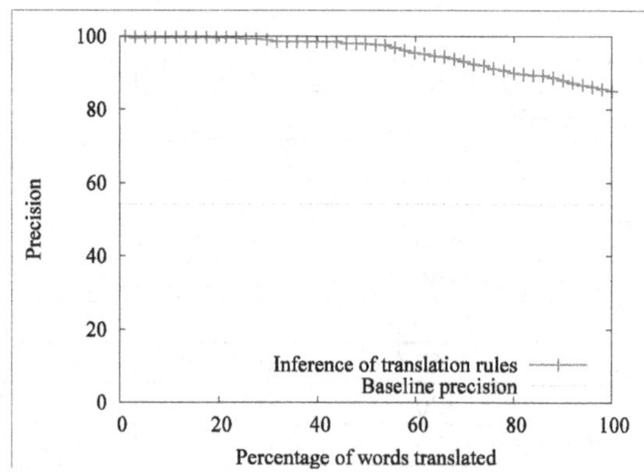

Figure 6. Performances of translation from Portuguese into English

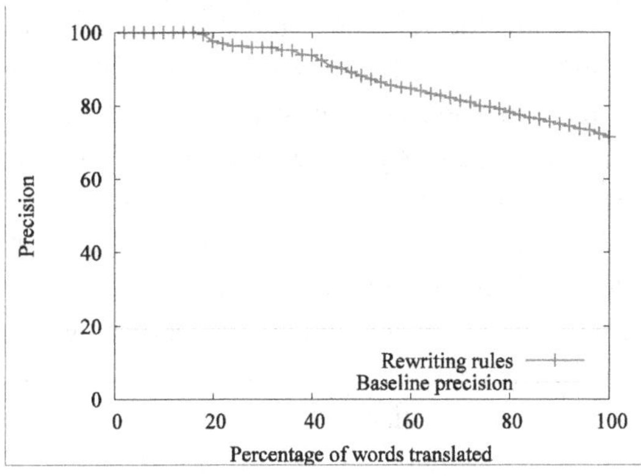

Figure 7. Performances of translation from Spanish into English

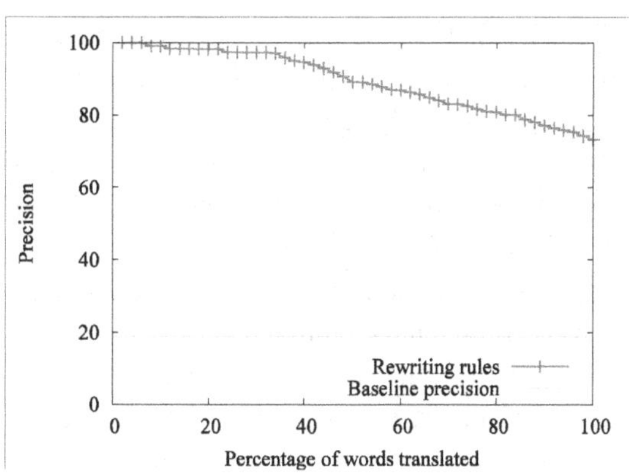

Figure 8. Performances of translation from Italian into English

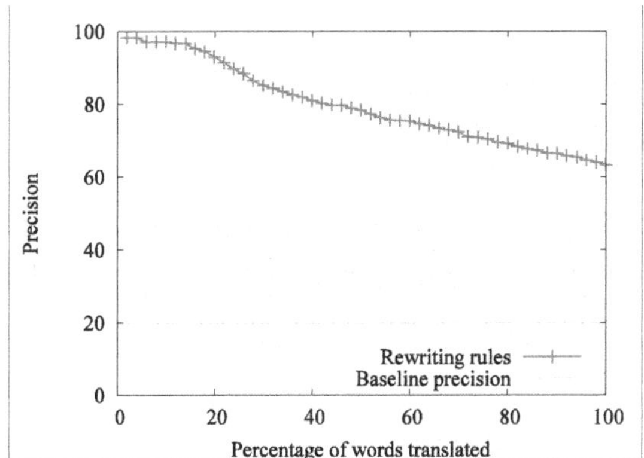

Figure 9. Performances of translation from Czech into English

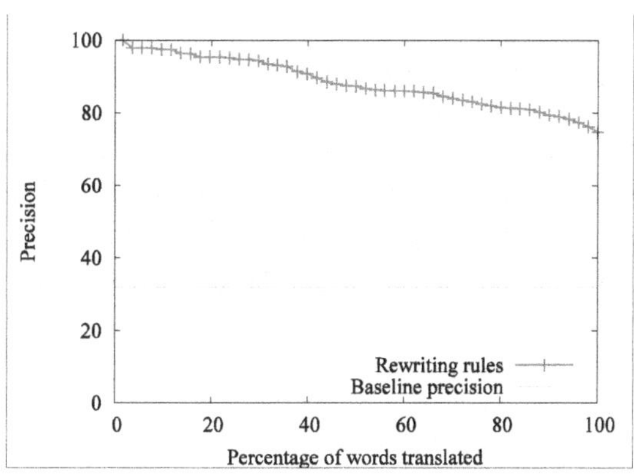

Figure 10. Performances of translation from German into English

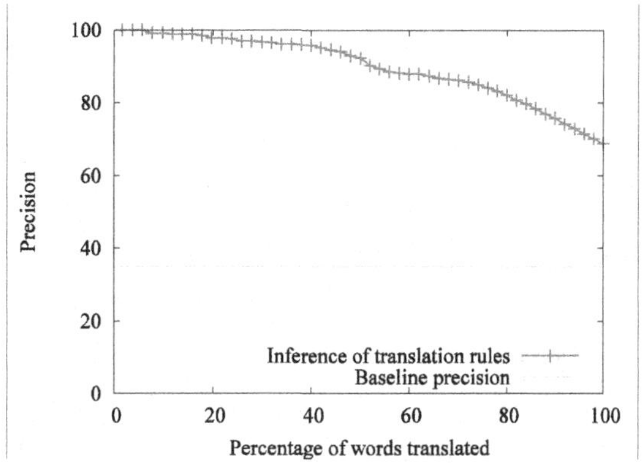

& Zweigenbaum (2005a), the approach described in this paper can be easily used with languages that do not share the same alphabet but show some regularity that can be learnt. Figures 11 and 12 present the results we obtain. Due to the different alphabets, the baseline is 0 in this case. The minimal precision rates (i.e., when every word is translated) are 57.5% for English into Russian and 64.5% for Russian into English.

These translation performances are surprisingly good given the apparent difficulty of the task. Of course, they are a bit lower than those of the other language pairs we examined but could be useful enough for many applications. It also proves if needed that most of the biomedical terms in Russian are built from Cyrillic transliterations of the same Latin and Greek morphemes used in English, French or Italian...

Common Causes of Errors

Our translation technique automatically captures existing regularities between biomedical terms in different languages. For this reason and unsurprisingly, when examining the results in detail, it appears that the main cause of error is due to the lack of morphological links between the source and the target term. Obviously, this is more often the case for the Russian-English language pair, but still occurs for languages known to be close (e.g. asimiento/grip for Spanish-Portuguese translation or embrochage/pinning for French-English). Besides these unavoidable errors, as already discussed, some errors are also due to similar forms with different part-of-speech or Semantic features; as it was shown for the French/English experiments, most of these errors could be avoided if we had at our disposal the part-of-speech of Semantic information. After all, the experiments tend to show that these cases are rare enough to make our approach yield good precision rates (though they are variable according to the considered languages).

APPLICATION TO A CLIR EXPERIMENT

Our translation approach is now evaluated within a simple cross-language information retrieval

Figure 11. Performances of translation from Russian into English

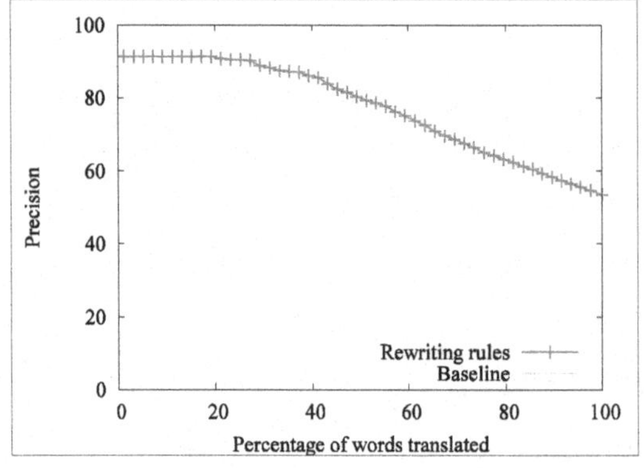

Figure 12. Performances of translation from English into Russian

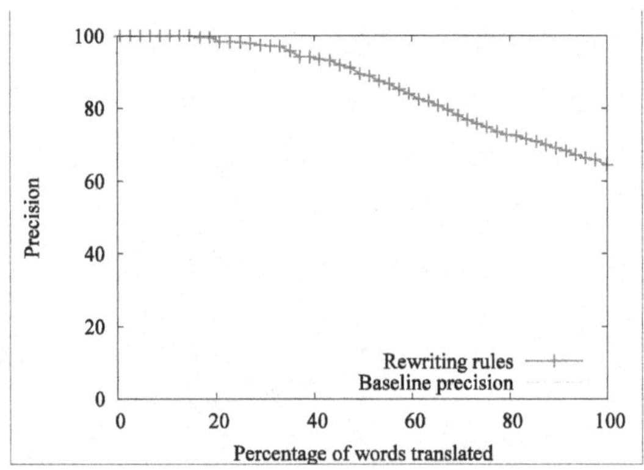

framework. More precisely, our technique is used to translate terms used to query a collection of biomedical documents.

Experimental Framework

The information retrieval collection used comes from the TREC 9 "Filtering Task" (derived itself from the OHSUMED collection). It consists in 350 000 abstracts from MEDLINE and more than 4000 queries in English with their relevance judgment. These queries are made up of two fields: the subject, usually a biomedical term, and a definition of this term.

Initially developed for a filtering task, we use these data as a standard information retrieval collection. The actual queries we use only correspond to the subject field of the original queries. In order to use these data in a cross-language framework, the queries are manually translated from English into another language with the help of the UMLS Metathesaurus. Since some terms are not translated in the UMLS (which is a motivation of this work), we only keep queries whose translations are present. The resulting number of query varies from one language to another, but remains important in practice (e.g. 2300 queries for French).

Finally, we thus have a collection of documents in English and a large set of queries in another language. Our translation technique can now be used to translate the queries back from the considered language into English; the query is then sent to a standard information retrieval system (we use Lemur with its parameters set to copy the well-known Okapi system (Robertson et al., 1998)). Of course, to avoid any bias in the results, no term from the queries is used as training data for our translation system.

Results

Results are classically presented by recall-precision curves. For comparison purpose, we indicate for each experiment the results obtained when using the same query set in their original English version. We also report the results obtained when the queries are translated by a non-specialized tool: Systran BabelFish (http://babelfish.altavista.com).

Hereafter, we only give the results for a few languages for which BabelFish can provide a comparison basis. Figures 13, 14, 15, 16 and 17 respectively present the recall-precision curves for French, Italian, Spanish, Portuguese and Russian queries.

Unsurprisingly, the queries translated with our system perform distinctly worse than the original ones. Yet, the results are respectable, in particular when compared with those of BabelFish. From other experiments, it clearly appears that the CLIR results are closely related with the translation performances presented in the previous section. It is also noteworthy that only a part of the queries are mainly responsible for making the results not as good as the reference's ones; this is due to the presence of non specialized terms in these queries which our specialized translation system is not designed to handle. Moreover, when examining the results, it clearly appears that most of the errors made by our approach are due to these unspecialized terms while most of the errors made by BabelFish are caused by very specialized terms (too rare to be in the BabelFish dictionary). This fact points up all the benefits that would be gained in combining our system with a non-specialized translation system in real-world biomedical applications.

CONCLUDING REMARKS AND PERSPECTIVES

Cross-language information retrieval is a thorny yet important issue in the biomedical domain. The original method presented in this chapter makes it possible to translate efficiently simple biomedical terms between various languages. It

Figure 13. Results of the French into English CLIR experiment

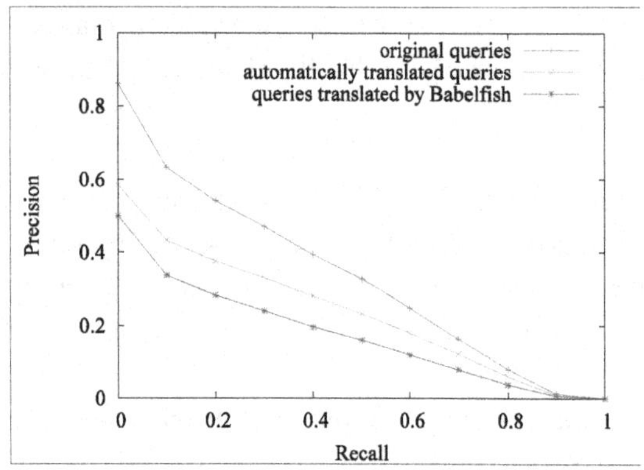

Figure 14. Results of the Italian into English CLIR experiment

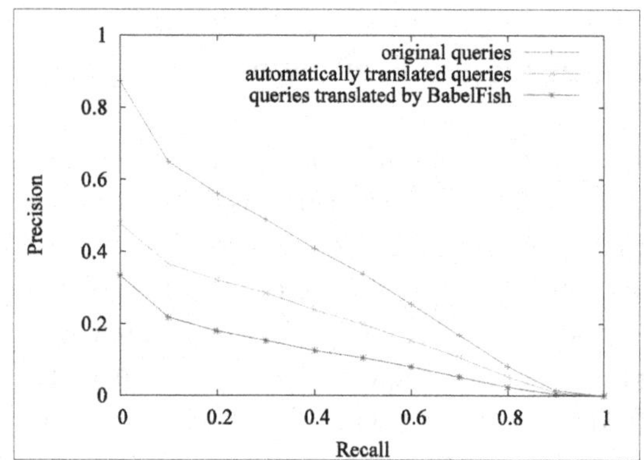

Figure 15. Results of the Spanish into English experiment

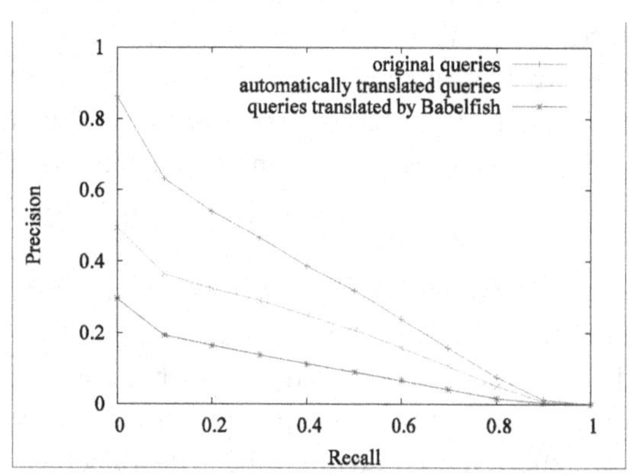

Figure 16. Results of the Portuguese into English CLIR experiment

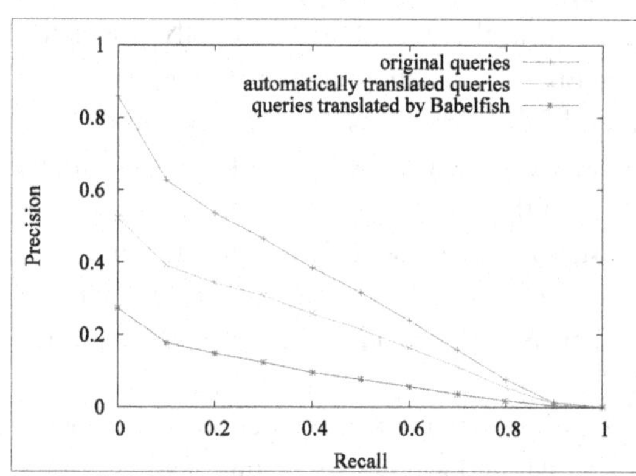

Figure 17. Results of the Russian into English CLIR experiment

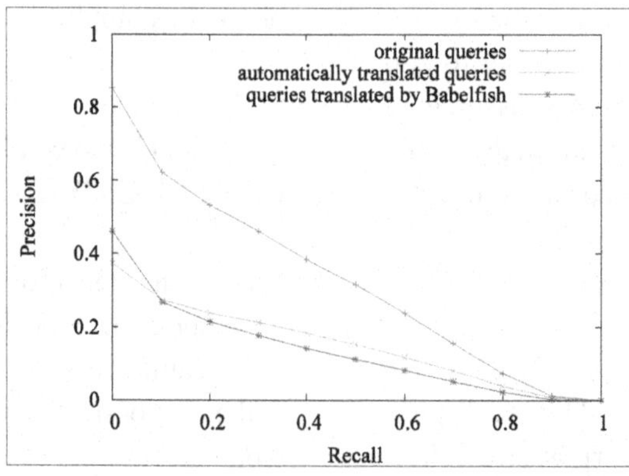

relies on a machine-learning technique inferring rewriting rules from examples of a list of bilingual term pairs and on a letter-based language modeling. These examples can be found easily in the existing—yet incomplete—multilingual terminologies; no other external knowledge or human intervention is needed. The approach is efficient and successful for translating unseen terms with a high precision, depending on the languages, and can thus be used to overcome problems due to incomplete multilingual language resources. The simple CLIR experiments carried out with this translation approach underline the validity of such an approach. But they also show that our term-to-term translation technique should only be considered as an element among others in a broader translation system if one wants to handle real-world data mixing specialized terms with general language.

Many perspectives are foreseen for this work including technical enhancements and applications of our translation approach and its use in a cross-language framework. For instance, the translation of complex terms (terms composed of more than one word) is currently closely examined. These terms are widely used in the biomedical domain (for instance, 50% of the MeSH terminology are complex terms), and some of them are not compositional, meaning that they cannot undergo the word-by-word translation our approach proposes. Moreover, even compositional terms would certainly necessitate a syntactic analysis to identify the head-modifier relations and thus translate it accordingly to these dependency relations.

Lastly, our translation system bears numerous similarities with the standard statistical machine translation approach based on a translation model and a language model (Brown et al., 1993). The parallel between the two approaches could lead to interesting insights. Moreover, in the experiments presented in this chapter, only one translation was kept–the one with the best language model score. But in this particular CLIR settings, instead of the LM or in conjunction with it, one could also use the index to check that the proposed translation exist, as it is done in transliteration studies (Qu et al., 2003; Al-Onaizan & Knight, 2002b, for example).

REFERENCES

AbdulJaleel, N., & Larkey, L. S. (2003). Statistical transliteration for English-Arabic cross language information retrieval. In *Proceedings of the 12th International Conference on Information and Knowledge Management, CKIM'03*, (pp. 139–146), New Orleans, United-States of America.

Ahrenberg, L., Andersson, M., & Merkel, M. (2000). *A knowledge-lite approach to word alignment,* (pp. 97–138). In Véronis.

Al-Onaizan, Y., & Knight, K. (2002a). Machine transliteration of names in arabic text. In *Proceedings of ACLWorkshop on Computational Approaches to Semitic Languages*, Philadelphia, United-States of America.

Al-Onaizan, Y., & Knight, K. (2002b). Translating named entities using monolingual and bilingual resources. In *Proceedings of the Conference of the Association for Computational Linguistics, ACL'02*, (pp. 400-408), Philadelphia, United-States of America.

Bodenreider, O. (2004). The unified medical language system (UMLS): Integrating biomedical terminology. *Nucleic Acids Research*, *32*(D267-D270).

Brown, P. F., Cocke, J., Stephen A., Della Pietra, V. J. D. P., Jelinek, F., Lafferty, J. D., Mercer, R. L., & Roossin, P. S. (1990). A statistical approach to machine translation. *Computational Linguistics*, *16*(2).

Brown, P. F., Pietra, V. J. D., Pietra, S. A. D., & Mercer, R. L. (1993). The mathematics of statistical machine translation: Parameter estimation. *Computational Linguistics, 19*(2).

Claveau, V. & Zweigenbaum, P. (2005a). Automatic translation of biomedical terms by supervised transducer inference. *In Proceedings of the 10th Conference on Artificial Intelligence in Medicine, AIME 05, Lecture Notes of Computer Science*, Aberdeen, Scotland, UK. Springer.

Claveau, V., & Zweigenbaum, P. (2005b). Traduction de termes biomédicaux par inférence de transducteurs. In *Actes de la conférence Traitement automatique des langues naturelles, TALN'05*, Dourdan, France.

Deléger, L., Namer, F., & Zweigenbaum, P. (2007). Defining medical words: Transposing morphosemantic analysis from French to English. In *Proceedings of MEDINFO 2007*, volume 129 of Studies in Health Technology and Informatics, Amsterdam, Netherlands.

Eichmann, D., Ruiz, M. E., & Srinivasan, P. (1998). Cross-language information retrieval with the UMLS metathesaurus. In *Proceedings of the 21st International Conference on Research and Development in Information Retrieval, SIGIR 98*, (pp. 72–80), Melbourne, Australia.

Erjavec, T., & Dzeroski, S. (2004). Machine learning of morphosyntactic structure: Lemmatizing unknown Slovene words. *Applied Artificial Intelligence, 18*(1), 17–41.

Fluhr, C., Bisson, F., & Elkateb, F. (2000). Parallel text alignment using crosslingual information retrieval techniques, chapter 9. In (Véronis, 2000).

Fontelo, P., Liu, F., Leon, S., Anne, A., & Ackerman, M. (2007). PICO linguist and BabelMeSH: Development and partial evaluation of evidence-based multilanguage search tools for Medline/Pubmed. *Studies of Health Technology and Informatics, 129.*

Fung, P., & McKeown, K. (1997a). Finding terminology translations from non-parallel corpora. In *Proceedings of the 5th Annual Workshop on Very Large Corpora*, Hong Kong.

Fung, P., & McKeown, K. (1997b). A technical word and term translation aid using noisy parallel corpora across language groups. *Machine Translation, 12*(1/2), 53–87.

Gale, W., & Church, K. (1991). Identifying word correspondences in parallel texts. In *Proceedings of the 4th DarpaWorkshop on Speech and Natural Language*, (pp. 152–157), Pacific Grove, CA, United-States of America.

Gaussier, E. (1999). Unsupervised Learning of Derivational Morphology from Inflectional Corpora. In *Proceedings of Workshop on Unsupervised Methods in Natural Language Learning, 37th Annual Meeting of the Association for Computational Linguistics, ACL 99*, (pp. 24–30), Maryland, United-States of America.

Herskovic, J. R., Tanaka, L. Y., Hersh, W., & Bernstam, E. V. (2007). A day in the life of PubMed: Analysis of a typical day's query log. *Journal of American Medical Informatics Association, 14*, 212–220.

Knight, K., & Graehl, J. (1998). Machine transliteration. *Computational Linguistics, 24*(4), 599–612.

Langlais, P., & Carl, M. (2004). General-purpose statistical translation engine and domain specific texts: Would it work? *Terminology, 10*(1), 131–152.

Langlais, P., Yvon F., & Zweigenbaum, P. (2007). What analogical learning can do for terminology translation? In *Proceedings of Computational Linguisitics in Netherlands*, CLIN'07, Nijmegen, Netherlands.

Langlais, P., & Patry, A. (2007). Translating unknown words by analogical learning. In *Proceed-*

ings of the 2007 Joint Conference on Empirical Methods in Natural Language Processing and Computational Natural Language Learning (EMNLP-CoNLL), Prague, Czech Republic.

Markó, K., Stefan Schulz, O. M., & Hahn, U. (2005). Bootstrapping dictionaries for crosslanguage information retrieval. In *Proceedings of the 28th International Conference on Research and Development in Information Retrieval, SIGIR 05*, (pp. 528–535), Salvador, Brasil.

Moreau, F., Claveau, V., & Sébillot, P. (2007). Automatic morphological query expansion using analogy-based machine learning. In *Proceedings of the 29th European Conference on Information Retrieval, ECIR 2007*, Roma, Italy.

Oflazer, K., & Nirenburg, S. (1999). Practical bootstrapping of morphological analyzers. In *Proceedings of EACL Workshop on Computational Natural Language Learning, CONLL 99*, Bergen, Norway.

Qu, Y., Grefenstette, G., & Evans, D. A. (2003). Automatic transliteration for Japanese-to-English text retrieval. In *Proceedings of the 26th International Conference on Research and Development in information Retrieval, SIGIR 03*, Toronto, Canada.

Robertson, S. E., Walker, S., & Hancock-Beaulieu, M. (1998). Okapi at TREC-7: Automatic ad hoc, filtering, VLC and interactive. In *Proceedings of the 7th Text Retrieval Conference, TREC-7*, Gaithersburg, United-States of America.

Schulz, S., Markó, K., Sbrissia, E., Nohama, P., & Hahn, U. (2004). Cognate mapping - A heuristic strategy for the semi-supervised acquisition of a Spanish lexicon from a Portuguese seed lexicon. In *Proceedings of the 20th International Conference on Computational Linguistics, COLING'04*, (pp. 813–819), Geneva, Switzerland.

Tiedemann, J. (2004). Word to word alignment strategies. In *Proceedings of the 20th International Conference on Computational Linguistics, COLING 04*, (pp. 212–218), Geneva, Switzerland.

Tran, T. D., Garcelon, N., Burgun, A., & Le Beux, P. (2004). Experiments in cross-language medical information retrieval using a mixing translation module. In *Proceeding of the World Congress on Health and Medical Informatics MEDINFO*, San Francisco, CA, United-States of America.

Tsuji, K., Daille, B., & Kageura, K. (2002). Extracting French-Japanese word pairs from bilingual corpora based on transliteration rules. In *Proceedings of the Third International Conference on Language Resources and Evaluation LREC'02*, (pp. 499–502), Las Palmas de Gran Canaria, Spain.

Tuttle, M., Sherertz, D., Olson, N., Erlbaum, M., Sperzel, D., Fuller, L., & Neslon, S. (1990). Using Meta-1 – the 1st version of the UMLS metathesaurus. In *Proceedings of the 14th annual Symposium on Computer Applications in Medical Care (SCAMC)*, Washington, D.C.

Véronis, J., (Ed.) (2000). *Parallel text processing*. Dordrecht: Kluwer Academic Publishers.

Wagner, R. A., & Fischer, M. J. (1974). The string-to-string correction problem. *Journal of the Association for Computing Machinery, 21*(1), 168–173.

Chapter VII
Lexical Enrichment of Biomedical Ontologies

Nils Reiter
Heidelberg University, Germany

Paul Buitelaar
DERI - NLP Unit, National University of Ireland Galway, UK

ABSTRACT

This chapter is concerned with lexical enrichment of ontologies, that is how to enrich a given ontology with lexical information derived from a semantic lexicon such as WordNet or other lexical resources. The authors present an approach towards the integration of both types of resources, in particular for the human anatomy domain as represented by the Foundational Model of Anatomy and for the molecular biology domain as represented by an ontology of biochemical substances. The chapter describes our approach on enriching these biomedical ontologies with information derived from WordNet and Wikipedia by matching ontology class labels to entries in WordNet and Wikipedia. In the first case the authors acquire WordNet synonyms for the ontology class label, whereas in the second case they acquire multilingual translations as provided by Wikipedia. A particular point of emphasis here is on selecting the appropriate interpretation of ambiguous ontology class labels through sense disambiguation, which we address by use of a simple algorithm that selects the most likely sense for an ambiguous term by statistical significance of co-occurring words in a domain corpus. Acquired synonyms and translations are added to the ontology by use of the LingInfo model, which provides an ontology-based lexicon model for the annotation of ontology classes with (multilingual) terms and their linguistic properties.

INTRODUCTION

As information systems become more and more open, i.e. by including web content, as well as more complex, e.g. by dynamically integrating web services for specific tasks, data and process integration becomes an ever more pressing need - in particular also in the context of biomedical information systems. A wide variety of data and processes must be integrated in a seamless way to provide the biomedical professional with fast and efficient access to the right information at the right time.

A promising approach to information integration is based on the use of ontologies that act as a formalized inter-lingua onto which various data sources as well as processes can be mapped. An ontology is an explicit, formal specification of a shared conceptualization of a domain of interest as defined by Gruber (1993), where 'formal' implies that the ontology should be machine-readable and 'shared' that it is accepted by a community of stakeholders in the domain of interest. Ontologies represent the common knowledge of this community, allowing its members and associated automatic processes to easily exchange and integrate information as defined by this knowledge.

For instance, by mapping a database of patient radiology reports as well as publicly accessible scientific literature on related medical conditions onto the same ontological representation a service can be build that provides the biomedical professional with patient-specific information on up-to-date scientific research. Scenarios like these can however only work if data can be mapped to ontologies on a large-scale, which implies the automation of this process by automatic semantic annotation. As a large part of biomedical data is available only in textual form (e.g. scientific literature, diagnosis reports), such systems will need to have knowledge also of (multilingual) terminology in order to correctly map text data to ontologies.

This chapter is therefore concerned with the enrichment of ontologies with (multilingual) terminology. We describe an approach to enrich biomedical ontologies with WordNet (Fellbaum, 1998) synonyms for ontology class labels, as well as multilingual translations as provided by Wikipedia. A particular point of emphasis is on selecting the appropriate interpretation of ambiguous ontology class labels through sense disambiguation. Acquired synonyms and translations are added to the ontology by use of the LingInfo model, which provides an ontology-based lexicon model for the annotation of ontology classes with (multilingual) terms and their linguistic properties.

Related work to this chapter is on word sense disambiguation and specifically domain-specific word sense disambiguation as a central aspect of our algorithm lies in selecting the most likely sense for ambiguous labels on ontology classes. The work presented here is based directly on Buitelaar & Sacaleanu (2001) and similar approaches (McCarthy et al., 2004a; Koeling & McCarthy, 2007). Related to this work is the assignment of domain tags to WordNet synsets (Magnini & Cavaglia, 2000), which would obviously help in the automatic assignment of the most likely synset in a given domain – as shown in Magnini et al. (2001). An alternative to this idea is to simply extract that part of WordNet that is directly relevant to the domain of discourse (Cucchiarelli & Velardi, 1998; Navigli & Velardi, 2002).

However, more directly in line with our work on enriching a given ontology with lexical information derived from a semantic lexicon is presented in Pazienza and Stellato (2006). In contrast to Pazienza and Stellato (2006), the approach we present in this chapter uses a domain corpus as additional evidence for statistical significance of a synset.

Finally, some work on the definition of ontology-based lexicon models (Alexa et al., 2002; Gangemi et al., 2003; Buitelaar et al., 2006) is of (indirect) relevance to the work presented here as the derived lexical information needs to be represented in such a way that it can be easily accessed and used by natural language processing components as well as ontology management and reasoning tools.

There is also some work in the field of lexical semantics on linking lexical resources such as WordNet or FrameNet to general, upper model ontologies. Niles & Pease (2003) link WordNet to the Suggested Upper Merged Ontology (SUMO); Scheffczyk (2006) and Reiter (2007) link FrameNet, a resource containing event prototypes based on frame semantics, to the SUMO ontology.

LEXICAL ENRICHMENT OF BIOMEDICAL ONTOLOGIES WITH WORDNET

In this section we describe our approach in enriching a given ontology with additional lexial information (words) derived from a semantic lexicon such as WordNet. The assumption here is that an ontology represents domain knowledge with less emphasis on the words that can be associated with such knowledge objects, whereas a semantic lexicon such as WordNet rather defines words with less emphasis on the domain knowledge associated with these. An integration of both types of resources therefore seems appropriate and needed as outlined in the previous section.

Sense Disambiguation

A central aspect of our approach lies in the definition of a simple but effective sense disambiguation algorithm for selecting the appropriate interpretation of ambiguous ontology class. By ambiguous, we mean that the label of the ontology class appears in more than one synset in WordNet.

The sense disambiguation algorithm is shown in Figure 1. It iterates over every synonym of every synset in which the label of the ontology class appears. It calculates the χ^2 values of each synonym and adds them up for each synset.

χ^2 is often used as a measure of corpus similarity (Kilgariff & Rose, 1998). Its intuition is to look at corpora as random samples of the same population If they really were random samples, we would expect similar frequencies for most of the words. But as we know, corpora are not at all random samples. Especially if we compare a domain corpus with a reference corpus, we can expect the domain corpus to contain a lot of terms relatively much more often than reference corpus. These terms can be seen as domain terms.

We calculate the χ^2 scores according to Manning & Schütze (1999):

$$\chi^2 = \frac{N(O_{11}O_{22} - O_{12}O_{21})^2}{(O_{11} + O_{12})(O_{11} + O_{21})(O_{12} + O_{22})(O_{21} + O_{22})}$$

In this formula, O_{11} and O_{12} represent the frequencies of a term and of all other terms in a domain corpus, while O_{21} and O_{22} represent the frequencies of the same term and of all other terms in the reference corpus. N is the size of both the domain and reference corpus taken together. The χ^2 value then is higher when the token occurs relatively more often in the domain corpus than in the reference corpus.

The term "gum", for instance, has six noun senses with on average 2 synonyms. The χ^2 value of the synonym "gum" itself is 6.22. Since this synonym occurs obviously in every synset of the term, it makes no difference for the rating. But the synonym "gingiva", which belongs to the second synset and is the medical term for the gums in the mouth, has a χ^2 value of 20.65. Adding up the domain relevance scores of the synonyms for each synsets, the second synset gets the highest weight and is therefore selected as the appropriate one.

The algorithm as shown in Figure 1 uses the synonyms found in WordNet. Since WordNet contains a lot more relations than just synonymy,

Figure 1. Sense disambiguation algorithm

```
function getWeightForSet(set) {
        elements = all elements of set
          weight = 0
          foreach elem in elements
             c = chi-square(elem)
          weight = weight + c
          end foreach
          return weight
}

s = synsets to which t belongs
highest_weight = 0
best_synsets = {}
foreach synset in s
          synonyms = all synonyms of synset
          weight = getWeightForSet(synset)
          if (weight == highest_weight)
             best_synsets = best_synsets + { synset }
          else if (weight > highest_weight)
             best_synsets = { synset }
    end if
end foreach
return best_synsets
```

Figure 2. Improved sense disambiguation algorithm – as in Figure 1 but including WordNet relations

```
r = WordNet relations
s = synsets to which t belongs
highest_weight = 0
best_synsets = {}
foreach synset in s
          weight = getWeightForSet(synset)
          related = with r related synsets
          foreach rsynset in related
             weight += getWeightForSet(rsynset)
          end foreach
          if (weight == highest_weight)
             best_synsets = best_synsets + { synset }
          else if (weight > highest_weight)
             best_synsets = { synset }
          end if
end foreach
return best_synsets
```

we refined our algorithm to take other relations into account. Figure 2 shows the modified algorithm. The main difference is that we calculate and add the weights for each synonym of each synset to which a synset containing the ontology class label is related.

Lexical Enrichment of a Human Anatomy Ontology with WordNet

In an empirical experiment that was first described in Reiter and Buitelaar (2008), the Foundational Model of Anatomy (FMA) ontology has been enriched with lexical information (synonyms) derived from WordNet using a domain corpus of Wikipedia pages on human anatomy and the British National Corpus (BNC) as reference corpus. The FMA describes the domain of human anatomy in much detail by way of class descriptions for anatomical objects and their properties – see Rosse and Mejino Jr (2003) for details. Additionally, the FMA lists terms in several languages for many classes, which makes it a lexically enriched ontology already. However, our main concern here is to extend this lexical representation further by automatically deriving synonyms from WordNet.

The FMA consists of 120,417 classes. 1,631 of them have a direct counterpart in WordNet, which can be identified using the class label, 250 are polysemous and therefore their class labels occur in more than one synset. A vast majority of the remaining 118,786 ontology classes are multi-word expressions like "precentral branch of left first posterior intercostal artery", which cannot be expected to be included in WordNet. In Reiter and Buitelaar (2008) we therefore focused only on single word expressions.

In our current work we extend the algorithm presented in Reiter and Buitelaar 2008 with a head extraction heuristic. For expressions like "precentral branch of left first posterior intercostal artery", the WordNet synset "branch" seems to be appropriate. We use a simple heuristic to extract the head of the multiword expressions:

1. If the multi-word expression contains one or more prepositions, remove everything from the first preposition to the end, including the preposition itself.
2. Until the remaining string can be found in WordNet: Remove the first word (space-separated token).

Using this heuristic, we can, for instance, link the ontology class "lateral epicondyle of right femur" to the WordNet synset "lateral epicondyle". To be exact, we do not extract the syntactic head of the expression (at least not on purpose). In fact, we try to find a substring that is as long as possible and thus as specific (and as unambiguous) as possible but still included in WordNet. Nevertheless, this heuristic increases the number of classes whose (reduced) labels appear in more than one synset: In addition to the 250 labels that are already ambiguous, 79,761 of the multiword class labels are reduced to one of 581 ambiguous substrings. Overall, 582 different phrases and words need to be disambiguated.

Evaluation

Our benchmark (gold standard) for the disambiguation task consists of 50 randomly selected ontology classes with ambiguous labels. Four classes have been removed from the test set because none of their senses belong to the domain of human anatomy. The system was evaluated with respect to precision, recall and f-score. Precision is the proportion of the synsets predicted by the system that are correct. Recall is the proportion of correct synsets, which are predicted by the system. Finally, the f-score is the harmonic mean of precision and recall, and is the final measure to compare the overall performance of systems. We calculated precision, recall and f-score separately for WordNet relations and test items. The test item

Table 1. Evaluation results for the different WordNet relations, using the FMA ontology

Relation	Precision	Recall	F-Measure
Baseline (first sense)	58.7	46.6	51.9
Only Synonyms	56.3	60.7	58.4
Hypernym	65.2	53.1	58.5
Hypernym (instance)	54.0	54.2	54.1
Hyponym	62.3	56.0	59.0
Holonym (substance)	57.4	60.7	59.0
Holonym (part)	71.0	65.0	67.9
Meronym (member)	55.3	58.5	56.8
Meronym (substance)	55.1	56.3	55.7
Meronym (part)	63.6	66.1	64.8
Topic (domain)	58.5	62.9	60.6
All Other	56.3	60.7	58.4
Holonym (part), Meronym (part), Hypernym	80.4	66.1	72.6
Meronym (part), Holonym (part), Topic	73.2	67.2	70.1

"jaw", for instance, was manually disambiguated to the first or second noun synset containing the word "jaw". Our algorithm, using the hyponymy relation, returned only the first noun synset. For this item, we calculate a precision of 100% and a recall of 50%.

Results

Table 1 shows the results averaged over all 46 test items for the different relations. The relations not shown did not return other results than the algorithm without using any of the relations (results for "all other" are exactly the same as "only synonyms"). The two lines at the bottom of the table are combinations of relations. In the first line, we use the three relations with the highest precision together (hypernym, holonym (part) and meronym (part)). The last line shows the three relations with the highest recall taken together (topic, holonym (part) and meronym (part)).

Discussion

Our results show – in most configurations – a clear improvement compared to the baseline. Using just the synonyms of WordNet and no additional relation(s), we observe an increase in recall (around 15%) and a relatively small decrease in precision (around 2%). The increase in recall can easily be explained by the fact that our baseline takes only the first (and therefore: only one) synset – most of the terms are disambiguated to only one synset and therefore contribute a high recall only if the algorithm selects only one synset. Using only synonyms, however, the algorithm selects more than one synset in a number of cases.

This behavior also explains the decrease in precision. In several cases our algorithm is not able to decide which synset is the appropriate one – several synsets get the same weight and are therefore all returned. Obviously, a few of these synsets are not correct, thus decreasing the precision. The lemma "jaw", for instance, is contained in three different WordNet synsets. Unfortunately, none of them does contain additional synonyms; "jaw" is therefore the only lemma for which we can calculate □2 values. But since every synset does contain this lemma, every synset gets the same weight. Even if one of the synsets does contain more synonyms, they only contribute to our calculation of domain relevance scores if they are contained in the corpora. We are looking for positive evidence for the right synset – our algorithm is not equipped to deselect certain synsets based on the non-occurrence of synonyms in the corpus.

The vast majority of the 29 different WordNet relations lead to the same results than taking only synonyms, because only nine of them contribute to the set of lemmas for which we calculate relevance ratings. Most of the WordNet relations simply do not appear in our test set, these relations relate none of the synset in which an ontology class label is contained to another synset. The WordNet relations leading to the best results are holonymy (part) and meronymy (part) – this represents basically the part-of-relation in both directions. Intuitively, it is clear that using the part-of-relation increases the performance of our algorithm, since we can expect the parts or wholes of a thing to be in the same domain than the thing itself: The part holonym of one synset containing "elbow" is a synset containing "arm", which is contained in the corpora and in the ontology. Using parts and wholes, we find strong positive evidence for a given synset. It is interesting that the hypernymy relation also performed very well, because we cannot be sure in general that the hypernym synset belongs to the same domain than the original. The hypernym of a concept is usually more general than the concept itself and may be a generalization across domains. However, in our test set, the items seem to be so deep in the WordNet hierarchy, that the hypernym synset still belongs to the same domain. And since every synset has a hypernym, we get additional lemmas for every test item. It follows intuitively, that the combination of relations of already good discriminators further improves the results. We confirmed that expectation in the two lines at the bottom of Table 1.

We also investigated the general coverage of the different WordNet relations on our test set. Table 2 shows the number of lemmas that were included in the calculation of the relevance measure for each relation. The four relations that were used in combinations are highlighted. As the table shows, on average we look at 6.56 different lemmas for each term in question without using any

Table 2. Average number of lemmas per relation

Relation	Average Number of Lemmas
Only Synonyms	6.56
Hypernym	14.80
Hypernym (instance)	6.76
Hyponym	32.80
Holonym (substance)	6.66
Holonym (part)	9.76
Meronym (member)	6.74
Meronym (substance)	6.96
Meronym (part)	9.68
Topic (domain)	6.94

additional WordNet relations. The use of WordNet relations obviously increases the number of lemmas. However, the "richest" relation, hyponymy, is not the one that performed best. Using hyponymy increases the number of lemmas to 32.8. The performance measures reflect that increase to a certain extent: The precision increased when using hyponymy, but the recall decreased. This decrease is caused by the fact that the ranking calculated by the system is much clearer, when more lemmas are included – there are fewer cases in which two synsets are ranked equally. If more lemmas are included in the calculation of the summed fi 2 values it gets unlikelier that two synsets are assigned exactly the same score. The Topic relation adds only few new lemmas, but it seems that they have a very good influence on the relevance ranking. They seem to contribute high relevance ratings, such that the results improve in both precision and recall.

Our evaluation uses a very strict notion of recall. The benchmark set contains 14 ontology class labels with more than one associated synsets. A specific test item returns a recall of 100% only if all of the associated synsets are selected. The way the algorithm works, this is extremely hard. The algorithm generates a list of synsets that are ranked according to the added fi 2 values of all lemmas contained in or related with the synset. The only way to return two different synsets as appropriate for the ontology class is to assign them exactly the same weight and rank them equally on the first rank. Using the relation with the highest recall, this happened only in cases where lemmas were not found in a corpus and the set of lemmas used for the calculation is exactly the same for different synsets. On the other hand, it is generally questionable, whether the algorithm should select all synsets annotated in the benchmark, since some of these cases are caused by differences in granularity between WordNet and the FMA ontology. We therefore argue that precision is the important performance measure for this algorithm.

Lexical Enrichment of a Molecular Biology Ontology with WordNet

The Substance[1] ontology is part of the "Bio Tutorial" by the CO-ODE project and describes a selection of biochemical substances. The ontology contains 80 classes in a rather shallow hierarchy. WordNet contains a direct counterpart for 60 ontology class labels (4 of them are multi-word expressions), which can easily be looked up. Of the remaining 20 ontology class labels are 14 multi-word expressions. 13 of these multi-word expressions can be reduced to a substring contained in WordNet, using the head extraction heuristic as in the previous section. The algorithm is unable to find a matching WordNet lemma for a single multi-word expression and six single-word expressions. In total, our list of ontology class labels contains 73 labels that appear in WordNet, out of which 10 appear in more than one synset. In order to test our approach in a different scenario, we apply the same algorithm to this ontology. As a domain corpus, we use a number of Wikipedia pages from the category "Molecular Biology" and several sub categories, consisting of 485,580 tokens and 24,128 types.

Table 3 shows the results based on a manually annotated benchmark (all 10 ambiguous terms have been annotated). As the table shows, using only synonyms scores clearly below the baseline. This is due to the fact that we use a relatively small corpus, in which most of the synonyms just do not appear. Most of the WordNet relations do not score differently than using only synonyms, because they simply are not present in our sample. In these cases, we were not able to pick one specific synset and deselect the others, so all of the synsets are selected. This is why the precision (the proportion of synsets predicted by the system, which are correct) is lower than the baseline, while the recall (the proportion of correct synsets, which are predicted by the system) is relatively high.

Table 3. Evaluation results for the different WordNet relations, using the Substance ontology

Relation	Precision	Recall	F-Measure
Baseline (first sense)	50%	43.8%	46.7%
Only Synonyms	37.5%	62.5%	46.9%
Hypernym	43.8%	43.8%	43.8%
Hyponym	68.9%	68.9%	68.9%
Meronym (member)	31.2%	50.0%	38.5%
All Other	37.5%	62.5%	46.9%

The inclusion of three relations however produces other results than taking only the synonyms. We will now discuss them in some detail.

- **Meronym (member):** When using the meronym (member) (which is similar to "part-of") relation, precision and recall dropped even below the results of using only synonyms. The algorithm is able to make one additional decision (for the ontology class with the label "glycine"), but it is an inappropriate one. Using only synonyms, both synsets containing the lemma "glycine" were ranked equally, because the only other synonym, appearing in one synset containing "glycine", "genus_Glycine", is not contained in the domain corpus. But the meronym (member) relation relates this synset with the one containing the lemma "soybean" (among others). The synset gets selected because there are several occurrences of "soybean" in our corpus.
- **Hypernym:** Using hypernymy increases precision and decreases recall. This is basically what can be expected (and it is in line with the observations we made using the FMA ontology), because every synset has a hypernym, thus we include more lemmas in our calculation of domain relevance, resulting in an increased decisiveness. In fact, there are only two ontology classes, for which we still cannot decide between two synsets ("Purine" and "K").
- **Hyponym:** The hyponymy relation performs with almost 70% precision and recall by far best for this ontology and corpus. The lemma "alcohol", for instance, appears in two synsets. Using only synonyms, we cannot decide which one is the appropriate one. But if we include hyponyms, we include – for the correct synset – a lot of domain terms in our calculation (like "methanol", "amyl alcohol", …). For the incorrect synset, we include terms like "wine" or "liquor" which are clearly less important in our domain.

In general, we observe a relatively clear cut in our test data. For some test items, the algorithm presented above works reasonably well, but for others it does not. We assume that this is due to the fact that this ontology includes out-of-domain terms. In order to describe the behavior and properties of certain substances on a molecular level, the need for classes like (electrical) charge – with the subclasses positive, negative and neutral – is obvious. As the basic assumption of our approach is that the ontology classes in a domain ontology all belong to that domain, the algorithm is unable to cope with out-of-domain classes. Out-of-domain classes therefore significantly decrease the efficiency of the approach presented here.

Further, it can be argued that such classes should be defined in another ontology and imported through namespace mechanisms.

LEXICAL ENRICHMENT OF BIOMEDICAL ONTOLOGIES WITH WIKIPEDIA TRANSLATIONS

In this section, we present an approach to enrich ontologies with multilingual labels, i.e., with translations of ontology class labels in different languages. We use a completely automatic approach based on the inter-language links found in Wikipedia. Mediawiki, the software running the Wikipedia webpage, provides the facility to include so-called inter-language links. These are links, found directly in the page source, that link the article to an article in another language about the same concept. The article "Democracy" in the English Wikipedia is linked to the article "Demokratie" in the German Wikipedia, for instance. In the page source of the English article, we find the link [[de:Demokratie]].

There are two kinds of special pages in Wikipedia that we need to take into account: Redirect pages and disambiguation pages. Redirect pages simply redirect the user to another page. This is used to allow different spellings, synonyms or paraphrasing. On the pages "Chair (academic)" and "Prof", for instance, we find redirects to the page "Professor".

Wikipedia also contains disambiguation pages. They are used to differentiate meanings of a lemma. For the lemma "Corpus", for instance, Wikipedia knows ten different meanings, which are all described in a separate article. The disambiguation page lists the different meanings of a lemma and usually provides a short description (similar to the glosses in WordNet). Sometimes, disambiguation pages are marked in their title (as in "Chair (disambiguation)"), sometimes not (the page "Corpus"). All disambiguation pages include the template {{disambig}} in their source code, by which they can be identified.

Since the class labels of most ontologies are provided in English, we link the ontology classes to articles from the English Wikipedia (We use the Java Wikipedia API provided by Zesch et. al. (2007)). The initial linking is done straightforwardly, using the class labels of the ontology and some string preprocessing if necessary (class labels in the substance ontology are defined in CamelCase, for instance). While making the linking, the algorithm differentiates four different cases:

1. Wikipedia contains a page with that name and this page is neither a disambiguation nor a redirect page.
2. Wikipedia contains a page with that name, but it is a redirect page.
3. Wikipedia contains a disambiguation page with that name.
4. Wikipedia does not contain a page with that name.

Figure 3. General algorithm to assign an appropriate page to a ontology class

```
t = class label in the ontology
page = Wikipedia(t)
while(page.isRedirect()) {
   page = page.followRedirect()
}
if (! page.isDisambiguation()) {
   return page
} else {
   return page.disambiguation()
}
```

In the first case, we simply extract the inter-language links of the page found and attach the translations of the article title to the class. In the second case, we follow the redirect and extract the inter-language links of the article we were redirected to as translations. In principle, we would follow several redirects in a chain, but this case did not occur in our data. In the third case, we have to disambiguate between Wikipedia pages. We will describe our algorithm below. In the fourth case, we do nothing. Figure 3 shows the algorithm schematically in a pseudo object oriented syntax. In lines 3-5, we follow redirects as long as necessary. In lines 6-10, we distinguish between disambiguation and article pages. For simplicity, we do not show the handling of the fourth case here.

Disambiguation

In the following, we will take Wikipedia articles as sense descriptions and all the articles listed on a disambiguation page as the sense inventory for this lemma. Even though there are conceptual differences between the synsets used by WordNet and the articles written by Wikipedia contributors, both of them represent concepts and provide useful information to be included in an ontology. Furthermore, Mihalcea (2007) shows that Wikipedia articles provide a valid sense inventory for word sense disambiguation approaches.

Our disambiguation algorithm is shown in Figure 4. Here, we iterate over all links found in the page (lines 4-12). The gloss is extracted by heuristics and regular expressions for each link. It is then tagged with parts of speech using the

Figure 4. Basic disambiguation algorithm

```
function getWeightForSet(set) {
        elements = all elements of set
          weight = 0
          foreach elem in elements
            c = chi-square(elem)
          weight = weight + c
          end foreach
          return weight
}
method disambiguation() {
   weight = 0
   best_pages = {}
   foreach(page : page.getAllLinks()) {
      text = page.getGloss()
      nouns = text.getNouns()
      if (getWeightForSet(nouns) > weight) {
         best_pages = { page }
      } else if (getWeightForSet(nouns) == weight) {
         best_pages = best_pages + { page }
      }
   }
   return best_pages
}
```

TreeTagger (Schmid, 1994). The algorithm then calculates the domain relevance score for each noun, using the same method as described in section 2. Finally, we add up the domain relevance scores for each link and select the link with the highest domain relevance. We return the article defined by this link as the appropriate one.

Unfortunately, this rather simple approach has a major drawback: The glosses on disambiguation pages in Wikipedia are not very uniform. Some disambiguation pages contain a lot of glosses of different lengths, but some only contain the links themselves. In some cases, it is even very hard to actually extract the gloss, since the gloss itself contains another link. In general, the glosses are not reliable. In order to use the glosses in an automatic disambiguation approach, we would need them to be much more reliable.

We therefore modified our algorithm, such that we have more reliable texts to work with. Instead of using the half-sentence descriptions on the disambiguation pages, the first paragraph of the page itself is extracted. As first paragraph, everything between the start of the page and the first headline, marked by two equal signs (e.g. ==Classification== on the page "Epithelium") is used. The modified algorithm can be seen in Figure 5.

Using this heuristic, the number of lemmas on which the algorithm bases its relevance measure jumps for the FMA from 13.5 tokens per link (using only the glosses) to 344.9 tokens per link. For the Substance ontology, the number of tokens per link jumps from 16.0 to 398.6.

Again, the TreeTagger is used to identify the nouns in the first paragraph. Also, the same domain relevance score (□2) as before is applied. The algorithm retrieves a sorted list of links, from which it selects the highest weighted one.

Simple regular expressions can be used to extract the translations from the target article. At this point, additional information can naturally be extracted from the articles. We will point out several possibilities later in section 5.

Results for FMA and Substance Ontologies

The FMA ontology contains 120,409 classes. 4,665 of them have counterparts in Wikipedia of which 287 are disambiguation pages. Translations to 4,378 ontology classes of the FMA can

Figure 5. Refined disambiguation algorithm

```
method disambiguation() {
  weight = 0
  best_pages = {}
  foreach(page : page.getAllLinks()) {
    text = page.getFirstParagraph()
    nouns = text.getNouns()
    if (getWeightForSet(nouns) > weight) {
      best_pages = { page }
    } else if (getWeightForSet(nouns) == weight) {
      best_pages = best_pages + { page }
    }
  }
  return best_pages
}
```

be assigned by a simple lookup, without using any head extraction heuristics or disambiguation algorithms. On average, translations in 4.5 different languages can be attached to every ontology class. The rather low average number of inter-language links is caused by the fact that a lot of pages in the human anatomy domain are either stubs (incomplete pages) or do not exist in other languages. Since the inter-language links are not distributed uniformly across the different languages in which Wikipedia is available, it is possible to increase their coverage by triangulation, i.e., by viewing the inter-language links as relations and calculating their transitive closure. This has been done and evaluated by Wentland et al. (2008) for pages describing named entities, but we can expect this to work equally well for other kinds of Wikipedia pages.

Of the 80 classes in the substance ontology, 59 have a direct counterpart in Wikipedia, which is not a disambiguation page. 5 are ambiguous in the sense that the Wikipedia pages with their labels as titles are disambiguation pages. The remaining 14 classes have labels that cannot be found in Wikipedia. On average, every class label can be translated into 23 different languages. The majority of the labels can be translated in more than 20 languages, but there are a few concepts that have very few translations ("H2O" is translated in 7 languages, "Cerebroside" in only 3).

In order to evaluate this disambiguation approach, we manually disambiguate two test sets. For the FMA ontology, we randomly select 15 ontology classes whose labels link to disambiguation pages. We simply use all five ambiguous terms for the substance ontology. There are several items in both benchmark sets that are disambiguated to more than one appropriate Wikipedia article (On the disambiguation page for "Charge", for instance, we find both "Electric charge" and "Charge (physics)"). Since both of them represent to some extent an appropriate concept, we include both in the benchmark set. We count the portion of ontology classes that are successfully disambiguated to at least one appropriate Wikipedia page as accuracy measure.

FMA

The algorithm selects one of the appropriate articles for exactly two third of the ontology classes in the FMA test set (accuracy is 66.6%). We will now discuss a few cases in detail.

The algorithm selects the Wikipedia article "H-4 visa" for the ontology class labeled "H4". "H-4 visa" talks about the visa issued by the U.S. Citizenship and Immigration Service to immediate family members of holders of visa of some other kind. The appropriate article ("Histone H4") is ranked second. Unfortunately, the article about H-4 visa does not contain any headings, so the heuristic to extract the first paragraph fails and returns the complete article. This results in using four paragraphs of textual material for the visa page, as opposed to only one short paragraph for the histone H4. And since this algorithm does not take the number of nouns that are used to calculate the domain relevance score into account, the wrong page is selected.

Substance Ontology

We observe similar difficulties as before in the WordNet linking when linking the classes of the substance ontology to Wikipedia. Most of the ontology class labels are unambiguous, but the ambiguous ones are very general terms that do not perfectly fit in the domain of molecular biology. However, the algorithm is able to assign an appropriate Wikipedia article in 4 of the 5 test cases (80%).

The case where the algorithm is unable to assign an appropriate page is the class label "Charge". For "Charge", the highest ranked page is "Psychology". This is somewhat surprising, since psychology is of course not even a sense of the lemma "Charge". Unfortunately, the disambiguation pages in Wikipedia do not differentiate between the actual targets of the disambiguation and other, informative links. The disambiguation page for "Charge" contains over 30 different links, structured in several categories. Some of the category descriptions contain links like "Psychology" as a domain for the senses in this category (This can be seen in the version from July 5, 2007, 05:53, the version from April 2008 has changed and does not include this link). The algorithm is not capable to differentiate automatically between the senses of the ambiguous term and arbitrary links on the disambiguation page. We simply follow every link on the page and therefore include pages like "Psychology". The appropriate article "Electric charge", however, is ranked second.

REPRESENTING LEXICAL KNOWLEDGE IN ONTOLOGIES WITH LINGINFO

After the senses for an ambiguous term t have been ranked by the algorithms discussed above, we can select the top one or more to be included as (additional) lexical/terminological information in the ontology, i.e., the synonyms that are selected can be added as (further) terms for the ontology class c that corresponds to term t.

Here, we propose to extend the ontology with the ontology-based lexicon model LingInfo[2], which has been developed for this purpose in the context of previous work (Buitelaar et al., 2006). By use of the LingInfo model we will be able to represent each synonym for t as a linguistic object l that is connected to the corresponding class c. The object l is an instance of the LingInfo class of such linguistic objects that cover the representation of the orthographic form of terms as well as relevant morpho-syntactic information, e.g. stemming, head-modifier decomposition, part-of-speech.

The LingInfo model consists of the following main classes:

- The LingInfo class is the base class of the LingInfo model and is used to associate a term to a class in a domain ontology, e.g. the class Alcohol from the Substance ontology can be associated with the German term "Alkohol". Properties used are term, lang (language) and morphoSyntacticDecomposition (specified by one or more objects of class PhraseOrWordForm).
- The PhraseOrWordForm class is the superclass of all linguistic surface structures, whether phrasal ("muscular branch") or (un)inflected word forms ("branch", "branches").
- The Phrase class is a sub-class of the PhraseOrWordForm class and is used to describe the syntactic (phrasal) structure of complex terms such as "right third posterior intercostal artery".
- The WordForm class is a sub-class of the PhraseOrWordForm class and is used to describe the morphological structure of complex terms such as "third posterior intercostal artery".
- The InflectedWordForm class is a subclass of the WordForm class and is used to describe an inflected word form such as "hydrophilic". Properties that can be used include inflection (specified by one or more objects of class Affix) partOfSpeech, case, gender and semantics (specified by a backlink to a domain ontology class).
- The Stem class is a sub-class of the WordForm class and is used to describe a stem such as "hydrophile".

An example application of the model as used in Protégé editing of the lexically enriched version of the Substance ontology is shown in Figure 6.

We are currently working on the development of a complete lexical enrichment system that will allow for the automatic generation of LingInfo instances on the basis of the work presented in this chapter. The idea is to develop a service that

Figure 6. Application of the LingInfo model to the Substance ontology

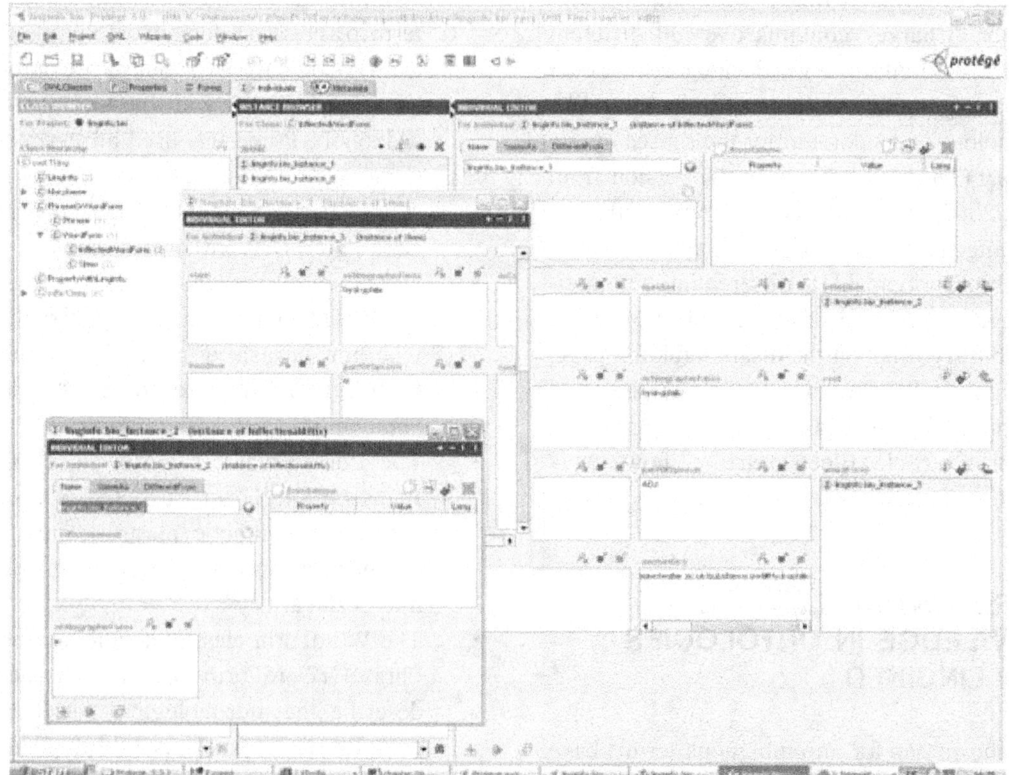

will be able to generate a LingInfo based lexicon for a given ontology, in combination with external resources such as WordNet, Wikipedia and possible others.

CONCLUSIONS AND FUTURE WORK

We presented a corpus-based approach to the lexical enrichment of ontologies, i.e. enriching a given ontology with lexical entries derived from a semantic lexicon. The presented algorithm extracts synonyms from WordNet and multilingual translations from Wikipedia. The main issue here is the disambiguation between different senses provided by WordNet, Wikipedia respectively. We therefore developed a domain-specific approach that exploits the statistical distribution of senses over domain corpora based on previous work. Our approach was empirically tested by a set of experiments on the disambiguation of ambiguous classes in two ontologies (the Foundational Model of Anatomy; the Substance ontology on biochemical substances) with WordNet and Wikipedia.

Results show that the approach performs better than a most-frequent sense baseline in the case of linking ontology class to WordNet synsets. Further refinements of the algorithm that include the use of WordNet relations such as hyponymy, hypernymy, meronymy etc. show a much improved performance, which again improve drastically by combining the best of these relations. In the case of linking ontology class to Wikipedia articles, the algorithm obtains a performance of over 60% and 80% accuracy on a sample of ambiguous class names in the FMA and Substance ontology respectively.

In summary, we achieved good performance on the defined tasks with relatively cheap methods. This will allow us to use our approach in large-scale automatic enrichment of biomedical and other ontologies with WordNet derived lexical information, i.e. in the context of the OntoSelect[3] ontology library and search engine. In this context, lexically enriched ontologies will be represented by use of the LingInfo model for ontology-based lexicon representation.

A detailed analysis of the algorithm presented above shows strengths and weaknesses of the approach. The algorithm performs very well in detecting synsets or articles from the domain of human anatomy or molecular biology, respectively. Linking ontology classes to Wikipedia articles, there are several cases in which this is not enough, because Wikipedia knows more than one different article that is part of the domain. In order to differentiate between multiple domain articles, the algorithm would need to do a more fine-grained analysis on both sides.

On the one hand, the algorithm as presented above makes very little use of the information encoded in the ontology. Apart from the subclass relation, mature ontologies such as the FMA contain a lot more information such as part-of, has-mass, sometimes non-English equivalents or even definitions. On the other hand, we would expect this information to be contained in the Wikipedia article about the concept. But by using very shallow frequency based domain relevance measures, the algorithm can only make little use of this information. Future work will therefore be concerned with a more fine-grained analysis of the ontologies and the WordNet and Wikipedia information. In a two-tiered approach, for instance, we would make a ranking based on shallow (and cheap) domain relevance measures in the first tier. An in-depth analysis of the candidates resulting from the first tier would then be used on top, in a second tier. Since in this tier we would have much less data to process, extensive processing such as deep parsing might be possible.

ACKNOWLEDGMENT

This research has been supported in part by the THESEUS Program in the MEDICO Project, which is funded by the German Federal Ministry of Economics and Technology under the grant number 01MQ07016. The responsibility for this publication lies with the authors. We thank Hans Hjelm of Stockholm University (Computational Linguistics Dept.) for making available the FMA term set and Thomas Eigner for making available the Wikipedia anatomy and biology corpora.

REFERENCES

Alexa, M., Kreissig, B., Liepert, M., Reichenberger, K., Rostek, L., Rautmann, K., Scholze-Stubenrecht, W., & Stoye, S. (2002). The Duden Ontology: An Integrated Representation of Lexical and Ontological Information. In K. Simov, N. Guarino, & W. Peters, (Eds.), Proceedings of the OntoLex Workshop at LREC (pp. 1-8). Spain.

Buitelaar, P., & Sacaleanu, B. (2001). Ranking and selecting synsets by domain relevance. In D. Moldovan, S. Harabagiu, W. Peters, L. Guthrie, & Y. Wilks, (Eds.), *Proceedings of the Workshop on WordNet and other Lexical Resources: Applications, Extensions and Customizations at NAACL*. Pittsburgh, U.S.A.

Buitelaar, P., Sintek, M., & Kiesel, M. (2006). A Lexicon Model for Multilingual/Multimedia Ontologies. In Y. Sure & J. Domingue (Eds.), *The Semantic Web: Research and Applications. Proceedings of the 3rd European Semantic Web Conference (ESWC).* Budva, Montenegro.

Cucchiarelli, A., & Velardi, P. (1998). Finding a domain-appropriate sense inventory for semantically tagging a corpus. *Natural Language Engineering, 4*(4), 325–344.

Fellbaum, C. (1998). WordNet. *An Electronic Lexical Database.* Cambridge, USA: MIT Press.

Gangemi, A., Navigli, R., & Velardi, P. (2003). The OntoWordNet Project: extension and axiomatization of conceptual relations in WordNet. In *Proceedings of ODBASE 2002.*

Gruber, T. R. (1993). A translation approach to portable ontology specifications. *Knowledge Acquisition, 5*(2), 199–220.

Kilgariff, A., & Rose, T. (1998). Measures for corpus similarity and homogenity. In *Proceedings of the 3rd Conference on Empirical Methods in Natural Language Processing* (pp. 46-52). Granada, Spain.

Koeling, R., & McCarthy, D. (2007). Sussx: WSD using Automatically Acquired Predominant Senses. *In Proceedings of the Fourth International Workshop on Semantic Evaluations* (pp. 314–317). Association for Computational Linguistics.

Magnini, B., & Cavaglia, G. (2000). Integrating subject field codes into WordNet. *In Proceedings of the International Conference on Language Resources and Evaluation* (pp. 1413–1418).

Magnini, B., Strapparava, C., Pezzulo, G., & Gliozzo, A. (2001). Using domain information for word sense disambiguation. *In Proceeding of Second International Workshop on Evaluating Word Sense Disambiguation Systems* (pp. 111–114).

Manning, C., & Schütze, H. (1999). *Foundation of Statistical Natural Language Processing.* Cambridge, MA.

McCarthy, D., Koeling, R., Weeds, J., & Carroll, J. (2004). Finding predominant senses in untagged text. *In Proceedings of the 42nd Annual Meeting of the Association for Computational Linguistics,* (pp. 280–287).

Mihalcea, R. (2007). Using Wikipedia for Automatic Word Sense Disambiguation. *In Proceedings of the North American Chapter of the Association for Computational Linguistics.* Rochester, U.S.A.

Niles, I., & Pease A. (2003). Linking Lexicons and Ontologies: Mapping WordNet to the Suggest Upper Merged Ontology. *In Proceedings of the Conference on Information and Knowledge Engineering.*

Pazienza, M., & Stellato, A. (2006). An environment for semi-automatic annotation of ontological knowledge with linguistic content. In Y. Sure & J. Domingue (Eds.), *The Semantic Web: Research and Applications. Proceedings of the 3rd European Semantic Web Conference (ESWC).* Budva, Montenegro.

Reiter, N. (2007). *Towards a Linking of FrameNet and SUMO.* Diploma thesis, Saarland University, Saarbrücken, Germany.

Reiter, N., & Buitelaar, P. (2008). Lexical Enrichment of a Human Anatomy Ontology using WordNet. In A. Tanács, D. Csendes, V. Vincze, C. Fellbaum, & P. Vossen, (Eds.), *Proceedings of the 4th Global WordNet Conference* (pp. 375-387). Szeged, Hungary.

Rosse C., & Mejino J. L. V. Jr (2003). A reference ontology for biomedical informatics: the foundational model of anatomy. *Journal of Biomedical Informatics, 36*(6), 478–500.

Schmid, H. (1994). Probabilistic Part-of-Speech Tagging Using Decision Trees. *In Proceedings of the International Conference on New Methods in Language Processing.* Manchester, United Kingdom.

Wentland, W., Knopp, J., Silberer, C., & Hartung, M. (2008). Building a Multilingual Lexical Resource for Named Entity Disambiguation, Translation and Transliteration. *In Proceedings of the 6th Language Resources and Evaluation Conference*. Marrakech, Morocco.

Zesch, T., Gurevych, I., & Mühlhäuser, M. (2007). Analyzing and Accessing Wikipedia as a Lexical Semantic Resource. In G. Rehm, A. Witt, & L. Lemnitzer (Eds.), *Data Structures for Linguistic Resources and Applications* (pp. 197-205), Tübingen, Germany.

ENDNOTES

1. http://www.co-ode.org/ontologies/bio-tutorial/sources/SUBSTANCE.owl
2. http://olp.dfki.de/LingInfo/
3. http://olp.dfki.de/ontoselect/

Chapter VIII
Word Sense Disambiguation in Biomedical Applications:
A Machine Learning Approach

Torsten Schiemann
Humboldt-Universität zu Berlin, Germany

Ulf Leser
Humboldt-Universität zu Berlin, Germany

Jörg Hakenberg
Arizona State University, USA

ABSTRACT

Ambiguity is a common phenomenon in text, especially in the biomedical domain. For instance, it is frequently the case that a gene, a protein encoded by the gene, and a disease associated with the protein share the same name. Resolving this problem, that is, assigning to an ambiguous word in a given context its correct meaning is called word sense disambiguation (WSD). It is a pre-requisite for associating entities in text to external identifiers and thus to put the results from text mining into a larger knowledge framework. In this chapter, we introduce the WSD problem and sketch general approaches for solving it. The authors then describe in detail the results of a study in WSD using classification. For each sense of an ambiguous term, they collected a large number of exemplary texts automatically and used them to train an SVM-based classifier. This method reaches a median success rate of 97%. The authors also provide an analysis of potential sources and methods to obtain training examples, which proved to be the most difficult part of this study.

INTRODUCTION

Ambiguity, i.e., words with multiple possible meanings, is a common phenomenon in natural languages (Manning & Schütze 1999). Which of the different meanings of a word is actually meant in a concrete text depends on the context the word appears in and cannot be judged based only on the appearance of the word itself. For instance, the terms 'sin' and 'soul' both are common English words – but they are also names of proteins. If a person only sees one of these two words on a piece of paper, he cannot decide which of the two meanings (or senses) the paper tries to convey. However, given a phrase such as "Salvation from sins", humans immediately recognize the correct sense of the ambiguous word.

From a linguistics point of view, the term ambiguity in itself has different senses. The most common form is homonymity, that is, words that have multiple, possibly unrelated meanings. 'Sin' and 'soul' both are homonyms. However, there are also more complex forms of ambiguity, such as polysemy, which describes cases where a word has different yet closely related senses. Examples in the life sciences are identical names for a gene, the protein it encodes, and the mRNA in which it is transcribed.

Word sense disambiguation (WSD) is the problem of assigning to an ambiguous term in

Figure 1. Screenshot of the Ali Baba main window after searching PubMed for the term 'soul'. Colored boxes represent biological entities. One can see that various Meanings of 'soul' are intermixed in the display – mentioning of the immortal soul by the Greek poet Homer, results from a large international study called 'Heart and Soul', and facts describing the protein 'soul'.

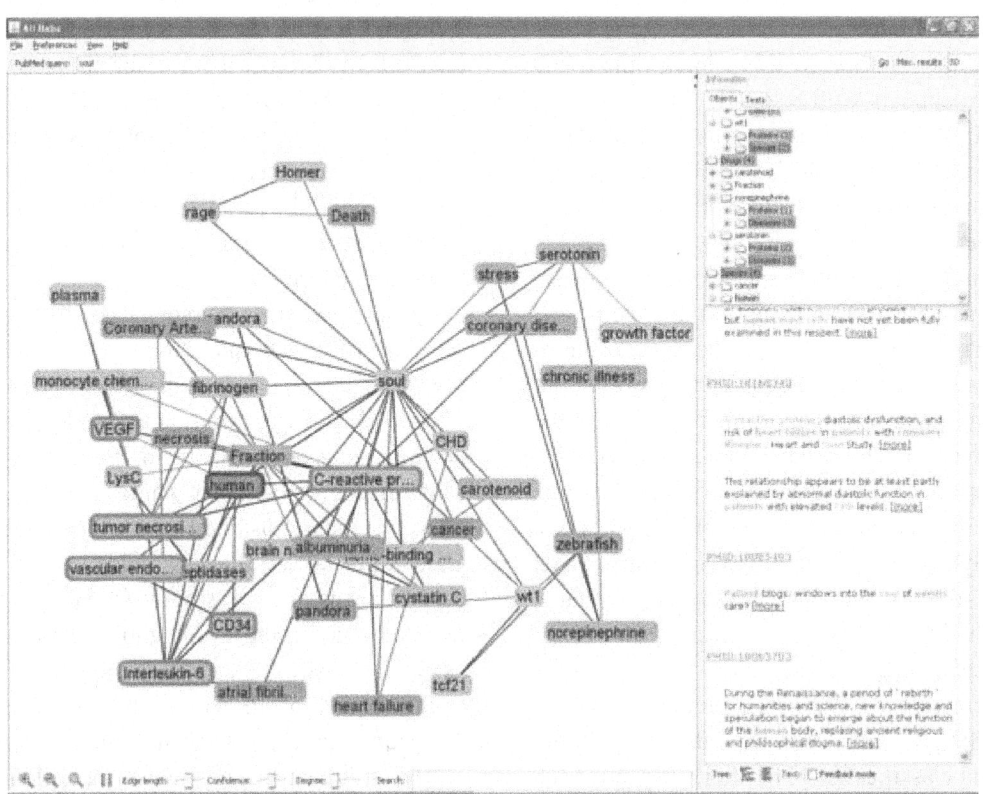

a given context its correct sense (Ide & Veronis 1998). Although humans usually have no problem in disambiguating terms, the problem is challenging for computers due to the necessity to capture the context of a word in a text, which, in general, not only encompasses the preceding and following words, but also background knowledge on the different senses of the word that might apply in the topic of the text. Obviously, WSD is the more difficult the more related the different senses are. It should be rather simple to distinguish the senses *mtg gene* and *particular tube announcement* of the term 'mind the gap', but much more difficult to tell the senses *gene* and *drug* from the term 'oxytocin'.

However, solving the WSD-problem is a prerequisite for high-quality named entity recognition and, in particular, entity normalization (Leser & Hakenberg 2005, Cohen 2005). As an example, consider the AliBaba system described in (Plake et al. 2005). AliBaba extracts occurrences of cells, diseases, drugs, genes/proteins, organisms, and tissues from PubMed abstracts using class-specific dictionaries. In this context, the WSD problem appears with terms that are contained in multiple dictionaries, and whose occurrences therefore indicate entities from different classes. Note that such terms are more frequent than one might expect. In a small study, we found 175 terms indicating both a species and a protein, 67 terms indicating a drug and a protein, and 123 terms indicating a cell and a tissue. Furthermore, names of biological entities often are homonym with common English word, like the above mentioned 'sin' and 'soul', but also terms such as 'black', 'hedgehog', or 'mind the gap', which are all names of genes in Drosophila (see http://flybase.bio.indiana.edu/). Some terms even appear in more than two classes, such as 'dare', which may indicate a *protein*, an *organism*, or the English verb.

There are three classical approaches to tackle the WSD problem: Clustering, dictionary look-ups, and classification. The clustering approach gathers all occurrences of an ambiguous word and clusters them into groups, with the hope that each cluster eventually will represent one sense. Its advantage is that no external resources are necessary, but only the problematic passages. However, clustering does not provide sense tagging, i.e., it is not able to tag a word with one of a set of predefined senses; instead, it discovers senses. In a sense, it can tell were problematic words are, but it cannot really help to resolve the problem automatically. Dictionary-based methods rely on the existence of a dictionary of senses, where each sense is explicitly described in some way, such as an explanatory text or an example. Such descriptions can be matched with the textual context of an ambiguous word. Though intuitively appealing, this method has the drawback that such dictionaries do not exist in specialized domains such as the Life Sciences – there simply is no dictionary describing all senses of gene symbols. Finally, the classification-based approach gathers many examples for all senses of an ambiguous term and learns a model from those, which is later used to predict a sense for ambiguous occurrences. This approach is the most beneficial in targeted information extraction, where both the set of ambiguous terms is fixed and the different senses are fixed. However, the problem remains to gather sufficient examples for each sense of a problematic term.

We present in this chapter the results of a study on WSD using a classification approach based on the one--sense--per--discourse assumption (Gale et al. 1992). This assumption says that, whenever an ambiguous term appears multiple times in the same discourse (abstract, paragraph, text, etc.), all occurrences most likely share the same sense. Gale et al. showed that this holds in 98% of all cases. For instance, it is not very likely to find a text that contains the term 'lamb' both in its sense as *species* and in its second sense, the abbreviation of the *gene* "laminin subunit beta-1 precursor". Consequently, one can use the entire discourse of a term as indicator for its sense. We build on this observation by learning a model for word senses from entire texts. Given an ambiguous term with unknown sense, we use an SVM to classify the term to its sense using the model learned before. In our study, we achieved a median success rate of 93.7% on 304 terms. We also discuss several extensions of the method. For instance, we show that an enrichment of the training set using abstracts from different terms of the same sense not only increases the reach of the method, but also considerably improves its performance.

The rest of this chapter is organized as follows. In the next section, we give a short introduction into the problem of word sense disambiguation and highlight its impact for natural language processing in the Life Sciences. Classical approaches to solving the problem are presented with their strength and weaknesses. In Section 3 we present our own classification approach to the WSD-problem. We describe and evaluate the method in detail and specifically focus on how a sufficient set of examples to learn from can be obtained. We conclude the chapter in Section 4.

In the remainder of this chapter, we use the following notations. A word in single quotation marks ('cancer') refers to an ambiguous term as it might be encountered in a text. Words in double quotation marks refer to compounds words or short text snippets ("posterior vena cava"). Words in italics refer to a sense (*disease*), which is usually one out of many possibilities. Exceptions (e.g., data shown in tables) will be indicated in the text.

WORD AMBIGUITY IN THE LIFE SCIENCES

In this section, we give a brief introduction into word ambiguity and approaches to word sense disambiguation. More specifically, we focus on lexical ambiguity, i.e., ambiguous terms, where a term is a semantic unit in a text. A term may be single word or a sequences or words. For instance, a gene name is considered as a term, even though it comprises multiple tokens. For other forms of ambiguity, such as ambiguous parses of a sentence ("The man saw the woman with the telescope" – who has the telescope?), see, for instance, Manning & Schütze (1999) or Hausser (2001).

Ambiguity of Terms

Terms that have multiple possible senses are called ambiguous. Word sense disambiguation is about assigning to an ambiguous term its correct senses in a given context, such as a sentence or a paragraph. Ambiguity of terms is very common in natural language; if one thinks long enough, the majority of English words (at least nouns) are ambiguous. The different senses may be semantically far apart, such as 'bass' – a *particular species* and *class of sounds*, or closely related, such as the many meanings of 'title' – a *header* for a book or film, a *legal ownership*, or the *document stating a legal ownership*. Ambiguity may also span word classes, such as 'bank' – a *financial institute* and a *verb indicating support* for someone. Finally, there may be many more than just two senses for a term. For instance, the Oxford Dictionary lists ten different senses of the term 'take' as a verb, and another three as a noun.

Ambiguous terms are generally called homonyms. Homonyms that derive from the same lemma are called polysemes. Other forms of ambiguity include metonymy, which are terms that can be used both in a direct and a metaphoric form (like "Hannibal sieged Rome" -- obviously, Rome was not sieged by Hannibal himself, but by his troops), and real metaphors (like "I get it", meaning that I understood something). Another frequent source of ambiguity is abbreviations, i.e., acronyms abbreviating a long term. In general, one distinguishes between common, generally accepted acronyms (such as AIDS), and local acronyms which are introduced once in a text to enable a more concise style of writing. According to a study by Liu et al (2002), more than 80% of all abbreviations that are encountered in Medline are ambiguous, i.e., the same abbreviation is used for different long forms. Acronyms for genes are often polyseme, depicting the gene in itself, the protein a gene encodes, and the mRNA which is the result of transcription of this gene. For genes showing differential splicing, the very same name may even represent all existing splice forms, i.e., a set of different proteins.

Two further observations are important for any approach to solve the WSD problem. First, as highlighted by Gale et al. (1992), multiple occurrences of an ambiguous term in a given context usually all have the same sense. This is called the "One sense per discourse" assumption (OSPDA). Using this assumption greatly facilitates WSD, because one may use all occurrences of a term in a text to resolve its one sense, i.e., one is able to use more context, indications, and evidences to tell senses apart. However, it is in general not clear what a discourse or a context exactly is. Surely, the OSPDA usually holds within scientific abstracts, but it is not clear if it still holds when extending the scope to full papers.

The second observation is that even humans sometimes do not agree in sense disambiguation. Several studied reported a surprisingly low inter-annotator agreement for various flavors of the WSD task (Ng et al. 1999, Veronis 1999). As a consequence, evaluating WSD approaches is not trivial, as it usually depends on hand-annotated gold standard corpora. Such corpora should always come along with a measure of the inter-annotator agreement during its creation. However, this disagreement is the higher the more similar two senses are from a semantic point-of-view.

Approaches to Solving the WSD Problem

There are three main approaches to solving the WSD problem: (a) the knowledge-based approach using definitions of senses, (b) the classification-based approaches using examples of, and (c) the clustering-based approach which helps to find different senses. In the following, we shortly explain each of these methods; for more details, see, for instance, Agirre & Edmonds (2006). We assume that we are trying the associate an ambiguous term T to one of its senses, where T is contained at least once in a document D.

Knowledge-Based WSD

The knowledge-based approach, also called dictionary-based WSD, depends on the existence of a machine readable dictionary containing descriptions of all senses of an ambiguous term. Tagging the sense of T then works a follows. First, extract a local context of T in D. This could be a window of N words around T, or the sentence or paragraph containing T. Next, match all words in this context against all words in the definition of the different senses, one sense after the other. Assign T the sense where the context matches best its definition. Therein, matches between two sets of words are usually performed using cosine distance of the vector representation of the words or the Jaccard coefficient (see later in this chapter for details). Usually, it is beneficial to first stem all words. Further improvements are possible when the senses of occurrences of T in a document are considered together, i.e., by exploiting the OSDP assumption. Finally, it is also possible to match the senses of all different terms in a document together, since these senses usually will be semantically close to each other. This approach is called sense chaining (Galley & McKeown 2003).

The main drawback of this approach is that it assumes a high-quality and complete dictionary. While such dictionaries exist for common English (e.g. the Oxford Dictionary etc.), the situation is different for Life Science – specific terms. In such cases, less stringent resources such as UMLS may help, as they can also provide semantically close words for a given sense. However, for highly productive areas, such as genes and proteins, where new terms (= gene names) are invented all the time, a knowledge-based approach is hard to follow.

Classification-Based WSD

In this approach, also called supervised WSD, the problem is perceived as a classification task: Classify T in D to one of its potential senses using any of the many existing classification algorithms, such as decision trees, naïve Bayes, or Support Vector Machines (see, for instance, Mitchell (1997)). We shall describe one such method in detail in Section 3 of this chapter, and therefore only give a very short account here. In general terms, classification-based WSD works as follows. First collect a set of documents which contain T such that the particular sense of T is known. From the set of examples for each sense, learn a model for the sense; this could be as simple as counting the distribution of word frequencies in each example set to complex statistical methods. Given a new occurrence of T in a document D, we compare the sense models with the context of T in D and assign to T that sense whose model fits best.

Given a sufficient number of examples for each sense, classification-based WSD usually achieves very good accuracy and therefore is the method of choice in most applications. However, collecting many pre-classified examples is a laborious and expensive task. To collect such examples automatically, one has to cope with the problem that for each example the sense must be assured; thus, performing a simple full-text search is not enough.

While the number of examples is of outstanding importance, the particular choice of a classifier method is not; usually, the differences in accuracy are only small. Lee & Ng (2002) performed an exhaustive empirical study of different learning algorithms and knowledge sources applied to WSD on the well established Senseval data sets (http://www.senseval.org). They showed that support vector machines using part-of-speech information on the ambiguous term, surrounding words, collocations and syntactic relations as input outperformed other methods, but often only by a few percent. This best system yielded 79.2% accuracy on the Senseval-2 data set. For this reason, we also chose to use SVMs as the learning algorithm in our experiments. Furthermore, combining different classifiers into ensembles has proven to improve sense-tagging accuracy (Florian & Yarowsky, 2002).

Clustering-Based WSD

Clustering-based or unsupervised WSD is different from the previous two methods because it actually doesn't really solve the WSD problem. Instead, it is a method to detect senses from examples, rather than deciding which sense a particular occurrence of T should have. It works as follows: Given a set of examples of texts each containing a particular term T, cluster those into groups of similar texts. Any text clustering method, such as hierarchical clustering or k-Means clustering, are applicable. The distance measure between two texts which is necessary for clustering may, again, use cosine distance or the Jaccard coefficient (or any other). As a result, each cluster should contain only occurrences of T with the same sense; i.e., there should emerge as many clusters as senses for T exist.

The distinctive feature of clustering-based WSD is that one does not have to predefine the set of potential senses for each term. However, as already said, it doesn't directly help to assign a sense to a term, though the clusters may be seen as examples and thus may be used to train a classifier in a second step. The problem with this approach is that the clusters usually are not good enough to result in a high-quality classifier. Furthermore, to actually assign a sense, one also need to chose a name for each cluster, which is a very difficult task for a computer.

WSD IN LIFE SCIENCE TEXTS

Term ambiguity is a problem both for general language and for domain-specific languages, such as that used in the Life Sciences. A text in this domain typically mentions many concepts and objects that are not usually used in English texts, such as genes and proteins, diseases, chemical objects, highly specialized biological terms to describe gene function and biological processes, etc.

The number of such objects is actually quite large. For instance, there are approximately 20,000 genes in the human genome, many of which have a name that is formed by common English words. Most of these genes have an extensive set of synonyms or terms depicting closely related objects, such as a UniGene cluster. About the same number of genes exist in mice, but names are often shared with human (and other mammal) genes. The fruit fly Drosophila has approximately 18,000 genes, which often are named after a particular phenotype found in evolutionary studies (Brookes 2001). Since such studied have a century-long tradition, fly gene names often are quite old and tend to use more common English names than in mouse or humans. There are also many gene names from other organisms which use English terms, although the majority of gene names still are artificial, encoding, e.g., the chromosomal location of a gene or number of EST clusters which gave first hints to the existence of a gene. However, genes are only a small fraction of all specialized terms. Another class of domain-specific words consists of scientific terms, such as those collected in biomedical ontologies, such as the Gene Ontology (Gene Ontology Consortium 2001) or the Mammalian Phenotype Ontology (Smith et al. 2005). Finally, large collections of biomedical terms, such as UMLS, comprise Millions of terms, many of which are highly specialized and rarely used in texts others than scientific publications. To add the problem, these collections might themselves contain ambiguous terms: UMLS itself contains more than 8000 terms with more than one meaning.

Thus, when domain-specific jargon comes into play, one may differentiate between different types of ambiguity: (1) Ambiguity between common English terms, (2) ambiguity between the domain-specific terms, and (3) ambiguity between common English and domain-specific terms. In this work, we only consider the latter two cases, as these are specific to the domain we study.

Approaching the WSD problem for Life Science texts to our knowledge has first been pursued by the MetaMap project (see Aronson 2006). Later, a number of systems for solving the WSD problem have been proposed in the biomedical and other domains (see Schuemie et al. 2005) for a detailed overview). Gaudan et al. (2005) presented a system for disambiguating abbreviations occurring in PubMed abstracts. Their method automatically builds a dictionary of abbreviation/sense--pairs. For each abbreviation with different senses, they train a Support Vector Machine (SVM) that takes the context of each instance as input. The system yielded a precision of 98.9% for a recall of 98.2% (98.5% accuracy). Andreopoulos et al. (2007) tackled the problem of Gene Ontology terms that also have a different, non-GO sense, such as 'development' or 'spindle' – i.e., problems of type (3) from the classification above. They compared different methods using clustering and co-occurrence graphs. Depending on the term, precision was between 82% and 93% at recall levels of 75% and 92%, respectively. Widdows et al. (2003) compared several knowledge-based methods using the UMLS metathesaurus. Their best system yielded a precision of 79%. Leroy and Rindflesch (2004) evaluated a naïve Bayes classifier on the disambiguation of words from the UMLS WSD corpus (see later in this section). They selected the 15 terms for which the most frequent sense was correct in less than 65% of the instances, and tested each using eight different input data, such as main word, part-of-speech tag, and phrase type. Using all semantic types, their averaged accuracy for all 15 terms was 66%, a 10%-increase compared to the baseline (voting for the sense the majority of all respective instances shared.).

Some specialized approaches, dealing with the disambiguation of gene names (also called gene mention normalization) have also been proposed (for an overview, see Morgan et al. 2008). In many cases, disambiguation based on known synonyms and string similarity measures provides good results already (Fundel & Zimmer, 2007). However, best performance can be achieved only when including the local context of an ambiguous gene name (see, for instance, Hakenberg et al. 2008). Results for gene mention normalization currently range from 80 to 90% in f-measure when restricted to a single species (e.g., only human genes), and 80% for the inter-species problem. Farkas (2008) presented an approach based on a co-authorship network of publications as the single type of knowledge. The assumption underlying this approach is that most researchers in the biomedical field study only a few genes or diseases during their career; every publication they write will thus likely deal with one of these genes (although they might use different names over time) and unlikely with a completely different gene having the same name. Although the coverage of the method usually is low, a precision above 95% can be achieved.

There are also a couple of works which tackled polysemy. Hatzivassiloglou et al. (2001) tested a naïve Bayes classifier, decision trees, and a rule-based approach to tell apart names referring to proteins, genes, and mRNA. They reached 75% for gene/protein and 67% for gene/mRNA disambiguation using an automatically derived corpus. An SVM-based approach for the disambiguation of proteins and genes was described by Pahikkala et al. (2005), reaching 85.5% accuracy on a data set of 2000 abstracts.

A CLASSIFICATION-BASED APPROACH TO THE WSD PROBLEM

"WSD is essentially a task of classification: word senses are the classes, the context provides the evidence, and each occurrence of a word is assigned to one or more of its possible classes based on the evidence" (Agirre & Edmonds 2007). Classification, as a supervised approach, relies on labeled examples as input for training models. In the case of word sense disambiguation, labeled examples are text fragments containing an ambiguous terms and labels are possible senses of a term. Note that it is necessary to train one classifier per ambiguous term. Usually, such labeled samples are provided by human domain experts; see, for instance, the collection of examples for 50 biomedical terms provided by Weeber et al. (2001). In this chapter, we present a method which does not rely on costly human annotation of texts. Thereby, we can treat WSD on a much larger scale than when we would rely on annotated corpora, few of which are available. Furthermore, circumvent the problem of the typical low inter-annotator agreement in WSD tagging (see Section 2.1). As an example, Hatzivassiloglou et al. (2001) reported that the inter-annotator agreement in between three experts was only 78% for telling the senses "mRNA" and "gene".

In this section, we first present an overview of (text) classification in the biomedical domain. We continue with a description of our methods to automatically collect a labeled data set for an arbitrary set of biomedical terms of a fixed set of classes. We evaluate our system on test sets derived from these data, and present quantitative and qualitative results.

Introduction to Classification in Biomedical Text Mining

Classification algorithms work on sets of features describing the objects to be classified. To be applied to textual objects, text fragments must be transformed into feature sets. This is usually accomplished by considering each possible word in a corpus as one feature. Words here can be single tokens or compound words (if previously identified as such). Most often, a bag-of-words semantic is used, i.e., the order of words in a text is ignored. Features can be binary (word present or not) or weighted using word frequency counts (TF, term frequency), possibly normalized with the frequency of a word in the overall data set (resulting in TF*IDF, where IDF is the inverse document frequency). TF*IDF gives high weights to words that occur often in a text, but not very often in the whole collection, the idea being that such words are highly representative for this text. Words can also be replaced (or augmented) with higher level concepts: on the one hand, these can be word stems or lemmas; on the other hand, these can be concepts derived from hierarchical terminologies or ontologies. Consider, for example, the words `drug' and `drugs'. A straight-forward implementation of a bag-of-words feature set would map them to two different features. Reduction to the word stem `drug' helps to i) reduce the dimensionality of the feature space, ii) map different word forms to the same feature, adjusting their weights, and iii) map different word forms occurring in different texts to the same feature.

Based on such a representation of a label corpus, classification algorithms, such as Naïve Bayes, decision tree induction, Support Vector Machines, or Nearest Neighbor classifiers, learn models of the data which they can later use to classify unlabeled texts. We will not discuss machine learning techniques in this section; see, for instance, (Mitchell 1999). Classification of text has, apart from WSD, various applications in the biomedical domain. We describe three of them for illustration.

First, Poulter et al. (2008) presented the MScanner system which supports information retrieval. It essentially classifies all Medline abstracts as relevant or not, given a set of relevant documents. Users of the system thus build their own `classifier' by providing a set of input documents. MScanner achieves a precision of up to 92%, depending on the task and size of the input, and retrieves results from currently 17 million abstracts in less than two minutes.

Second, the BioCreative 2 challenge included a task for classifying biomedical abstracts as to whether or not they contain evidence for protein-protein interactions (Krallinger & Valencia 2007). Among 19 different methods proposed for this task, top-scoring systems achieved an f-score of 78% (75% accuracy). Among the best systems was the one by Lan et al. (2007), which investigated different text representations (which terms should become features) and weighing schemes. Using 900 features weighted by TF*RF (Lan et al. 2006) proved the best combination, resulting in an f-score of 78%.

Third, classification can be used to rank documents for containment of evidence for annotating genes with Gene Ontology terms (http://www.geneontology.org/). This task, which was put as a challenge in the TREC Genomics track (http://ir.ohsu.edu/genomics/), simulates a part of the curation process for biological databases usually performed by human experts, scanning documents for evidence for annotations. The system by Camous et al. (2007) achieved significant improvements in classification accuracy for this task by not only considering words as features, but also other types of information which is derived from the text using semantic analysis. In particular, they used the MeSH vocabulary and its inter-concept relationships to represent documents, thus extending existing MeSH annotations of Medline articles. For instance, an existing annotation "Neoplastic Process" would lead to adding the annotation "Neoplasm" as a higher level concept. Using support vector machines as classifier, this enrichment improves performance by about 17% to 58% in the normalized utility value, U_{norm} (f-score of up to 40%), as compared to the baseline (original annotations only). The system was at TREC with a test set consisting of 6043 documents with 518 positive instances. The task is to

General Description of the Method

The first step in classification-based approaches is to identify the set of ambiguous terms. For each combination of an ambiguous term and one of its senses, texts that function as labeled examples have to be collected. We propose strategies to automatically collecting likely positive and likely negative samples of different levels of reliability. Using this collection, a binary classifier is trained for each sense of each term. To assess the performance of the classifier, the collection can be split into training and test sets, and evaluation carried out with cross-validation. In this section, we describe each of these steps in more detail.

Identification of Ambiguous Terms

In our study, we distinguish between terms from six classes of biomedical entities: *cells*, *diseases*, *drugs*, *organisms*, *proteins*[1] and *tissues*. As many terms of objectes of those classes are also *common* English words, we included "common" as 7th class or sense. For each sense, we compiled a dictionary of all known members according to a number of databases/vocabularies (see Table

Table 1. Sources for terms from each entity class. The last column contains the number of terms in each class.

Sense	Source	Field	Count
Cell	MeSH, tree A11	Heading, entry term	1,074
Disease	MeSH, tree C	Heading, entry term	18,100
Drug	MedlinePlus	Entry name, brand names, other names	14,177
Species	NCBI Taxonomy	Entry name, synonym, common names	208,143
Protein	UniProt/SwissProt	Protein/gene names, synonyms	234,497
Tissue	MeSH, tree A10	Heading, entry term	595
Common English	British Nat. Corpus	most frequent words	7,700

Table 2. Numbers of terms contained in two classes

	Cell	Disease	Drug	Species	Protein	Tissue	Common	Sum
Cell		5	2	0	0	123	0	130
Disease	5		5	18	4	3	3	37
Drug	2	5		9	67	1	15	99
Species	0	8	9		175	4	38	239
Protein	0	4	67			2	55	300
Tissue	123	3	1	4	2		2	134
Common	0	3	15	38	55	2		108

1). The set of English words was based on the most frequent common English words (Leech et al. 2001).

To identify terms contained in more than one dictionary, i.e., to find ambiguous terms, we compared all entries to each other allowing for minor spelling variations. This means that we also treat such terms as ambiguous that have slight syntactic differences, for instance, singular/plural variations and capitalization. The reason for the inclusion of spelling variations is that we later need to identify entity names in text (before disambiguating them) using a so-called dictionary tagger. Those taggers usually allow for minor variations in entity names to cope with ad-hoc spelling variations, which may lead to ambiguity. For instance, the *protein* name `Thi' becomes critical only in its artificial plural form, `This', which resembles a *common* English word. The *organism* `Dares' could be confused with the gene name (*protein*) `dare' or the *common* words `dare' and `dares'. However, allowing for these variations in general helps a dictionary tagger to recognize a larger amount of mentions (higher recall). Altogether, our data set contains 531 ambiguous terms. Table 2 shows the number of ambiguous terms between each pair of classes.

Collection of Samples

Rich sources for finding textual examples for each term and each of its senses are the Medline citation index for biomedical terms, and the Reuters corpus for common English words (http://about.reuters.com/researchandstandards/corpus/). We used two different methods to collect examples for term/sense pairs. One was based on known synonyms (Synsets), and the other on local explanations (see below). Both methods work completely automatic and identify samples for each sense of each term with high accuracy. In addition, sometimes manually curated texts for each term and sense are available, for instance, descriptions of a drug from MedlinePlus.

Synsets

The first way to identify occurrences of given senses of terms was to search for texts containing unambiguous synonyms. If such a text was found, we assigned it to the original term for the corresponding sense, although it does not in itself contain the original term. Consider the term `cat', which has distinctive sets of synonyms for each respective sense:

- *organism*: Felis domesticus, Felis silvestris catus, Felis catus, feline, felid, domestic cat
- *protein*: chloramphenicol acetyltransferase, catB, catB2, catB7, catD, catP, catQ, Cat-86, carnitine acetyltransferase, CrAT, CAT2, YCAT

If a text contained at least one of the synonyms (and none of the synonyms of the other sense), we added it to the positive training examples for either *organism* or *protein.*

Local Explanations

The second method to obtain training examples searches for locally resolved abbreviations or explanations. We consider local resolutions of the form "unambiguous synonym (term)" or "term (unambiguous synonym)". These forms occur, for instance, in cases where an abbreviation for a long term is defined, such as in "chloramphenicol acetyltransferase (CAT)". Other examples are enumerations with alternatives, like "posterior vena cava of a rabbit (cat)", or explanations, like "dog, fox, cat (Carnivora)". We checked whether the bracketed expression matched one of our ambiguous terms and whether the term before the brackets matched one of the synonyms known for this term and its senses, or vice versa. We used all other terms within the same sense and their respective synonyms as synonyms for the current term.

As we will show later in this chapter, we use a machine learner (SVM) to model the texts available for each term and sense pair. Using synsets and local explanations constitute (simple but effective) approaches to WSD in themselves. Thus, a bias may be introduced where the learner learns to imitate the methods for collecting the data set. In the case of local explanations, for instance, a learner could be biased to search for (words in) the long form of an ambiguous abbreviation, which initially is present in training and test data. To reduce this bias, we replaced all synonyms and local explanations (all long and short forms) used for finding a text with the term under consideration.

Other Resources

We retrieved additional examples from knowledge bases dedicated to the specific types of biomedical objects used in our study. UniProt contains textual descriptions in form of plain, comments descriptions of protein function and implications for diseases. Each *protein* entry also contains a number of references to publications (most of them indexed by PubMed.) MedlinePlus describes prescriptions, precautions, and other conditions for each *drug*.

Overlapping Meanings

Some terms that appear to have multiple senses essentially share the same sense. For example, 'cat' occurs among the 7700 most frequent English words (in both singular and plural form) and thus is considered as a common term. However, the meaning of 'cat' in *common* English is the very same than that of the term 'cat' in the class *organism*. Thus, in this case, we would not need to disambiguate between *organism* and *common*. To identify such overlaps (which can only appear between a biomedical class common English), we checked the categorization of the word given by an online dictionary (in our case, http://dict.leo.org). Whenever we found a category associated to a term that hint on a biomedical meaning (anatomy, botany, medicine, zoology), we treated the common English and the biomedical sense as equal.

Enrichment of Sparse Training Data

Our combination of synsets and local explanations could identify at least four examples for 304 of the 531 ambiguous terms we studied. For 227 terms, we found only three or less example texts, which we considered as insufficient for training. We hypothesized that an enrichment of those sparse sets with examples assigned to other terms of the same sense could *i)* increase the coverage of our proposed method and *ii)* increase the overall disambiguation performance, both simply because more training data for more terms were available. We identify terms that have at least one example for each of its senses and added to those abstracts from other terms of the same class. These other terms were replaced by the term under consideration to avoid side-effects. The drawback was that this method potentially decreased the quality of the data set. This can be dealt with using two heuristics. First, one should, as discussed previously, only use terms from the same sense that are themselves unambiguous. Next, one may include a degree of relatedness between the two terms; this is given, for instance, in hierarchically organized vocabularies such as MeSH (cells, diseases, drugs, tissues) and the NCBI Taxonomy (organisms). As an example, consider the term 'cancer', which can refer to a *disease* or an *organism*. Using the hierarchical information on the two senses (MeSH and NCBI Taxonomy, respectively), we may include texts discussing 'diseases' (more general term) or various forms of neoplasms (more specific terms) for the *disease* sense, and texts discussing 'crustacea' (more general) or various species in the genus 'cancer' (more specific) for the *organism* sense.

Feature Generation

We built the feature vector for each term by including all word stems occurring in a window of variable size around the current term. Therein, we tested different settings: i) different window sizes; ii) different amounts of stop words to be filtered from the window; iii) different weighting schemes as features. For stop words, we used the list of most frequent English terms provided by Leech et al. (2001), which consists of 7700 words. Weights were calculated either as binary (term does/does not occur in the window), term frequency in the current window (TF), or weighted term frequency (TF*IDF). We used the Porter stemmer (Porter, 1980) to reduce dimensionality of the vectors.

Application of SVM

As classification method, we used the SVM*light* implementation of support vector machines (Joachims, 1999). For each sense, we calculated a one-versus-all model to distinguish the given sense from all others. We used a linear kernel with default parameters, a setting which repeatedly has been shown to yield good results in text classification (Joachims, 1998; Hakenberg et al., 2004).

Evaluation

Evaluation was performed using leave-one-out cross-validations for each term. We calculated the accuracy for all such tests, which yielded overall disambiguation accuracy. Because for many terms sizes of training samples for either sense differ largely, we also calculated also the F1-measure for each test.

Results

The comparison of our seven dictionaries yielded 531 ambiguous terms. Four terms have three senses, and all others have two. The terms with three senses are `mum', `dare', `this' (*common, organism, protein*), and `axis' (*common, organism, tissue*). Table 2 shows the overlaps between senses in detail. For our first experiment, we used only terms for which we could gather at least four example texts for either meaning. This limitation left 304 ambiguous terms. Later, we successfully relaxed these requirements to classify 118 additional terms (see below). The full data set is available at http://alibaba.informatik.hu-berlin.de/corpora/.

In the first experiment, the system yields an average accuracy of 87.2%, evaluated for all seven senses versus all others on terms for which at least eight examples were available. We used

Table 3. Inter-class accuracies (average accuracy of protein versus organism disambiguation and so on). In brackets: number of tests available for each pair. The last column gives the average over all senses.

	Organism	Drug	Disease	Tissue	Cell	Common	All
Protein	88% (101)	85% (54)	95% (4)	17% (1)	(0)	89% (55)	88%
Organism		97% (6)	95% (4)	80% (9)	24% (5)	84% (7)	86%
Drug			93% (5)	(0)	92% (1)	98% (12)	89%
Disease				99% (1)	91% (1)	97% (4)	90%
Tissue					73% (33)	95% (1)	75%

the full abstract to obtain features, TF-weighting, and filtering with 100 stop words; the impact of changing these settings is discussed below. Table 3 shows the accuracies for each pair of senses. As Figure 2a shows, the average accuracy is largely influenced by a few outliers. Accordingly, the median accuracy is much higher at 93.7%. Table 4 shows the most extreme outliers, whereas Table 5 contains terms that could be disambiguated best.

As a concrete example, we discuss the term `cat' in more detail. The accuracy for the disambiguation of 'cat' is 98%, as determined on 762 texts for each sense (*organism* and *protein*). Figure 2b shows the predicted p-values for each of the 2*762 cases. The majority of examples have a p-value of more than +/-0.5, which is consistent with results presented for similar settings (Gaudan et al., 2005). Setting the decision boundary to a threshold of 0.5 would result in an average accuracy of 95% (+7.8%; F1: 97%, +8%), but leave almost 40% of the cases unsolved.

We also analyzed the correlation between disambiguation accuracy and the number of training examples (see Figure 3). Clearly, terms with more examples in general have a higher chance of being disambiguated well; however, the relative low correlation coefficient ρ=0.27 shows that this relationship is not linear and that also terms with few training examples may have high disambiguation accuracy[2].

Enrichment of Training Data

For 118 out of the 531 terms under consideration, we found only between one and three examples. Enriching the set of texts using the method described previously for these 118 examples so that at least eight examples were available each yielded an average accuracy of 93% (an increase of 5.8%; median accuracy increased by 3.3% to 97%); this confirms our hypothesis that the addition of theoretically less reliable examples would (a) increase the overall performance and (b)

Figure 2. (a) Accuracies for all 304 terms (left column) and plot of each respective accuracy (right column); each red square corresponds to one (or more) terms. (b) Values of the decision function for classifying the term 'cat', including both senses (organism and protein). Red, real sense for each case; blue, opposite sense (false sense); squares, right prediction; crosses, wrong prediction.

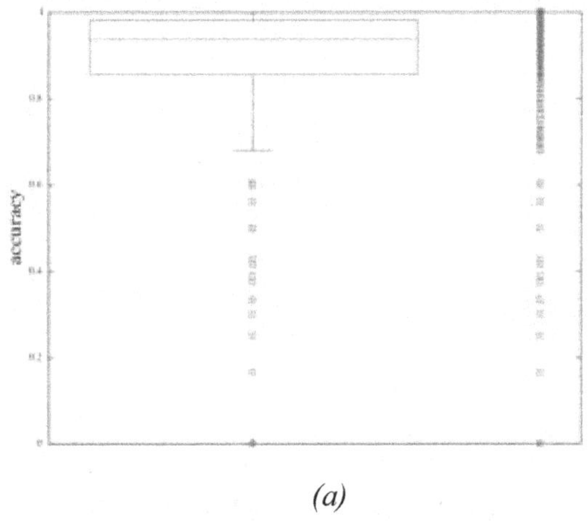

(a)

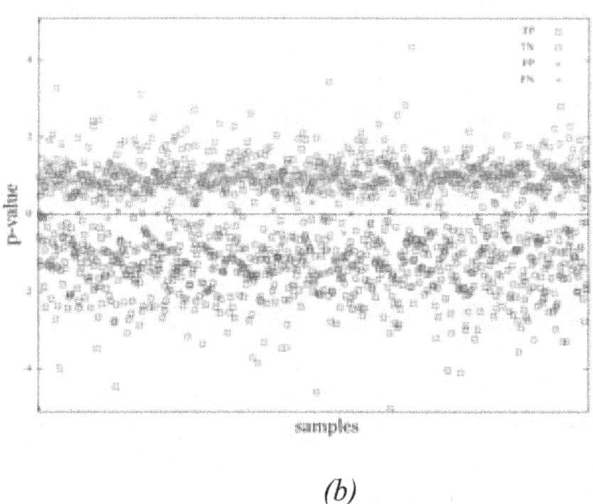

(b)

Figure 3. Dependency of accuracy on the number of training examples (logarithmic scale).

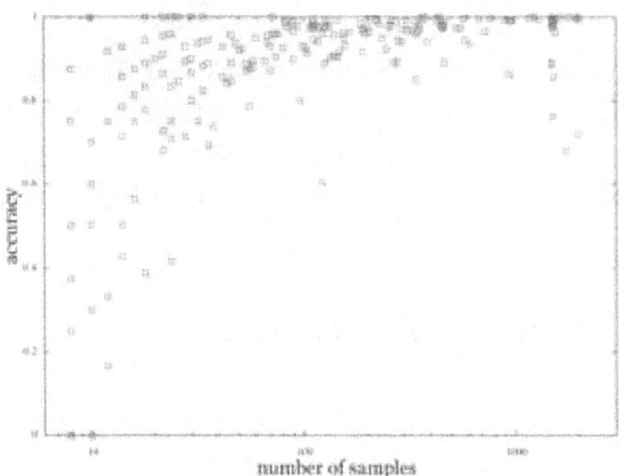

Figure 4. Comparison of results for normal (left) and artificially enriched data sets (right).

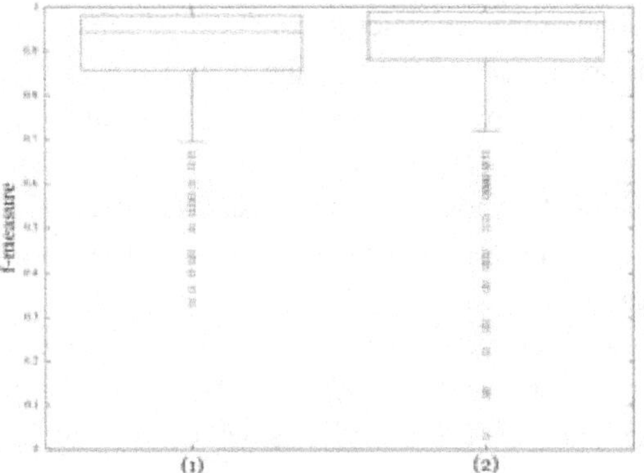

Table 4. Terms with a disambiguation accuracy of less than 60%. The third column contains the number of PubMed abstracts available in the corpus.

Term	Accuracy	Abstracts	Sense 1	Sense 2
pine	56%	16	Common	Protein
taxi	50%	8	Common	Protein
scot	50%	14	Common	Protein
pikas	50%	10	Protein	Organism
aeh1	50%	8	Protein	Organism
bike	43%	14	Common	Protein
paca	43%	14	Protein	Organism
pas	39%	18	Protein	Drug
ahf	30%	10	Protein	Drug
cis	25%	8	Protein	Organism
man	17%	12	Common	Organism
enterocytes	12%	10	Tissue	Cell
chromaffin granules	0	8	Tissue	Cell
microglia	0	8	Tissue	Cell
liz	0	8	Common	Protein

increase the overage of our method considerably. The average F1-score increased to 90%, median to 97%. Figure 4 shows the comparison for the base and enriched data sets.

Impact of Feature Set

Table 6 shows the impact of window size and stop word filtering on disambiguation performance.

Table 5. Terms with the best disambiguation accuracy

Term	Accuracy	Abstracts	Sense 1	Sense 2
ribes	100%	96	Protein	Organism
ca2	99%	1504	Protein	Drug
pan	99%	1534	Common	Organism
cat	98%	1524	Protein	Organism
podophyllum	97%	308	Drug	Organism
cage	96%	154	Common	Protein
oxytocin	95%	584	Protein	Drug
pig	96%	1558	Protein	Organism
puma	95%	100	Protein	Organism
acre	94%	72	Common	Protein
leo	93%	100	Protein	Organism
cancer	93%	250	Organism	Disease

Table 6. Impact of window size (N) and stop word filtering (sw) on accuracy (average/ median) for TF weighting, with average number of resulting features per term (f).

N	sw	Average	Median	f
10	7700	85%	91%	730
20	7700	87%	92%	986
infinity	7700	88%	93%	1900
infinity	100	90%	96%	2234

Table 7. Time performance for single classification events, dependent on different settings for window size (N), stop word filtering (numbers of stop words, sw), and term weighting (weight). Generating a feature vector takes 88-90ms.

N	sw	Weight	ms
10	7700	TF	45.2
20	7700	TF	55.6
20	100	TF	82.0
infinity	7700	TF	123.6
infinity	100	TF	301.6
infinity	7700	binary	122.9
infinity	7700	TF*IDF	128.6

The best performance was achieved using only 100 stop words and all available text. All figures are for TF weights. The performance of binary features or TF*IDF was consistently worse (in the range of 1-2%).

The set of features largely influences the time required to classify ambiguous terms, which is an important issue for applications performing online disambiguation, for instance to tag entities in search results. Table 7 shows the necessary time per classification (one event for terms with two sense, three for three senses.) Given these figures, it is clear that such applications might have to trade some accuracy for speed.

Error Analysis

Manual inspection of errors revealed five main sources: *i)* semantically close senses, *ii)* additional, unconsidered senses, *iii)* failures of the short/long form collection method, *iv)* too few training examples, which also adds to *v)*, cases having atypical contexts. An example for semantically close senses is `IL-2', as short-form of the protein Interleukin-2, which is also the name of a *drug* (Aldesleukin, Proleukin(R)). The same happens for *cells* and *tissues*, where the *cells* are named after the encompassing *tissue*; for instance, `enterocytes' are the *cells* of the intestinal mucosa *tissue* and occur in three different branches of the MeSH tree.

The system was always forced to decide on one of the seven input classes, without the possibility to reject all. This restriction caused errors when we encountered additional, unconsidered senses. In the case of `cat', "k(cat)" would not refer to any of our seven classes, but rather to a enzymatic reaction rate, and thus should be rejected. Such cases can be attributed to the method of collecting the data set. A similar type of error occurs with the local explanations. When we encountered an ambiguous term right before or within parentheses, we checked for any synonym from any term sharing the same sense. This included potentially ambiguous synonyms (like in "codon (CAT)", where `codon' could be, but in this case it not, an *organism*). Restrictions to closer synonyms (for instance exploiting the hierarchical structure of MeSH terms and the NCBI taxonomy) resulted in fewer data sets and did not improve the overall performance significantly.

DISCUSSION

WSD is a major building block for high-quality text extraction and analysis systems in biomedical science. It is especially important in this domain, where a substantial number of objects under study share names, leading to a high level of ambiguity. Based on our experience, we estimate that 68% of all PubMed abstracts contain at least one ambiguity concerning our seven entity classes. This coincides roughly with the findings of Xu et al. (2006), who found that in a set of 89,922 PubMed abstracts that were known to be related to mouse genes, 99.7% contained a gene name that is also a common English word, and 99.8% contained an ambiguity between gene and non-gene UMLS concepts. The higher numbers of Xu et al. can be explained by the selection procedure of the abstracts, i.e., abstracts containing a gene name have a higher chance of also containing an ambiguous term than abstracts drawn purely by chance.

We presented a classification-based approach to the WSD problem. Our system is able to correctly assign senses to many ambiguous terms from seven biomedical classes with a median success rate of 97%. Particular effort was put into the automatic collection of high-quality training examples. The methods we implemented harvest a whole range of data sources. Furthermore, we showed that enriching training data with unrelated texts that stems from the same semantic class is a promising approach to deal with terms/senses without examples. Our best results were achieved for disambiguating terms of the senses *diseases* and *drugs* from all others (90 to 98%). Terms sharing senses between the classes *protein* and *tissue* and between *cell* and *organism* were the toughest to disambiguate (17 and 24%, respectively). This confirms the assumption that WSD is the more difficult the more related the senses of terms are. Note that most of these difficult terms are metonyms rather than polysemous words, like *proteins* that are named after the *tissue* they were first found in or in which *cells* they are exclusively expressed, or like *cell* types named after the *organism* they occur in. Making an error in such cases seldom is regarded as severe.

We envisage that applications using our WSD method will apply a threshold to tell confident from less confident sense tags. This threshold should directly be applied to the value of the decision function of the SVM, as shown in Figure 2b. Any prediction below this threshold (in our experiments, we found 0.5 a good boundary) would result in keeping all potential senses, that is, to confront the user with an unresolved ambiguity rather than presenting a potentially faulty disambiguation.

There are a number of areas where our method could be improved. Knowledge about the capitalization of names should be exploited, because many occurrences of ambiguity result from inexact, case insensitive dictionary matching[3]. In particular, protein names often bear a distinctive capitalization pattern: `AttA', `attA', `guaR', or `BIKe' could all be assigned to *protein* instead of *organism* or *common*; `Bike', on the other hand, remains to be disambiguated, because it could also appear as first word of a sentence. Background knowledge about the a-priori probability of a particular sense could be included, and also the time of publication of a text containing an ambiguous term can be instructive (Hofmann & Valencia, 2003; Tamames & Valencia, 2006). We also believe that the classification model itself could be improved by including POS-tags and the distance of words from the term under classification, as shown in Pahikkala et al. (2005). Finally, it is clear that our method currently is not capable of disambiguating between terms in the same class, such as genes in different species sharing the same name. Addressing also this problem would require a more targeted search for examples, but would at the same time have to cope with an expected lower numbers of examples.

REFERENCES

Agirre, E., & Edmonds, P. (Eds.). (2006). *Word Sense Disambiguation - Algorithms and Applications*: Springer.

Andreopoulos, B., Alexopoulou, D., & Schroeder, M. (2007). Word Sense Disambiguation in Biomedical Ontologies with Term Co-occurrence Analysis and Document Clustering. *Int J Data Mining Bioinf*, Special Issue on Biomedical Text Retrieval and Mining.

Aronson, A. R. (2006). *MetaMap: Mapping Text to the UMLS Metathesaurus*: National Library of Medicine.

Brookes, M. (2001) *Fly - the Unsung Hero of Twentieth Century Science*: Ecco.

Camous, F., Blott, S., & Smeaton, A.F. (2007). Ontology-based MEDLINE document classification. In: *Proc BIRD*, 439-452.

Cohen, A. M., & Hersh, W. R. (2005). A survey of current work in biomedical text mining. *Briefings in Bioinformatics, 6*(1), 57-71.

Farkas, R. (2008) The strength of co-authorship in gene name disambiguation. *BMC Bioinformatics, 9*(1), 69.

Florian, R., & Yarowsky, D. (2002). *Modeling Consensus: Classifier Combination for Word Sense Disambiguation.* Paper presented at the Conference on empirical methods in natural language processing.

Fundel, K., & Zimmer, R. (2007) *Human Gene Normalization by an Integrated Approach including Abbreviation Resolution and Disambiguation.* In: *Proc Second BioCreative Challenge Evaluation Workshop*, Madrid, Spain.

Gale, W. A., Church, K. W., & Yarowsky, D. (1992). *One sense per discourse.* Paper presented at the Workshop on Speech and Natural Language Harriman, New York.

Galley, M., & McKeown, K. (2003). *Improving word sense disambiguation in lexical chaining.* Paper presented at the 18th Int. Joint Conference on Artificial Intelligence, Acapulca, Mexico.

Gaudan, S., Kirsch, H., & Rebholz-Schuhmann, D. (2005). Resolving abbreviations to their senses in Medline. *Bioinformatics, 21*(18), 3658-3664.

GeneOntology Consortium, T. (2001). Creating the gene ontology resource: design and implementation. *Genome Research, 11*(8), 1425-1433.

Hakenberg, J., Schmeier, S., Kowald, A., Klipp, E., & Leser, U. (2004). Finding Kinetic Parameters Using Text Mining. *OMICS: A Journal of Integrative Biology*, *8*(2), 131-152. Special issue on Data Mining meets Integrative Biology - a Symbiosis in the Making.

Hausser, R. (2001). *Foundations of Computational Linguistics: Human-Computer Communication in Natural Language.* Heidelnerg, Berlin, New York: Springer-Verlag.

Hofmann, R., & Valencia, A. (2003). Life cycles of successful genes. *Trends in Genetics*, *19*, 79-81.

Ide, N., & Veronis, J. (1998). Word Sense Disambiguation: The State of the Art. *Computational Linguistics, 14*(1), 1-40.

Joachims, T. (1998). Text Categorization with Support Vector Machines: Learning with Many Relevant Features. *Proc ECML.*

Joachims, T. (1999). Making Large-Scale SVM Learning Practical. In: B. Schoelkopf, C. J. C. Burges, & A. J. Smola (Eds.), *Advances in Kernel Methods - Support Vector Learning*, Cambridge, MA, USA.

Krallinger, M., & Valencia, A. (2007). Evaluating the Detection and Ranking of Protein Interaction relevant Articles: the BioCreative Challenge Interaction Article Sub-task (IAS). In: *Proc 2nd BioCreative Challenge Evaluation Workshop*, Madrid, Spain, (pp. 29-39).

Lan, M., Tan, C. L., & Low, H. B. (2006). Proposing a New Term Weighting Scheme for Text Classification. In: *Proc 21st AAAI,* (pp. 763-768).

Lan, M., Tan, C. L., & Su, J. (2007). A Term Investigation and Majority Voting for Protein Interaction Article Sub-task (IAS). In: *Proc 2nd BioCreative Challenge Evaluation Workshop*, Madrid, Spain, (pp. 183-185).

Lee, Y. K., & Ng, H. T. (2002). *An empirical evaluation of knowledge sources and learning algorithms for word sense disambiguation.* Paper presented at the Conference on empirical methods in natural language processing.

Leech, G., Rayson, P., & Wilson, A. (2001). *Word Frequencies in Written and Spoken English: based on the British National Corpus*: Longman, London.

Leroy, G., & Rindflesch, T. C. (2004). Using Symbolic Knowledge in the UMLS to Disambiguate Words in Small Datasets with a Naive Bayes Classifier. In: M. Fieschi et al. (Eds), *MEDINFO.* IOS Press.

Leser, U., & Hakenberg, J. (2005). What Makes a Gene Name? Named Entity Recognition in the Biomedical Literature. *Briefings in Bioinformatics, 6*(4), 357-369.

Liu, H., Aronson, A. R., & Friedman, C. (2002). *A study of abbreviations in MEDLINE abstracts.* Paper presented at the AMIA Symposium.

Manning, C., & Schütze, H. (1999). *Foundations of Statistical Natural Language Processing.* Cambridge, Massachusetts: MIT Press.

Mitchell, T. (1997). *Machine Learning*: McGraw Hill.

Morgan, A., Lu, Z., Wang, X., Cohen, A., Fluck, J., Ruch, P., Divoli, A., Fundel, K., Leaman, R., Hakenberg, J., Sun, C., Liu, H-H., Torres, R., Krauthammer, M., Lau, W., Liu, H., Hsu, C-N., Schuemie, M., Cohen, K. B., & Hirschman, L. (2008) Overview of BioCreative II Gene Normalization. *Genome Biology*, Special Issue on BioCreative Challenge Evaluations.

Ng, H. T., Lim, C. Y., & Foo, S. K. (1999). *A Case Study on Inter-Annotator Agreement for Word Sense Disambiguation.* Paper presented at the ACL SIGLEX Workshop: Standardizing Lexical Resources.

Pahikkala, T., Ginter, F., Boberg, J., Jarvinen, J., & Salakoski, T. (2005) Contextual weighting for Support Vector Machines in Literature Mining: An Application to Gene versus Protein Name Disambiguation. *BMC Bioinformatics, 6*, 157.

Plake, C., Schiemann, T., Pankalla, M., Hakenberg, J., & Leser, U. (2006). AliBaba: PubMed as a graph. *Bioinformatics, 22*(19), 2444-2445.

Porter, M. F. (1980). An algorithm for suffix stripping. *Program, 14*(3), 130-137.

Poulter, G. L., Rubin, D. L., Altman, R. B., & Seoighe, C. (2008). MScanner: a classifier for retrieving Medline citations. *BMC Bioinformatics, 9*, 108.

Schuemie, M. J., Kors, J. A., & Mons, B. (2005). Word Sense Disambiguation in the Biomedical Domain: An Overview. *Journal of Computational Biology, 12*(5), 554-565.

Smith, C. L., Goldsmith, C. A., & Eppig, J. T. (2005). The Mammalian Phenotype Ontology as a tool for annotating, analyzing and comparing phenotypic information. *Genome Biol, 6*(1), R7.

Tamames, J. & Valencia, A. (2006). The success (or not) of HUGO nomenclature. *Genome Biology, 7*(5), 402.

Véronis, J. (1999). *A study of polysemy judgements and inter-annotator agreement.* Paper presented at the Advanced Papers of the SENSEVAL Workshop Sussex, UK.

Weeber, M., Mork, J. G., & Aronson, A. R. (2001). Developing a Test Collection for Biomedical Word Sense Disambiguation. *Proc AMIA.*

Widdows, D., Peters, S., Cederberg, S., Chan, C. K., Steffen, D., & Buitelaar, P. (2003). Unsupervised monolingual and bilingual word-sense disambiguation of medical documents using UMLS. *Proc. ACL Workshop NLP in Biomed*, 9-16.

Xu, H., Markatou, M., Dimova, R., Liu, H., & Friedman, C. (2008). Machine learning and word sense disambiguation in the biomedical domain: design and evaluation issues. *BMC Bioinformatics, 7*(1), 334.

ENDNOTES

1 In this chapter, we do not differentiate between genes, proteins, and mRNAs.

2 A value of 1 for ρ and most examples lying on the diagonal would correspond to a strong positive correlation

3 Case-insensitive matching is needed to ensure high recall of named entity recognition components.

Section II

Going Beyond Words:

NLP Approaches Involving the Sentence Level

Chapter IX
Information Extraction of Protein Phosphorylation from Biomedical Literature

M. Narayanaswamy
Anna University, India

K. E. Ravikumar
Anna University, India

Z. Z. Hu
Georgetown University Medical Center, USA

K. Vijay-Shanker
University of Delaware, USA

C. H. Wu
Georgetown University Medical Center, USA

ABSTRACT

Protein posttranslational modification (PTM) is a fundamental biological process, and currently few text mining systems focus on PTM information extraction. A rule-based text mining system, RLIMS-P (Rule-based LIterature Mining System for Protein Phosphorylation), was recently developed by our group to extract protein substrate, kinase and phosphorylated residue/sites from MEDLINE abstracts. This chapter covers the evaluation and benchmarking of RLIMS-P and highlights some novel and unique features of the system. The extraction patterns of RLIMS-P capture a range of lexical, syntactic and semantic constraints found in sentences expressing phosphorylation information. RLIMS-P also has a second phase that puts together information extracted from different sentences. This is an important feature since it is not common to find the kinase, substrate and site of phosphorylation to be mentioned in the same sentence. Small modifications to the rules for extraction of phosphorylation information have also allowed us to develop systems for extraction of two other PTMs, acetylation and methylation. A thorough evaluation of these two systems needs to be completed. Finally, an online version of RLIMS-P with enhanced functionalities, namely, phosphorylation annotation ranking, evidence tagging, and protein entity mapping, has been developed and is publicly accessible.

INTRODUCTION

Protein post translational modification (PTM), a molecular event in which a protein is chemically modified during or after its being translated, is essential to many biological processes. Protein phosphorylation is one of the most common PTMs, which involves the addition of a phosphate group to serine, threonine or tyrosine residues of a protein, and is fundamental to cell metabolism, growth and development. Many cellular signal transduction pathways are activated through phosphorylation of specific proteins that initiate a cascade of protein-protein interactions, leading to specific gene regulation and cellular response. It is estimated that one third of the mammalian genome coding sequences code for phosphoproteins. The phosphorylation state of cellular proteins is also highly dynamic, detection, quantification and functional analysis of the dynamic phosphorylation status of proteins, and the kinases involved are essential for understanding the regulatory networks of biological pathways and processes, which are under extensive investigation by researchers of many areas of biological research.

While PTMs are fundamental to our understanding of cellular processes, the experimental PTM data are largely buried in free-text literature. For example, a recent PubMed query for protein phosphorylation returned 103,478 papers. Although PTMs, especially phosphorylation, are among the most important protein features annotated in protein databases, currently only limited amount of data are annotated in a few resources, such as UniProt Knowledgebase (UniProtKB) (Wu et al., 2006), and specialized databases including Phospho.ELM and PhosphoSite, which can not keep up with the fast-growing literature. With the increasing volume of scientific literature now available electronically, efficient text mining tools will greatly facilitate the extraction of information buried in free text. Information extraction of PTM information on specific proteins, sites/residues being modified, and enzymes involved in the modification are particularly useful not only to assist database curation for protein site features and related pathway or disease information, but also to allow users to quickly browse and analyze the literature, and help other bioinformatics software to integrate text mining component into pathway and network analysis.

There are many BioNLP relation extraction systems that have been developed in the past few years. Some of these employ special rule/pattern based approaches (e.g., Blaschke et al., 1999; Pustejovsky et al., 2002). Other approaches for extracting protein-protein interactions include detecting co-occurring proteins (Proux et al., 2000; Stapley and Benoit, 2000; Stephens et al., 2001), or using a text parser tailored for the specialized language typically found in the biology literature (e.g., Friedman et al., 2001; Daraselia et al., 2004). The rule-based approach involves designing patterns to extract specific types of information, while the parser approach requires development of grammars, methods for disambiguation and further effort to provide methods that map parse information to objects involved in the relation. More modern approaches employ machine learning for relation extraction (e.g., Bunescu and Mooney, Gioliana et al). Such methods require an annotated corpus, where the sentences are marked with the relation and related objects manually. Machine learning techniques are then employed to learn a model that will extract from unseen text.

THE RLIMS-P EXTRACTION SYSTEM

We have developed the RLIMS-P (Rule-based LIterature Mining System for Protein Phosphorylation) system for extracting protein phosphorylation information from MEDLINE abstracts. Most of the BioNLP systems extract interactions between two proteins. RLIMS-P has some unique features that distinguishe it from the others. It is exclusively devoted to extraction of a specific biochemical reaction, i.e., phosphorylation. We are not aware of other systems that are devoted to extraction of protein PTMs information from text. Another distinguishing feature of RLIMS-P is that it extracts three objects involved in protein phosphorylation—the protein kinase, the protein substrate (phosphorylated protein), and the residue/position being phosphorylated (phosphorylation site). This contrasts with most existing systems which extracted two related objects. Further, these two objects are typically found in the same sentence. As we shall see later, rarely are the 3 objects that we extract found in the same sentence. Hence we employ techniques to combine pieces of information that are found in different sentences.

Before we describe the RLIMS-P system, we wish to note that each of the three objects that are extracted provide critical information. Clearly with the extraction of the residue at a particular position (which shall be called "site" in the description of the system) which gets phosphorylated must also require the extraction of the protein substrate (which will be called the "theme" in RLIMS-P's description) to which it belongs. The extraction of the residue information is motivated by the fact that phosphorylation of certain residues may activate certain function of that substrate while that of other sites in the same substrate may trigger different responses. Further, the kinase (which will be called "agent" in the description of RLIMS-P) involved may be site specific; i.e., while several kinases may catalyze the phosphorylation of a protein, some kinases may be able to phosphorylate certain sites only and others may catalyze the phosphorylation of other sites in the same substrate. For this reason, we believe it is important to go beyond the extraction of the two proteins only.

RLIMS-P has several components that will be discussed in detail below. Its major components include a shallow parser, a classifier of terms into semantic categories (e.g., protein, residue or site, cell), a syntactic simplifier and matching of patterns for extraction from individual sentences and a component for combining information obtained from different sentences.

Shallow Parsing

Rather than fully parse a sentence that may contain phosphorylation-related information, we employ shallow parsing. Our shallow parser identifies simple constituents such as noun phrases and verb groups in a sentence. The pipeline of processing starts with simple text processing including dividing the text (currently Medline abstracts) into sentences and identifying the title. Next the sentences are input to a part of speech tagger (currently, the system uses the Brill's tagger (Brill, 1995)), supplemented with a few rules to correct common errors it makes in the biology domain. The system has been designed to easily replace the current POS tagging system with the more recent taggers specialized for the BioNLP domain. Once each word is tagged with a POS tag, using simple non-recursive grammar rules certain simple types of phrases are recognized using simple non-recursive grammar rules.

The most crucial type of phrases is the so-called BaseNP—simple noun phrases that do not involve any recursion. BaseNPs play an important role in information extraction as they often refer to named entities. In our case, the objects that are extracted (agent, theme or site) will be BaseNPs. In Ex 1 below, three BaseNPs are detected (the underlined phrases). We also chunk verb groups and determine their voice. The following example illustrates the utility of chunking verb groups.

Ex 1: "Active p90Rsk2 was found to be able to phosphorylate histone H3 at Ser10."

The verb group sequence "was *found to be able to phosphorylate"* is recognized and identified as containing 3 separate verb groups. The last verb group "to phosphorylate" is detected to have active form in contrast to the first verb group "was found", which is in passive form. The detection of active form of the "to phosphorylated" verb group will allow the assignment of agent role to the subject (while, in contrast, if the verb group had been in the passive form the subject noun phrase must be assigned the theme role).

The next aspect of our shallow parsing approach is to detect other syntactic constructions related to noun phrases. These include coordination of entity names, relative clauses and appositives. The detection of constructs such as the appositives is mainly to correctly identify the location of the arguments. Consider, for example, the following sentence:

EX2: In the yeast Saccharomyces cerevisiae, Sic1, an inhibitor of Clb-Cdc28 kinases, must be phosphorylated and ...

We consider appositives and relative clauses as intervening parenthetical material that can appear between the arguments. As parentheticals, we assume they may contain extra information that need not be directly related the verb and its arguments. Once the parser detects and annotates such parenthetical constructs, our pattern matching method (see below) will treat the sentence as though the parenthetical did not appear in the sentence and hence, as far as the pattern matcher is concerned, it will consider EX2 to be equivalent to "In the yeast Saccharomyces cerevisiae, Sic1, must be phosphorylated and ..." in terms of extraction of information.

Semantic Classification

We employ more than syntactic processing for extraction of phosphorylation information. One of the key components of the RLIMS-P system is the assignment of semantic types to noun phrases that refer to the phosphorylation objects of interest (i.e., arguments <AGENT> <THEME> and <SITE>). Semantic type assignment (also employed in information extraction systems such as those outlined in Rindflesch *et al.*, 2000, Pustejovsky *et al.*, 2002) plays a fundamental role in pattern specifications. It simplifies the pattern specifications and improves the precision. Consider the underlined phrases in the following examples:

EX3: ATR/FRP-1 also phosphorylated p53 in Ser 15 ...

EX4: Active Chk2 phosphorylated the SQ/TQ sites in Ckk2 SCD ...

EX5: cdk9/cyclinT2 could phosphorylate the retinoblastoma gene (pRb) in human cell lines

These three sentences roughly correspond to a surface form of "X phosphorylated Y in Z". While all three examples match this same syntactic pattern, the relation extracted will depend on what matches Y and Z (the underlined phrases). These two terms would correspond to the theme and site in the first example, and site and theme in the second example, while in the third example only theme is present. Thus the theme and site cannot be disambiguated simply by using a pattern that is based only on syntax/surface form. If the patterns were merely syntactic and didn't include type information, then the relation extracted would be correct in only in the first of examples above and incorrect in the other two.

In RLIMS-P system, NPs are classified as proteins (or genes), as protein part (site) or as "other". For example, the two underlined terms in the first sentence will be classified as protein and protein part respectively, as protein part and protein in the second sentence and as protein/gene and others in the third sentence. This classification is based on methods that we employed in our previously developed name entity extraction system (Narayanaswamy at al. 2003). In order to perform such classification, the system uses a dictionary of common well-known common names, as well as uses information of words appearing in the term itself as well as neighboring words. When words appearing in the name are taken into account, it is the words that are taken into consideration. For example, in the name "mitogen activated protein kinase", our system will use the word kinase to assign the protein type to the name. Other such type bearing words include "protein", "gene", "factor", and "enzyme". In addition, we use suffix information as well as phrases appearing immediately to the left or right of a name. For more details on our classification method, we refer the reader to Narayanaswamy et al. 2003. While the initial list of suffixes, words and neighboring phrases were manually maintained in this system originally, subsequently this list was extended by using the automatically learned list discussed in (Torii, 2004).

Patterns and Pattern Matching

The three key phosphorylation objects are next extracted by matching text with manually designed pattern templates. The patterns cover the verbal inflected forms such as "phosphorylated/phosphorylating/phosphorylates" as well as nominal forms. An example of a pattern for the verbal form is:

Pattern 1: <AGENT> <VG-active-phosphorylate> <THEME> (in/at <SITE>)?

Here "VG-active-phosphorylate" denotes a verb group in active form that is headed by an inflected form of the verb "phosphorylate". Almost every rule will have a lexical basis involving some word related to phosphorylation and is called the lexical trigger. Given a sentence, to verify whether it matches a pattern, we first verify whether the lexical trigger of the pattern can be found. Returning to the discussion of the above pattern, <AGENT> can be matched by any noun phrase which is of type appropriate for an agent (i.e., protein). If the pattern is matched successfully for a sentence, then the noun phrase that matches the <AGENT> is extracted and assigned the AGENT (i.e., kinase) role. Next, <THEME> can be matched by any noun phrase which is of type protein (the type appropriate for the substrate in a protein phosphorylation). <SITE> refers to a noun phrase that has been classified to be of type, protein part. When the pattern is matched, the noun phrase that matches <SITE> will provide the site of phosphorylation information. Note that this pattern requires that the site phrase appear after the lexical words "in" or "at". The symbol "?" denotes that the entire site information is an optional argument.

Clauses matched by this pattern include "*ATR/FRP-1 also phosphorylated p53 in Ser 15*" (EX 3 above). The pattern also describes "*The recombinant protein was shown to phosphorylate Kemptide*" where the site is not present. As noted earlier, <VG-active-phosphorylate> requirement of Pattern 1 is met here because of the second (rightmost) of the two verb groups contains the "phosphorylate"verb in active form. The clause "*Active Chk2 phosphorylated the SQ/TQ sites in Ckk2 SCD*" does not match this pattern due to the order of the site and the theme information. Pattern 1 requires a noun phrase of type protein to follow the phosphorylate verb group and this is not the case in the sentence. Instead, there is another pattern that expresses this order of <SITE> and <THEME>, and that pattern will apply and be used to obtain the arguments in the correct manner. There are several more patterns for <VG-active-phosphorylate>. In contrast, the patterns for the passive form capture the fact that the subject of the clause gives the theme and/or site. For example, one of the patterns is:

Pattern 2: <THEME> <VG-passive-phosphorylate> (by <AGENT>)? (at <SITE>)?

Here both the agent and the site are optional arguments. It is quite common for the subject to provide the site information rather than the theme information. This is captured by the following pattern:

Pattern 3: <SITE > (in/of <THEME>)? <VG-passive-phosphorylate> (by <AGENT>)?

Here the theme and/or agent can be optional. This rule is matched by

EX 6: ... all three sites in c-jun were phosphorylated.

A large number of patterns are not based on "phosphorylate" appearing in the verbal form but rather in the nominal form.

Pattern 4: phosphorylation of <THEME> (by <AGENT>)? (in/at <SITE>)?

This pattern applies and captures the theme and agent (note site is optional) from the sentence fragment

EX 7: … phosphorylation of CFTR by protein kinase A (PKA)

The patterns for phosphorylation are diverse and include examples such as:

Pattern 5: <AGENT> <VG-active> <THEME> by/via phosphorylation at (<SITE>)?

Note here the first VG is only required to be in active form and does not require it to be a inflected form of phosphorylate. The pattern matches with

EX 8: Both kinases also inactivate spinach sucrose phosphate synthase via phosphorylation at Ser-15,"

The pattern captures the fact that "inactivation" and "phosphorylation" here have the same arguments (i.e., *both kinases*) because inactivation is the result of phosphorylation. (A simple anaphora resolution program has been implemented that will attempt to resolve anaphoric expressions such as "both kinases".)

Some of the patterns have other trigger words including "phosphate group" as well as words with prefix "phospho". For example, the following pattern extracts the amino acid component of the site information from the trigger word specified as "phospo<amino acid>:

Pattern 6: phospho<amino acid> (of <THEME>)?

This pattern matches the following fragment and extracts the theme (substrate) as skeletal muscle phosphorylase kinase and extracts partial information of the site by obtaining the amino acid part of the site information.

EX 9: Localization of phosphoserine residues in skeletal muscle phosphorylase kinase…

Notice that the theme is optional in the above pattern. Just the presence of a term matching the pattern "phospho<amino acid>" itself is enough to indicate a phosphorylation of a residue whose amino acid component is being specified. For example, the term "phosphoserine" indicates that a serine residue has been phosphorylated.

In addition to these patterns, we introduced a heuristic to improve the recall of the site information. This rule is applied after all patterns are considered. Sometimes, the site information was found to not fit any systematic pattern. But in most of these cases, any residue information mentioned in a sentence mentioning phosphorylation turned out to be usually the site of phosphorylation. Based on this observation, we introduced a heuristic:

Site Rule (SR)

This rule is used to identify site information and is triggered by the use of a pattern that does not provide the site information. The rule is applied to see if the site information can be located within the same sentence. As an example, consider the sentence:

EX 10: Phosphorylation of bovine brain PLC-beta by PKC in vitro resulted in a stoichiometric incorporation of phosphate at serine 887, without any concomitant effect on PLC-beta activity.

For this sentence, a pattern is invoked which extracts the theme and the agent. But the site information is not extracted as none of our patterns expresses such a surface form. On the other hand, since a pattern has been invoked and some partial information extracted, and since there is a residue mentioned elsewhere in the sentence, SR applies and identifies this residue (serine 887) as the site of phosphorylation. SR can also be applied to extract the site information even in cases where conceivably a general patterns may exist. One such example is the extraction of the position information from the sentence:

EX 11: The phosphoserine was located at position 2.

In this case, Pattern 6 would apply to get the partial site information which gets completed with the application of SR.

Extra-Clausal Processing

The processing discussed above involves extraction of phosphorylation objects by matching the patterns against the text. Given the nature of these patterns, these patterns will typically be matched by phrases that appear in a clause. Now, we will consider some rules that allow us to extract arguments that are not mentioned in the same clause or sentence.

As we noted above, we are interested in not only extracting the two proteins (the kinase, i.e., agent; and the substrate, i.e., theme) involved in phosphorylation but also the site of phosphorylation. It is uncommon to see all the three objects mentioned in the same sentence let alone the same clause. Given that many of the patterns we deploy are matched against constituents of a clause, this implies that patterns would not be sufficient to extract the three objects. For example, with the verbal use of "phosphorylate" (e.g., *"phosphorylated", "phosphorylates", "to phosphorylate"*) it is not uncommon to see only the two of the objects mentioned in the clause (e.g., the agent and theme the active form). However, with the nominal usage (e.g., using the word "phosphorylation"), the focus seems to be more on the theme or site and the agent may not be mentioned. And there are cases as exemplified by EX 11 above where only one of the three objects is mentioned in the sentence. Since, we wish to extract all three arguments, we believed it was necessary to apply discourse-based rules to combine pieces of information that are expressed in different sentences.

We first discuss the rules to include the theme information. Quite often in a sentence the site of phosphorylation or the kinase involved is mentioned without the theme being mentioned (in that sentence). Clearly, the authors could not have indicated the site or kinase without divulging the substrate (theme) information. Consider the EX 11 sentence again. It is obvious that the authors must believe that the substrate/theme is obvious from context. We further assume that not only is the protein substrate previously mentioned in the abstract, but also assume in the first of the Theme Rules (TR), that protein is a substrate of phosphorylation and has also been mentioned in this discourse (abstract) previously. Thus the first TR is applied when the site or agent is extracted from a sentence (using pattern and/or SR) and yet the theme was not extracted. In that case, the closest previously mentioned theme of phosphorylation is used for the current extraction. As an example, from the sentence:

EX 12: The site, identified as Ser378, is also the site of phosphorylation by protein kinase C (PKC) in vitro.

From this sentence, the pattern will extract the agent (PKC). SR is applied to extract the site (Ser 378) information. At this point, there is no theme information known. However, there is a previous sentence which had mention of phosphorylation and had a mention of theme. This sentence is in fact the previous sentence in the abstract.

EX 13: We also show that stimulation of HeLa cells with the phorbol ester TPA enhances phosphorylation of PTP1B.

The pattern applied for this sentence would have extracted the theme as PTP1B. The TR now combines the theme information from this sentence with the other two pieces from EX 12 to eventually yield for EX 12, the triple

< protein kinase C (PKC), PTP1B, Ser378>

Another example of its use are exemplified by EX 14 and previously occurring sentence (EX 15) in the abstract.

Ex 14: The primary site of phosphorylation by protein kinase C was also near the amino terminus at Ser-27.

Here, SR recovers the site and patterns extract the agent from this sentence. Next TR is (correctly) applied and recovers the theme from a preceding sentence:

EX 15: Lipocortin I was phosphorylated near the amino terminus at Tyr-21 by recombinant c-src.

It is interesting to note that the theme is picked as same for the two, despite the fact that they are two distinct relations with different agents.

The second theme rule is also similar and is again applied when the site and/or agent is extracted but not the theme. Further, we assume that no substrate has been extracted so far (otherwise the first TR will trigger). In this case, we take the theme to be protein mentioned in the title of the abstract (as long as it does not follow the word "by"). The rough idea behind this rule is that what is phosphorylated (i.e. the theme) is probably more central and more important information than what does the phosphorylation (agent). Thus the protein in the title is taken to be the theme rather than the agent.

Fusion

By the time the patterns, SR and TR rules are applied, we expect that any site or agent extractions would also include the extraction of the theme. However, it is still possible that two separate extractions, one containing agent and them and other containing theme and site, are obtained from different sentences and that they need to be combined to give the three objects together. To do so, we developed an operation called *fusion* that merges two extracted records provided there is overlapping information but no incompatibilities. Notice that fusion is an operation on extracted information records rather than applied on text/

sentences. An example of application of fusion is given from the following two pieces extracted from text (PubMed ID (PMID) - 1985907):

R1: <casein kinase II, skeletal muscle calsequestrins, UNK>

R2: <UNK, skeletal muscle calsequestrins, <threonine, 363>>

The fused information is given by the triple <casein kinase II, skeletal muscle calsequestrins, <threonine, 363>>. Fusion is also useful because it allows us to detect redundancy and subsumption of information. An illustration of the latter can be seen when we attempt to fuse the following two records:

R3: <Syk, PLC-gamma1, UNK>

R4: <Syk, PLC-gamma1, <Tyrosine, 771>>

Since the resulting fused record is the same as R4, one of the original records, we can note that R3's information is contained in R4. Our web-based online version of RLIMS-P (see below) uses fusion to detect redundancy and information subsumption in order to make a decision of which extracted records to display.

EVALUATION

We have conducted two separate evaluations of RLIMS-P during the course of its development. For both studies, the system was evaluated based on the following performance measures:

precision = TP/(TP + FP); recall = TP/(TP + FN)

where TP is true positive, FP is false positive, and FN is false negative.

The first of these used data sets for testing and benchmarking the RLIMS-P literature mining system that were derived from data sources in iProLINK (Hu et al., 2004) of the Protein Information Resource (PIR). Specifically, we used the annotation-tagged literature corpora that were developed for evidence attribution of experimental phosphorylation features (http://pir.georgetown.edu/pirwww/iprolink/ftcorpora.shtml). Evidence tagging involves tagging the sentences providing experimental phosphorylation evidence in the abstract and/or full-text of the paper, which may include information of <THEME>, <SITE> and <AGENT>. For example, the tagged sentence:

EX 16: Phosphorylation of bovine brain PLC-beta by PKC in vitro resulted in a stoichiometric incorporation of phosphate at serine 887, without any concomitant effect on PLC-beta activity.

contains information on <THEME>*bovine brain PLC-beta*, <AGENT>*PKC* and <SITE>*serine 887*, thereby, providing evidence for the experimental feature line where the site is *phosphate (Ser)* at sequence position *887*, the enzyme is *protein kinase C* (i.e., PKC), and the feature is for the PIR-Protein Sequence Database (PSD) entry "*A28822*" for "*1-phosphatidylinositol-4,5-bisphosphate phosphodiesterase I*" (also known as *Phospholipase C-beta-1*) from "*bovine*" (i.e., brain PLC-beta).

In this study (see (Hu et al. 2005) for additional details), we used only MEDLINE abstracts (titles included) obtained using PMIDs in the data sets. Those papers were deemed to be *positive* papers contain information on the phosphorylation process along with at least one of the three arguments (<AGENT>, <THEME>, <SITE>). Therefore, abstracts mentioning kinases or phosphoproteins without associating with the process of phosphorylation did not constitute positive papers. For example, abstract describing "Growth-associated protein (GAP)-43 is a neuron-specific *phosphoprotein* whose expression is associated with axonal outgrowth" [PMID: 2153895] was not considered as positive paper. Furthermore, papers containing no relevant phosphorylation information in the abstracts regardless of information in full-text were regarded as negative data for program evaluation (as RLIMS-P was applied only to abstracts in this study).

In this first evaluation, the RLIMS-P system was evaluated both for retrieval of phosphorylation positive papers (IR) as well as for phosphorylation information extraction (IE). For the IR evaluation, a data set with 370 abstracts was used, including 110 positive and 260 negative papers. 116 abstracts were detected as positives, with 106 true positives, giving a precision of 91.4%. Four positive papers were missed, yielding a recall of 96.4%.

To better evaluate how the RLIMS-P system can assist database annotation of phosphorylation features, we further analyzed the performance of the program on phosphorylation information extraction using the PIR evidence-tagged abstracts as the benchmark standard. As shown above, the tagged sentences provide experimental evidence for the corresponding features—kinases (<AGENT>) and phosphorylated residues and their positions (<SITE>)—in the feature lines of the PIR-PSD protein entries (substrates or <THEME>). Since only 47 of the (43%) of the 110 *positive* abstracts from the benchmarking data set contained the kinase (agent) information, in this IE performance evaluation, we focused on <SITE> and <THEME>, with information on both amino acid residues and their sequence positions in the context of protein substrates.

Among the 110 positive papers used in the IR benchmarking study, 59 abstracts were tagged for experimental site features, covering site residue and sequence position information for a total of 129 sites. Among the tagged sites, the positions of 21 sites were based on implicit information such as sequence patterns rather than explicit residue numbers. An example of derivable residue position information in tagged sentences is:

EX 17: sequence patterns such as "phosphopeptide AT(P)S(P)NVFAMFDQSQIQEFK" (which indicates phosphorylation of both threonine and serine residues)

In such cases, annotators need to verify sequence positions of the phosphorylated residues by mapping the sequence patterns onto the protein sequences in the database. Such implicit phosphorylation positions were excluded for IE evaluation because current version of the program does not provide sequence mapping. Thus, the benchmark standard to evaluate RLIMS-P for site feature extraction consists of tagged abstracts for 108 sites (i.e., <SITE>-<THEME> pairs), where *explicit* sequence position is given for each site residue in the substrate. The results showed that 95 of the 108 phosphorylation sites were extracted for site residues and positions as well as the protein substrates, giving a recall of 88.0%. The RLIMS-P system had a high precision (97.9%) with only two false positives.

Our second evaluation was conducted on a larger scale. Further, we wanted to also evaluate our ability to extract all three pieces of information and not just the site and theme information. For this evaluation of RLIMS-P and in particular the effectiveness of the extra-clausal processing it performs, we used annotated data from Phospho.ELM database. This database contains a collection of experimentally verified Serine, Threonine and Tyrosine phosphorylation sites in eukaryotic proteins. The entries are manually annotated and based on scientific literature. Each entry contains the phosphorylated amino acid and position (site), the substrate (theme) and the kinase responsible for the modification (agent) and links to bibliographic references. More details regarding this database and the entire dataset can be found at http://phospho.elm.eu.org/.

Our evaluation was based on extraction from 386 abstracts from the Phospho.ELM data set. This set constitutes an *unseen* test data set, which is distinct from the abstracts we had used for development of our system, its patterns and the extra-clausal rules we evaluate here. We refer the readers for the details of this evaluation in (Narayanaswamy et al. 2005), in particular on how the annotated data was extracted from the PhosphoELM database. We now summarize the evaluation results here.

To evaluate the aspects of our system, we consider three versions: the first where only patterns are applied but no extra-clausal processing is applied, second corresponding to the application of SR and the TRs to the basic patterns based system and finally the complete system.

The first set of numbers (ATS) corresponds to the extraction of the entire relation (i.e., the ternary relationship between the agent, theme and site). While the precision of all three systems is in 93 to 95% range (the full set of numbers may be found in (Narayanaswamy et al. 2005)), the recall rises from 24.2% to 77.4% for the patterns-only to the full system. The second system is around the middle with recall of 57.2%. This shows that fusion also has a significant role in improving the recall.

To further investigate where the gains of the use of the extra clausal processing are we looked at the improvements in the extraction of agent-theme (AT) relation and the theme-site relations. The AT relation extraction is similar to extraction of protein-protein interactions and might be of interest to those who are only interested in the interactions between pairs of proteins. The TS relation might be of interest to those researchers who are more interested in the biological consequence of phosphorylation (where the identity of the kinase catalyzing the modification is not as important). The recall for both relations is significantly better than that for the composite ternary relation. The precision is also higher (in the 97-98%) region for all systems and for both these binary relations. As should be expected, the second and third systems have identical numbers for AT and TS evaluation, since fusion should help with improved recall of ATS only. The recall of the first system is poor for the TS (25.1%) and better for the AT (64.9%) showing the protein-protein interaction like relation (i.e., AT) is easier to extract with patterns only. These numbers increase significantly with use of SR and TR to 82.4% and 82.6% respectively. Since we expect most of the gain in recall for TS relation to be from use of SR we considered how much the patterns based system augmented with SR alone (i.e., without TR) helped. We noticed that the recall moves up from 25.1% with patterns only to 61.5% with the use of SR. Of course augmenting patterns-only system with SR alone will not make a difference in the numbers of AT relation.

DEVELOPMENT OF ONLINE RLIMS-P TOOL

We have developed an online version of RLIMS-P (Yuan et al., 2006) that is freely available for any user (http://pir.georgetown.edu/iprolink/rlimsp/). A user can specify 1 or more PMID's as input, and returns a summary table for all PMIDs (Figure 1A) with links to full reports (Figure 1B). The summary table lists the PMID of each phosphorylation-related abstract that the tool finds along with its top-ranking annotation result, followed by a list of remaining PMIDs for abstracts containing no phosphorylation information. Full reports can be retrieved from the summary table using hypertext links (from "text evidence") or by selecting one or more PMID(s) in the list.

In producing its output, the online system not only extracts all the agent, theme and site of phosphorylation that might be mentioned in an abstract, it also post-processes the output three additional functionalities— phosphorylation annotation ranking, evidence tagging, and protein entity mapping.

Figure 1. Online RLIMS-P text-mining results in (A) summary table and (B) full report. The summary table lists PMIDs with top-ranking phosphorylation annotation. The full report provides detailed annotation results with evidence tagging and automatic mapping to UniProtKB entry containing the citation (KPB1_RABIT shown here).

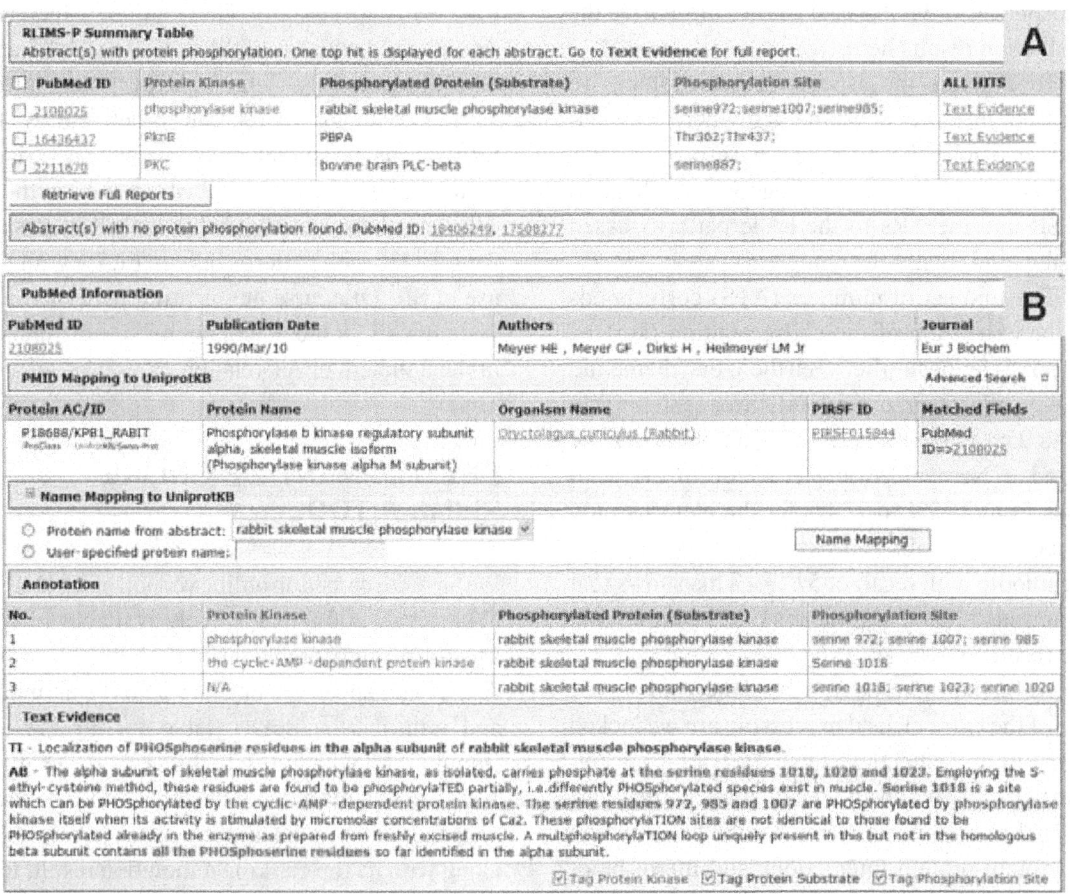
RLIMS-P Summary Table
Abstract(s) with protein phosphorylation. One top hit is displayed for each abstract. Go to Text Evidence for full report.
A
PubMed ID
Protein Kinase
Phosphorylated Protein (Substrate)
Phosphorylation Site
ALL HITS
2108025
phosphorylase kinase
rabbit skeletal muscle phosphorylase kinase
serine972;serine1007;serine985;
Text Evidence
16436437
PknB
PBPA
Thr362;Thr437;
Text Evidence
2211670
PKC
bovine brain PLC-beta
serine887;
Text Evidence
Retrieve Full Reports
Abstract(s) with no protein phosphorylation found. PubMed ID: 18406249, 17508277
PubMed Information
B
PubMed ID
Publication Date
Authors
Journal
2108025
1990/Mar/10
Meyer HE , Meyer GF , Dirks H , Heilmeyer LM Jr
Eur J Biochem
PMID Mapping to UniprotKB
Advanced Search
Protein AC/ID
Protein Name
Organism Name
PIRSF ID
Matched Fields
P18688/KPB1_RABIT
Phosphorylase b kinase regulatory subunit alpha, skeletal muscle isoform (Phosphorylase kinase alpha M subunit)
Oryctolagus cuniculus (Rabbit)
PIRSF015844
PubMed ID=>2108025
Name Mapping to UniprotKB
Protein name from abstract: rabbit skeletal muscle phosphorylase kinase
User-specified protein name:
Name Mapping
Annotation
No.
Protein Kinase
Phosphorylated Protein (Substrate)
Phosphorylation Site
1
phosphorylase kinase
rabbit skeletal muscle phosphorylase kinase
serine 972; serine 1007; serine 985
2
the cyclic-AMP -dependent protein kinase
rabbit skeletal muscle phosphorylase kinase
Serine 1018
3
N/A
rabbit skeletal muscle phosphorylase kinase
serine 1018; serine 1023; serine 1020
Text Evidence
TI - Localization of PHOSphoserine residues in the alpha subunit of rabbit skeletal muscle phosphorylase kinase.
AB - The alpha subunit of skeletal muscle phosphorylase kinase, as isolated, carries phosphate at the serine residues 1018, 1020 and 1023. Employing the S-ethyl-cysteine method, these residues are found to be phosphorylaTED partially, i.e.differently PHOSphorylated species exist in muscle. Serine 1018 is a site which can be PHOSphorylated by the cyclic-AMP -dependent protein kinase. The serine residues 972, 985 and 1007 are PHOSphorylated by phosphorylase kinase itself when its activity is stimulated by micromolar concentrations of Ca2. These phosphorylaTION sites are not identical to those found to be PHOSphorylated already in the enzyme as prepared from freshly excised muscle. A multiphosphorylaTION loop uniquely present in this but not in the homologous beta subunit contains all the PHOSphoserine residues so far identified in the alpha subunit.
Tag Protein Kinase
Tag Protein Substrate
Tag Phosphorylation Site

Phosphorylation Annotation Ranking

For a given phosphorylation-related abstract, RLIMS-P produces one or multiple annotation results, each consisting of up to three phosphorylation objects (kinase, phosphorylated protein and site). The multiple annotation results are ranked based on the number of objects and sites extracted (see Figure 1B). Annotations with phosphorylated protein information take precedence over protein kinase information. Therefore, annotation with three objects and with the most sites will rank first, while annotation with site and phosphorylated protein will precede one with site and kinase.

Evidence Tagging

To provide evidence attribution for the annotation results, the online RLIMS-P tags each individual object with an internal identifier during its shallow parsing, and uses it subsequently for color-tagging phosphorylation objects in the abstract for web display.

Protein Entity Mapping

The online RLIMS-P provides a mapping of phosphorylated proteins to UniProtKB entries based on PubMed ID (PMID) and/or proteins names.

PMID Mapping

UniProtKB contains extensive bibliographic information for each protein entry via the UniProtKB-PMID mapping that includes reference citations annotated in UniProtKB and collected from curated databases such as SGD, MGD and GeneRIF (Wu *et al.*, 2006). For an abstract that already exists in the PMID mapping, the online RLIMS-P automatically associates the phosphorylated protein with the UniProtKB protein entry.

Name Mapping

If the abstract has no PMID mapping in UniProtKB, the phosphorylated protein can be mapped based on protein names using the web-based BioThesaurus (Liu *et al.*, 2006). BioThesaurus provides a comprehensive collection of gene/protein names from multiple molecular databases with associations to UniProtKB protein entries. The online BioThesaurus allows the retrieval of synonyms of a given protein and the identification of protein entries sharing a given name. The online RLIMS-P integrates these BioThesaurus functions, allowing users to select the corresponding protein entry for the phosphorylated protein from a list of UniProtKB entries retrieved by BioThesaurus.

CONCLUSIONS AND FUTURE ENHANCEMENTS

We have developed RLIMS-P that extracts a targeted type of information: the extraction of substrate and site of phosphorylation with the kinase involved. An online version is also available that has enhanced functionalities for easy access of extracted information. RLIMS-P uses shallow parsing, entity type classification and an extensive set of manually developed patterns for extraction. Additional rules have been developed that allow the combination of information obtained from different sentences. RLIMS-P has been evaluated and shown to have high precision as well as recall.

Plans to extend RLIMS-P in different ways. In particular, more work is needed to see how the system can generalize from its current application on abstracts to application of full length articles. Application of machine learning methods to mining other biological information associated with protein phosphorylation in the text, such as biological signals leading to and subsequent effects of phosphoryaltion, will also be explored. Additionally, we are exploring how the system including its patterns can be generalized to extract other PTMs such as methylation and acetylation.

REFERENCES

Blaschke, C., Andrade, M. A., Ouzounis, C., & Valencia, A. (1999). Automatic extraction of biological information from scientific text: Protein-protein interactions. *Proc Int Conf Intell Syst Mol Biol*, (pp. 60-67).

Daraselia, N., Yuryev, A., Egorov, S., Novichkova, S., Nikitin, A., & Mazo, I. (2004). Extracting human protein interactions from MEDLINE using a full-sentence parser. *Bioinformatics*, *20*, 604-11.

Donaldson, I., Martin, J., de Bruijn, B., Wolting, C., Lay, V., Tuekam, B., Zhang, S., Baskin, B., Bader, G. D., Michalickova, K., Pawson, T., & Hogue, C. W. (2003). PreBIND and Textomy--mining the biomedical literature for protein-protein interactions using a support vector machine. *BMC Bioinformatics*, *4*(1), 11.

Friedman, C., Kra, P., Yu, H., Krauthammer, M., & Rzhetsky, A. (2001). GENIES: A natural-langauge processing system for the extraction of molecular pathways from journal articles. *Bioinformatics*, *17*(Suppl 1), 74-82.

Hu, Z. Z., Mani, I., Hermoso, V., Liu, H., & Wu, C. H. (2004). iProLINK: an integrated protein resource for literature mining. *Comput Biol Chem*, *28*, 409-416.

Hu, Z. Z., Narayanaswamy, M., Ravikumar, K. E., Vijay-Shanker, K., & Wu, C. H. (2005). Literature mining and database annotation of protein phosphorylation using a rule-based system. *Bioinformatics*, *21*, 2759-65.

Koike, A., Kobayashi, Y., & Takagi, T. (2003). Kinase pathway database: an integrated protein-kinase and NLP-based protein-interaction resource. *Genome Res.*, *13*, 1231-43.

Liu, H., Hu, Z. Z., & Wu, C. H. (2006a). BioThesaurus: a web-based thesaurus of protein and gene names. *Bioinformatics, 22*, 103-105.

Liu, H., Hu, Z. Z., Torii, M., Wu, C., & Friedman, C. (2006b). Quantitative Assessment of Dictionary-based Protein Named Entity Tagging. *J Am Med Inform Assoc, 13*, 497-507.

Mika, S., & Rost, B. (2004). Protein names precisely peeled off free text. *Bioinformatics*, *20*(Suppl 1), I241-I247.

Narayanaswamy, M., Ravikumar, K. E., & Vijay-Shanker, K. (2005). Beyond the clause: Extraction of phosphorylation information from Medline abstracts. *Bioinformatics,* (Suppl 1), i319-i327.

Proux, D., Rechenmann, F., & Julliard, L. (2000). A Pragmatic Information Extraction Strategy for Gathering Data on Genetic Interactions. *Proc Int Conf Intell Syst Mol Biol*, *8*, 279-285.

Pustejovsky, J., Castaño, J., Zhang, J., Kotecki, M., & Cochran, B. (2002). Robust relational parsing over biomedical literature: Extracting inhibit relations. *Pac Symp Biocomput*, (pp. 362-373).

Shatkay, H., & Feldman, R. (2003). Mining the biomedical literature in the genomic era: an overview. *J Comput Biol.*, *10*(6), 821-55.

Stapley, B. J., & Benoit, G. (2000). Bio-bibliometrics: information retrieval and visualization from co-occurrences of gene names in Medline abstracts. *Pac Symp Biocomput*, (pp. 529-540).

Stephens, M., Palakal, M., Mukhopadhyay, S., Raje, R., & Mostafa, J. (2001). Detecting gene relations from Medline abstracts. *Pac Symp Biocomput*, (pp. 483-495).

Wu, C. H., Apweiler, R., Bairoch, A., Natale, D. A., Barker, W. C., Boeckmann, B., Ferro, S., Gasteiger, E., Huang, H., Lopez, R. et al. (2006). The Universal Protein Resource (UniProt): an expanding universe of protein information. *Nucleic Acids Res, 34*(Database issue), D187-191.

Yeh, A., Morgan, A., Colosimo, M., & Hirschman, L. (2005). BioCreAtIvE task 1A: gene mention finding evaluation. *BMC Bioinformatics*, *6*(Suppl 1), S2.

Yuan, X., Hu, Z. Z., Wu, H. T., Torii, M., Narayanaswamy, M., Ravikumar, K. E., Vijay-Shanker, K., & Wu, C. H. (2006). An online literature mining tool for protein phosphorylation. *Bioinformatics, 22*(13), 1668-9.

Zhou, G., Zhang, J., Su, J., Shen, D., & Tan, C. (2004). Recognizing names in biomedical texts: a machine learning approach. *Bioinformatics*, *20*, 1178-90.

Chapter X
CorTag: A Language for a Contextual Tagging of the Words Within Their Sentence

Yves Kodratoff
University Paris-Sud (Paris XI), France

Jérôme Azé
University Paris-Sud (Paris XI), France

Lise Fontaine
Cardiff University, UK

ABSTRACT

This chapter argues that in order to extract significant knowledge from masses of technical texts, it is necessary to provide the field specialists with programming tools with which they themselves may use to program their text analysis tools. These programming tools, besides helping the programming effort of the field specialists, must also help them to gather the field knowledge necessary for defining and retrieving what they define as significant knowledge. This necessary field knowledge must be included in a well-structured and easy to use part of the programming tool. In this chapter, we present CorTag, a programming tool which is designed to correct existing tags in a text and to assist the field specialist to retrieve the knowledge and/or information he or she is looking for.

INTRODUCTION AND MOTIVATION

In this paper we present a new programming language, called CorTag, which is devoted to tagging words within the boundaries of the sentence in which they are contained. The context we are concerned with here is therefore limited to the sentence and the words within it. The tagging process in CorTag includes syntactic, functional and semantic tags. Ultimately CorTag is designed to correct the existing tags in highly specialised or technical texts.

Our primary aim is to contribute to the creation of a system which is able to find interesting pieces of knowledge within specialised texts. There is no attempt being made towards the broader understanding of natural language. Our ambition is to be able to spot parts of the texts that may be of particular interest to the specialist of a given technical domain. As we shall see, the process does nevertheless require a kind of 'primitive' understanding of the text.

In creating this new language, we have been motivated by two facts which, despite being intuitively obvious, are challenging when used as a base for the building of a computer system.

The first of these is that the number of genre specific texts is increasing exponentially. It follows that humans can no longer handle these masses of texts and the whole process has to be automated. The scientific community is certainly aware of this need as it is exemplified by the large number of competitions and challenges, dealing with many topics expressed in many different languages. This has led to the development of software solutions devoted to solving at least one of the problems encountered for each step of the overall process. In order to make these steps explicit, let us propose a tentative list of the main steps involved. The text mining process starts by gathering the texts of interest, what we will refer to as 'text gathering'. The process ends when the desired information has been found in the text. This final step is identified here as 'information extraction'. There is a large set of intermediate steps which take place between these two steps, and the precise set of steps depends on the state of the retrieved texts and the nature of the information sought. The following sequence shows one possible ordering of the necessary intermediate steps:

text gathering → sorting → standardization → creation/improvement of lexicon → tagging and/or parsing → terminology → concept recognition → co-reference resolution → finding the relations among concepts → information extraction.

In the following, when speaking of any step in particular, we will always assume that all n-k steps have been executed before the current $step_n$. We shall not, however, assume that they have been correctly completed. One of the main difficulties is that these different levels of Natural Language (NL) processing are mutually dependent. In general, the context independent processes can be performed quite satisfactorily, while the context dependent ones are very challenging as we shall exemplify. Unfortunately, the users (and sometimes even the creators) of the '$step_n$ specialized software' are not aware that this software is absolutely unable to function properly if some of $step_{n-k}$ has not been properly completed. For example, 'sorting', a step which will be described later in the paper, illustrates well the dependencies amongst steps. Sorting is not really context-dependent, as we shall explain, and therefore it is a step which should be completed relatively easily. However, an improperly performed $step_n$ causes mistakes at $step_{n+k}$ which then spread throughout the process. It is the context dependent steps which are most greatly affected by this. Since many of the context dependent mistakes of $step_{n-k}$ cannot be detected before $step_n$, we need a language to backtrack and correct them. This defines the first primary constraint placed on CorTag's development.

The second motivating fact is that each specific genre tends to develop its own lexical and grammatical tendencies, often considered as jargon outside of the genre. As researchers, we cannot be put off because of the difficulties and challenges presented as the texts become more highly specialised or because they diverge from standard written English. Linguists, whether working on learner English texts, SMS texts, or other instances of 'non-standard' language, will analyse the data in an "as is" state and it is precisely this state that is of utmost interest to linguists – how speakers use language *really*. As Stubbs [Stubbs, 1993] stresses, whole texts must be analysed since the distribution of linguistic features is not regular throughout any given text and further, the main object of linguistic analysis must be "actual, attested, authentic instances of use" [Stubbs, 1993, p 8]. The problem for the linguist is how to handle a very large volume of texts. The problem for the computer scientist is developing systems to automatically process texts produced within a highly specialised subject field. The cost of having to refine the syntax and lexicon is computationally expensive. In a sense, the approach taken here is similar to the story of the importance of teaching a person how to fish rather than giving them the fish. We are not yet at the point technologically speaking where we can build a system that can extract information from many different types of highly specialised texts. What we can do is build tools that will enable the extraction of information from within the specialised community. We propose CorTag as a language which can be used to program the specific needs of the field specialist in order to extract significant information. In a sense, this implies that most linguists and computer scientists lack the complete qualification to build a system that extract information from genre specific texts.

In computer science terms, CorTag is a Perl regular expression translator. Anyone can write down such regular expressions, although it does become difficult when a large number of complex expressions need to be written. When users want to experiment on the effect of a regular expression on a text, they have to write tentative rules which may be modified depending on effect they have. Thus, CorTag is essential for the research phase during which the user must focus more on the effect of the rules rather than on their syntax.

We shall now provide an informal specification of CorTag that fulfills at least partially the two primary constraints we defined above. The entire paper will show in detail how our implementation respects this specification which may seem to be mere good sense.

CorTag's primary feature is that the programs are written in such a way that they are almost self commentary. When a new user wishes to start from an old program (or when a given programmer re-uses old programs), the commentaries, however still useful, can be very short. This is why a CorTag program is a sequence of easy to read rules of the classical form: IF (condition) THEN (action). These rules apply in their sequential ordering. The commentaries can then be reduced to pointing out the possible effect of rule number n on rule $n+p$, if any.

CorTag treats the sentence in the order in which the words are entered between two 'end of sentence' marks. Each word encountered in this way is looked upon as the current sentence's pivot, its index is 0 and the other words are indexed relative to the current pivot. When the action of a rule modifies the position of a word, the indexing of all the words is modified as a consequence. This kind of side effect is usually hard to control within a language of actions such as CorTag. Every effort has been made to reduce the number of side effects. It is impossible to avoid all of them, but since there are only a relatively small number, we have been able to document all of them in detail.

The remainder of the paper is organised as follows. Following a brief section describing existing systems and the main functionalities of CorTag, a more detailed section is presented which explains how CorTag works by discussing two positive results and three limitations from using our approach. The positive results were firstly how we were able to improve the morpho-syntactical and functional contextual tagging and secondly how CorTag assists in the discovery of relations among concepts (see [Fontaine and Kodratoff, 2004] for a more detailed presentation of the discovery of concepts in texts). The limitations concern semantic contextual tagging, co-reference resolution, and sorting. Finally the paper closes with our conclusions.

A BRIEF OVERVIEW OF RELATED SYSTEMS AND CORTAG

Other Systems

The UNITEX system (http://igm.univ-mlv.fr/~unitex/index.htm) is a very complete tool which works on raw texts and selects parts of the text which are interesting to the user. This tool provides the facility (which is as well a constraint) of using the grammars and dictionaries associated to it and it can be applied to several languages. The system uses transductors, which amount to a graphical language to write regular expression, in order to put in evidence various lexical units of the text, viz. the beginning and end of sentences, or the marker 'STOP' when it has been introduced in the text, a lexical tag, or a sequence on contiguous letters, alphabetic or not. Other grammars can be introduced provided they are written in the Unitex format, but this is not trivial. It enables its user to extract from a text any part of it, or as well as modifying this part, showing a given pattern which is a regular expression written as a transductor. CorTag rules differ from the formalism used by Unitex in the sense that the transductors need solid training before being properly handled. It cannot, however, work on a text that has already been tagged, therefore it is not adapted to correcting existing tags. Although it is a powerful system, it pays for this power in memory and running time.

The tool GATE (http://gate.ac.uk) is also very powerful system that offers to the user a toolbox containing different predefined tools enabling the user to perform basic tasks on text. If specific applications have to be developed, the user can write them through a simple JAVA plugin. In doing so, however, the user must write the corresponding JAVA program. Another difference with CorTag is that GATE reduces the 'context' to the words that are adjacent to the word under study. An interesting extension of GATE is OLLIE [Tablan et al., 2003] which enables several specialists to collaborate in tagging the same corpus through a web applet.

POSEDIT (Nov. 2007, http://elearning.unistrapg.it/corpora/posedit.html) is a very recent system but since it is so new, it is still very poorly documented. Therefore it will not be included in this brief review.

CorTag

CorTag has been designed to work with any type of technical text since its two theoretical limitations are genre independent. Since CorTag corrects a text's tags, ('Cor(rects the) Tags'), the texts it works on have to be tagged, possibly with dummy tags if none are known beforehand. Furthermore, it works successively on each sentence of the text, therefore the end and the beginning of each sentence must be accurately recognized. In practice, we have developed CorTag in order to apply it to the English as used in the field of macromolecular biology. The examples given in this paper all come from the corpus provided to the competitors of TREC'2005. The specialists of this domain seem to have developed a genre-specific use of language which is efficient in the sense that field specialists seem to cope perfectly well with its specialised grammar. The phenomena they describe are so complex that they seem to have developed grammatical patterns that would be considered rare at best. This leads to an extra layer of difficulty as the non specialist reader, who does not understand the meaning of these sentences, will find it very difficult to correctly analyse the syntactic structure of the sentences. Consequently it is of no surprise that an automated parser is unable to work properly on such sentences, as we shall illustrate later. The goal of CorTag is to enable someone who does understand these sentences - not a linguist or computer scientist who may not understand them– to make decisions about the morpho-syntactic, functional and semantic tags that need to be attached to the terms of the text in order to be able to extract significant knowledge from it. Since none of the authors of this paper is a specialist of this field, we make no claims concerning finding such significant knowledge. Our claim is that we provide a simple and useful tool to the domain specialist to be able to do so.

Although we have concentrated our efforts on molecular biology, we have also checked the applicability of using CorTag with other corpora. In particular, we worked on another corpus, believed to be less technical, namely the *Acquaint* newspaper corpus of TREC'2004. *Acquaint* certainly requires less in-depth knowledge but it is actually highly specialised nevertheless on many different topics, including for example baseball, American politics, American religious rights, etc.

As stated above, decisions concerning tagging are made by the user, however for our purposes, the basic tags we used are those of the project Penn Treebank - see http://www.cis.upenn.edu/~treebank/. The user can then decide to introduce functional or semantic tags. For example, in a given text, a chemical compound, say NaCl, may play a specific role and be referred to by the expression NaCl but it will tend to be referred to as 'salt' when its chemical properties are not very relevant. Suppose, on the contrary, that a user is interested in finding relations among chemical products that may be a possible cause for some sickness, it then becomes very important to give special tags to these chemical compounds in order to select the proper relations. This also illustrates one possible iterative use of Cortag. The users can find in the literature a list of the compounds known for having an action of this sickness. These compounds are thus tagged in a special way and, as shown in section 4, the users can find the relations that exist between these compounds. In turn, they can then find the not yet specially tagged compounds that show the same relationships among them, and set up lists of products yet unknown for having a potential action.

The field specialist is also asked to provide some kind of linguistic knowledge specific to the field in the form of 'ontologies' that are nothing but simple ISA trees, the leaves of which can have common elements. The simplicity of this representation has enabled us to optimize retrieval within these ontologies. For instance, we currently use a nominal and a verbal ontology describing around 150 possible semantic tags of nouns, and verbs containing some 30 000 words. This does not significantly change the execution speed of our programs. In its normal use, these taxonomies enable the specialist to provide the knowledge necessary to disambiguate the functional role of various grammatical forms as we will show in next section. Nevertheless, as already stated, we cannot claim that the examples we will provide are an 'exact' solution that would satisfy the needs of a biologist. Our purpose here is to show how CorTag could be used by a real biologist to get a right answer.

CorTag handles the effects of the context of the current word within the sentence, for each word in sequence. It has been conceived for efficiency in that respect. It is then easy to write an efficient and easy to understand rule to change a tag and word. The execution speed of CorTag is linear in the size of the corpus, linear in the number of rules executed, but non linear in the complexity of each rule. Therefore there is a "CorTag programming style" which may look initially very poor to the astute programmer but which in fact optimizes the execution speed. For instance, we also optimized the detection of sequences of letters within a word (for instance, the word ends with 'ed') because there are conditions in which a given context can be significant. These internal properties are normally a part of the 'condition' of CorTag's rules. Inversely, when the 'action' modifies the part of a word without changing the whole word, the rules to be written are not optimal. In these relatively simple cases, it is much better to directly write a Perl regular expression. For example, orthographic corrections may be handled by a rule or they may be very difficult and costly. In this example, a spelling error that can be recovered from the local context, as in *he talk fast* where the person agreement marker has been omitted, are easily repaired with CorTag. Non-contextual errors such as finding *adress* rather than *address* in the text are not.

An important step in dealing with technical texts is dealing with terminology since specialists use terms specific to them and they tend to create a large number of them. They will therefore produce sentences that look incomprehensible because they are read by non-specialists as containing general non-technical single word terms. The terms actually being used are composed of several words, perhaps better seen as multi-word expressions or even formulaic expressions (see for example [Wray, 2002]), and consequently, the problem of tagging them is not trivial. In many cases, the last word of the term is a useful indicator for a good tag, as for example in 'heterodimeric_transmembrane' which is an obvious noun. There are many cases where this choice is not obvious. It may be that the last word of the term is itself grammatically ambiguous. For instance, in the case of an "open_reading frame" 'reading' could be a present participle, a noun or an adjective. The various contexts in which this term is found show that 'open_reading' is only used as a premodifier that behaves as modifier in the sentence. The case of "dose_related lethality" is even more ambiguous since 'dose_related' is most often used as noun would be. In other words, *dose related* is a type of nominal compound where *dose* rather than *related* functions as the head of the compound expression. This is problematic since typically in nominal compounds it is the right-most lexical element which classifies the term. We must accept that these are challenging areas for the analyst who does not have specialist knowledge and a near impossible task for any automated tagging system. These problems have been analyzed elsewhere [Amrani et al., 2004]. A good definition of the existing terms is obviously important in parsing the sentence. Another less expected effect of a bad terminology is that it can increase the difficulty in spotting significant relationships up to the point of making them impossible to find. A particularly simple example of this is illustrated by the sentence: "The salm_gene acts independently of abd_A". If the term 'salm_gene' was not introduced, either the system of relation detection would become so complex that its running time becomes unbearable, or it would find that 'a gene acts independently of something', which cannot be significant since a large corpus would lead to thousands of similar relationships.

MORPHO-SYNTACTIC AND FUNCTIONAL CONTEXTUAL TAGGING

The Problem

A typical example of the need for a functional tagging is the case of the English past participle forms. They have the same morphology as most active past forms (except in the case of irregular verbs, such as 'chose' and 'chosen'). This introduces an obvious possible confusion in their role which is marked in the Penn Treebank notation by tagging the past forms with a /VBD and the participles with a /VBN. In canonical English, according to [Quirk et al., 1985], they also can have the role, as adjectives would, of pre or postmodifiers of a noun. Even though their 'normal' use is the one of a passive meaning, premodification is possible when the word in the past participle form indicates a permanent or characteristic feature [Quirk et al., p 1325-29]. They can also be postmodifiers especially when they are followed by a 'by-agent'.

It is even possible to find them in postposition without any prepositional construction, but only in fixed expressions. It happens that this feature of standard English has been stretched very far in the way of writing results of molecular biology that systematically use postmodifying past participle forms. Consider the relatively simple sentence:

"the tyrosine phosphorylation of FRS2_SNT was examined in AP20187 treated iFGFR1 transduced nih3t3 fibroblasts to determine if iFGFR1 activation can signal through this pathway."

The form *examined* is not at all ambiguous, it is the past participle form of the verb examine expressed in a passive voice construction. The two forms *treated* and *transduced*, inversely, are ambiguous in their use, although clearly either in the simple past tense or past participle form, and in order to be correctly tagged, the understanding of the whole sentence is needed. This sentence calls for two very different comments. Firstly, the embedded sentence "AP20187 treated iFGFR1" is not semantically ambiguous since it means that *iFGFR1* has been treated by *AP20187* but it is syntactically ambiguous since *treated* can be either an active past form or a postmodifier of *AP20187*. Since a clause can contain only one main verb, and *examined* is unambiguously the main verb, *treated* must be a postmodifier. There are further linguistic arguments to support this analysis but since this is not the purpose here, we will not discuss it further. Secondly, the segment "iFGFR1 transduced nih3t3 fibroblasts" has no immediate meaning. The same argument as before eliminates the past tense case, but *transduced* can be either a postmodifier of *iFGFR1* or a premodifier of *nih3t3 fibroblasts*. Field knowledge will determine the ambiguity by identifying which one can be 'transduced', i.e. *iFGFR1* or some kind of fibroblasts. Clearly we have simplified the full reasoning in order to avoid overly lengthy explanations. Our point here is simply to exemplify the fact that a normal tagger or a normal parser will not function properly on these types of sentences.

Note that we have used the vocabulary of grammar to discuss this, where one is supposed to be able to know at once if a word ending with an *-ed* is in the form of simple past tense or past participle. This is obviously impossible for a machine, which is why, in the following, we will not speak of *–ed* forms of the verb, and instead refer specifically to the morphological suffix (e.g. "*–ed* endings" *-ed* for brevity), regardless of what type of verb form is being expressed.

When any *–ed* is both preceded and followed by a noun, the same problems will occur. We estimate that this problem is encountered more than 15 000 times in our corpus. We have used CorTag to solve one of the subproblems of the one just presented: what happens when the sentence is even more complex because it contains a sequence of a noun, followed by two *–ed* word forms, followed by a noun. This configuration is less common. We found 359 instances of it.

Solution of the *–ed –ed* Case

Basic general rule: All verbs can be marked with an *–ed* ending which can be a postmodifying *–ed* form.

Specific Rule:

WHEN two *–ed* follow each other in between two nouns,
THEN the first *–ed* is normally a past tense (tagged VBD) and the second one is a premodifying *–ed* form,
EXCEPT IF the first *–ed* ending is a postmodifier because it fulfils **Condition** 1.
IN THIS CASE, the second *–ed* ending is
EITHER a past form if **Conditions** 2, 3 or 5 are true
OR it is a premodifying *–ed* form IF **Conditions** 5' or 4 are true.

Condition 1: the noun before the first *-ed* cannot be the actor of the action supposed to be described by the verb (if it were a past tense). What follows are several lists of such impossible forms:

List 1:{aberrations, properties, species, tissues, types, yeast, etc.} DO NOT {examine, analyze, identify, list, observe, study, survey, etc.}

List 2: {sample, samples, eEF1A_2_S1 (peptide_elongation_factor), etc.} DO NOT {hybridize, infect, etc.} SOMETHING

List 3: {tyrosine etc.} DO NOT {phosphorylate, etc.} SOMETHING

List 4: {model, models, reporters, reporter, etc.} DO NOT {use, etc.} SOMETHING

List 5: {mother, mothers, we, etc.} {feed (in the present tense only} SOMETHING. This strange rule means that, in our corpus at least, when a female animal 'fed' it always means that she received some food, never that she gave it to her progeny.

Condition 2: the second –ed belongs to a list we call 'inclusion', including:{comprise, contain, include, involve, etc.}

Condition 3: the second *–ed* belongs to -ed that cannot be premodifiers such as {showed}. [No other instance in our corpus]

Condition 4: the first *-ed* belongs of the –ed forms that are always pre or postmodifiers: {misfolded} [No other instance in our corpus]

Condition 5: A clause contains one and one only process. This rule is useful only when a –ed is unambiguously recognizable within the same clause.

Condition 5': Some sequences of words are not sentences at all, for example: titles, citations, authors' lists, figure captions, authors addresses etc.

Such a complex rule is much easier to discover for a field specialist than for us. Nevertheless, starting from the assumption that sentences in texts accepted for publication in a scientific review would not be ambiguous, we were able to suppose that some kind of rule, such as the one above, was in action. The role of CorTag, for us, as it would be for a field specialist, is to allow us to build a hypothesis from very few (usually only one) examples, and checking its validity on the entire corpus. We isolated some of the '*noun –ed –ed noun*' sequences and tried to find a rule that explained the tagging. Once this is done, it is then quite easy and quick to write this rule in CorTag and check that the whole corpus is in agreement with it.

DISCOVERING RELATIONS AMONG CONCEPTS

There are two obvious sources for the difficulty of finding significant relationships among entities. One is that these relationships are manifold (for instance a slight negative interaction is completely different from a strong positive one) and each of them can be expressed in a large variety of styles. The second is that no known list of 'interesting' compounds can exist since they differ for each specific application. Following the specifications of CorTag, as given above, it is designed for a field specialist needing to experiment many variations in the text, thus well adapted to the present problem. To be more precise, we will describe the typical problems met in this case, and the typical solutions the user can find.

At first, the user has to obtain a text from a relatively well tagged corpus by using one of the classical taggers such as Brill's tagger [Brill, 1994], SVM POS taggers (see, for instance, http://www.lsi.upc.es/~nlp/SVMTool/) or even taggers based on Logical Programming [Cussens, 1997]. Using

CorTag, it is possible to improve it. No mistake can be tolerated when it involves interesting compounds and the verbs expressing a potential interesting interaction. This seems trivial but it deeply affects the tagging strategy. For instance the word 'uses' can be either a plural noun, tagged NNS, or a verb present 3rd person, tagged VBZ. When dealing with knowledge extraction in general, it may well be useless to make such a difference between the two forms since something is used in both cases. Inversely, if it expresses a relation of interest (discovering what uses what in which way, for example), making the difference between the nominal forms (use, uses), the verbal forms (use, uses, using, used) and the pre and postmodifiers (used), it may be very important.

Most often, these confusions can be avoided by using the context, provided this context is properly tagged. For example, in 'that use' 'use' is obviously a verb if 'that' is a conjunction introducing a new clause, but it is obviously a singular noun if 'that' is a determiner. The tagging of the word 'that' is by itself a hard problem which recursively depends on the tagging of its context, that is, in the example above, 'that' is tagged as a determiner or a conjunction depending on the next word being a noun or a verb. This problem is often considered secondary because of the high success of learning systems on the tagging problem. However, this success is obtained on a previously tagged example corpus which does not exist for most technical fields. Furthermore, the measurements are measured by the precision on the whole set of tags of the learning corpus. A 99% precision on millions of tags means an error on tens of thousands. If these tens of thousands errors are specialized to the difficult cases (which should not surprise anyone) such as verb/noun and 'that' confusions, this means that tens of thousands of relationships among concepts could be missed. Since a field specialist looks for hundreds of significant relations – otherwise the topic studied is too general to be of interest – it is easy to understand that a special effort must be made to reach a 99% precision on the difficult cases. Using CorTag, we have been able to see that this tagging depends on many factors including a context which is not only relative to the tags but also relative to the words themselves. This fact requires the creation of lists of words that constitute a special context. For example, we have built lists of (non ambiguous) verbs that are normally followed by a subordinative 'that', tagged /IN. These lists are efficient in various contexts that can be tested with a relative ease using CorTag. The existing list can be improved by the user; it is included as a part of the program and can be found in *ontology_verbale.xml*, in *<VerbThatIN>*.

In the next section, we shall discuss the problem of semantic tagging, for which more work is needed by the user. In order to continue illustrating how we can discover relations, let us suppose that the user has been able to obtain a list of the words and terms designating an interesting concept. For example, consider the sentence: *rux acts genetically to negatively regulate CycA*. In spite of being short, this sentence is very complex since the 'action' of *rux* is described by the clause *to negatively regulate CycA*. This problem is solved if the user has tagged rux and CycA as 'interesting compounds' and, for example, that the verb *to act* is not interesting while *to regulate* is. The tagged sentence may be as follows where adverbs are tagged /RB and to is tagged /TO: "rux/NNinterest acts/VBZ genetically/RB to/TO negatively/RB regulate/VBinterest CycA/NNinterest ./." A simple CorTag rule can spot the cases where the sentence contains two '/NNinterest' around a '/VBinterest' and it will notice that this verb is modified by 'negatively'. If the user is not interested by the negative interactions, this relation will be rejected. Otherwise, the system can then either bring back a summary: "rux … negatively regulate CycA" or everything in between the two

/NNinterest, as it should during the experimentation phase. There are many ways of expressing a negative interaction. The user can now write a rule that will bring back all sentences containing the sequence "rux … to regulate … CycA. In this way, new ways of expressing an interaction are found and those considered as negative by the user can be added to a list of 'negative modifiers'. Suppose the user is interested by everything that negatively regulates CycA. It is then easy to write another rule that will return all sentences containing the verb to regulate together with a negative modifier, thus enriching the list of /NNinterest showing this behavior. By successive increase of both lists, the user will reach (actually quite fast, as we observed) exhaustive lists of /NNinterest that repress each other.

It is also important to identify the really significant terms within the text. Consider the sentence: "expression of odd is repressed by ectopic eve expression." Notice that 'odd' and 'eve' do not have their usual meaning here, and should be tagged accordingly beforehand. Suppose they have been tagged /NNinterest. CorTag will bring back the summary "odd/NNinterest repressed/VBNpassive eve/NNinterest". Note in passing that the VBNpassive (tagged with a 100% accuracy by using CorTag) indicates that *eve* represses *odd.* If the user is interested by the fact that they interact through their expressions, then the fastest way to find it is to rewrite the corpus by introducing the terms expression_of_odd and eve_expression. If *ectopic* is of interest, the term ectopic_eve_expression should be introduced. Clearly then, the necessity for creating these terms does not depend at all on the frequency of the simultaneous occurrences of the words composing the term, but on the problem addressed.

More generally, as soon as the user introduces problem specific tags such as /NNinterest, then terms of interest should also be introduced, with their proper tag. In this way, a corpus of general interest will become a corpus specialized in the solution of a given problem. Since these modifications are done using CorTag rules, it becomes trivial to transform new texts into 'this problem specific texts' in order to keep the corpus up to date.

A NON CONTEXTUAL PROBLEM: SORTING

Whatever the topic, a really 'raw' text is a juxtaposition of different topics that do not use the same linguistic resources. In the TREC'2004 journalistic corpus, the different topics that had to be dealt with included the various references of the paper and to other papers, the sentences in foreign language, the slogans reported. For example, "GOD IS POWERFUL!" introduces the problem of sentences only written in capitals.

The first point, (usually non context dependent), is that the whole chain will fail if a preliminary sorting text is not properly done. In the TREC'2005 molecular biology corpus, entirely written in an English, which is, in principle, controlled by the referees and the publisher, we could observe an even larger number of differing registers or linguistic styles. We observed a significant level of linguistic variation within the same paper, viz., publisher's references and tags, title of the paper, summary and 'body' of the text, references to other papers, citations in foreign language within the text, titles, list of authors, bibliography, authors' physical and email addresses, figure and tables captions, comments inside tables, description of experiments performed, material used in these experiments, list of the abbreviations and acronyms used in the paper. As a simple example of the impossibility of treating all these problems with a unique system, consider the case of the acronyms used to designate the chemical elements as K for potassium etc. In the body of the text, the letter 'K' being an acronym, a rule will say that the form 'K.' is the end of sentence. In a list of authors, the inverse rule applies. More generally, a system that learns from texts that must be interpreted by logically contradictory rules will perhaps show a good precision on the learning set but cannot converge when presented more examples. It will lead to 100% error rates on some parts of the text, that is, it will be much less efficient than any random drawing.

It is actually very difficult to spot these contradictory rules which are usually lost in a mass of coefficients while it is very easy for a human and for a machine to recognize when the semantics of the linguistic objects varies. For example, the dots of a list of names, of a list of web addresses, of a list of numbers mean completely different things even though they have the same graphical representations. These mistakes tend to spread over the whole text with a surprising readiness. For example, the biologists named two genes as IS and ARE. Read the sentence in capitals just above, and you will see that if IS is a gene, then this sentence says, in bad English, that it is a powerful God. No one will write these genes as 'is' or 'are' but we did meet 'Is' and 'Are'. This is possible because biologists do not ask questions in their papers and therefore no sentence will begin with either of these words as verbs. However, this can be very dangerous in view of an automated knowledge extraction. In order to test how far it went, we tagged our corpus with the same Brill's tagger as usual with the one tiny change that the lexicon included an 'is' that could be also a noun. We obtained a surrealistic effect by having tens of thousands of 'is' badly tagged, and the errors propagated to other words, making the texts totally obscure.

Once this problem is acknowledged, it can be easily solved by providing to any learning system a few examples of the needed sorting. This solution does not need to take into account the context of the words in any way.

A 'NEGATIVE' RESULT: BUILDING ONTOLOGIES FROM TEXTS

We have set out to build ontologies that reflect exactly what is said by the authors. It seemed to us to be a necessary tool for co-reference resolution. We, however, quickly obtained a disheartening solution to this usually difficult problem. There is a simple and efficient rule to solve co-references in molecular biology. A slightly simplified, but essentially exact, version of it is: "In order to solve a co-reference, spot the general term that seems to refer to a particular case. Scan the text which is before this general term. Then, the first word which is not in the Worldnet corpus is the one it refers to." The simplicity of this rule is due to the following facts. Firstly, the vocabulary of molecular biology is so particular and so vast that Worldnet cannot take it into account and, secondly, that cataphora are almost inexistent except, rarely, in the introduction when no precise results are reported. This rule will only need to be made a bit more complex when several objects are referred to together.

This simplicity, however, is not very useful for building ontologies from texts because the real problem is in the complexity of the structure of these 'general terms' which reflects the complexity of the knowledge of molecular biology itself. This means that building huge lists of proteins or genes from texts is certainly an easy task. Finding the relationships among subgroups of such lists is as difficult as molecular biology is.

We are obviously unable to solve this problem ourselves since only a biologist aware of this knowledge is able to do so. We would however like to provide a few hints on how CorTag could be used to ease this formidable task. We have shown how it can be used to create lists of words playing a similar functional role in the sentence. This property could be used to gather groups of biological objects linked to each other by special relationships. As we already explained in section 4, this is possible when the user is able to provide a starting collection of semantic tags and of types of verbal relations. CorTag is well adapted to help complete both types of information.

CONCLUSION

We have described a new system, CorTag, which aims to correct the existing tags in texts in order to discover rules that will then lead to the extraction of significant information for the specialist. Despite the difficulty of working with these highly specialised texts, we have shown how CorTag can improve both the morpho-syntactic and functional contextual tags in a large corpus of specialised and highly technical texts.

This paper has detailed the two main principles upon which CorTag is based. Firstly, it is important to do more than simply include a field expert in the linguistic process. We claim that, due to the complexity and specificity of the technical language, the field expert must be central to the process of a computer-based text understanding. The linguist's and computer scientist's role should be 'reduced' to producing intelligent tools which the field specialist can use to solve his or her problems. We also have shown that this role is more complex than what has been assumed in the past by language and computer specialists. Therefore we believe we have defined an enhancement, rather than a reduction of their role. Secondly, a necessary condition for actualising our first principle, if not a sufficient one, is the need for developing special languages to be used by the field specialist to encode the knowledge held by the members of the scientific community (genre-specific knowledge). These languages must maintain intuitively simple properties. They should be self-commenting – that is, old programs should be easily re-used, and, in spite of describing 'actions' to be done to change the text, they must be conceived in such a way that they minimise the number of side-effects.

CorTag and its notice of use are available on the web, at http://www.lri.fr/~aze/CorTag/ . The list of words identified as having a specific role in the sentence, such as the verbs that usually introduce a subordinate clause, is available with the program. Creating more accurate lists specialised to other technical fields should then be possible in the future.

REFERENCES

Amrani, A., Azé, J., Heitz, T., Kodratoff, Y., & Roche, M. (2004). From the texts to the concepts they contain: a chain of linguistic treatments. In *Proc. TREC'04* (Text REtrieval Conference), National Institute of Standards and Technology, Gaithersburg Maryland USA, (pp. 712-722).

Brill, E. (1994). Some Advances in Transformation-Based Part of Speech Tagging. *AAAI, 1*, 722-727.

Cussens J. (1997). Part-of-speech tagging using Progol. In S. Dzeroski and N. Lavrac, editors. *Proc. of the 7th International Workshop on Inductive Logic Programming, LNCS, 1297*, 93-108.

Fontaine, L., & Kodratoff, Y. (2002). Comparaison du rôle de la progression thématique et de la texture conceptuelle chez des scientifiques anglophones et francophones s'exprimant en Anglais. *Asp, La revue du GERAS*, n° 37-38, 2002, pp. 59 - 83, Bordeaux, France. [English version available online; The role of thematic and concept texture in scientific text http://www.lri.fr/~yk/fon-kod-eng.pdf].

Quirk, R., Greenbaum, S., Leech, S., & Svartvik, J. (1985). *A comprehensive grammar of the English language*. London: Longman.

Stubbs, M. (1993). British Traditions in Text Analysis: From Firth to Sinclair. In M. Baker, G. Francis, & E. Tognini-Bonelli (Eds.), *Text and Technology: In honour of John Sinclair* (pp. 1-33). Amserdam: John Benjamins Publishing Company.

Tablan, V., Bontcheva, K., Maynard, D., & Cunningham, H. (2003). OLLIE: On-Line Learning for Information Extraction. *HLT-NAACL 2003 Workshop: Software Engineering and Architecture of Language Technology Systems (SEALTS).* Edmonton, Canada.

Wray, A. (2002). *Formulaic language and the lexicon.* Cambridge: Cambridge University Press.

Chapter XI
Analyzing the Text of Clinical Literature for Question Answering

Yun Niu
Ontario Cancer Institute, Canada

Graeme Hirst
University of Toronto, Canada

ABSTRACT

The task of question answering (QA) is to find an accurate and precise answer to a natural language question in some predefined text. Most existing QA systems handle fact-based questions that usually take named entities as the answers. In this chapter, the authors take clinical QA as an example to deal with more complex information needs. They propose an approach using Semantic class analysis as the organizing principle to answer clinical questions. They investigate three Semantic classes that correspond to roles in the commonly accepted PICO format of describing clinical scenarios. The three Semantic classes are: the description of the patient (or the problem), the intervention used to treat the problem, and the clinical outcome. The authors focus on automatic analysis of two important properties of the Semantic classes.

INTRODUCTION

The vast increase in online information brings new challenges to the area of information retrieval (IR) in both query processing and answer processing. To free the user from constructing a complicated boolean keywords query, a system should be able to process queries represented in natural language. Instead of responding with some documents relevant to the query, the system should actually answer the questions accurately and concisely. Systems with such characteristics are *question-answering* (QA) systems, which take advantage of high-quality natural language processing and mature technologies in IR. The task of a QA system is to find the answer to a particular natural language question in some predefined text. In this paper, we propose an approach that aims to automatically find answers to clinical questions.

Clinicians often need to consult literature on the latest information in patient care, such as side effects of a medication, symptoms of a disease, or time constraints in the use of a medication. The published medical literature is an important source to help clinicians make decisions in patient treatment (Sackett & Straus, 1998; Straus & Sackett, 1999). For example:

- **Q:** In a patient with a suspected MI does thrombolysis decrease the risk of death if it is administered 10 hours after the onset of chest pain?

An answer to the question can be found in *Clinical Evidence* (CE) (Barton, 2002), a regularly updated publication that reviews and consolidates experimental results for clinical problems:

- **A:** Systematic reviews of RCTs have found that prompt thrombolytic treatment (within 6 hours and perhaps up to 12 hours and longer after the onset of symptoms) reduces mortality in people with AMI and ST elevation or bundle branch block on their presenting ECG.

Studies have shown that searching the literature can help clinicians answer questions regarding patient treatment (Cimino, 1996; Gorman, Ash, & Wykoff, 1994; Mendonça, Cimino, Johnson, & Seol, 2001). It has also been found that if high-quality evidence is available in this way at the point of care—e.g., the patient's bedside—clinicians will use it in their decision making, and it frequently results in additional or changed decisions (Sackett & Straus, 1998; Straus & Sackett, 1999). The practice of using the current best evidence to help clinicians in making decisions on the treatment of individual patients is called *evidence-based medicine* (EBM).

Clinical questions usually represent complex information needs and cannot be answered using a single word or phrase. For a clinical question, it is often the case that more than one clinical trial with different experimental settings will have been performed. Results of each trial provide some evidence on the problem. To answer such a question, all this evidence needs to be taken into account, as there may be duplicate evidence,

Figure 1. Example of a clinical question, with corresponding evidence from Clinical Evidence

Clinical question: Are calcium channel blockers effective in reducing mortality in acute myocardial infarction patients?

Evidence 1: … calcium channel blockers do not reduce mortality, may increase mortality.

Evidence 2: … verapamil versus placebo … had no significant effect on mortality.

Evidence 3: … diltiazem significantly increased death or reinfarction.

Evidence 4: … investigating the use of calcium channel blockers found a non-significant increase in mortality of about 4% and 6%.

partially agreed-on evidence, or even contradictions. A complete answer can be obtained only by synthesizing these multiple pieces of evidence, as shown in Figure 1. In our work, we take EBM as an example to investigate clinical QA. Our targets are questions posed by physicians in patient treatment.

Our task is to find answers to clinical questions automatically. Our work is part of the EPoCare project ("Evidence at Point of Care") at the University of Toronto. The goal of EPoCare is to develop methods for answering clinical questions automatically with CE as the source text. (We do not look at primary medical research text.)

BACKGROUND

Many advances have been made to answer *factoid* questions that have named entities such as a person or location as answers; this is factoid question answering (FQA). For example, the answer to the question *Who was the U.S. president in 1999?* is *Bill Clinton*. However, much less has been understood in finding answers to complex questions that demand synthesis of information, such as clinical QA, which is *non-factoid* QA (NFQA).

We observe two distinct characteristics that differentiate *factoid* QA and *non-factoid* QA.

- Non-factoid questions usually cannot be answered using a word or phrase, such as named entities. Instead, answers to these questions are much more complex, and often consist of multiple pieces of information from multiple sources.
- Compared to *factoid* QA, in which an answer can be judged as *true* or *false*, *non-factoid* QA needs to determine what information is *relevant* in answer construction.

Non-factoid QA is attracting more and more research interest (Diekema, Yilmazel, Chen, Harwell, He, & Liddy, 2004; Niu, Hirst, McArthur, & Rodriguez-Gianolli, 2003; Stoyanov, Cardie, & Wiebe, 2005; DUC, 2005). Unlike FQA, in which the main research focuses on *wh-* questions (e.g. *when, where, who*) in a rather general domain, most work in NFQA starts with a specific domain, such as terrorism, or a specific type of question, such as opinion-related questions. The complexity of NFQA tasks may account for this difference. In this section, current work in NFQA is reviewed according to different research problems in the QA task that it addresses.

Because the information needs are more complex, some work puts more effort into understanding questions. Hickl et al. (2004), Small et al. (2004) and Diekema et al. (2004) suggest answering questions in an interactive way to clarify questions step by step. In addition, Hickl et al. argue that decomposition of complex scenarios into simple questions is necessary in an interactive system.

Following that work, Harabagiu et al. (2004) derived the intentional structure and the implicatures enabled by it for decomposing complex questions, such as *What kind of assistance has North Korea received from the USSR/Russia for its missile program?* The authors claim that intentions that the user associates with the question may express a set of *intended questions*; and each intended question may be expressed as *implied questions*. The intended questions of this example include *What is the USSR/Russia? What is assistance? What are the missiles in the North Korean inventory?* Then, these intended questions further have implied questions, such as *Is this the Soviet/Russian government? Does it include private firms, state-owned firms, educational institutions, and individuals? Is it the training of personnel? What was the development timeline of the missiles?*

The system HITIQA (High-Quality Interactive Question Answering) (Small, Strzalkowski, Liu, Ryan, Salkin, Shimizu, et al., 2004) also emphasizes interaction with the user to understand their information needs, although it does not attempt to decompose questions. During the interaction, the system asks questions to confirm the user's needs. After receiving *yes* or *no* from the user, the goal of searching is clearer. The interaction is data-driven in that questions asked by the system are motivated by the previous results of information searching (which form the answer space).

Diekema et al. (2004) also suggest having a question-negotiation process for complex. Their QA system deals with real-time questions related to reusable launch vehicles. For example, broad-coverage questions like *How does the shuttle fly?*, and questions about comparison of two elements such as *What advantages/disadvantages does an aluminum alloy have over Ti alloy as the core for a honeycomb design?* are typical in the domain. A question-answering system architecture with a module for question negotiation between the system and the questioner is proposed in the paper.

Berger et al. (2000) describe several interesting models to find the connection between question terms and answer terms. Soricut and Brill (2006) extend Berger's work to answer FAQ-like questions. In their work, although FAQ question and answer pairs are used as training data, the goal is to extract answers from documents on the Web, instead of pairing up existing questions and answers in FAQ corpora. Taking questions and answers as two different languages, a machine translation model is applied in the answer extraction module to extract three sentences that maximize the probability $p(q|a)$ (where q is the question and a is the answer) from the retrieved documents as the answer.

In the system HITIQA, frame structure is used to represent the text, where each frame has some attributes. For example, a general frame has *frame type*, *topic*, and *organization*. During the processing, frames will be instantiated by corresponding named entities in the text. In answer generation, text in the answer space is scored by comparing their frame structures with the corresponding goal structures generated by the system according to the question. Answers consist of text passages from which the zero conflict frames are derived. The correctness of the answers was not evaluated directly. Instead, the system was evaluated by how effective it is in helping users to achieve their information goal. The results of a three-day evaluation workshop validated the overall approach.

Cardie et al. (2004) aim to answer questions about opinions (multi-perspective QA), such as: *Was the most recent presidential election in Zimbabwe regarded as a fair election?* and *What was the world-wide reaction to the 2001 annual U.S. report on human rights?*. They developed an annotation scheme for low-level representation of opinions, and then proposed using opinion-oriented scenario templates to act as a summary representation of the opinions. Possible ways of using the representations in multi-perspective QA are discussed. In related work, Stoyanov, Cardie, and Wiebe (2005) analyzed characteristics of opinion questions and answers and showed that traditional FBQA techniques are not sufficient for multi-perspective QA. Results of some initial experiments showed that using filters that identify subjective sentences is helpful in multi-perspective QA.

The typical work discussed here shows the state-of-the-art in NFQA. Most systems are investigating complex questions in specific domains or of particular types. Although interesting views and approaches have been proposed, most work is at the initial stage, describing the general framework or potential useful approaches to address characteristics of non-factoid QA.

Our work on NFQA is in the medical domain. Clinical QA as an NFQA task presents challenges similar to those of the tasks described in this section. Our work is to investigate these challenges by addressing a key issue: *what information is relevant?* We do not attempt to elicit such information by deriving additional questions, such as performing question decomposition (Hickl et al., 2004) or through interactive QA (Small et al, 2004). Instead, we aim to identify the best information available in a designated source to construct the answer to a given question. To achieve these goals, we propose to use Semantic class analysis in non-factoid QA and use frame structure to represent Semantic classes.

OUR APPROACH FOR CLINICAL QA: SEMANTIC CLASS ANALYSIS

As discussed in the introduction, answers to clinical questions are not named entities and often consist of multiple pieces of information. In response to these major characteristics, we propose frame-based Semantic class analysis as the organizing principle to answer these questions.

Representing Scenarios Using Frames

Clinical questions often describe scenarios. For example, they may describe relationships between clinical problems, treatments, and corresponding clinical outcomes, or they may be about symptoms, hypothesized diseases, and diagnosis processes. To answer these questions, essentially, we need an effective schema to understand scenario descriptions.

Semantic Roles

The Semantics of a scenario or an event are expressed by the Semantic relationships between its participants, and such Semantic relationships are defined by the role that each participant plays in the scenario. These relationships are referred to as *Semantic roles* (Gildea & Jurafsky, 2002), or *conceptual roles* (Riloff, 1999). This viewpoint dates back to frame Semantics, posed by Fillmore (1976) as part of the nature of language. Frame Semantics provides a schematic representation of events or scenarios that have various participants as roles. In our work, we use frames as our representation schema for the Semantic roles involved in questions and answer sources.

Research on Semantic roles has proposed different sets of roles ranging from the very general to the very specific. The most general role set consists of only two roles: PROTO-AGENT and PROTO-PATIENT (Dowty, 1991; Valin & Robert, 1993). Roles can be more domain-specific, such as perpetrators, victims, and physical targets in a terrorism domain. In question-answering tasks, specific Semantic roles can be more instructive in searching for relevant information, and thus more precise in pinpointing correct answers. Therefore, we take domain-specific roles as our targets.

The Treatment Frame

Patient-specific questions in EBM usually can be described by the so-called **PICO** format (Sackett, Straus, Richardson, Rosenberg, & Haynes, 2000). In a *treatment scenario*, **P** refers to the *status of the patient (or the problem)*, **I** means an *intervention*, **C** is a *comparison intervention* (if relevant), and **O** describes the *clinical outcome*. For example, in the following question:

- **Q:** In a patient with a suspected myocardial infarction does thrombolysis decrease the risk of death?

the description of the patient is *patient with a suspected myocardial infarction*, the intervention is *thrombolysis*, there is no comparison intervention, and the clinical outcome is *decrease the risk of death*. Originally, PICO format was developed for therapy questions describing treatment scenarios, and was later extended to other types of clinical questions such as diagnosis, prognosis, and etiology. Representing clinical questions with PICO format is widely believed to be the key to efficiently finding high-quality evidence (Ebell, 1999; Richardson, Wilson, Nishikawa, & Hayward, 1995). Empirical studies have shown that identifying PICO elements in clinical scenarios

Table 1. The treatment frame

P:	a description of the patient (or the problem)
I:	an intervention
O:	the clinical outcome

improves the conceptual clarity of clinical problems (Cheng, 2004).

We found that PICO format highlights several important Semantic roles in clinical scenarios, and can be easily represented using the frame structure. Therefore, we constructed a frame based on it. Since **C** mainly indicates a comparison relation to **I**, we combined the comparisons as one filler of the same slot *intervention* in the frame, connected by a specific relation. We focused on therapy-related questions and built a *treatment frame* that contains three slots, as shown in Table 1.

A slot in a frame designates a *Semantic class* (corresponding to a *Semantic role* or a *conceptual role*), and relations between Semantic classes in a scenario are implied by the design of the frame structure. The treatment frame expresses a cause-effect relation: the *intervention* for the *problem* results in the *clinical outcome.*

When applying this frame to a sentence, we extract constituents in the sentence to fill in the slots in the frame. These constituents are *instances of Semantic classes.* In this paper, the terms *instances of Semantic classes* and *slot fillers* are used interchangeably. Some examples of the instantiated treatment frame are as follows.

- **Sentence**: One RCT [randomized clinical trial] found no evidence that low molecular weight heparin is superior to aspirin alone for the treatment of acute ischaemic stroke in people with atrial fibrillation.
  P: acute ischaemic stroke in people with atrial fibrillation
  I: low molecular weight heparin vs. aspirin
  O: no evidence that low molecular weight heparin is superior to aspirin
- **Sentence**: Subgroup analysis in people with congestive heart failure found that diltiazem significantly increased death or reinfarction.
  P: people with congestive heart failure
  I: diltiazem
  O: significantly increased death or reinfarction
- **Sentence**: Thrombolysis reduces the risk of dependency, but increases the risk of death.
  P: —
  I: thrombolysis
  O: reduces the risk of dependency, but increases the risk of death

The first example states the result of a clinical trial, while the second and third depict clinical outcomes. We do not distinguish the two cases in this study, and treat them in the same manner.

Relationship to Information Extraction

Our approach of Semantic class analysis has a close relation to *information extraction* (IE), in which domain-specific Semantic roles are often explored to identify predefined types of information from text (Riloff, 1999). Our approach shares the view with IE that Semantic classes/roles are the keys to understanding scenario descriptions. Frames are also used in IE as the representation scheme. Nevertheless, in our work, as shown by the above examples of treatment frames, the syntactic constituents of an instance of a Semantic class can be much more complex than those of traditional IE tasks, in which slot fillers are usually named entities (Riloff, 1999; TREC, 2001). Therefore, approaches based on such Semantic classes go beyond named-entity identification, and thus will better adapt to clinical QA. In addition, extracting instances of Semantic classes from text is not the ultimate goal of QA. Frame representation of Semantic classes provides a platform for matching questions to answers in our QA system.

Main Components of a QA System Guided by Semantic Class Analysis

With Semantic class analysis as the organizing principle, we identify four main components of our QA system:

- Detecting Semantic classes in questions and in answer sources
- Identifying properties of Semantic classes
- Question-answer matching: exploring properties of Semantic classes to find relevant pieces of information
- Constructing answers by merging or synthesizing relevant information using relations between Semantic classes

To search for the answer to a question, the question and the text in which the answer may occur will be processed to detect the Semantic classes. A Semantic class can have various properties. These properties can be extremely valuable in finding answers, which we will discuss in detail in the following sections. In the matching process, the question scenario will be compared to an answer candidate, and pieces of relevant information should be identified by exploring properties of the Semantic classes. To construct the answer, relevant information that has been found in the matching process will be merged or synthesized to generate an accurate and concise answer. The process of synthesizing scenarios relies on comparing instances of Semantic classes in these scenarios; for example, two instances might be exactly the same or one might be the hypernym of the other.

In the following sections we will discuss our approaches to automatically detecting two properties of the Semantic classes in the treatment scenario: the cores of the classes and the polarities of clinical outcomes.

CORES OF SEMANTIC CLASSES

In a frame structure, the slots in question and answer frames can be filled with either *complete* or *partial* information. Consider the following example, where parentheses delimit each instance of a Semantic class (a slot filler) and the labels **P** (problem description), **I** (an intervention), **O** (the clinical outcome) indicate the type of the instance:

- **Sentence**: Two systematic reviews in (people with AMI)$_P$ investigating the use of (calcium channel blockers)$_I$ found a (non-significant increase in mortality of about 4% and 6%)$_O$.
  Complete slot fillers:
  P: people with AMI
  I: calcium channel blockers
  O: a non-significant increase in mortality of about 4% and 6%
  Partial slot fillers:
  P: AMI
  I: calcium channel blockers
  O: mortality

The partial slot fillers in this example contain the smallest fragments of the corresponding complete slot fillers that exhibit information rich enough for deriving a reasonably precise answer. We use the term *core* to refer to such a fraction of a slot filler (instance of a Semantic class).

Importance of Cores

As mentioned in the introduction, before the matching process, keyword-based document retrieval is usually performed to find relevant documents that may contain the answer to a given question. Keywords in the retrieval are derived from the question. Cores of Semantic classes can be extremely valuable in searching for such documents for complex question scenarios, as shown in the following example. (The scenario is an example used in usability testing in the EPoCare project at the University of Toronto.)

- **Question scenario**: A physician sees a 7-year-old child with asthma in her office. She is on Flovent and Ventolin currently and was recently discharged from hospital following her fourth admission for asthma exacerbation. During the most recent admission, the dose of Flovent was increased. Her mother is concerned about the impact of the additional dose of steroids on her daughter's growth. This is the question to which the physician wants to find the answer.

For a complex scenario description like this, the answer could be missed or drowned in irrelevant documents found by inappropriate keywords derived from the question. However, the search can be much more effective if we have the information of cores of Semantic classes, for example, *P: asthma, I: steroids, O: growth.*

Similarly, Semantics presented in cores can help filter out irrelevant information that cannot be identified by searching methods based on simple string overlaps.

1. In patients with **myocardial infarction**, do **β blockers** reduce all cause **mortality** and **recurrent myocardial infarction** without adverse effects?
2. In someone with **hypertension** and **high cholesterol**, what management options will decrease his risk of **stroke** and **cardiac events**?

In question 1, the first occurrence of *myocardial infarction* is a disease but the second occurrence is part of the clinical outcome. In question 2, *stroke* is part of the clinical outcome rather than a disease to be treated, as it usually is. Obviously, string matching cannot distinguish between the two cases. By identifying and classifying cores of Semantic classes, the relations between these important Semantic units in the scenarios are very clear. Therefore, documents or passages that do not contain *myocardial infarction* or *stroke* as clinical outcomes can be discarded.

In addition, identifying cores of Semantic classes in documents can facilitate the question-answer matching process. Some evidence relevant to the above question scenario on *asthma* is listed below, where boldface indicates a core:

- **Evidence 1**: A more recent systematic review (search date 1999) found three RCTs comparing the effects of **becolmetasone** and **non-steroidal medication** on linear **growth** in children with **asthma** (200μg twice daily, duration up to maximum 54 weeks) suggesting a short-term decrease in linear **growth** of –1.54 cm a year.
- **Evidence 2**: Two systematic reviews of studies with long-term follow up and a subsequent long-term RCT have found no evidence of **growth retardation** in **asthmatic children** treated with inhaled **steroids**.

The evidence sentences here are from CE (Barton, 2002). The clinical outcomes mentioned in the evidence have very different phrasings — yet both pieces of the evidence are relevant to the question. The pieces of evidence describe two distinct outcomes — that short-term decrease in growth is found and that there is no effect on growth in some long-term studies. Missing either of the outcomes will lead to an incomplete answer for the physician. Here, cores of the Semantic classes provide the only clue that both pieces of evidence are relevant to this question and should be included in the answer. Hence, a complete description of Semantic classes does not have to be found. In fact, such a description with more information could make the matching harder to find because of the different expressions of the outcomes.

Finally, cores of Semantic classes in a scenario are connected to each other by the relations embedded in the frame structure. The frame of the treatment scenario contains a cause–effect relation: an intervention used to treat a problem results in a clinical outcome.

In this section, we propose a method to automatically identify and classify the cores of Semantic classes according to their context in a sentence. We take the treatment frame as an example, in which the goal is to identify cores of *interventions*, *problems*, and *clinical outcomes.* For ease of description, we will use the terms *intervention-core*, *disease-core*, and *outcome-core* to refer to the corresponding cores. We work at the sentence level, i.e., we identify cores in a sentence rather than a clause or paragraph. Two principles are followed in developing the method. First, complete slot fillers do not have to be extracted before core identification. Second, we aim to reduce the need for expensive manual annotation of training data by using a semi-supervised learning approach.

Architecture of the Method

In our approach, we first collect candidates of the target cores from sentences under consideration. For each candidate, we classify it as one of the four classes: *intervention-core*, *disease-core*, *outcome-core*, or *other.* In the classification, a candidate will get a class label according to its context, its UMLS Semantic types, and the syntactic relations in which it participates. Figure 2 shows the architecture of the approach.

Preprocessing

In the preprocessing, all words in the data set are examined. The first two steps are to reduce noise, in which some of the words that are unlikely to be part of real cores are filtered out. Then, the rest are mapped to their corresponding concepts, and these concepts are candidate target cores.

PoS tagging Our observation is that cores of the three types of slot fillers are usually nouns or noun phrases. Therefore, words that are not nouns are first removed from the candidate set. PoS tags are obtained by using Brill's tagger (Brill, 1993).

Filtering out some *bad* nouns This step is the second attempt to remove noise from the candidate set. Nouns that are unlikely to be part of real cores are considered as *bad* candidates. Two research options of measures are used to evaluate how *good* a noun is.

- Extended *tf.idf.* After the *tf.idf* value is calculated for a noun in each document, the highest value of all the documents is taken as the final score of the noun. Nouns with scores lower than a threshold are removed from the candidate set. The threshold was set manually after observing the scores of some nouns that frequently occur in the text. CE text is used to get the score of a noun. For this, 47 sections in CE are segmented to 143 files of about the same size. Each file is treated as a document. This measure is referred to as *tf.idf* in later description.
- Domain specificity. We calculate the conditional probability $p(c|n) = p(c,n) / p(n)$, where c is the medical class, and n is a noun. It is the probability that a document is in the medical domain c given it contains the noun n. Intuitively, *intervention-cores*, *disease-cores*, and *outcome-cores* are domain-specific, i.e., a document that contains them is very likely to be in the medical domain. For example, *morbidity, mortality,*

Figure 2. Architecture of the approach of core identification

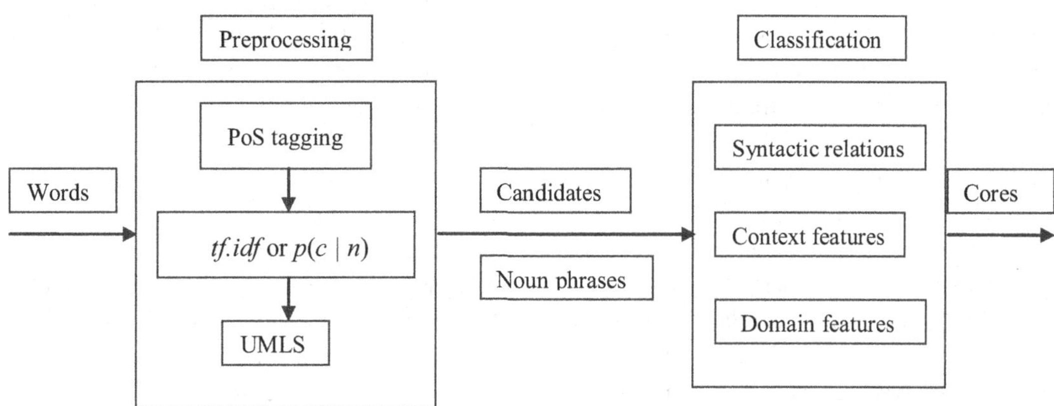

aspirin, and *myocardial infarction* are very likely to occur in a medicine-related context. This measure intends to keep highly medical domain-specific nouns in the candidate set. A noun is a better candidate if the corresponding probability is high. Text from two domains is needed in this measure: medical text, and non-medical text. In our experiment, we used the same 47 sections in *CE* as the medical class text (separated into 143 files of about the same size). For the non-medical class, we used 1000 randomly selected documents from the Reuters-21578 newswire text collection, because newswire stories are mainly in the general domain. Nouns whose probability values are below a threshold (determined in the same manner as in the *tf.idf* measure) are filtered out.

Mapping to concepts To this point, the candidate set consists of nouns. In many cases, nouns are part of noun phrases (concepts) that are better candidates of cores. For example, the phrase *myocardial infarction* is a better candidate of a disease-core than the noun *infarction*. Therefore, the software MetaMap (Aronson, 2001) is used to map a noun to its corresponding concept in the Metathesaurus. All the concepts form the candidates of cores to be classified.

Representing Candidates Using Features

We expect that candidates in the same Semantic class will have similar behavior. Therefore, the idea of the classification is to group together similar candidates. The similarity is characterized by syntactic relations, context information, and Semantic types in UMLS. All features are binary features, i.e., a feature takes value 1 if it is present; otherwise, it takes value 0.

Syntactic Relations

Previous researchers have explored syntactic relations to group similar words (Lin, 1998) and words of the same sense in word sense disambiguation (Kohomban & Lee, 2005). Lin (1998) inferred that *tesguino* is similar to *beer*, *wine*, etc., i.e., it is a kind of drink, by comparing syntactic relations in which each word participates. Kohomban and Lee (2005) determined the sense of a word in a context by observing a subset of all syntactic relations in the corpus that the word participates in. The hypothesis is that different instances of the same sense will have similar relations.

In our work, we need to group cores of the same Semantic class. Such cores may participate in similar syntactic relations while those of different classes will have different relations. For example, intervention-cores often are subjects of sentences, while outcome-cores are often objects.

Candidates in our task are phrases, instead of words as for Lin and Kohomban and Lee. Thus, we extend their approaches of analyzing relations between two words to extract relations between a word and a phrase. This is done by considering all relations between a candidate noun phrase and other words in the sentence. To do that, we ignore relations between any two words in the phrase when extracting syntactic relations. Any relation between a word not in the phrase and a word in the phrase is extracted. We use the Minipar parser (Lin, 1994) to get the syntactic relations between words. After a sentence is parsed, we extract relevant syntactic relations from the output of the parser. A relation is represented using a triple that contains two words (one of them is in the noun phrase and the other is not) and the grammatical relation between them. Figure 3 shows relevant triples extracted from a sentence. Because long-distance relations are considered, the relation between *thrombolysis* and *increases* is captured.

In the feature construction, a triple is taken as a feature. The set of all distinct triples is the syntactic relation feature set in the classification.

Local Context

Context of candidates is also important in distinguishing different classes. For example, a disease-core may often have *people with* in its left context. However, it is very unlikely that the phrase *people with mortality* will occur in the text.

We considered the two words on each side of a candidate (stop-words were excluded). When extracting context features, all punctuation marks were removed except the sentence boundary. The window did not cross boundaries of sentences. We evaluated two representations of context: with and without order. In the ordered case, local context to the left of the phrase is marked by *-L*, and *R-* marks that to the right. The symbols *-L* and *R-* are used only to indicate the order of text. For the candidate *dependency* in Figure 3, the context features with order are: *reduces-L*, *risk-L*, *R-increases*, and *R-chance*. The context features without order are: *reduces*, *risk*, *increases*, and *chance*.

Figure 3. Example of dependency triples extracted from output of Minipar parser

Sentence:

Thrombolysis reduces the risk of dependency, but increases the chance of death.

Candidates:

thrombolysis, dependency, death

Relations:

(thrombolysis subj-of increase), (thrombolysis subj-of reduce)

(dependency pcomp-n-of of)

(death pcomp-n-of of)

This example shows a case where ordered context helps distinguish an intervention-core from an outcome-core. If order is not considered, candidates *thrombolysis* and *dependency* have overlapped context: *reduces* and *risk*. When taking order into account, they have no overlapped features at all — *thrombolysis* has features *R-reduces* and *R-risk*, while *dependency* has features *reduces-L* and *risk-L*.

Domain Features

As described in the *mapping to concepts* step in the preprocessing, at the same time of mapping text to concepts in UMLS, MetaMap also finds their Semantic types. Each candidate has a Semantic type defined in the Semantic Network of UMLS. For example, the Semantic type of *death* is **organism function**, that of *disability* is **pathologic function**, and that of *dependency* is **physical disability**. These Semantic types are used as features in the classification.

Data Set

Two sections of *CE* were used in the experiments. A clinician labeled the text for intervention-cores and disease-cores. Complete clinical outcomes are also identified. Using the annotation as a basis, outcome-cores were labeled by the author. The number of instances of each class is shown in Table 2.

The Model of Classification

Because our classification strategy is to group together similar cores and the cluster structure of the data is observed, we chose a semi-supervised learning model developed by Zhu, Ghahramani, and Lafferty (2003) that explores the cluster structure of data in classification. The general hypothesis of this approach is that similar data points will have similar labels.

A graph is constructed in this model. In the graph, nodes correspond to both labeled and unlabeled data points (candidates of cores), and an edge between two nodes is weighted according to the similarity of the nodes. More formally, let $(x_1,y_1), \ldots, (x_l,y_l)$ be labeled data, where $Y_L = \{y_1, \ldots, y_l\}$ are corresponding class labels. Similarly, let $(x_{l+1},y_{l+1}), \ldots, (x_{l+u},y_{l+u})$ be unlabeled data, where $Y_U = \{y_{l+1}, \ldots, y_{l+u}\}$ are labels to be predicted. A connected graph $G = (V,E)$ can be constructed, where the set of nodes V correspond to both labeled and unlabeled data points and E is the set of edges. The edge between two nodes i, j is weighted. Weights w_{ij} are assigned to agree with the hypothesis; for example, using a radial basis function (RBF) kernel, we can assign larger edge weights to closer points in Euclidean space.

Zhu, Ghahramani, and Lafferty formulated the intuitive label propagation approach as a problem of energy minimization in the framework of Gaussian random fields, where the Gaussian field is over a continuous state space instead of over a discrete label set. The idea is to compute a *real-valued* function $f\colon V \rightarrow R$ on graph G that minimizes the energy function $E(f) = \frac{1}{2}\sum_{ij} w_{ij}(f(i) - f(j))^2$, where i and j correspond to data points in the problem. The function $f = \operatorname{argmin}_f E(f)$ determines the labels of unlabeled data points. This solution can be efficiently computed by direct matrix calculation even for multi-label classification, in which solutions are generally computationally expensive in other frameworks.

Table 2. Number of instances of cores in the whole data set

Intervention-core	Disease-core	Outcome-core	Total
501	153	384	1038

This approach propagates labels from labeled data points to unlabeled data points according to the similarity on the edges, thus it follows closely the cluster structure of the data in prediction. We expect it to perform reasonably well on our data set. It is referred to as *SEMI* in the following description. We use SemiL (Huang, Kecman, & Kopriva, 2006), an implementation of the algorithm using Gaussian random fields in the experiment (default values are used for the parameters unless otherwise mentioned).

Results and Analysis

We first evaluate the performance of the semi-supervised model on different feature sets. Then, we compare the two candidate sets obtained by using *tf.idf* and domain specificity, respectively. Finally, we compare the semi-supervised model to a supervised approach to justify the usage of a semi-supervised approach in the problem.

In all experiments, the data set contains all candidates of cores. Unless otherwise mentioned, the result reported is achieved by using the candidate set derived by $p(c|n)$, the feature set of the combination of syntactic relations, ordered context, and Semantic types, and the distance measure of cosine distance. The result of an experiment is the average of 20 runs. In each run, labeled data is randomly selected from the candidate set, and the rest is unlabeled data whose labels need to be predicted. We make sure all classes are present in labeled data. If any class is absent, we redo the sampling. The evaluation of the Semantic classes is very strict: a candidate is given credit if it gets the same label as given by the annotator and the tokens it contains are exactly the same as marked by the annotator. Candidates that contain only some of the tokens matching the labels given by the annotators are treated as the *other* class in the evaluation.

Experiment 1: Evaluation of Feature Sets

This experiment evaluates different feature sets in the classification. As described above, two options are used in the second step of preprocessing to pick up *good* candidates. Here, as our focus is on the feature set, we report only results on candidates selected by $p(c|n)$. The number of instances of each of the four target classes in the candidate set is shown in Table 3 (the performance of candidate selection will be discussed below).

Figure 4 shows the accuracy of classification using different combinations of four feature sets: syntactic relations, ordered context, un-ordered context, and Semantic types.

We set a baseline by assigning labels to data points according to the prior knowledge of the distribution of the four classes, which has accuracy of 0.395. Another choice of baseline is to assign the label of the majority class, *others* in this case, to each data point, which produces an accuracy of 0.567. However, all the three classes of interest have accuracy 0 according to this baseline. Thus, this baseline is not very informative in this experiment.

It is clear in the figure that incorporating new kinds of features into the classification resulted in a large improvement in accuracy. Using only syntactic relations (*rel* in the figure) as features, the best accuracy is a little lower than 0.5, which is much higher than the baseline of 0.395. The addition of ordered context (*orderco*) or no-order context features (*co*) improved the accuracy by about 0.1. Adding Semantic type features (*tp*) further improved 0.1 in accuracy. Combining all three kinds of features achieved the best performance. With only 5% of data as labeled data, the whole feature set achieved an accuracy of 0.6, which is much higher than the baseline of 0.395. Semantic type seems to be a very powerful feature set, as it substantially improves the performance on top of the combination of the

Table 3. Number of instances of target classes in the candidate set

Intervention-core	Disease-core	Outcome-core	Others	Total
298	106	209	801	1414

Figure 4. Classification results of candidates

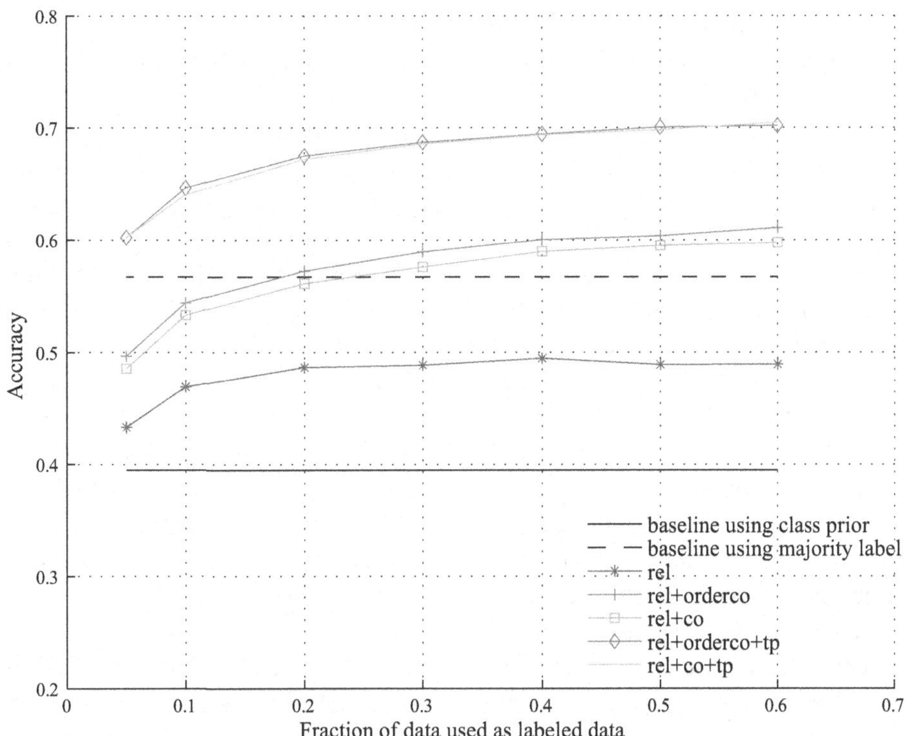

other two kinds of features. Therefore, we took a closer look at the Semantic type feature set by conducting the classification using only Semantic types, and found that the result is even worse than using only syntactic relations. This observation reveals interesting relations among the feature sets. In the space defined by only one kind of features, data points may be close to each other, hence hard to distinguish. Adding another kind sets apart data points in different classes toward a more separated position in the new space. It shows that every kind of feature is informative to the task. The feature sets characterize the candidates from different angles that are complementary in the task. We also see that there is almost no difference between ordered and unordered context in distinguishing the target classes, although ordered context seems to be slightly better when Semantic types are not considered.

Experiment 2: Evaluation of Candidate Sets

In the second step of preprocessing, one of two options can be used to filter out some *bad* nouns

— using the *tf.idf* measure or the domain specificity measure $p(c \mid n)$. This experiment compares the two measures in the core identification task. A third option using neither of the two measures (i.e., skip the second step of preprocessing) is evaluated as the baseline. The first three rows in Table 4 are numbers of instances remaining in the candidate set after preprocessing. The last row shows the numbers of manually annotated true cores, which has been listed in Table 2 and is repeated here for comparison.

tf.idf and Domain Specificity vs. Baseline

As shown in Table 4, there are many fewer instances in the *others* class in the sets derived by *tf.idf* and the probability measure as compared to those derived by the baseline, which shows that the two measures effectively removed some of the *bad* candidates of intervention-core, disease-core, and outcome-core. At the same time, a small number of real cores were removed. Compared to the baseline method, the probability measure kept almost the same number of intervention-cores and disease-cores in the candidate set, while omitting some outcome-cores. It indicates that outcome-cores are less domain-specific than intervention-cores and disease-cores. Compared to the *tf.idf* measure, more intervention-cores and outcome-cores were kept by the conditional probability measure, showing that the probability measuring the domain-specificity of a noun better characterizes the cores of the three Semantic classes. The probability measure is also more robust than the *tf.idf* measure, as *tf.idf* relies more on the content of the text from which it is calculated. For example, if an intervention is mentioned in many documents of the document set, its *tf.idf* value can be very low although it is a good candidate for being an intervention-core.

The precision, recall, and F-score of the classification shown in Table 5 confirm the above analysis. The domain specificity measure gets substantially higher F-scores than the baseline for all the three classes that we are interested in, using different amounts of labeled data. Compared to *tf.idf*, the performance of the domain specificity measure is much better on identifying intervention-cores (note that $p(c|n)$ picked up more real intervention-cores than *tf.idf*), and slightly better on identifying outcome-cores, while the two are similar on identifying disease-cores.

Baseline vs. the Set of Manually Annotated Cores

As mentioned at the beginning of this subsection, the baseline candidate set was derived by the first (PoS tagging) and third step (mapping from nouns to concepts) in the preprocessing. As shown by Table 4, 62.3% of manually annotated cores are kept in the baseline. We roughly checked about one-third of the total true cores (manually annotated cores) in the data set and found that 80% of lost cores are because MetaMap either extracted more or fewer tokens than marked by the annotator, or it failed to find the concepts. 10% of missing cores are caused by errors of the PoS tagger, and the rest are because some cores are not nouns.

Experiment 3: Comparison of the Semi-Supervised Model and SVMs

In the semi-supervised model, labels propagate along high-density data trails, and settle down at low-density gaps. If the data has this desired structure, unlabeled data can be used to help learning. In contrast, a supervised approach makes use only of labeled data. This experiment compares SEMI to a state-of-the-art supervised approach; the goal is to investigate how well unlabeled data contributes to the classification using the semi-supervised model. We compare the performance of SEMI to support-vector machines (SVMs) when different amounts of data are used as labeled data.

Table 4. Number of candidates in different candidate sets

Measures	Intervention-core	Disease-core	Outcome-core	Others
tf.idf	243	108	194	785
$p(c\|n)$	298	106	209	801
baseline	303	108	236	1330
true cores	501	153	384	—

Table 5. Results of classification on different candidate sets

INT: intervention-core; DIS: disease-core; OUT: outcome-core.

Fraction of		1%			5%			10%			30%			60%		
labeled data		P	R	F	P	R	F	P	R	F	P	R	F	P	R	F
INT	baseline	.44	.69	.53	.51	.83	.63	.53	.87	.66	.58	.90	.70	.59	.92	.72
	tf.idf	.44	.62	.51	.52	.74	.61	.55	.77	.64	.59	.84	.69	.60	.87	.71
	$p(c\|n)$	.51.	.65	**.57**	.60	.83	**.69**	.62	.86	**72**	.65	.90	**.75**	.67	.91	**.77**
DIS	Baseline	.16	.63	.25	.25	.68	.36	.31	.73	.43	.34	.84	.48	.35	.86	.49
	tf.idf	.20	.55	**.29**	.31	.64	**.41**	.34	.70	.46	.39	.82	**.53**	.41	.86	**.55**
	$p(c\|n)$	.18	.56	.27	.30	.66	**.41**	.34	.73	**.47**	.39	.83	**.53**	.41	.87	**.55**
OUT	Baseline	.22	.42	.28	.33	.53	.41	.39	.61	.48	.44	.66	.53	.46	.69	.55
	tf.idf	.30	.43	.35	.43	.56	**.49**	.47	.61	.53	.53	.66	.59	.55	.70	.61
	$p(c\|n)$	.31	.46	**.37**	.43	.56	**.49**	.48	.62	**.54**	.54	.69	**.60**	.56	.71	**.63**

Support Vector Machines

In SVMs, the process of classification given a set of training examples is an optimization procedure searching for the optimal rule that predicts the label of unseen examples with minimum errors. The goal of SVMs is to find an optimal hyperplane so that examples on the same side of the hyperplane will have the same label. The classification task is then to determine on which side of the hyperplane a data point lies. The optimal hyperplane that SVMs chose is the one with the largest margin.

In this experiment, we use OSU SVM (Ma, Zhao, Ahalt & Eads, 2003), a toolbox for Matlab built on top of LIBSVM (Chang & Lin, 2001). LIBSVM is an implementation of SVMs. We use RBF as the kernel method, and set the Sigma value heuristically using labeled data. SVM addresses the problem of unbalanced data using a parameter, which assigns weights to each class in the task. A class with larger weight will get a greater penalty when finding the optimum hyperplane. We set the parameter according to the prior knowledge of the class distribution and give larger weight to a class that contains fewer instances. Default values are used for other parameters.

Comparison of SEMI to SVMs

As shown in Table 6, when there is only a small amount of labeled data (less than 5% of the whole data set), which is often the case in real-world applications, SEMI achieves much better performance than SVMs in identifying all the three classes. For intervention-cores and outcome-cores, with 5% data as labeled data, SEMI outperforms SVMs with 10% data as labeled data. With less than

Table 6. F-score of classification using different models

Candidate set: produced by p(c|n) (see Table 4)
INT: intervention-core; DIS: disease-core; OUT: outcome-core.

Fraction of	labeled data	1%	5%	10%	30%	60%
INT	SEMI	.57	.69	.72	.75	.77
	SVM	.33	.60	.68	.74	.77
DIS	SEMI	.27	.41	.47	.53	.55
	SVM	.33	.60	.68	.74	.77
OUT	SEMI	.37	.49	.54	.60	.63
	SVM	.07	.27	.44	.56	.62

60% data as labeled data, the performance of SEMI is either superior to or comparable to SVMs for intervention-cores and outcome-cores. This shows that SEMI effectively exploits unlabeled data by following the manifold structure of the data. The promising results achieved by SEMI show the potential of exploring unlabeled data in classification.

Related Work

The task of named entity (NE) identification, similar to the core-detection task, involves identifying words or word sequences in several classes, such as proper names (locations, persons, and organizations), monetary expressions, dates, and times. NE identification has been an important research topic ever since it was defined in Message Understanding Conference (MUC, 2003). In 2003, it was taken as the shared-task in the Conference on Computational Natural Language Learning (Erik, Sang & Meulder, 2003). Most statistical approaches use supervised methods to address the problem (Chieu & Ng, 2003; Florian, Ittycheriah, Jing & Zhang, 2003; Klein, Smarr, Nguyen, & Manning, 2003). Unsupervised approaches have also been tried in this task. Cucerzan and Yarowsky (1999) use a bootstrapping algorithm to learn contextual and morphological patterns iteratively. Collins and Singer (1999) tested the performance of several unsupervised algorithms on the problem: modified bootstrapping (DL-CoTrain) motivated by co-training (Blum & Mitchell, 1998), an extended boosting algorithm (CoBoost), and the Expectation Maximization (EM) algorithm. The results showed that DL-CoTrain and CoBoost perform about the same, and both are superior to EM.

Much effort in entity extraction in the biomedical domain has gene names as the target. Various supervised models including naive Bayes, support vector machines, and hidden Markov models have been applied (Ananiadou & Tsujii, 2003). The work most related to our core-identification in the biomedical domain is that of Rosario and Hearst (2004), which extracts *treatment* and *disease* from MEDLINE and examines seven relation types between them using generative models and a neural network. They claim that these models may be useful when only partially labeled data is available, although only supervised learning is conducted in the paper. The best *F*-score of identifying *treatment* and *disease* obtained by using the supervised method is .71. Another piece of work extracting similar Semantic classes is by Ray and Craven (2001), who report an *F*-score of about .32 for extracting *proteins* and *locations* and about .50 for *gene* and *disorder*.

A difficulty of using this approach, however, is in detecting boundaries of the targets. A segmentation step that pre-processes the text is needed. This will be our future work, in which we aim to investigate approaches that perform the segmentation precisely.

As a final point, we want to emphasize the difference between cores and named entities. While the identification of NEs in a text is an important component of many tasks including question answering and information extraction, its benefits are constrained by its coverage. Typically, it is limited to a relatively small set of classes, such as *person*, *time*, and *location*. However, in sophisticated applications, such as the non-factoid medical question answering that we consider, NEs are only a small fraction of the important Semantic units discussed in documents or asked about by users. As shown by the examples in this section, cores of clinical outcomes are often not NEs. In fact, many Semantic roles in scenarios and events that occur in questions and documents do not contain NEs at all. For example, the *test method* in *diagnosis* scenarios, the *means* in a *shipping* event, and the *manner* in a *criticize* scenario may all have non-NE cores. Therefore, it is imperative to identify other kinds of Semantic units besides NEs. Cores of Semantic classes are one such extension that consist of a more diverse set of Semantic units that goes beyond simple NEs.

POLARITY OF CLINICAL OUTCOMES

One of the major concerns in patient treatment is the clinical outcomes of interventions in treating diseases: are they positive, negative or neutral? This polarity information is an inherent property of clinical outcomes. An example of each type of polarity taken from CE is shown below.

- **Positive**: Thrombolysis reduced the risk of death or dependency at the end of the studies.
- **Negative**: In the systematic review, thrombolysis increased fatal intracranial haemorrhage compared with placebo.
- **Neutral**: The first RCT found that diclofenac plus misoprostol versus placebo for 25 weeks produced no significant difference in cognitive function or global status.

Sentences that do not have information on clinical outcomes form another group: no outcome.

- **No outcome**: We found no RCTs comparing combined pharmacotherapy and psychotherapy with either treatment alone.

Polarity information is crucial to answering questions related to clinical outcomes. We have to know the polarity to answer questions about benefits and harms of an intervention. In addition, knowing whether a sentence contains a clinical outcome can help filter out irrelevant information in answer construction. Furthermore, information on negative outcomes can be crucial in clinical decision making. In this section, we discuss the problem of automatically identifying outcome polarity in medical text (Niu, et al., 2005). More specifically, we focus on detecting the presence of a clinical outcome in medical text, and, when an outcome is found, determining whether it is positive, negative, or neutral. We observe that a single sentence in medical text usually describes a complete clinical outcome. As a result, we perform sentence-level analysis in our work.

Related Work

The problem of polarity analysis is also considered as a task of sentiment classification (Pang, Lee & Vaithyanathan, 2002; Pang & Lee, 2003) or Semantic orientation analysis (Turney, 2002): determining whether an evaluative text, such as a movie review, expresses a "favorable" or "unfavorable" opinion. All these tasks are to obtain the orientation of the observed text on a discussion topic. They fall into three categories: detection of the polarity of words, of sentences, and of documents. Among them, as Yu and Hatzivassiloglou (2003) pointed out, the problem at the sentence level is the hardest one.

Turney (2002) has employed an unsupervised learning method to provide suggestions on documents as *thumbs up* or *thumbs down*. The polarity detection is done by averaging the Semantic orientation (SO) of extracted phrases (phrases containing adjectives or adverbs) from a text. The document is tagged as *thumbs up* if the average of SO is positive, and otherwise is tagged as *thumbs down*. In more recent work, Whitelaw, Garg, and Argamon (2005) explore *appraisal groups* to classify positive and negative documents. Similar to phrases used in Turney's work, *appraisal groups* consist of coherent words that together express the polarity of opinions, such as "extremely boring", or "not really very good". Instead of calculating the mutual information, a lexicon of *adjectival appraisal groups* (groups headed by an appraising adjective) is constructed semi-automatically. These groups are used as features in a supervised approach using SVMs to detect the sentiment of a document. Pang et al. (2002) also deal with the task at document level. The sentiment classification problem was treated as a text classification issue and a variety of machine-learning techniques were explored to classify movie reviews into positive and negative. A series of lexical features were employed on these classification strategies in order to find effective features. Pang et al. found that support vector machines perform the best among three classification strategies. The main part of Yu and Hatzivassiloglou's work (2003) is at the sentence level, and hence is closest to our work. They first separate facts from opinions using a Bayesian classifier, then use an unsupervised method to classify opinions as positive, negative, and neutral by evaluating the strength of the orientation of words contained in a sentence.

The polarity information we are observing relates to clinical outcomes instead of the personal opinions studied by the work mentioned above. Therefore, we expect differences in the expressions and the structures of sentences in these two areas. For the task in the medical domain, it will be interesting to see whether domain knowledge will help. These differences lead to new features in our approach.

A Supervised Approach for Clinical Outcome Detection and Polarity Classification

Since SVMs have been shown also very effective in many other classification tasks, we investigate SVMs in sentence-level analysis to detect the presence of a clinical outcome and determine its polarity.

In our approach, each sentence as a data point to be classified is represented by a vector of features. In the feature set, we use words themselves as they are very informative in related tasks such as sentiment classification and topic categorization. In addition, we use contextual information to capture changes described in clinical outcomes, and use generalized features that represent groups of concepts to build more regular patterns for classification.

We use binary features in most of the experiments except for the *frequency* feature in one of our experiments. When a feature is present in a sentence, it has a value of 1; otherwise, it has a value of 0. Among the features in our feature set, UNIGRAMS and BIGRAMS have been used in previous sentiment classification tasks, and the rest are new features that we developed.

Unigrams

A sentence is composed of words. Distinct words (unigrams) can be used as the features of a sentence. In previous work on sentiment classification (Pang et al., 2002; Yu & Hatzivassiloglou, 2003) unigrams are very effective. Following this work, we also take unigrams as features. We use unigrams occurring more than 3 times in the data set in the feature set, and they are called UNIGRAMS in the following description.

Context Features

Our observation is that outcomes often express a change in a clinical value (Niu and Hirst, 2004). In the following example, *mortality* was *reduced.*

- In these three postinfarction trials ACE inhibitor versus placebo significantly *reduced mortality, readmission for heart failure, and reinfarction.*

The polarity of an outcome is often determined by how a change happens: if a **bad** thing (e.g., mortality) was **reduced**, then it is a positive outcome; if a **bad** thing was **increased**, then the outcome is negative; if there is no change, then we get a neutral outcome. We tried to capture this observation by adding context features – BIGRAMS, two types of CHANGE PHRASES (MORE/LESS features and POLARITY-CHANGE features), and NEGATIONS.

Bigrams

Bigrams (two adjacent words) are also used in sentiment classification. In that task, they are not so effective as UNIGRAMS. When combined with UNIGRAMS, they do not improve the classification accuracy (Pang et al., 2002; Yu & Hatzivassiloglou, 2003). However, in our task, the context of a word in a sentence that describes the change in a clinical value is important in determining the polarity of a clinical outcome. Bigrams express the patterns of pairs, and we expect that they will capture some of the changes. Therefore, they are used in our feature set. As with UNIGRAMS, bigrams with frequency greater than 3 are extracted and referred to as BIGRAMS.

Change Phrases

We developed two types of new features to capture the trend of changes in clinical values. The collective name CHANGE PHRASES is used to refer to these features. To construct these features, we manually collected four groups of words by observing several sections in CE: those indicating **more** (*enhanced, higher, exceed, ...*), those indicating **less** (*reduce, decline, fall, ...*), those indicating **good** (*benefit, improvement, advantage, ...*), and those indicating **bad** (*suffer, adverse, hazards, ...*).

- **MORE/LESS features**. This type of feature emphasizes the effect of words expressing "changes". The way the features are generated is similar to the way that Pang et al. (2002) add negation features. We attached the tag _MORE to all words between the **more**-words and the following punctuation mark, or between the **more**-words and another **more** (or **less**) word, depending on which one comes first. The tag _LESS was added similarly. This way, the effect of the "change" words is propagated.
    - The first systematic review found that ß blockers significantly reduced_LESS the_LESS risk_LESS of_LESS death_LESS and_LESS hospital_LESS admissions_LESS.
    - Another large RCT (random clinical trial) found milrinone versus placebo increased_MORE mortality_MORE over_MORE 6_MORE months_MORE.
- **POLARITY-CHANGE features.** This type of feature addresses the co-occurrence of **more/less** words and **good/bad** words, i.e., it detects whether a sentence expresses the idea of "change of polarity". We used four features for this purpose: MORE GOOD, MORE BAD, LESS GOOD, and LESS BAD. As this type of feature aims for the "changes" instead of "propagating the change effect", we used a

smaller window size to build these features. To extract the first feature, a window of four words on each side of a **more**-word in a sentence was observed. If a **good**-word occurs in this window, then the feature MORE GOOD was set to 1. The other three features were set in a similar way.

Negations

Most frequently, negation expressions contain the word *no* or *not*. We observed several sections of CE and found that *not* is usually used in a way that does not affect the polarity of a sentence, as shown in the following examples, so it is not included in the feature set:

- However, disagreement for uncommon but serious adverse safety outcomes has **not** been examined.
- The first RCT found fewer episodes of infection while taking antibiotics than while **not** taking antibiotics.
- The rates of adverse effects seemed higher with rivastigmine than with other anticholinesterase drugs, but direct comparisons have **not** been performed.

The case for *no* is different: it often suggests a neutral polarity or no clinical outcome at all:

- There are **no** short or long term clinical benefits from the administration of nebulised corticosteroids ...
- One systematic review in people with Alzheimer's disease found **no** significant benefit with lecithin versus placebo.
- We found **no** systematic review or RCTs of rivastigmine in people with vascular dementia.

We develop the NEGATION features to take into account the evidence of the word *no*. To extract the features, all the sentences in the data set are first parsed by the Apple Pie parser (Sekine, 1997) to get phrase information. Then, in a sentence containing the word *no*, the noun phrase containing *no* is extracted. Every word in this noun phrase except *no* itself is attached by a *_NO* tag.

Semantic Types

Using category information to represent groups of medical concepts may relieve the data sparseness problem in the learning process. For example, we found that diseases are often mentioned in clinical outcomes as **bad** things:

- A combined end point of death or disabling stroke was significantly lower in the accelerated-t-PA group...

Thus, all names of specific diseases in the text are replaced with the tag DISEASE.

Intuitively, the occurrences of Semantic types, such as **pathologic function** and **organism function**, may be different in different polarity of outcomes, especially in the *no outcome* class as compared to the other three classes. To verify this intuition, we collect all the Semantic types in the data set and use each of them as a feature. They are referred to as SEMANTIC TYPES. Thus, in addition to the words contained in a sentence, all the medical categories mentioned in a sentence are also considered. The Unified Medical Language System (UMLS) is used as the domain knowledge base for extracting Semantic types of concepts. The software MetaMap (Aronson, 2001) is incorporated for mapping concepts to their corresponding Semantic types in the UMLS Metathesaurus.

Experiments

We carried out several experiments on two text sources: CE and Medline abstracts. Compared to CE text, Medline has a more diverse writing style as different abstracts have different authors. The performance of the supervised classification approach on the two sources was compared to find out if there is any difference. We believe that these experiments will lead to better understanding of the polarity detection task.

Outcome Detection and Polarity Classification in CE Text

Experimental Setup

The data set of sentences in all the four classes was built by collecting sentences from different sections in CE (sentences were selected so that the data set is relatively balanced). The number of instances in each class is shown in Table 7. The data set was labeled manually by three graduate students, and each sentence was labeled by one of them. We used the OSU SVM package (Ma et al., 2003) with an RBF kernel for this experiment. The σ value was set heuristically using training data. Default values were used for other parameters in the package.

Results and Analysis

Table 8 shows the results of the five feature sets used for classification. The accuracy is the average of 50 runs of the experiment. In each run, 20% of the data is selected randomly as the test set, and the rest is used as the training set. With just UNIGRAMS as features, we get 76.9% accuracy, which is taken as the baseline. The addition of BIGRAMS in the feature set results in an increase of about 2.5% in accuracy, which corresponds to 10.8% of relative error reduction. CHANGE PHRASES lead to a very small improvements and NEGATIONS do not improve the performance on top of BIGRAMS. Note that CHANGE PHRASES tend to capture the impact of context, and bigrams also contain context information. It could be that some effect of CHANGE PHRASES has already been captured by bigrams. Also, since the target classes are different in the two tasks, CHANGE PHRASES may be more important in distinguishing positive from negative outcomes. The SEMANTIC TYPES features further improve the performance on top of the combination of other features, which shows that generalization is helpful.

Which class is the most difficult to detect, and why? To answer these questions, we further examine the errors in every class. The precision, recall and *F*-score of each class are shown in Table 9 (it is the result of one run of the experiment). It is clear in the table that the negative class has the lowest precision and recall. A lot of errors occur in distinguishing negative from no-outcome classes. We studied the incorrectly classified sentences and found some interesting cases. Some of the errors occur because descriptions of diseases in the no-outcome class are often identified as negative. These sentences are difficult in that they contain negative expressions (e.g., *increased risk*), yet do not belong to the negative class:

- Lewy body dementia is an insidious impairment of executive functions with Parkinsonism, visual hallucinations, and fluctuating cognitive abilities and increased risk of falls or autonomic failure.

Negative samples are sometimes assigned a positive label when a sentence has phrasings that seem to contrast, as shown in the following example:

Table 7. Number of instances in each class (CE)

Positive	Negative	Neutral	No-outcome	Total
472	338	250	449	1509

- The mean increase in height in the budesonide group was 1.1 cm less than in the placebo group (22.7 vs 23.8 cm, P= 0005); ...

In this sentence, the clinical outcome of impaired growth is expressed by comparing height increase in two groups, which is less explicit and hard to capture.

Outcome Detection and Polarity Classification in Medline

With Medline abstracts, we evaluate two tasks: the first one is two-way classification that aims to detect the presence of clinical outcomes. In this task, a sentence is classified into two classes: containing a clinical outcome or not. The second task is the four-way classification, i.e., identifying whether an outcome is positive, negative, neutral, or the sentence does not contain an outcome.

Experimental Setup

We collected 197 abstracts from Medline that were cited in CE. The number of sentences in each class is listed in Table 10. The data set was annotated with the four classes of polarity information by two graduate students. Each single sentence was annotated by one of them.

In this experiment, again, 20% of the data was randomly selected as test set and the rest was used as the training data. The averaged accuracy was obtained from 50 runs. We again used the OSU SVM package for this experiment; parameters were set in the same manner.

Results and Analysis

Results of the two tasks are shown in Table 11. Not surprisingly, the performance on the two-way classification is better than on the four-way task. For both tasks, we see a similar trend in accuracy as for CE text (see Table 8). The accuracy goes up as more features are added, and the complete feature set has the best performance. Compared to UNIGRAMS, the combination of all features significantly improves the performance in both tasks (paired *t*-test, *p* values <0.0001). With just UNIGRAMS as features, we get 80.1% accuracy for the two-way task. The addition of BIGRAMS in the feature set results in an increase of 1.6 percentage points in accuracy, which corresponds to 8.0% of relative error reduction as compared to UNIGRAMS. Similar improvements are observed in the four-way task. The SEMANTIC TYPES features also slightly reduce the error rate.

Compared to the results on CE text in Table 8, the four-way classification task tends to be more difficult on Medline text. This can be observed by comparing the improvement of adding all other features to UNIGRAMS. As we mentioned in section 5.3, Medline abstracts have a more diverse writing style because they are written by different authors. This could be a factor that makes the classification task more difficult. However, the general performance of features on Medline abstracts and

Table 8. Results of the four-way classification with different feature sets in CE

Features	Accuracy (%)	Relative Error Reduction (%) (to UNIGRAMS)
(1) UNIGRAMS	76.9	—
(1)+(2) BIGRAMS	79.4	10.8
(1)+(2)+(3) CHANGE PHRASES	79.6	11.7
(1)+(2)+(3)+(4) NEGATIONS	79.6	11.7
(1)+(2)+(3)+(4)+(5) SEMANTIC TYPES	80.6	16.0

Table 9. Classification results of each class on CE data

	Positive	Negative	Neutral	No Outcome
Precision (%)	86.8	73.1	79.2	76.8
Recall (%)	83.2	73.1	76.0	82.0
F-score (%)	85.0	73.1	77.6	79.3

Table 10. Number of instances in each class (Medline)

Positive	Negative	Neutral	No Outcome	Total
469	122	194	1513	2298

Table 11. Results of two-way and four-way classification with different feature sets (Medline)

RER=Relative Error Reduction (compared to unigrams)

	two-way		four-way	
Features	Accuracy (%)	RER (%)	Accuracy (%)	RER (%)
(1) UNIGRAMS	80.1	—	75.5	—
(1)+(2) BIGRAMS	81.7	8.0	77.4	7.8
(1)+(2)+(3) CHANGE PHRASES	82.0	9.5	77.6	8.6
(1)+(2)+(3)+(4) NEGATIONS	81.9	9.0	77.6	8.6
(1)+(2)+(3)+(4)+(5) SEMANTIC TYPES	82.5	12.1	78.3	11.4

CE text is similar, which shows that the feature set is relatively robust. In our outcome detection and polarity classification task, UNIGRAMS are very effective features, as has been previously shown in the context of sentiment classification problems. This shows that information in words is very important for the polarity detection task. Context information represented by BIGRAMS and CHANGE PHRASES is also valuable in our task (see Table 8 and Table 11). The effectiveness of BIGRAMS is different from the results obtained by Pang et al. (2002) and Yu & Hatzivassiloglou (2003). In their work, adding bigrams does not make any difference in the accuracy, or even is slightly harmful in some cases. This indicates the difference in the expression of polarity in clinical outcomes and the polarity in opinions. Generalization features (SEMANTIC TYPES in Table 8 and Table 11) are also helpful in our task.

Discussion

The Performance Bottleneck in Polarity Classification

As described in section 5.1, supervised approaches have been used in sentiment classification. Features used in these approaches usually include: *n*-grams, PoS tags, and features based on words with Semantic orientations (e.g., adjectives such as *good, bad*). In all such studies, a common observation is that unigrams are very effective, while adding more features does not gain much.

- In the task of detecting polarity of documents (Pang et al., 2002), the best performance is obtained using unigrams.
- In the sentence-level opinion/fact classification task (Yu & Hatzivassiloglou, 2003), various features based on Semantic orientation of words are tried, including counts of Semantically oriented words, the polarity of the head verbs and the average Semantic orientation score of the words in the sentence. A gold standard set is built which includes 400 sentences labeled by one judge. In the opinion class, the only result better than the performance of unigrams is obtained by combining all features, which results in only 0.01 improvement in precision. Similarly, not much is achieved by adding all other features in detecting facts.
- In the work of Whitelaw, Garg, and Argamon (2005), the best performance of the approach is achieved by the combination of unigrams with the appraisal groups, which is 3% higher in accuracy than using unigrams alone.

From all this work, we observe a *performance bottleneck* problem in the polarity classification task: various features have been developed; however, adding more features does not gain much in classification accuracy, and it may even hurt the performance. In our task, although the context and generalization features significantly improve the performance compared to unigrams, we observe a similar *performance bottleneck* problem.

Analysis of the Problem

The bottleneck problem shows that additional features have much overlap with unigram features, and they may add noise to the classification. We further analyzed the data, and found that most words in a sentence do not contribute to the classification task. Instead, they can be noise that cannot be removed by adding more features. This could be a crucial reason of the bottleneck discussed above.

To verify this hypothesis, we conducted some additional experiments on the Medline data set of 2298 sentences. From each sentence in the data set, we manually extracted some words that fully determine the polarity of the sentence. We refer to these words by *extractions* in the following description. For those sentences that do not contain outcomes, nothing is extracted. The following examples are some sentences with different polarity and the extractions from them. These extractions form another data set, which we call the *extraction set.*

- **Sentence**: Treatment with reperfusion therapies and achievement of TIMI 3 flow are associated with increased short- and medium-term survival after infarction.
  Extraction: Increased short- and medium-term survival
- **Sentence**: In all three studies, a significant decrease in linear growth occurred in children treated with beclomethasone compared to those receiving placebo or non-steroidal asthma therapy.
  Extraction: Decrease in linear growth occurred
- **Sentence**: The doxazosin arm, compared with the chlorthalidone arm, had a higher risk of stroke.
  Extraction: A higher risk of stroke
- **Sentence**: Prednisolone treatment had no effect on any of the outcome measures.
  Extraction: No effect
- **Sentence**: There was no significant mortality difference during days 0–35, either among all randomised patients or among the prespecified subset presenting within 0–6 h of pain onset and with ST elevation on the electrocardiogram in whom fibrinolytic treatment may have most to offer.
  Extraction: No significant mortality difference

We performed the four-way classification task on this extraction set. We constructed UNIGRAM features based on the extraction set and used them in the classification. Using 80% of the data as the training data and the rest as the test data, we achieved an accuracy of 93.3%, which is much higher than the accuracy of the four-way classification task on the original sentence set (75.5%).

The fact that we do not extract any words from no-outcome sentences may make the task easier. Therefore, we removed from the extraction set all sentences that do not contain an outcome, and reran the experiment. This task has three target classes: positive, negative or neutral. We obtained an accuracy of 82.2%. However, performing the three-way classification on the original sentence set only achieves 70.7% accuracy.

The results clearly show that irrelevant words actually introduce a lot of noise in the polarity detection task. Therefore, a new direction of research on the task is to conduct feature selection to remove words that do not contribute to the classification.

We took a closer look at the extraction set and found that the extractions usually form a sequence or several sequences in a sentence. Because hidden Markov models and conditional random fields are effective models for sequence detection, they will be explored in the future work of this research.

Summary

In this section, we discussed a supervised approach to identifying an inherent property of clinical outcomes — their polarity. Polarity information is important to answer questions related to clinical outcomes. We analyzed this problem from various aspects:

- We developed features to represent context information and explored domain knowledge to get generalized features. The results show that adding these features significantly improves the classification accuracy.
- We showed that the feature set has consistent performance on two different text sources, CE and Medline abstracts.
- We compared outcome polarity detection to sentiment classification according to different performance of context features on the two tasks. We found that although bigram features have almost no effect on the sentiment classification task, they improve the classification accuracy of identifying presence and polarity of clinical outcomes.
- We identified a *performance bottleneck* problem in the polarity classification task using a supervised approach. In both the sentiment classification and the outcome polarity detection, we observed that adding more features on top of the unigram features does not lead to major improvement in accuracy. We found a crucial reason for this — the noise in the feature set is not removed by adding more features. We proposed to use hidden Markov models or conditional random fields to conduct feature selection and thus to remove noise from the feature set.

CONCLUSION

Clinical question-answering is a complex task in which multiple pieces of information are often needed to construct a complete answer. We have proposed a novel approach guided by Semantic class analysis to deal with the complicated information needs. This approach consists of four major components:

- Detecting Semantic classes in questions and answer sources
- Identifying properties of Semantic classes
- Question-answer matching: exploring prop-

erties of Semantic classes to find relevant pieces of information
- Constructing answers by merging or synthesizing relevant information using relations between Semantic classes

We focused on three Semantic classes that correspond to roles in the commonly accepted PICO format of describing clinical scenarios. The three classes are: the problem of the patient, the intervention used to treat the problem, and the clinical outcome. In this paper, we have described our approach to automatically identifying two important properties of the three Semantic classes.

ACKNOWLEDGMENT

This project is supported by grants from Bell University Laboratories at the University of Toronto and by a grant from the Natural Sciences and Engineering Research Council of Canada.

REFERENCES

Ananiadou, S., & Tsujii, J. (Eds.) (2003). *Proceedings of the ACL 2003 Workshop on Natural Language Processing in Biomedicine.* Stroudsburg, PA, USA: Association for Computational Linguistics.

Aronson, A. R. (2001). Effective mapping of biomedical text to the UMLS Metathesaurus: the MetaMap program. In S. Bakken (Ed.), *American Medical Informatics Association Symposium* (pp. 17–21). Bethesda, MD, USA: American Medical Informatics Association.

Barton, S. (Ed.). (2002). *Clinical Evidence.* London, England: BMJ Publishing Group.

Berger, A., Caruana, R., Cohn, D., Freitag, D., & Mittal, V. (2000). Bridging the lexical chasm: statistical approaches to answer-finding. In N. J. Belkin, P. Ingwersen, & M. Leong (Eds.), *23rd International Conference on Research and Development in Information Retrieval* (pp. 192–199). New York, NY, USA: Association for Computing Machinery Press.

Blum, A., & Mitchell, T. (1998). Combining labeled and unlabeled data with co-training. In *Proceedings of the 11th Annual Conference on Computational Learning Theory* (pp. 92–100). New York, NY, USA: Association for Computing Machinery Press.

Brill, E. (1993). A *corpus-based approach to language learning.* Unpublished doctoral dissertation, University of Pennsylvania, Philadelphia, PA.

Cardie, C., Wiebe, J., Wilson, T., & Litman, D. (2004). Combining low-level and summary representations of opinions for multi-perspective question answering. In L. Greenwald, Z. Dodds, A. Howard, S. Tejada, & J. Weinberg (Eds.), *AAAI Spring Symposium: New Directions in Question Answering* (pp. 20–27). Menlo Park, CA, USA: AAAI Press.

Chang, C. C., & Lin, C. J. (2001). *LIBSVM — A library for support vector machines.* http://www.csie.ntu.edu.tw/~cjlin/libsvm/.

Cheng, G. Y. (2004). A study of clinical questions posed by hospital clinicians. *Journal of the Medical Library Association, 93*(4), 445–458.

Chieu, H. L., & Ng, H. T. (2003). Named entity recognition with a maximum entropy approach. In W. Daelemans & M. Osborne (Eds.), *7th Conference on Computational Natural Language Learning* (pp. 160–163). Stroudsburg, PA, USA: Association for Computational Linguistics.

Cimino, J. J. (1996). Linking patient information systems to bibliographic resources. *Methods of Information in Medicine, 35*(2), 122–126.

Collins, M., & Singer, M. (1999). Unsupervised models for named entity classification. In *Proceedings of the 1999 Joint SIGDAT Conference on Empirical Methods in Natural Language Processing and Very Large Corpora* (pp. 189–196). Stroudsburg, PA, USA: Association for Computational Linguistics.

Cucerzan, S., & Yarowsky, D. (1999). Language independent named entity recognition combining morphological and contextual evidence. In *Proceedings of the 1999 Joint SIGDAT Conference on Empirical Methods in Natural Language Processing and Very Large Corpora* (pp. 90–99). Stroudsburg, PA, USA: Association for Computational Linguistics.

Diekema, A., Yilmazel, O., Chen, J., Harwell, S., He, L., & Liddy, E. D. (2004). What do you mean? Finding answers to complex questions. In L. Greenwald, Z. Dodds, A. Howard, S. Tejada, and J. Weinberg (Eds.), *AAAI Spring Symposium: New Directions in Question Answering* (pp. 87–93). Menlo Park, CA, USA: AAAI Press.

Dowty, D. R. (1991). Proto-roles and argument selection. *Language*, *67*(3), 547–619.

DUC. (2005). *Document Understanding Conference.* http://duc.nist.gov/duc2005.

Ebell, M. H. (1999). Information at the point of care: answering clinical questions. *Journal of the American Board of Family Practice*, *12*(3), 225–235.

Fillmore, C. J. (1976). Frame Semantics and the nature of language. *Annals of the New York Academy of Sciences: Conference on the Origin and Development of Language and Speech*, *280*, 20–32.

Florian, R., Ittycheriah, A., Jing, H., & Zhang, T. (2003). Named entity recognition through classifier combination. In W. Daelemans & M. Osborne (Eds.), *7th Conference on Computational Natural Language Learning* (pp. 168–171). Stroudsburg, PA, USA: Association for Computational Linguistics.

Gildea, D., & Jurafsky, D. (2002). Automatic labeling of Semantic roles. *Computational Linguistics*, *28*(3), 245–288.

Gorman, P., Ash, J., & Wykoff, L. (1994). Can primary care physicians' questions be answered using the medical journal literature? *Bulletin of the Medical Library Association*, *82*(2), 140–146.

Harabagiu, S., Maiorano, S., Moschitti, A., & Bejan, C. (2004). Intentions, implicatures and processing of complex questions. In S. Harabagiu and F. Lacatusu (Eds.), *Human Language Technology Conference of the North American Chapter of the Association for Computational Linguistics, Workshop on Pragmatics of Question Answering* (pp. 31–42). Stroudsburg, PA, USA: Association for Computational Linguistics.

Hickl, A., Lehmann, J., Williams, J., & Harabagiu, S. (2004). Experiments with interactive question answering in complex scenarios. In S. Harabagiu & F. Lacatusu (Eds.), *Human Language Technology Conference of the North American Chapter of the Association for Computational Linguistics, Workshop on Pragmatics of Question Answering* (pp. 60–69). Stroudsburg, PA, USA: Association for Computational Linguistics.

Huang, T. M., Kecman, V., & Kopriva, I. (2006). *Kernel based algorithms for mining huge data sets.* Berlin, Germany: Springer.

Klein, D., Smarr, J., Nguyen, H., & Manning, C. D. (2003). Named entity recognition with character-level models. In W. Daelemans & M. Osborne (Eds.), *7th Conference on Computational Natural Language Learning* (pp. 180–183). Stroudsburg, PA, USA: Association for Computational Linguistics.

Kohomban, U. S., & Lee, W. S. (2005). Learning Semantic classes for word sense disambiguation.

In *Proceedings of the 43rd Annual Meeting of the Association for Computational Linguistics* (pp. 34–41). Stroudsburg, PA, USA: Association for Computational Linguistics.

Lin, D. (1994). Principar — an efficient, broad-coverage, principle-based parser. In *Proceedings of the 15th International Conference on Computational Linguistics* (pp. 482–488). Stroudsburg, PA, USA: Association for Computational Linguistics.

Lin, D. (1998). Automatic retrieval and clustering of similar words. In *Proceedings of the 17th International Conference on Computational Linguistics* (pp. 768–774). Stroudsburg, PA, USA: Association for Computational Linguistics.

Ma., J., Zhao, Y., Ahalt, S., & Eads, D. (2003). *OSU SVM classifier Matlab toolbox*. http://svm.sourceforge.net/docs/3.00/api/.

Mendonça, E. A., Cimino, J. J., Johnson, S. B., & Seol, Y. H. (2001). Accessing heterogeneous sources of evidence to answer clinical questions. *Journal of Biomedical Informatics, 34*, 85–98.

MUC. (2003). Message Understanding Conference. http://www.cs.nyu.edu/cs/faculty/grishman/muc6.html

Niu, Y. (2007). *Analysis of Semantic classes: toward non-factoid question answering*. Unpublished doctoral dissertation, University of Toronto, Toronto, Canada.

Niu, Y., & Hirst, G. (2004). Analysis of Semantic classes in medical text for question answering. In D. Mollá & J. L. Vicedo, *42nd Annual Meeting of the Association for Computational Linguistics, Workshop on Question Answering in Restricted Domains* (pp. 54–61). Stroudsburg, PA, USA: Association for Computational Linguistics.

Niu, Y., & Hirst, G. (2007). Identifying cores of Semantic classes in unstructured text with a semi-supervised learning approach. In *Proceedings of Recent Advances in Natural Language Processing 2007* (pp. 418–424).

Niu, Y., Zhu, X.D., & Hirst, G. (2006). Using outcome polarity in sentence extraction for medical question-answering. In Daniel Masys (Ed.), *American Medical Informatics Association 2006 Annual Symposium* (pp. 599–603). Bethesda, MD, USA: American Medical Informatics Association.

Niu, Y., Zhu, X., Li, J., & Hirst, G. (2005). Analysis of polarity information in medical text. In C. P. Friedman (Ed.), *American Medical Informatics Association 2005 Annual Symposium* (pp. 570–574). Bethesda, MD, USA: American Medical Informatics Association.

Niu, Y., Hirst, G., McArthur, M., and Rodriguez-Gianolli, P. (2003). Answering clinical questions with role identification. In Ananiadou, S., & Tsujii, J. (Eds.), *41st Annual Meeting of the Association for Computational Linguistics, Workshop on Natural Language Processing in Biomedicine* (pp. 73–80). Stroudsburg, PA, USA: Association for Computational Linguistics.

Pang, B., & Lee, L. (2003). A sentimental education: sentiment analysis using subjectivity smmarizaiton based on minimum cuts. In *Proceedings of the 42th Annual Meeting of the Association for Computational Linguistics* (pp. 271–278). Stroudsburg, PA, USA: Association for Computational Linguistics.

Pang, B., Lee, L., & Vaithyanathan, S. (2002). Thumbs up? sentiment classification using machine learning techniques. In *Proceedings of 2002 Conference on Empirical Methods in Natural Language Processing* (pp. 79–86). PA, USA: Association for Computational Linguistics.

Ray, S., & Craven, M. (2001). Representing sentence structure in hidden Markov models for information extraction. In B. Nebel (Ed.), *17th International Joint Conferences on Artificial*

Intelligence (pp. 1273–1279). San Fransisco, CA, USA: Morgan Kaufmann Publishers Inc.

Richardson, W. S., Wilson, M. C., Nishikawa, J., & Hayward, R. S. (1995). The well-built clinical question: a key to evidence-based decisions. *ACP Journal Club, 123*(3), 12–13.

Riloff, E. (1999). Information extraction as a stepping stone toward story understanding. In A. Ram & K. Moorman (Eds.), *Computational Models of Reading and Understanding.* Cambridge, MA, USA: The MIT Press.

Rosario, B., & Hearst, M. A. (2004). Classifying Semantic relations in bioscience texts. In *Proceedings of 42nd Annual Meeting of the Association for Computational Linguistics* (pp. 431–438). Stroudsburg, PA, USA: Association for Computational Linguistics.

Sackett, D. L., & Straus, S. E. (1998). Finding and applying evidence during clinical rounds: the "evidence cart". *Journal of the American Medical Association, 280*(15), 1336–1338.

Sackett, D. L., Straus, S. E., Richardson, W. S., Rosenberg, W., & Haynes, R. B. (2000). *Evidence-based medicine: How to practice and teach EBM.* Edinburgh: Harcourt Publishers Limited.

Sekine, S. (1997). *Apple Pie Parser.* http://nlp.cs.nyu.edu/app/.

Small, S., Strzalkowski, T., Liu, T., Ryan, S., Salkin, R., Shimizu, N., Kantor, P., Kelly, D., Rittman, R., Wacholder, N., & Yamrom, B. (2004). HITIQA: Scenario based question answering. In S. Harabagiu and F. Lacatusu (Eds.), *Human Language Technology Conference of the North American Chapter of the Association for Computational Linguistics, Workshop on Pragmatics of Question Answering* (pp. 52–59). Stroudsburg, PA, USA: Association for Computational Linguistics.

Soricut, R., & Brill, E. (2006). Question answering using the Web: Beyond the factoid. *Information Retrieval — Special Issue on Web Information Retrieval, 9*, 191–206.

Stoyanov, V., Cardie, C., & Wiebe, J. (2005). Multi-perspective question answering using the OpQA Corpus. In *Proceedings of Human Language Technology Conference/Conference on Empirical Methods in Natural Language Processing* (pp. 923–930). Stroudsburg, PA, USA: Association for Computational Linguistics.

Straus, S. E., & Sackett, D. L. (1999). Bring evidence to the point of care. *Journal of the American Medical Association, 281,* 1171–1172.

Tjong Kim Sang, E.F. & De Meulder, F. (2003). Introduction to the CoNLL-2003 shared task: language-independent named entity recognition. *Proceedings of Conference on Computational Natural Language Learning* (pp. 142–147). Stroudsburg, PA, USA: Association for Computational Linguistics.

TREC. (2001). *Text REtrieval Conference.* http://trec.nist.gov/.

Turney, P. (2002). Thumbs up or thumbs down? Semantic orientation applied to unsupervised classification of reviews. In *Proceedings of the 40th Annual Meeting of the Association for Computational Linguistics* (pp. 417–424). Stroudsburg, PA, USA: Association for Computational Linguistics.

Valin, V., & Robert, D. (1993). A synosis of role and reference grammar. In Robert, D., & Valin, V. (Ed.), *Advances in Role and Reference Grammar* (pp. 1–166). Amsterdam: John Benjamins Publishing Company.

Whitelaw, C., Garg, N., & Argamon, S. (2005). Using appraisal groups for sentiment analysis. In *Proceedings of the 14th ACM International Conference on Information and Knowledge management* (pp. 625–631). New York, NY, USA: Association for Computing Machinery Press.

Yu, H., & Hatzivassiloglou, V. (2003). Towards answering opinion questions: separating facts from opinions and identifying the polarity of opinion sentences. In *Proceedings of the 2003 Conference on Empirical Methods in Natural Language Processing* (pp. 129–136). Stroudsburg, PA, USA: Association for Computational Linguistics.

Zhu, X., Ghahramani, Z., & Lafferty, J. (2003). Semi-supervised learning using Gaussian fields and harmonic functions. In T. Fawcett & N. Mishra, (Eds.) *The 20th International Conference on Machine Learning* (pp. 912–919). Menlo Park, CA, USA: AAAI Press.

ENDNOTE

1 This chapter summarizes work that was published earlier in Niu, 2007; Niu & Hirst, 2004; Niu & Hirst, 2007; Niu, Hirst, McArthur & Rodriguez-Gianolli, 2003; Niu, Zhu, Li & Hirst, 2005; and Niu, Zhu & Hirst, 2006. Some con-tent in this chapter is reprinted from Niu & Hirst, 2004 and Niu, Hirst, McArthur & Rodriguez-Gianolli, 2003, with permission from the American Medical Informatics Association. Some content is reprinted from Niu, Zhu, Li & Hirst, 2005 and Niu, Zhu & Hirst, 2006 with permission from the Association for Computational Linguistics.

Section III

Pragmatics, Discourse Structures and Segment Level as the Last Stage in the NLP Offer to Biomedicine

Chapter XII
Discourse Processing for Text Mining

Nadine Lucas
GREYC CNRS, Université de Caen Basse-Normandie Campus 2, France

ABSTRACT

This chapter presents the challenge of integrating knowledge at higher levels of discourse than the sentence, to avoid "missing the forest for the trees". Characterisation tasks aimed at filtering collections are introduced, showing use of the whole set of layout constituents from sentence to text body. Few text descriptors encapsulating knowledge on text properties are used for each granularity level. Text processing differs according to tasks, whether individual document mining or tagging small or large collections prior to information extraction. Very shallow and domain independent techniques are used to tag collections to save costs on sentence parsing and semantic manual annotation. This approach achieves satisfactory characterisation of text types, for example reviews versus clinical reports, or argumentation-type articles versus explanation-type. These collection filtering techniques are fit for a wider domain of biomedical literature than genomics.

INTRODUCTION

In this chapter we address higher-levels of text processing, as related to text mining. The domain of biomedical language processing (BLP or bio-NLP) "encompasses the many computational tools and methods that take human generated texts as input, generally applied to tasks such as information retrieval, document classification, information extraction, plagiarism detection, or literature-based discovery" (Hunter & Bretonnel Cohen, 2006 p. 589).

Access to biomedical literature itself (primary sources) is provided since 2004 through PubMed Central established by the American National Library of Medicine (NLM) as a repository of free access articles. The search system Entrez PubMed offers abstracts from Medline along with on line full-text indexed by Mesh and access to databases (see NLM site). This has fostered a new circular situation where data and text bases feed literature in turn feeding databases and ontologies.

Related events are first, advances in genomics and the information deluge. A double exponential growth of published material is recorded in the biomedical field, creating in turn an increased amount of facts to be stored (Shatkay & Craven, 2007). Second, text mining techniques for specific purposes were developed in particular to help in database curation. Automats now directly fill a growing part of databases (Hunter & Bretonnel Cohen, 2006). Third, a new field called systems biology emerged at the frontier between data and text mining (Krallinger & Valencia, 2005). Text mining is used to back data interpretation. Computational processes are ubiquitous and the frontier between text and data mining is blurred as well as the frontier between human and automated processes. Integrated text mining systems inherit from expert systems (nomenclatures linked with inference rules) and from statistical data mining. They rely on what might be called tertiary sources of knowledge: unified nomenclatures, hand curated interaction databases and hand annotated corpora. These are sometimes grouped under the term "ontologies" (Ananiadou *et al.*, 2006). Last, users now take it for granted that raw information is quickly translated into secondary and tertiary sources, and rely on computer-manageable "concepts" (Rebholz-Schumann *et al.*, 2005). Recent developments can be watched by consulting the Biomedical Literature Mining Publication portal (Blimp) (2008).

Success in the genomics field opened the way for less specific purposes. As text mining is advertised in more publications, not only "omics" researchers, but also clinicians, general practitioners and medical librarians call for text processing (Fluck *et al.*, 2005; Hunter & Bretonnel Cohen, 2006; Mizuta *et al.*, 2006). One emerging trend in research is to take patients into consideration to best respond to users' needs (Leroy *et al.*, 2006). This implies a change in the way to produce results. While researchers can do with highly specialised words, evoking for them research trends, a wider public need full explanations, therefore lengthier passages of text. Robust text processing is needed but it is still in its infancy.

Another trend calls for semantic characterisation of texts in a collection. Most semantic oriented tasks, such as characterizing original findings on a topic, or eliciting hypotheses, require a wider context than the sentence. Valuable meta-information that could be used to qualify texts is still lacking. Some attempts at qualifying parts of them, like conclusions, e.g. tentative or definite are on the way. Yet, very few studies address text at a global level as a semantic unit. The gap between expectations and realisations is blatant.

The approach explained here relies on combining text mining characterisation techniques for collections and robust high-level discourse parsing techniques. We advocate a shift of paradigm from word-level description to text-level description. In the domain of biomedical text processing, text is characterized as "unstructured data" as compared to databases (Hunter & Bretonnel Cohen, 2006), or at best as semi-structured data (Hakenberg *et al.,* 2005). Yet, texts are structured by layout, a feature that has been overlooked. Academic articles in particular are highly structured. Scale issues are seldom addressed, although they are important for information retrieval and knowledge integration in biomedicine.

We consider layout structures in relation with rhetorical structures and discourse segments. A survey of the state of the art is provided in the background section. In the third section, original research on multi-scale text descriptors is thoroughly explained. Experiments for complex tasks in text mining are then introduced and future trends including evaluation is discussed in the following section. We conclude on these experiments and broaden perspectives in the last section.

BACKGROUND

Biomedical Language Processing

Text mining, also referred to as text data mining or literature mining, is a relatively new but very active and fast evolving part of bio-NLP. Text mining is widely relied upon for drug discovery, patent analysis and intelligent text processing. It was mentioned in relation with knowledge discovery, a trend prevalent in the United Sates of America. According to Shatkay & Feldman (2003, pp. 824-825):

Text mining is the combined, automated process of analyzing unstructured natural language text in order to discover information and knowledge that are typically difficult to retrieve [...]. It uses techniques from the general field of data mining [...], but since it handles unstructured data, a major part of the process deals with the crucial stage of pre-processing the document collections (using techniques such as text categorization [...], term extraction [...], and information extraction [...]).
In addition to pre-processing the documents, text mining also covers the storage of the intermediate representations, the techniques to analyze these intermediate representations, such as distribution analysis, clustering [...], trend analysis [...], association rules [...], and the visualization of the results [...].

Text mining in the bio-medical field is also (more soberly) described by three main tasks, information retrieval, information extraction and data mining (Ananiadou *et al.*, 2006 ; Krallinger & Valencia, 2005).

While statistical methods based on the "bag of words" approach did help in integrating knowledge, the need to grasp relations expressed in texts led to rely on natural language processing (NLP) techniques (de Bruijn & Martin, 2002; Roberts, 2006). However, mature techniques from the NLP field are dealing with sentences segmented in words. While offering access to tertiary sources of knowledge (ontologies and tagged corpora) through terms, they suffer from inaccuracies that cannot be solved at that level. Ambiguity resolution for instance would need a larger scope. Thus, the information deluge is handled at a very minute grain.

In the information extraction domain, a number of organized contests between systems exist. Among well-known competitive evaluation workshops are Biocreative (2004 and 2006), BioNLP and the Joint Workshop on Natural Language Processing in Biomedicine and its Applications JNLPBA, to which the Text Retrieval Conference (TREC) genomics track can be added (2003-2007). They have fostered and developed a homogeneous trend of research based on sentence screening for specific information. Techniques in the text processing pipeline include part of speech tagging, named entity recognition, filtering. They are well fit for precise information extraction at a fine grain but they also have limits explained in the last sub-section of this section.

Text Linguistics

Linguistic research is disconnected from computational linguistics, at least in the dominant Western sphere. In the field of text linguistics, theoretical work began anew at the wake of the 20th century. Starting with pioneer research in Russia, then the Prague Circle, it spread everywhere. Research developed with a wealth of aspects, from hermeneutics and semiotics to structural text grammar and layout description (De Beaugrande, 1991; Schiffrin *et al.*, 2003). Although many authors attempted to model text as a semiotic entity or as structured document in the latter part of the 20th century, their application was teaching and remained largely ignored in the computation world. Two theories stand as exceptions, the information theory (Harris, 1982, 2002) and, to a lesser degree, the Systemic Functional Linguistics theory after Halliday (1994).

Skipping research on news, and focussing on the academic genre, some useful books provide insights on scientific literature at large (Parsons, 1990; Fløttum & Rastier, 2002; Fløttum, 2007). Swales and colleagues extensively studied academic writing in English (Swales, 1990). Hyland and followers put emphasis on the sociological aspect of academic writing (Hyland, 2005; del Lungo & Tognini-Bonelli, 2006).

The domain of medicine and medical discourse in academic settings attracted early attention (Salager-Meyer, 1994; Skelton, 1994). Description of text structure and logical markers followed (Nwogu, 1997). Modality and epistemic markers were studied in English and in different languages (Rowley-Jolivet, 2007; Vold, 2006). Specialty language researches dealing with medicine were also conducted on the lexical and morphological side (Fleischman, 2003).

Apart from mainstream linguistic research, Harris and followers paid attention to the medical sublanguage in the mathematical linguistic approach (Harris *et al.*, 1989; Friedman *et al.*, 2002).

State of the Art in Text Mining as related to NLP

Pioneering research to bridge the gap between computational linguistics and text linguistics was conducted in Japan, later in Europe and America. Focussing on the academic writing subfield, Kando attempted an NLP-wise description of academic articles in Japanese for information retrieval (Kando, 1992, 1999) and later turned to summarization. For English, Teufel (1999) worked on discourse segmentation and markers then proceeded towards summarization (Teufel & Moens, 2002). The Systemic Functional Linguistics theory backs text mining experiments by Argamon and colleagues on academic writing (Argamon *et al.*, 2007). The Harris model (2002) has successfully been used in bio-NLP, as being related to the medical sublanguage (Friedman *et al.*, 2002; Grishman *et al.*, 2002; Rzhetsky *et al.*, 2004).

In contrast, most text mining techniques rely on medical vocabulary alone as the key to knowledge. This stems from the history of both fields of medicine and computer science. Medical literature has high exchange value, so nomenclatures and elaborate indexing systems were developed by hand for centuries (Lovis, 1998). In the field of expert systems, MYCIN was the first notable achievement as early as the 1970s (Buchanan & Shortliffe, 1984). Reliance on nomenclature allows direct relation between external resources (databases and ontologies) and processing of the text lexical content.

The dominant statistical lexical approach is called "bag of words" because texts are described by their words alone, irrespective of order. The natural language processing (NLP) approach is based on sentence parsing methods inherited from current computational linguistics trends and they are lexicon-dependent (therefore language dependent). Extraction of cue phrases and key sentences expressing relations between named entities is an important part of NLP engineering in the biomedical field. Key sentences are used to automatically index articles, to curate databases and to weight the relevance of articles against a query. Accuracy in this task is evaluated in shared tasks using recall, precision and F measure. Although results in information extraction have been improved by using redundancy and powerful machine learning techniques, they still are mediocre compared with information extraction from news (Hirshman *et al.,* 2005).

We present here some aspects of bio-NLP research on text explicitly stating discourse high level segments and discourse notions reflected at fine grain.

Text as Paragraph

Above sentence, the paragraph is also studied, either as a plain text unit, or as an implicit observation window containing so-called discourse or rhetorical relations. The most often cited frames, RST, SDRT, UDML, express relations inside and between sentences, relating short text segments (clauses). They are used for summarization or IR tasks, mainly on short news (Schilder, 2002). These models fail to express the entire text structure, notably for elaborate academic texts.

In bio-NLP, abstracts are favoured as observation windows (Ding *et al.*, 2002). Many reasons explain why abstracts are relied upon rather than text. First, only abstracts are widely and freely available (Wren, 2005). Second, full-text was until recently available in read-only format (image type PDF) and although document physical structure retrieval and conversion to computable formats has dramatically progressed, it still is not routinely integrated. Third, it might also be said that current NLP techniques can be applied at that scale only, on a few sentences. If starting from atomic words, upwards, it is a big enough unit.

Text as Higher Units

Most biomedical articles follow the IMRAD model (Introduction, Material and Methods, Results and Discussion) (Swales, 1990). In the bio-NLP field, sections and their role in discourse have been studied in relation with summarisation (Spyropoulos & Karkaletsis, 2005). They have been explored as the collocation space for terms in topic tracking by Perrin & Petry (1999, 2003).

Experiments on research articles following the IMRAD model show that some sections should be avoided or given more weight, for specific bio-NLP tasks (Schuemie *et al.*, 2004). Results in named entity recognition are improved when related to section (Shah *et al.*, 2003). Interesting sections depend on the objective, for instance Hakenberg *et al.* report that the *Material and Methods* section is useful for hereditary diseases classification while Shah *et al.* find it should be avoided for gene entity recognition (Hakenberg *et al.*, 2005).

When abstracts are compared to full-text, or to individual sections, the importance of abstracts is always recognised.

Projections of Text Models onto Smaller Units

Rhetorical zoning is a way of describing texts by discourse clues found at sentence or clause level. Although some authors restrict zoning to sub-sentence delimitation of named entities, Mizuta *et al.* (2006) apply the notion to rhetorical status of statements. They rely on Kando's and Teufel's work aimed at summarisation to argue that factoid extraction tasks should ignore background information or subsequently denied statements. This direction is also recommended for qualitative annotation of texts (Wilbur *et al.*, 2006).

Research reminiscent of the Hyland's "hedging" notion emerged under the term paradigm shift. The aim is to locate new ideas in text collections using cue phrases in sentences marking acceptation of previous work or dissent (Lisacek *et al.*, 2005).

Linguistics background related to current research in text mining is often underspecified. For instance, position of cue phrases inside the paragraph was used to select target information, in he GeneRIF task in TREC first Genomics track in 2003. it was aimed at automatically fill the "Gene references in function" template provided in the Locus link database. The winners in this task used positions of sentences in the paragraph to weight their importance (Jelier *et al.*, 2003). Using the entire text body as context, the winners in one of the first text mining competitions (KDD cup 2002) successfully used figure captions to facilitate entity recognition (Feldman *et al.*, 2003).

What these examples highlight is the usefulness of "context" at various degrees. It illustrates the importance of macro-syntax, articulating the relative position of a meaningful form in some span of text. Interestingly, such linguistic concepts, whether explicit or not, are easily related to machine learning algorithms (solvers). Departure from purely positive and normalised description towards more flexible text mining tools enables prediction, the main challenge for the scientific community.

To sum up this brief overview, it can be said that bio-NLP researchers use one text segment at a time, usually sentence and at best paragraph. These units are studied independently one by one and, like in classical NLP, a sub-sentence window of a few words is sequentially moved along the text in a linear fashion. Even when words or phrases are weighted by their larger context, the atomic unit is extremely small compared to the text and microscopic compared to a collection.

Problems in Biomedicine Text Processing

Results in information retrieval and information extraction in the biomedical domain are not quite satisfactory. The meaning of text is not captured when words are scrutinised at sentence-level. Moreover, on the practical side, annotation and processing costs at a very fine grain are high.

Since only abstracts were available for a long time, and still are the only free access part of the vast majority of articles, little research has been made at text-level. When full-text is used, it is mainly by statistical lexical techniques with the "bag-of-words" approach. High-value high-throughput techniques are called for, and use of full-text is the next challenge (Ananiadou *et al.,* 2006; Fluck *et al.,* 2005; Holmes & Peek, 2007).

A source of variation in the lexicon of scientific English has been spotted as related to the native language of authors (Netzel *et al.*, 2003). The same can be said on the ordering of arguments in articles. The importance of rhetorical status of statements has been shown in discussion sections, where a statement can be followed by a denial at some distance (Mizuta *et al.*, 2006). Another remark is that a clause, used in the context of premises, has not the same meaning as that same clause used in the context of a conclusion. Using only knowledge gained at sentence level is an obvious bias in the current approaches.

More generally, as researchers in content-based image retrieval have noted, the perceptive gap and the semantic gap are major problems. The perceptive gap means that computers organize data (pixels or character strings) that do not necessarily match with human perception. The semantic gap refers to the distance between low-level content and higher-level concepts. It can further be expressed as the distance between computerized value and semantic value as bestowed by users in different situations (Datta *et al.*, 2008). This is also the case in bio-NLP. Characters handled by computers are technically atomic but not atoms of meaning as perceived by humans.

Regarding information retrieval, the fact that a request is often expressed as isolated words by users or by a simple sentence in competitive evaluations does by no means entail that knowledge will be expressed in simple sentences in texts; on the contrary, it is well known that biomedical journals favour density in style (sentences are long and complex).

Robust text understanding is still an open problem. Whereas the semantic gap is recognized, the perceptive gap is seldom referred to in text-related tasks.. The main challenges are: how can the limits of memory-based NLP be overcome to facilitate adaptation to new domains and new languages; how can full texts be reasonably exploited; and how can texts be efficiently retrieved in large libraries for a specific aim. We propose some steps towards this goal by providing high-level segmentation and annotation of text.

We present an approach deliberately grounded in text linguistics and bent towards corpus characterisation. It is related to knowledge discovery in text databases, albeit this knowledge is related to biomedical literature itself, in terms of style and rhetorical disposition, rather than directly to the notions its conveys. This approach has similarities with Teufel's and Argamon's, because we concentrate on academic writing and relate low and high levels of analysis. It differs from Teufel's in that we do not annotate semantics by hand (Abdalla & Teufel, 2006). It differs from Argamon's in that we do not try and discover "hidden" relationships through text mining techniques but use knowledge on text relations to characterise collections (Argamon *et al.*, 2007).

Three main ideas are put forward. We advocate early pruning of collections or digital libraries, therefore bringing collection scale in scope; a document is an atom of the collection and should be described by a reasonable number of attributes to select relevant sub-collections. For document description, we use distributional principles: it is a grammar *more geometrico* by which we try and locate *where* information lies and not *what* information is. Last we advocate light-cost text processing informed by corpora.

We explain the general ideas in the next section devoted to discourse parsing and its relation with text characterisation, and proceed in the following section with experiments in text mining.

MULTI-SCALE TEXT PROCESSING

Texts are highly structured data from the text linguistics viewpoint. Text descriptors capture some text properties abstracted from text parsing. They help filter large corpora. Some examples will help understand the principles behind higher-level text description.

Text Parsing with a Specific Goal

Elaborate requests demand a high semantic characterisation. Suppose the task is to locate original findings on topic XXX. This is typically a task that involves qualitative differential judgement. It also concerns high-level relations, because original findings often bring new light on already known facts. Valuable answers would bring out a number of passages of text: sentences from an abstract, a few paragraphs or a whole section providing the rationale behind the finding. The following describes on going research exploiting more abstract rhetorical markers.

It might be useful to select articles with original findings and articles on the chosen topic separately. Next, it is necessary to translate the query into some set of observable characteristics

Figure 1. A. (left) Article with question statements B. (right) Article with outright statements

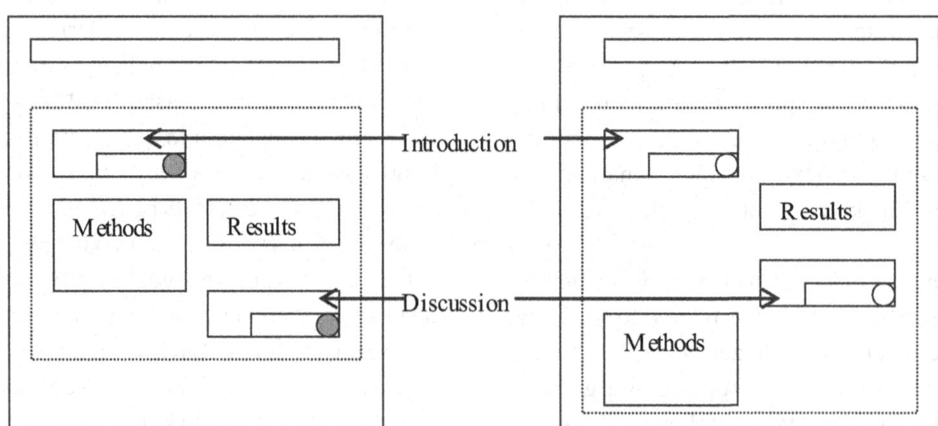

in text. "Original findings" should be related with assertion and completeness. Let us try and state on assertion. Compare two articles A (PII: S1 286-4579 (01) 01520-9) and B (doi: 10.1016/j.ccr.2006.10.020). Comments will probably be that in the first case, the authors are only half satisfied with their findings, while in the second they are fully satisfied. The difference does not lie in the phrasing in individual sentences, but in the disposition of text. Figure 1 shows where synthetic statements are made: in the last paragraph of the introduction and discussion sections. A positive statement reiterated at remarkable positions in text conveys a feeling of achievement, while a hued statement conveys a feeling of successful but un-terminated research (open question).

A positive statement is outright: it has no special linguistic mark, no question, no restriction nor negation. The grey dot in Figure 1 A represents a sentence expressing a question or "problem highlighting" sentence, while the white dot in B represents an assertion which is defined as no question (a zero mark).

Macro-syntax compares present and absent marking forms, and uses regularities but also differences in meaning to decide on which marks are useful at a given level. The open question feature is checked at text-body level. Rhetorical interrogative sentences or lexically marked "problem highlighting" sentences are usually located in introductions and conclusions. If examining the middle sections of an article, focussing on

Example 1. Text A with "problem highlighting" sentences (underlined)

> In the present study, we have examined the biological and ultrastructural effects of cysteine and serine protease inhibitors on the intracellular development of *Toxoplasma* tachyzoites. [...] However, cathepsin inhibitor III, TPCK and subtilisin inhibitor III, caused extensive swelling of the secretory pathway of the parasite leading to the breakdown of the parasite surface membrane and the disruption of secretory organelle formation. Nothing resembling lysosomal bodies was seen in any treated parasites, consistent with the absence of a well-defined autophagic-lysosomal pathway in the parasite. Nevertheless, the question of how the parasite recycles these organelles remains unanswered.
>
> [...]
>
> Lastly, one reason for this study was to see if using protease inhibitors could help elucidate how the parasites turn over the rhoptries and other cell organelles during daughter cell budding. [...] While the present results are consistent with observations showing that the mother cell organelles are not recycled by any form of bulk autophagic or lysosomal degradation, they leave the question of how the parasite recycles these organelles unanswered.

Example 2. Text B with assertion sentences

> We hypothesized that the downstream effects of the DCA-induced shift in metabolism will have beneficial effects in cancer therapy (Figure 1). We show that, as predicted, DCA changes the metabolism of cancer cells from the cytoplasm-based glycolysis to the mitochondria-based glucose oxidation. [...] We show that a metabolic-electrical remodeling regulates apoptosis resistance in cancer. Moreover, this abnormality is easily reversible by a simple drug that is already used in humans.
>
> [...]
>
> Our work identifies the mitochondria-NFAT-Kv channel axis and PDK as critical components of the metabolic electrical remodeling that characterizes many human cancers and offers a tantalizing suggestion that DCA may have selective anticancer efficacy in patients. The very recent report of the first randomized long-term clinical trial of oral DCA in children with congenital lactic acidosis (at doses similar to those used in our in vivo experiments) showing that DCA was well tolerated and safe (Stacpoole *et al.*, 2006) suggests a potentially easy translation of our work to clinical oncology.

each first paragraph, the description will rely on frequent features seen through a smaller window (the paragraph), like sentence conjunction by an adversative adverb (*Nevertheless*) or reinforcement adverb (*Moreover*).

The question in textual data mining can be expressed in the following way: does the difference observed between two research papers hold true for a whole collection, and what are the right conditions to maintain the reliability of the discourse markers just described?

Text Representation

Figure 2 shows the main granularity levels used to describe a text: text-body, sections, paragraphs, sentences, "comma-units". The latter refers to punctuated sub-segments of sentences and is also called period by some authors. They are called *selections* after the distributional linguistic frame and segments or *measures* when pragmatically mapped on layout. Remarkable positions are the beginning and the end of each layout measure, like position of prefix or suffix for a word (Hockett, 1958). For our purpose, the observation window for each text segment, from word upward to the entire article is called slot. For each measure, there are two slots or remarkable positions where some form-based textual hints are looked for.

It is important to separate out the surface hints from the slots they fill. Surface hints refer to form and are sometimes called morphological, when combined with position, irrespective of the granularity level (i.e. any character string is handled as a form, as related to a slot; we do not mean "morphology = word level"). Remarkable forms are annotated in the beginning and the end of the higher levels of analysis as well.

Cues for Detecting Judgments and Partial Conclusions

Now, let us try and state on completeness. Not all generic markers are found in a given article and some slots are filled while others remain empty. Assertion is not marked in English, like B above, so finding articles with no marks at text-body level do not provide sufficient clue that the article is indeed relevant. The general principle is zooming in the text. A good reason for having different markers for each grain of text is to express context and style constraints. The filled slots convey an idea of the best level of resolution for a given text: it may be the text body or the section. A collection is thus parsed according to filled slots and returns a number of classes representing the most reliable stylistic resolution level (because marked).

When taking a section into consideration, features best characterizing that granularity level are checked. Example 3 illustrates how discourse markers are used. Generic rhetorical features that can be found in a section are marked in bold: they indicate voice, mood or stance, such as indirect question, concession or impersonal statement. In the example below, impersonal statement + passive voice (grey) is detected at the beginning and end of a section (boxed paragraphs). The passive impersonal pattern is related to a section topic (section title, highlighted).

Coherence Check and Propagation Rules

Once the resolution level is labelled, here section, parsing is conducted at the next level with relaxed constraints. Local coherence is checked at paragraph level. For the first paragraph, the topical head (*cancer risks in mutation carriers*) is related to marked judgements highlighted as local conclusion. A second distant judgement is highlighted as complementary topic, though it is not marked at paragraph level (there is no discourse connector). Both paragraphs can be successfully related because they are located at beginning and end of the section.

Looking at a finer grain, inside the sentence, the distant paragraphs in grey share a similar chain (*be kept in mind*). As a conclusion, the

Figure 2. Segments at various granularity levels and remarkable positions in a document

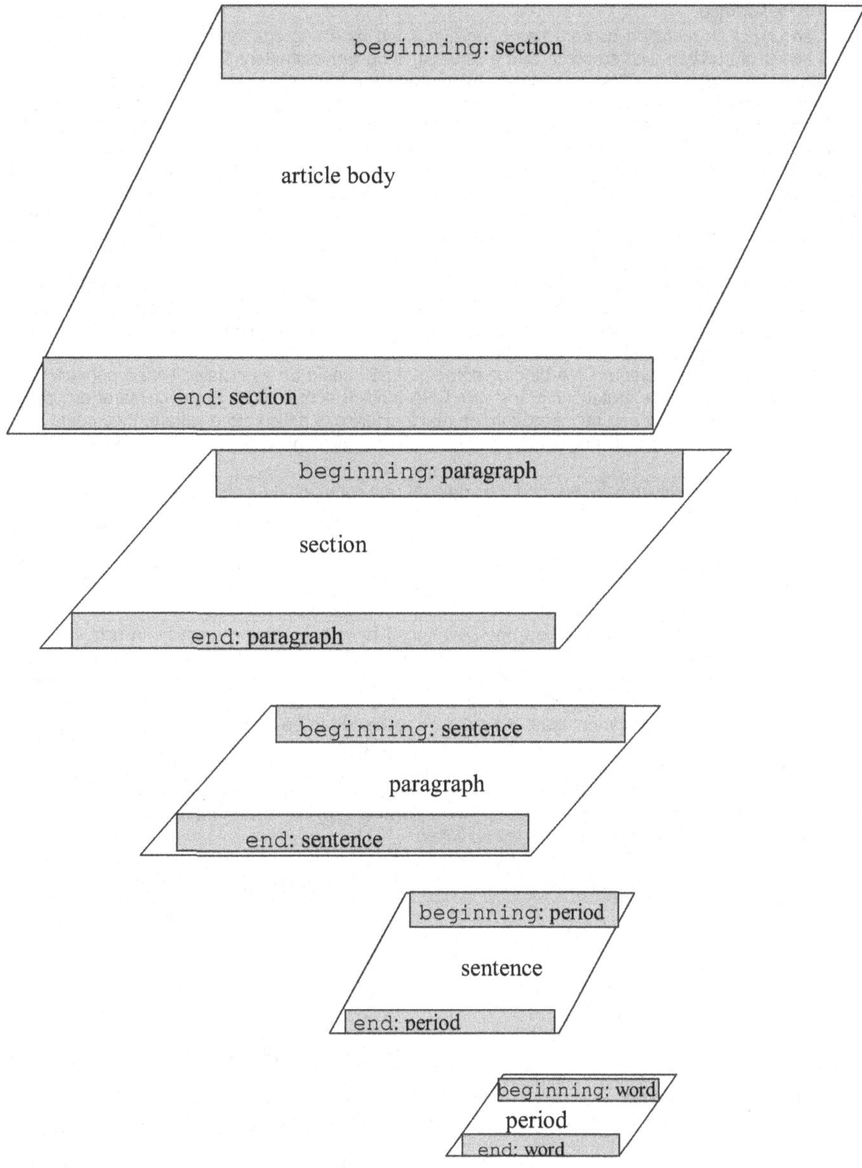

entire content of this section is deemed relevant for a query related with the major topic or the section title.

Parsing is elaborate. That is why it is not done at all times for every single text or every query-text pair, unless the task is information extraction on a small collection. Accordingly, discourse coherence is checked on a subset of a large collection, containing specific query keywords and screened according to text type.

Example 3. Section tagging

10. Penetrance

Cancer risk in mutation carriers has been evaluated by a segregation analysis in a hospital-based series of children with sarcoma and estimated to be approximately 50% by 40 years of age and 90% by 60 years of age. The age-specific penetrance was higher in women than in men because of the occurrence of breast cancer [14]. In another hospital-based series and using a method that takes into account the ascertainment bias, the risk was estimated to be about 15% before the age of 15, 41% in males and 84% in females at the age of 45. Lifetime risk was estimated to be 73% in males and nearly 100% in females, the difference almost entirely explained by breast cancer [30]. **It should** be kept in mind **that** individuals with LFS are also at very high risk of developing secondary cancers, especially if the first tumor occurred in childhood [80]. **It could** be firmly stated **that** penetrance is high, but incomplete particularly in males.

However, cancer incidence among family members of children with ADCC did not seem to be very high, suggesting that the inherited mutation represents a low-penetrance p53 allele which contributes in a tissue-specific manner to the development of ADCC in childhood [34,81]. Paradoxically, most of the LFS families displaying an ADCC carried a germline p53 mutation with a wide spectrum of mutations [27,29,35,56,63,66,82].

Mutations outside the core DNA-binding domain of p53 could be associated with a penetrance lower than that of missense mutations in the core DNA-binding domain [73]. Some cases of *de novo* mutations have been described and although the real incidence is difficult to evaluate, they could be not so rare [30,83,84]. This is not unexpected considering the high risk of death in childhood of mutation carriers.

One case of mosaïcism was reported [85]; **it must** be kept in mind for genetic counseling.

Example 4. Paragraph tagging

Cancer risk in mutation carriers has been evaluated by a segregation analysis in a hospital-based series of children with sarcoma and estimated to be approximately 50% by 40 years of age and 90% by 60 years of age. The age-specific penetrance was higher in women than in men because of the occurrence of breast cancer [14]. In another hospital-based series and using a method that takes into account the ascertainment bias, the risk was estimated to be about 15% before the age of 15, 41% in males and 84% in females at the age of 45. Lifetime risk was estimated to be 73% in males and nearly 100% in females, the difference almost entirely explained by breast cancer [30]. It should be kept in mind that individuals with LFS are also at very high risk of developing secondary cancers, especially if the first tumor occurred in childhood [80]. It could be firmly stated that penetrance is high, but incomplete particularly in males.

[...]

One case of mosaïcism was reported [85]; it must be kept in mind for genetic counseling.

Text Representation and Characterisation Algorithm

Unlike previous studies, the semantic value gained by manual annotation is not used, but rhetorical grammatical knowledge based on relations instead.

In our approach, knowledge on academic writing is used to avoid common pitfalls and to provide better characterisation of texts. The text characterisation task is performed by machine learning algorithms, called solvers as they gain in sophistication (Crémilleux *et al.*, 2008). It takes place before classification proper (in a dotted box in Figure 3). Characterisation output is also used to build collection filters to set apart those texts needing more elaborate annotation or parsing. In some cases, it also informs extraction templates hand-crafting for very specific tasks. Thus, text characterisation is an indirect way to access meaningful contents for users. Last, it allows machine learning bootstrapping and adaptation to varying corpora without costly manual annotations (Grishman *et al.*, 2002; Yangarber & Jokipii, 2005).

Texts are considered as items in a text collection. The document retrieval task is the first step in text mining. A collection is a library subset obtained by a query, typically using Entrez PubMed advanced search, following principles of sieving very large libraries by a keyword search. Filtering that collection to keep a relevant subset of documents is an intermediate step before information extraction. It often amounts to selecting the collection of texts in terms of text type or sub-genre, depending on the objective. Texts differ according to the kind of audience they target, so this task is also related to users profile.

In this new approach, text is described both sequentially and "vertically" at different grains altogether, from sentence or paragraph to text body in an attempt to show light on discourse (the whole article). Unlike the dominant trend, we do not suppose text is a tree of sentences or clauses. Different text descriptors are used at each level (multi-scale hierarchical descriptors), and their combination allows different queries.

Corpus

Different text collections were used for the experiments. The texts were always academic articles in English. The collections were fairly recent biomedicine articles retrieved from PubMed Central. One collection was covering a large number of disciplines from social sciences to chemistry and medicine, and one included older articles from 1970 on, which introduced the quality problem of digitalised documents with poor optical character recognition.

Collections varied according to document format, from text files (.doc) to HTML and PDF. Collections also varied in size, from small (36) to large (1038) as will be explained.

Pre-processing, i.e. text annotation, requires either shallow or elaborate discourse parsing, depending on the extent of the collection and the sophistication of the ultimate task. At the collection screening level, shallow descriptors are used e.g. to classify articles according to subgenre, e.g. reviews, research articles, clinical report etc. More elaborate descriptors are used for specific purposes e.g. to check correctness, select argumentative articles and extract main arguments or to track opinion on a specific topic.

From Discourse Markers to Text Descriptors

Best results in evaluation consistently show that taking due account of location of pieces of information within text has beneficial effects. Order plays an important role in sentence and in paragraph structure. We advocate this is true for any text unit, sentence, paragraph, section or text body. This means that position is represented as seen in Figure 2. The core of the method is providing representations at various text levels and using them all at a time to extract "transversal" information as well as sequential patterns for each level.

Variable Scale to Represent Context

Multi-scale descriptors were designed to reflect text hierarchy. The idea is the following: a single text is best represented by features describing a whole range of observation windows, or put in different terms, a text is described at different granularity levels. This is dubbed criss-crossing texts. This approach departs from intuitive representations of text. On a map, different items are represented, depending on scale, thus it is only natural that only large cities will be spotted on a map of Europe when single houses will be drawn on a detailed hiker's map. Human perception is limited to a representation at a time. Most researchers take it for granted that only one detailed representation at a very fine grain suffices for machine text processing.

On the contrary, machine learning allows heterogeneous data contributing to a more abstract representation of text. Although the term text hierarchy is used, it refers to the layout and does not imply that text is viewed in a strict inclusive perspective. It is both unpractical and useless to keep the same features to describe a text at various granularity levels. However, each level is not fully independent from the others. Redundancy is used as well.

The main reason why descriptors were explicitly linked with granularity level is because discourse markers have different functions and scopes in a given text. But it is also obvious that pre-processing by annotation on a very large collection of texts can be costly if it has to be carried at word or sentence level. Useful information on texts can be obtained at a fairly high granularity level.

Different observation windows were defined for a single document, proceeding from higher to lower: article, text-body, sections, sub-sections, paragraphs, sentences, "comma-units". The latter refers to punctuated sub-segments of sentences and is also called period by some authors. The windows depend on the actual layout of the document, while descriptors reflect organisation of text at a given text grammar level. Each grain has its own set of descriptors with some overlapping to accommodate for the difference between physical layout and logical macro-syntactic text structure (Lucas *et al.*, 2003, Lucas & Crémilleux, 2004).

Consequently, the first task is tokenisation in a number of different "tokens" (in the statistics meaning). To avoid confusion, because tokens in NLP are usually only words, they are called text "measures" and a text is described by a set of tables representing those measures.

Surface Hints and Co-Location Clues

To characterize texts, collective style descriptors are used. Collective style refers to the academic genre in English, in the life sciences for the corpus discussed here. Stable forms in medical literature are expressed as words, phrases or linguistic features such as tense or mood (caught through regular expression patterns). They are called surface hints or morphological bootstraps, because they are expected at remarkable positions. Surface hints include so-called "empty words" which are in a nearly finite list, called stop list by most authors who remove them because they have no lexical content. Discourse markers on the other hand, have rhetorical value for the linguist because they help establishing relations of varying scope: they are remarkable forms in macro-syntax (though of no semantic value for the biologist).

To exemplify scope in text elaboration, let's consider an example. Connectors for coordination are a small set, the most common is "*and*" inside a sentence. This word can also be used to connect sentences. But it is very seldom used to connect paragraphs. "*Additionally*" is a better choice in this case. In the same way tense, voice or mood have different scopes. Tense is used in research related with anaphora or topic segmentation, because it marks relatively small spans of text (Webber, 1988).

Discourse markers are most salient when they signal shifts between passages of texts at various levels. A difficult point in syntax in general and text grammar as well, is the fact that most relations are unseen because collocation and order are sufficient in morphologically poor languages like English. Another difficult point is that marks are very small compared to the marked segment. Most words do not have remarkable grammatical prefixes or suffixes at all: it is a basic principle in perception, well described in linguistics, that most forms in a selection are unmarked. By comparison with micro-syntax, when words have morphological marks, these are very small and usually scattered in the selection, thus delimiting a scope. We use that notion as well for higher levels of hierarchy in text. The principle of proportionality applies. The larger the scope is, the larger the selection. The surface form is also more extended, though it is still smaller than the marked segment. It is important to separate out the surface hints from the slots they may fill. Only *related* remarkable forms filling remarkable positions are used as discourse markers. Examples 5 and 6 show two measures, a paragraph and a section. The beginning and end slots are compared to prefix and

Figure 3. Machine-learning characterisation/adaptation step in the text mining loop

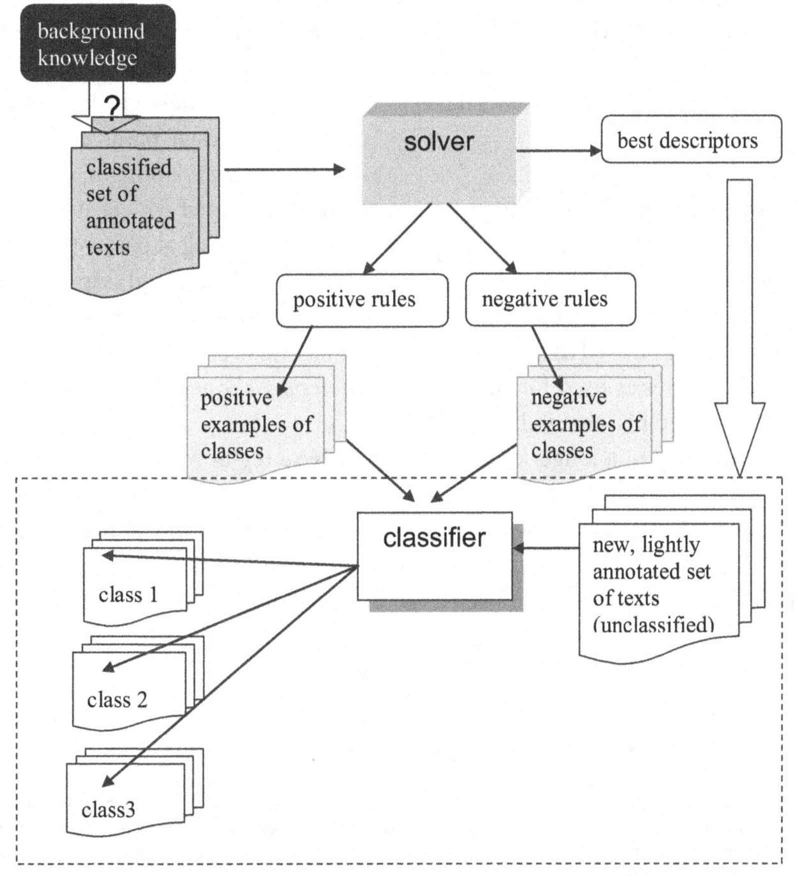

suffix for the selection. Marks found in the slots are in bold face.

This example shows that each level has its own marks. What is not visible is the theoretical frame by virtue of which marks are in correspondence. Text macro-syntax is a rather abstract matter and only the tip of the iceberg can be shown here. Suffice it to say what is at stake is relations, rather than forms *per se*.

What matters most is not the exact description of each section, in each article, but rather to capture meaningful differences between comparable sections and ultimately differences between types of articles. It is very easy to grasp the difference between an article that provides a synthesis *in the introduction*, and an article where the introduction ends with the announcement of the organization of the paper. To illustrate this contrast, example 7 shows a standard introduction for an expository article. Marks are distributed differently.

Descriptors

Descriptors are used in machine processing, so they are not the entire set of the linguist's hints but translations, some would say distorted, of what a human being is trained to see. In fact, they are nearer text linguistic features than self-explanatory markers. Yet, they are not pure features because they will be handled out of context as mere character strings + slot. A text collection is then seen as a multidimensional space meshed by a network of slots, some of which will remain empty, and some of which will be filled by character-strings of interest. The following points have to be kept in mind.

Reliability of Morphological Descriptors

Character strings used as morphological descriptors must be discriminative or reliable. The pronoun *I* for example cannot be used as a descriptor because it is the same letter as used for "one" in roman numeration *I*. Either this mark is discarded, either it has to be included in a longer character string, such as *I believe*.

It is important to note that the labels might retain some of the linguist's intent, but the character strings are simply character strings, and used as such. Consider for instance the voice in English. What is important in discourse parsing is the shift in voice (diathesis). Since it is not realistic to fully parse all texts in a collection, discourse-wise, only probes will be made on sections for strongly marked passive forms. The character string *is/are ... ed/ought ... by* (with some more variants deleted for clarity) captures something strongly hinting at passive voice, in a sentence or comma-unit slot, and skips eligible passive forms such as "*it has been presumed*" that brings too many false positives, such as "*it has many modified parasitophorous vacuoles*".

Adequacy of Morphological Descriptors

Descriptors vary with the aim of applications and with the type of mining performed. It is important to know if high frequency is requested, or if ex-

Example 5. Paragraph selection, prefix and suffix sentences

> *Toxoplasma gondii* **is** an obligate intracellular parasite capable of infecting and surviving in a wide range of nucleated cells [1]. [...]. **It is** not know**n** **what** happens to these structures, although it has been presumed that they are broken down and reabsorbed during the final stages of the budding process.

Example 6. PMID: 11880042 Section selection, prefix and suffix paragraphs

> 1. Introduction
>
> *Toxoplasma gondii* **is an** obligate intracellular parasite capable of infecting and surviving in a wide range of nucleated cells **[1]**. The invasive tachyzoite rapidly enters a host cell and become**s** established in a highly modified parasitophorous vacuole [2, 3]. Once established, the parasite replicate**s** by an unusual internal budding process **whereby** two new daughter cells are formed within each mother cell [4]. **While** much of the cytoplasm and organelles of the mother cell are incorporated into the two daughters, other parts (the apical complex and associated secretory organelles as well as parts of the subpellicular cytoskeleton) disappear. It is **not** known **what** happens to these structures, **although** it has been presumed that they are broken down and reabsorbed during the final stages of the budding process.
>
> [...]
>
> **In the present study, we have** examine**d** the biological and ultrastructural effects of cysteine and serine protease inhibitors on the intracellular development of *Toxoplasma* tachyzoites. **While** several protease inhibitors block**ed** parasite development, most caus**ed** only minor alterations to parasite morphology irrespective of the effects on the host cells. **However,** cathepsin inhibitor III, TPCK and subtilisin inhibitor III, caus**ed** extensive swelling of the secretory pathway of the parasite leading to the breakdown of the parasite surface membrane and the disruption of secretory organelle formation. Nothing resembling lysosomal bodies **was** seen in any treated parasites, consistent with the absence of a well-defined autophagic-lysosomal pathway in the parasite. **Nevertheless,** the question of **how** the parasite recycles these organelles remains unanswer**ed**.

ceptional features can be taken into consideration. This will be discussed in the next section.

Distribution of Morphological Descriptors

Statistical distribution has to be considered. Very frequent items, such as short grammatical words, have a shorter linguistic scope than less frequent grammatical phrases or patterns. This abides to the Zipf's law (1939). That is why search spaces are tested separately.

Example 8 shows an example of the character strings that will capture some features that are useful to characterize measures in a text.

Most probably, the text annotated with descriptors will look like a pointillist painting seen at a very short distance.

TEXTUAL DATA MINING EXPERIMENTS

Three experiments are reported. For the sake of clarity, text categorisation in sub genre, a generic and shallow task, is introduced first (predefined descriptors irrespective of specific lexical content). More specific tasks are introduced later (variable descriptors): text style characterisation of scientific English and argumentation screening. The steps of text processing informed by context are detailed for each task.

Text Categorisation in Sub-Genre

Sub-genre refers to biomedical articles categories such as review, research article, clinical report or editorial. The review label is one of the metadata that is most useful for on-line search, but some journals do not provide this distinction, and manual indexing has to be done. Automated characterisation of articles is therefore needed for bibliographic reasons, but also and ultimately to adapt search to the user's needs. Clinical reports for instance are valued by practitioners but discarded by system biologists. Sophisticated tasks such as detecting new trends or annotating protein-to-protein interactions suppose that the collection of retrieved articles is sieved to retain only relevant documents using the type of article, retaining research papers and excluding clinics.

Experiment Outline

An experiment was conducted to characterise texts distributed in three classes, reviews, research articles and clinical reports (Zerida *et al.*, 2006, 2007). Figure 4 shows the general overview, for a task aimed at finding the best descriptors for the classes.

Corpus

Texts were retrieved on a specific query related to cancer and genomics from PubMed Central.

Example 7. PMID: 17222789 Section selection, prefix and suffix paragraph

Background

The SYMBIOmatics Specific Support Action (SSA) **is a** European funded project. The main goal is to identify synergies between the bioinformatics (BI) and medical informatics (MI) research domains. **In addition** to experts that are approached through a survey, input will also be gathered from the analysis of scientific literature. **In this paper**, **we** focus on the analysis of scientific literature.

[...]

The rest of the document is organized as follows. The "Result" section reports on identified and shared topics between both domains and in the "Discussion" section **we** interpret the findings and discuss shortcomings of **our** approach. In the "Method" section **we** describe the generation of the corpus and the extraction of bigrams.

Example 8. PMID: 11880042 Descriptors for higher levels of text

Paragraph selection: prefix and suffix sentences

Toxoplasma gondii **is** an obligate intracellular parasite capable of infecting and surviving in a wide range of nucleated cells [1]. [...]. **It is** not known what happens to these structures, although it has been presumed that they are broken down and reabsorbed during the final stages of the budding process.

Section selection: prefix and suffix paragraphs

1. Introduction

Toxoplasma gondii **is an** obligate intracellular parasite capable of infecting and surviving in a wide range of nucleated cells [1]. The invasive tachyzoite rapidly enters a host cell and becomes established in a highly modified parasitophorous vacuole [2, 3]. Once established, the parasite replicates by an unusual internal budding process **whereby** two new daughter cells are formed within each mother cell [4]. **While** much of the cytoplasm and organelles of the mother cell are incorporated into the two daughters, other parts (the apical complex and associated secretory organelles **as well as** parts of the subpellicular cytoskeleton) disappear. It **is not** know**n what** happens to these structures, **although** it **has been** presum**ed** that they are broken down and reabsorbed during the final stages of the budding process.

[...]

In the present study, we have examined the biological and ultrastructural effects of cysteine and serine protease inhibitors on the intracellular development of *Toxoplasma* tachyzoites. **While** several protease inhibitors blocked parasite development, most caused only minor alterations to parasite morphology irrespective of the effects on the host cells. **However,** cathepsin inhibitor III, TPCK and subtilisin inhibitor III, caused extensive swelling of the secretory pathway of the parasite leading to the breakdown of the parasite surface membrane and the disruption of secretory organelle formation. Nothing resembling lysosomal bodies was seen in any treated parasites, consistent with the absence of a well-defined autophagic-lysosomal pathway in the parasite. **Nevertheless,** the question of how the parasite recycles these organelles remains unanswered.

Body selection: prefix and suffix sections

1. Introduction

[...] Once established, the parasite replicates by an unusual internal budding process **whereby** two new daughter cells are formed within each mother cell [4]. While much of the cytoplasm and organelles of the mother cell are incorporated into the two daughters, other parts (the apical complex and associated secretory organelles **as well as** parts of the subpellicular cytoskeleton) disappear. It **is not** known **what** happens to these structures, although it has been presumed that they are broken down and reabsorbed during the final stages of the budding process.

[...]

In the **present** study, **we have** examined the biological and ultrastructural effects of cysteine and serine protease inhibitors on the intracellular development of *Toxoplasma* tachyzoites. [...] Nevertheless, the question of how the parasite recycles these organelles remains unanswered.

4. Discussion

[...] The failure of some of these inhibitors to block parasite development and/or to induce changes in parasite morphology **may** indicate that such proteases are either absent or not essential to parasite survival, or that the inhibitors were unable to access the site(s) of proteolysis in the intracellular parasites.

[...] To this end **our** data add to accumulating evidence **suggest**ing that parasite proteases are a promising target for chemotherapeutic intervention.

[...] **It was** particularly **interesting** that treatment with cathepsin inhibitor III, an inhibitor of cathepsins B and L which, in eukaryotic cells, are localized to, and characteristic of, the lysosomal system, did not induce anything resembling a lysosome.

[...] At present **we know** little about the enzymes involved in the processing of secretory proteins in *Toxoplasma* or any apicomplexans.

[...] While **we cannot** exclude totally non-specific host cell effects, for some inhibitors the severity of drug-induced damage in the parasites did not correlate with changes in the host cells.

[...] While the **present results** are consistent with observations showing that the mother cell organelles are not recycled by any form of bulk autophagic or lysosomal degradation, they leave the question of how the parasite recycles these organelles unanswered.

Figure 4. General overview of text annotation and machine learning

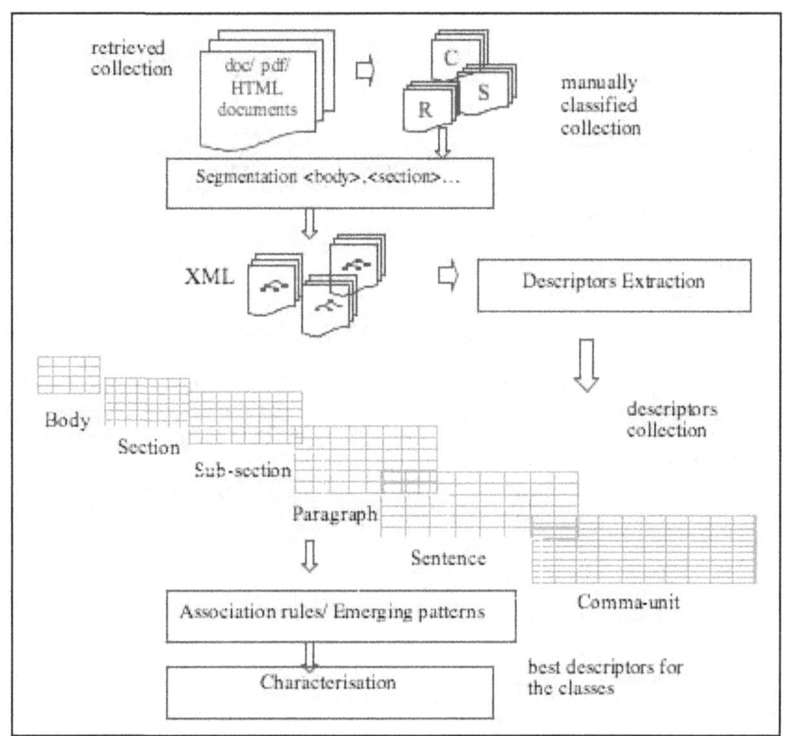

Most of them were in PDF format and for practical reasons only HTML documents were kept, which resulted in a small sample corpus of 47 articles. These articles were manually distributed in three classes, reviews, research articles and clinical reports.

Text Descriptors

The principle of multi-scale mining was used, with six text measures: text-body, section, subsection, paragraph, sentence, comma-unit (Fig. 5). Text grammar descriptors were coined to capture the relation between low-level descriptors and high-level descriptors (Figure 3). They were tagged at beginning and end of each measure and were called stylistic descriptors because they reflect collective style in sub-genres.

Apart from these descriptors, plan (main sections titles) and metrics on length of measures were tested. The bag of word approach was used as a baseline (Zerida *et al.*, 2006).

Results

The emerging patterns method was used to learn text type characterisation. A pattern X is an association of descriptors and a strong pattern is discriminative, with good contrast for a class against the others expressed by the growth rate (≥ 2). Lexical descriptors in the bag of words approach are uniformly distributed among the three classes, as expected. The contrasts expressed by the growth rate are weak. This family of descriptors alone does not discriminate the three classes.

Metric descriptors characterise only the reviews by a positive rule. One strong pattern is found, stating that X2= {number of sections > 5} supposes that the article is a review. Plan descriptors also provide a strong pattern X3= {Discussion,

Figure 5. Examples of stylistic descriptors as related to text level

<table>
<tr><th>Level</th><th>Descriptors</th></tr>
<tr><td><text body></td><td>Temporal : now, present, past, future, ever, current, often. Superpersonal : we, us, our, think, thought, believ(e|ed), sugges(t|ted), that, to, is, are, as Mode : can, may, should, would</td></tr>
<tr><td><main section></td><td>Index : citation call or figure call Epistemic: think, thought, believ(e|ed), sugges(t|ted) Voice : is, was, were, are, ed NegationList: do not, not, no FutureList: will, would PastList : was, were, had, might, could Aspect : do, has, -ed Determinants : These, This, Those, That, The, A, An Connectors : Moreover, Thus, Therefore, Indeed, in fact, -ly AnaphoraLink : This, These, Those, That, The, Thus Conjunctions : Because, If, However, Whether, Although, how, for this reason, though, as, as well as, as well, due to,</td></tr>
<tr><td><subsection></td><td>Conjunctions: why, because, if, how for this reason, although, though, as well, due to, however, while, when, which, where Perspective: even, they, it is, one, most, some, all, a number, several, few, first, second, third, its, their, such, only, other, otherwise, same</td></tr>
<tr><td><paragraph></td><td>Prepositions: In, At, For, From, to, with, by, of, by contrast, among, within AdverbPersp: inside, outside, though, after, before, meanwhile, while, despite, Indeed, in fact, in spite of Sing/plural : one, most, some, all, a number, several, few, first, second, third, fourth, fifth, it, they Negation : do not, no Determinants:this, that, the,a, an Coordination : and, but, also, or, instead, moreover Punctuation : ... ; : , Adverbs: generally, particularly, specifically, clearly, obviously , interestingly, accordingly</td></tr>
<tr><td><sentence></td><td>Coordination : and, but Reflexive : sel(f|ves)</td></tr>
<tr><td><comma-unit></td><td>Past : -ed, -ould, -ought Gerund: -ing Adverbs : -ly “s Form”: -s Determinants : the, a, an DemonstAnaph : this, these, those, that, there, thus, therefore, there is, there are, the other</td></tr>
</table>

Footnotes} {Abstract, Introduction, Material and Methods}. It characterises research articles very well and clinical articles to a lesser extent. On the other hand, this pattern is always absent in reviews, which means that when this pattern is found, the assumption that the article is a review is false. The characterisation of review articles is negative, expressing the fact that review papers do not follow the IMRAD disposition.

Text grammar (stylistic) descriptors are effective. The pattern X4 at the body level excludes the clinical papers, where X4 = {MOD_Fin, SUPPERS_Fin} indicating there is no speculation nor “hedging” in the last section of clinical papers. Some more patterns at the section and the sub-section levels discriminate in turn reviews and research articles, mostly by exclusion rules. Ultimately, each article falls in only one class.

This experiment shows that high-level descriptors are sufficient for attributing a class to articles: it is not useful to annotate paragraphs or sentences. This experiment also shows that our method based on plan and multi-scale stylistic descriptors often discriminates better the three classes of articles by *negative* characterisation, i.e., a pattern type X => NOT(class *i*).

Learning Scientific English

Scientific English has a variety of flavours related to the native language of writers. A comparison on scientific English relying on vocabulary alone was conducted for biomedical articles (Netzel *et al.*, 2003).

Experiment Outline

Scientific publishers tend to allow some variations in writing, provided readability is not impaired, in a pragmatic balance between high linguistic standards and correction costs. The experiment presented here started from this trade-off situation (Lucas *et al.*, 2003). The objective was to reduce costs by automatically highlighting erroneous passages in scientific papers. The corpus that was used to explore this question was a small set of manuscripts, after revision by the editorial board, and that same set hand corrected by the publisher's staff before print. It covered many disciplines, including biomedicine.

Unfortunately, very few pairs of articles were available to start with: only 18. It was not realistic to state on correctness and build a classifier on such a limited sample. Variability between correctors was high. Corrected articles presented many different types of grammatical or style errors, for instance lack of connector, misplacement of comma, adverb misplacement. Many corrected sentences looked correct if checked out of context, but modifications did improve clarity.

Nevertheless, this small sample was used to test what could be learnt from the bootstrapping sets. Therefore we hypothesised that unmodified articles or very lightly corrected articles would provide some clues on what is deemed legible scientific style in English. The idea was to learn some properties belonging to higher-level measures of texts that would be reflected as well in sentence construction. The subtask defined for machine learning was to characterise well-written articles versus badly written articles, relying on manual corrections to discriminate unmodified (0 correction) versus corrected articles (see details on the algorithms and parameters in Lucas *et al.*, 2003, Lucas & Crémilleux, 2004).

Descriptors

Text segments descriptors were defined for five observation windows from sections to comma-units where corrections could be detected by alignment and edition distance methods. The 36 texts were tokenised into 728 sections, 3 520 paragraphs, 10 643 sentences and 22 041 comma-units. These text measures were tagged with segment descriptors combining markers i.e. character strings detected by regular expressions and information on position (beginning, middle, end). A special segment descriptor described repetition of the same textual mark at the beginning and end of a text measure. It was called "isoperiphery" and signalled a kind of wrapping e.g. at the beginning and end of a paragraph there is a sentence marked by the word *is*.

Frequent items should not have more importance than less frequent items with a larger scope. An inheritance principle was designed to reflect higher-level descriptors that help or impair reading at a lower level. A sentence is thus defined by its sentence descriptors but also by its encapsulating paragraph descriptors and its section descriptors representing contextual information. This process applied to measures in a given text, tend to give weight to higher-level and scarcer text markers. Presence of related descriptors was computed one measure at a time by the frequent associations method and by the emerging patterns method. To that effect, thresholds have to be calculated for each measure.

Table 1. Examples of class characterisation rules concerning comma-delimited units (22,041 comma-units in the data) with contextual top-down inheritance

Characterisation rules	Class	Frequency	Confidence
P As well as S where	correct	229	1
P PASSIVE IMPERSO § ISOPERIPH S by	correct	837	0,96
P FUTURE § ISOPERIPH S THERE	correct	499	0,93
P ADV § CONJ § ISOPERIPH S semicolon	correct	295	0,89
S PARENTHESIS CU an CU the CU that	incorrect	47	0,37
S PARENTHESIS CU an CU the CU with	incorrect	36	0,37
S PARENTHESIS CU the CU for CU and	incorrect	27	0,36

Results

Results obtained by association rules showed reliability for characterising well-written articles, especially at higher levels. Rules extracted on comma-units but exhibiting a large span of inherited features do characterise well-written articles, as shown in Table 2.

The notation is somewhat difficult to read and needs to be translated, for example the first line reads "if a comma-unit belongs to a (complex) sentence including *where* and belongs to a section including a complex co-ordination *as well as*, then it is a correct segment". Line two reads "if a comma-unit belongs to a sentence showing the presence of *by*, and belongs to a paragraph characterised by isoperiphery, namely sentences containing the mark *is* at the beginning and end, and also belongs to a section characterised by the passive voice and the presence of impersonal pronouns, then it probably is a correct segment". It is particularly interesting to note that comma-units are not characterised by descriptors *sui generi* in well-written texts, but because they belong to a well-marked context. Section and subsections descriptors (noted P in the table) indicate good command of scientific English and are related with no corrections at sentence and comma-unit level. No reliable rules were found to characterise error-prone articles. This can be explained by the scarcity of corrections at higher level: human correctors do not rewrite articles in depth, e.g. by changing tense in an entire section. They seldom alter sections by fusing paragraphs together or moving them somewhere else.

The emerging patterns method, geared at discriminating classes, provided 118 valid patterns for characterising correct sections and 3 for incorrect sections, 216 patterns for correct paragraphs and 8 for incorrect paragraphs. Results obtained with strong rules (support threshold ≥ 4 and growth rate > 10) showed that in fact errors were well characterised. Errors were related with conflicting features. Mixture of retrospective and prospective in the same section, or lack of appropriate connectors, concluded on incorrect sections. Correct sections were related to homogeneous voice, homogeneity in personal versus impersonal features and to high-level connectors. Incorrect paragraphs lacked tense homogeneity while correct paragraphs were homogeneous and linked to context.

This experiment lacked a sufficient basis to overcome the variability between correctors and did not give a full picture of what a poorly written English text might be. What was learned, no withstanding, was the importance of context to decide on the value of a given discourse marker. No association rules were mined when the inheritance process was switched off. Another interesting outcome was that association rules performed well at the lowest levels, with well-populated measures, while emerging patterns were best fit to discover discriminative descriptors at high levels of text description.

Mining Argumentation

A frequently addressed question deals with argumentation. For most end-users this refers to high-level organization of text and implicitly refers to scientific requirements, such as sound grounding of conclusions, reflecting on possible biases in the experiments, referring to similar researches and so forth.

Widely different definitions of "argumentation" as expressed by NLP computer scientists are found in literature. Moreover, even in text linguistics, argumentation has various definitions. Two main schools can be found. The minimal requirement is that some sort of reflection (comparison) should be provided following exposition of facts. The maximal requirement abides to Aristotelian principles on thesis, antithesis and synthesis, with careful ponder and separation of arguments supporting the main proposal (thesis) and counter-arguments (antithesis).

Following the minimalist view, any academic paper in life sciences including biomedicine is "argumentative". The collective frame of discourse favours this disposition, contrary to computational sciences or physics following an expository frame. Following the maximal requirements, very few articles fall under the "argumentation" category. Pragmatically, users in the biomedicine field discriminate articles merely stating facts from those driven by a hypothesis and trying to demonstrate it. We report here on part of the experiment, concentrating on the linguistic characterisation.

Experiment Outline

The experiment was designed to test hypotheses and decide on a reasonable set of descriptors with maximum reliability to discriminate articles, particularly argumentative ones as set apart by human perception. After some sample tests, on section content and section titles, we wished to test the hypothesis that section titles could be sufficient to characterise a text at text-body level. A large amount of biomedicine titles are full-fledged sentences, and papers with sentential titles were prone to be judged "argumentative".

The MUSIC-DFS solver, based on emergent patterns techniques, ensures strict control on reliability. The idea is to automatically provide the best trade-off between discriminative value and a reasonable frequency of descriptors patterns (Soulet & Crémilleux, 2005; Crémilleux & Soulet, 2008).

The experiment was made on a collection of one thousand free access articles retrieved by a complex query about cancer and genomics via Entrez PubMed. Argumentation type was defined along logical and linguistic principles, as being a sequence of qualified judgements with pros and cons in an article. Other types included explanation, used in research and well structured review articles; proposals, referring to articles reporting facts put in perspective; and report typically for clinical reports or surveys of recent literature in the form of catalogues.

Articles were labelled manually for the first hundred or so, then with the help of automatic tools (grep). The distribution in classes was unbalanced, with few really argumentative articles and few purely descriptive catalogue articles. Some learning techniques are biased by too unbalanced effectives in categories. Since most articles fell into a huge middle class "proposals", it was subdivided into two (plain proposal, balanced proposal). "Balanced proposal" described a standard article putting forth a thesis with comparisons and reflection; "plain proposal" described less elaborate articles, typically when reporting an experiment with a judgement but no qualification for it.

The following examples can be produced, matching labelled articles with a corresponding list of their section and subsection titles (PMID is the reference in PubMed).

Report (hkm0512p452.pdf PMID: 16340021)

Introduction
Methods
Patient eligibility
Treatment regimen
Evaluation of response
Results
Discussion
References

Plain proposal (11631.pdf PMID: 16357174)

Introduction
Materials and Methods
Liposome preparation.
Preparation of monoclonal antibody fragments and immunoliposomes.
Pharmakokinetic studies.
Biodistribution studies.
In vivo uptake studies.
Tumor xenograft models.
Statistical analysis.
Results
Construction of immunoliposomal drugs targeted to EGFR.
Pharmacokinetics of anti–EGFR immunoliposome-doxorubicin.

Biodistribution of anti–EGFR immunoliposomes versus nontargeted liposomes.
Internalization of anti–EGFR immunoliposomes in xenografted tumor cells in vivo.
Efficacy of anti–EGFR immunoliposomal doxorubicin in EGFR–overexpressing tumor xenograft models.
Efficacy of anti–EGFR immunoliposome-epirubicin in an EGFR/EGFRvIII–overexpressing tumor xenograft model.
Efficacy of anti–EGFR immunoliposomes containing alternative chemotherapy drugs.
Discussion
Acknowledgments
References

Balanced proposal (476.pdf PMID: 12600941)

Results
Constitutive PDGF expression induces down-regulation of p190
Expression of p190 results in process extension
Role of p190 in glioma formation
Proviral insertion in p190RhoGAP
Discussion
Role of the p190 GAP domain
Oligodendrocyte differentiation and glioma formation—molecular similarities
Cross-talk between Rho and PDGF
Tumor suppressors on 19q and 1p
Implications for therapy
Materials and methods
Cell culture
Immunoprecipitation and immunoblotting
Constructs, transfections, and fluorescence microscopy
BRDU detection
RCAS vector construction
Infection of primary brain cultures
In vivo infection of tv-a transgenic mice
Tumor analysis
Tumor induction by MMLV/PDGF-B and genomic DNA preparation
Inverse polymerase chain reaction (IPCR)
Cloning and sequencing of IPCR fragments
Sequence analysis
Acknowledgments
References

Explanation (pnas-0509014102.pdf PMID: 16301525)

Materials and Methods
Cell Culture.
Western Blots.
Southern Analysis.
RNA Isolation and Microarray Analysis.
Patient Samples.
Matching of Human and Mouse Probes, Preprocessing, and Normalization.
NMF Dimension Reduction and Projection.
Gene Set Enrichment Analysis (GSEA).
Biplot.
Software.
Results
The Gene Expression Profile of Murine RTs Is Highly Related to That of Human RTs.
Snf5 Loss Leads to Transcriptional Activation.
A Subset of the MEF Snf5 Gene Sets Are Differentially Expressed in Human RT.
Inactivation of Snf5 Leads to Activation of E2F Targets but Decreased Growth of MEFs Due to Apoptosis, Growth Arrest, and Polyploidy.
Inactivation of p53 Synergizes with Snf5 Inactivation in Oncogenic Transformation.
Discussion
Validating Human Cancer Models.
Transcriptional Regulation by Snf5.

Stimulation of Cell Cycle Progression and Synergy with p53 Loss.

Argumentation (3675.pdf PMID: 9851974)

Results
Construction of Ntv-a transgenic mice
Development and characterization of a vector, RCAS–EGFR*, for expression of a mutant constitutively active EGF receptor
EGFR* gene transfer in vivo
Features of gliomas are induced by EGFR* gene transfer in INK4a –ARF-deficient mice
EGFR*-induced gliomagenesis requires disruption of cell-cycle arrest pathways and occurs more frequently after infection of Ntv-a than Gtv-a mice
bFGF gene transfer does not enhance EGFR*-induced glioma formation
CDK4 overexpression can cooperate with EGFR* and is required for EGFR*-induced gliomagenesis in p53+/– mice
Discussion
Infection of tv-a transgenic mice with RCAS vectors as a method for modeling human cancer
Gliomagenesis requires multiple mutations
Materials and methods
Constructs
Mice
Cell culture
Infection in cell culture
Immunoprecipitation, Western blot analysis, and immunoperoxidase staining of cultured cells
Infection of transgenic mice
Brain sectioning and immuno- and histochemical staining
Acknowledgments
Note added in proof
References

Collection Retrieval and Preprocessing

An advanced PubMed query on "glioblastoma, medulloblastoma, prostate cancer" returned 1427 free access articles (approximately 10% of the entire collection of relevant articles). The query returned documents in different formats, mainly html and pdf. They were all converted to XML using freeware tools, including a prototype to improve the pdf2xml extractor (Déjean & Giguet, 2008).

Pruning of this collection was done manually. We excluded: duplicate articles (same title and contents with different doc id), protected documents, and some irrelevant articles returned by keywords but not related to the intent (e.g. editorials, interviews with patients or epistemology papers). The pruned collection contained 1038 articles. Titles and subtitles were extracted with manual verification. They were grouped for each article between separators and lined (one title per line). The titles hierarchy was flattened subsequently by automatic processing. They were tagged with three sets of descriptors using a Python script for each.

Descriptors

79 linguistic features were selected to describe target strings, section and subsection titles. Target sentences are meaningful for the human eye and marked by negation versus assertion, and or marked by qualification (*is* + attribute). Since deep syntactic analysis at sentence level is not used, descriptors are much coarser. Yet, they are not ambiguous and since they are used in conjunction, they are reliable.

Descriptors were elaborated according to three viewpoints: lexical, grammatical and rhetoric. We make a distinction between "direct" descriptors, simply extracting words or expressions from titles; and "indirect" descriptors, obtained by patterns greps. The three sets were tested separately and all together.

- Lexical set. This set contains 36 direct descriptors that can be organized in categories somewhat similar to the headers in TREC Genomics.
    1. Words expressing changes and quantification of phenomena, such as *decrease, enhance.* Such clues have been used in previous studies related to cancer and genomics, (Feldman *et al.*, 2003).
    2. Words related to biological phenomena (*apoptosis, proliferation*);
    3. Words related to biological supports (*cell, tissue*);
    4. Words related to organisms (*mice*);
    5. Words related to techniques (*immunoblotting, cytometry, resection*).

    Example: *The G6PT inhibitor chlorogenic acid reduces proMMP-2 secretion in U-87 glioma cells*
    Chlorogenic acid inhibits G6PT-mediated U-87 glioma cell migration
- Grammatical set. This set contains 29 descriptors either direct or indirect. "Direct" refers to words or word-suffixes; "indirect" refers to descriptors capturing short patterns found in titles, such as attributive constructions, causal links. Tags are obtained after shallow parsing with regular expressions inside the line unit. To ensure reliability of forms without sentence parsing, only marked verbal forms were kept to express causal relations (*enhances, reduces,... causing*)
    Example: *The G6PT inhibitor chlorogenic acid reduces proMMP-2 secretion in U-87 glioma cells*
    Chlorogenic acid inhibits G6PT-mediated U-87 glioma cell migration
- Rhetorical set. This set contains 14 indirect descriptors obtained through patterns with large scope capturing relationships between titles including distant ones in the same article. Tags are obtained after shallow parsing with regular expressions in all lines for an article.

In the example below (doi:10.1186/1475-2867-6-7) a relation is detected between a comparative title and verbal titles (highlighted).

Background
Results
U-87 glioma cells express the highest levels of G6PT transcript among brain tumor-derived cell lines
The G6PT inhibitor chlorogenic acid reduces proMMP-2 secretion in U-87 glioma cells
Chlorogenic acid inhibits G6PT-mediated U-87 glioma cell migration
Chlorogenic acid inhibits sphingosine-1-phosphateinduced U-87 glioma cells migration
Chlorogenic acid inhibits sphingosine-1-phosphateinduced ERK phosphorylation in U-87 glioma cells
Intracellular ATP-depleting agents inhibit proMMP-2 secretion and antagonize S1P-induced ERK phosphorylation in U-87 glioma cells
Discussion
Methods
Materials
Cell culture and cDNA transfection method
Total RNA isolation and reverse transcriptase-polymerase chain reaction (RT-PCR) analysis
Gelatin zymography
Immunoblotting procedures
Cell migration assay
Statistical data analysis
Abbreviations
Acknowledgements
References

Six classes were set, the five positive listed above: report, plain proposal, balanced proposal, explanation, argumentation, plus one for non descript articles (irrelevant articles left over or difficult to read and class). The distribution was as follows.

report: 406; plain proposal: 343; balanced proposal: 40; explanation: 143; argumentation: 81; non descript: 27.

Results

The objective was to find which descriptors, or which combination of descriptors was best suited for the task of categorising biomedical articles according to the selected classes. The MUSIC-DFS solver produced very few patterns (i. e. subsets of descriptors). They were extracted as achieving the most reliable sorting of documents into one of the six classes. Rules use inclusion and exclusion to ensure the best discrimination of descriptors sets. Although the Argumentation class was small it was very well characterised by positive rules. The Report class is logically concluded upon by negative rules (if descriptors are not found, then the article is simply descriptive).

Combination of lexical and grammatical descriptors with positive and negatives rules give the best results. They suffice to discriminate the extreme classes on the ladder, respectively "Argumentation" and "Report", from the median group. They also conclude on the "Explanation" class. Most patterns were obtained with a single descriptor, sometimes two.

The most useful lexical descriptors to conclude on the "Argumentation" class are verbs (possibly adjectives) indicating change (*inhibit, reduce, promote*) and the best grammatical descriptors combine nouns derived from verbs (like *reduction, phosphorylation*) with comparative adjectives (*higher, lesser, more*). Grammatical descriptors concluding on the Explanation class are modal auxiliaries and relative clauses.

The "Plain proposal" class was on the contrary poorly defined by lexical or grammatical descriptors. Rhetorical and lexical rules are needed to discriminate plain proposal from balanced proposal. Since this distinction was created for technical reasons rather than motivated by obvious differences, it can be discarded. In this case, only grammatical and lexical descriptors are needed and the tagging process is extremely light.

The following excerpts from rules illustrate some of the strongest rules concluding on a class using lexical and grammatical descriptors only (support > 9% growth rate > 5, where support define representative rules and growth rate confidence in discrimination).

- An article with a negative verb or adversative adverb in a title falls in the argumentative class
- An article with no verb in titles falls in the descriptive class
- An article with no lexical change or cause mark falls in the descriptive class
- An article with no negative verb and with modal verb in title falls in the explanation class
- An article with lexical change or cause mark falls in the balanced proposal class
- An article with coordination and grammatical cause mark falls in the balanced proposal class
- An article with no biological and no change lexical marks falls in the non descript class

Rules do not express absolute truth but reflects tendencies in the corpus, both in style and vocabulary. Thus a negative rule associating *mice* and *increase* effectively excludes out of scope articles.

This trial showed that tagged section and subsection titles were effectively discriminating between classes for a reputedly difficult characterisation task. Some restrictions should be mentioned. Quality of parsing was not evaluated. Upon close investigation, older articles with poor character recognition quality caused some loss of information. Intrinsic evaluation of descriptors is not reported here. The fact is the lexical descriptors were (too) generic. Experiments are to be conducted with various descriptors sets, including highly user specific ones, to gain comparison advantage. It is also worth checking to which extent title extraction reduces the collection processing cost over full-text processing.

This experiment concluded on the discriminative value of section titles alone to categorise recent articles. Coarse though the descriptors were, they achieved the goal of sieving a collection. Very shallow parsing restricted to section titles provides qualitative information, i.e. clearly characterising argumentative articles and explanatory ones, the most interesting classes for our users.

FUTURE TRENDS

While experiments presented above concluded on the soundness of using few discriminative descriptors for higher-levels of text rhetorical organisation, a full-scale procedure for large collections has to be designed. Sieving expresses the relationship between users' need and the relevant text collection. Classifiers are needed to routinely sieve very large collections of texts obtained through lexical queries according to some text type (the bottom part of Figure 1).

We are currently exploring mining techniques best fit to convey meaningful relationships, in two directions. One direction is the blending of highly specialised lexicon with text stylistic properties, to overcome the reformulation bias: it is well known that some important notions are expressed in more than one word or phrase form in a text, all the more so in a collection. Since grammatical words and rhetorical phrases are repeated at key positions in a text, they could be used to hook interesting sequences. The second direction is to take full advantage of the geometrical representation of text to spot *where* important information is liable to be found in a document, without describing *what* precise form that information may take. This opens new ways for summarization.

Evaluation is a crucial problem as expressed by many researchers (Baumgartner *et al.*, 2008). In intrinsic evaluations, systems are evaluated independently or compared between them, irrespective of usage "for example, against a gold standard data set with named entities that are tagged by human annotators, judging the system on its ability to replicate the human annotations." (Caporaso *et al.*, 2008). The gold standard used in such evaluations is unique and might be completely out of reach for reproduction of tests at a later stage. The semantic gap is obvious. Extrinsic evaluations on the contrary try to measure usefulness of a system in real life. Evaluation is often expressed in terms of satisfaction, efficiency (time saved on a task), etc. Conditions for reproducing the tests at a later stage are also unstable.

It is probably too early to decide on which evaluation practices are relevant, since most researches are still evolving very quickly. Practical use often is serendipitous rather than calculated, some experiments get high recognition for a very short time, while others are repeated and gain value over time.

CONCLUSION AND PERSPECTIVES

We have advocated a shift of paradigm in text processing in the text mining field. This shift displaces attention from words to structure markers at higher level in text. While higher level text measures can still be handled as horizontally sliding windows on text, we stressed the usefulness of considering the logical vertical hierarchy between high and low levels of analysis in text. In many ways, other more subtle shifts have been made. From quantitative to qualitative and from heavily annotated to lightly annotated texts.

Text descriptors need not be homogeneous, and they need not be self-sufficient words. Tags obtained by checking relations, if only co-occurrence of some informative character strings in a definite window, are very useful. Context-sensitive descriptors at various scales are more effective for user oriented mining tasks. The core of the method is "criss-crossing" texts thus providing representations at various levels and using them all at a time to extract "transversal" information as well as sequential patterns for each measure.

A drawback of the approach introduced here is that multi-level text processing needs more care than in classical procedures. It is efficient when validated through powerful mining tools such as flexible constraints mining algorithms or "solvers". The descriptors choice and the set tuning for a task require expert knowledge on text and discourse. It should be kept in mind that variation parameters such as collective style, production period of the mined texts, tolerance to typing or grammatical errors in the corpus all play a role in text mining. In general, robust coverage on a heterogeneous corpus is achieved at the expense of precision.

The main advantage of the advocated method is qualitative value in results linked with low processing cost. Selection of relevant documents from a large collection can be achieved with very few descriptors with high discriminative value. A finer grain analysis can then be conducted on a smaller collection, a small subset of relevant sections, then on a small number of segments containing the precise information a group of users deems important.

As in other information retrieval tasks, the challenge in text-based knowledge retrieval lies in reducing the gap between computer scientists and users. Further research is needed on users' behaviour, but also on a variety of facets. Spyropoulos & Karkaletsis (2005) set the following objectives, still in order today:

- the scaling of existing research techniques to large size collections of documents;
- the use of more advanced techniques from the fields of natural language processing, machine learning, image processing, ontologies, as well as their effective combination in terms of the specific medical application;
- the handling of several languages;
- the development of techniques that can be easily adapted to new medical sub-domains;
- the provision of personalized access to information.

Scale problems call for effort to find the proper *resolution* for large or small collections of documents. This should be achieved through the proper balance between mining techniques, corpora and their automatic annotation at higher order text level.

Practitioners call for image processing and we advocate using titles, figure and table captions, along with image coarse processing, to enhance text information retrieval. Responding to practitioners' needs also calls for cross-lingual text linguistics, a very important domain we are keen to explore.

For computational linguists, many more challenges are offered. The objective in bio-NLP at large and in text mining in particular is to offer multiple views to users, including patients and their family, a growing concern as seen in recent conferences. Another exciting prospect is to use citation sequences available in most journals and on the Pub Med Central site (Ritchie *et al.*, 2007). This allows to characterize *shared interests* in the medical community, provided articles can be described as items of a set sharing some similarity expressing concern, against articles on the same topic but not cited.

Next, the above-mentioned research avenues need to be related together. There is growing concern to conduct research on ways to assess goal and search strategy for different groups of users. Collections filtering techniques including language, register and style, would efficiently reduce the size of retrieved collections. The long-term objective would be to make entirely transparent the process of translating the users' current concern into technical options bearing on constraints or on descriptors. This opens very exciting prospects for future research.

REFERENCES

Abdalla, R., & Teufel, S. (2006). A bootstrapping approach to unsupervised detection of cue phrase variants. In *21st international Conference on Computational Linguistics Coling06* (pp.921-928). Morriston, N.J.: Association for Computational Linguistics. doi: http://dx.doi.org/10.3115/1220175.1220291

Argamon, S., Whitelaw, C., Chase, P. J., Hota, S. R., Garg, N., & Levitan, S. (2007). Stylistic text classification using functional lexical features. *Journal of American Society for Information Science & Technology (JASIST), 58*(6), 802-822. doi: doi.org/10.1002/asi.20553

Ananiadou, S., Kell, D. B., & Tsujii, J. (2006). Text mining and its potential applications in systems biology. *Trends in Biotechnology, 24*(12), 571-579. doi:10.1016/j.tibtech.2006.10.002

Baumgartner, W. A. J., Bretonnel Cohen, K., & Hunter, L. (2008). An open-source framework for large-scale, flexible evaluation of biomedical text mining systems. *Journal of Biomedical Discovery and Collaboration, 3*(1). doi:10.1186/1747-5333-3-1

Biomedical Literature Mining Publication (BLIMP) website URL: http://blimp.cs.queensu.ca

Buchanan, B. G., & Shortliffe, E. H. (1984). Rule-based expert systems: The MYCIN experiments of the Stanford heuristic programming project. *Technical report from the Stanford Center for Biomedical Informatics Research.* (Electronic book) American Association for Artificial Intelligence http://www.aaaipress.org/Classic/Buchanan/buchanan.html.

Caporaso, G. J., Deshpande, N., Fink, L. J., Bourne, P. E., Bretonnel Cohen, K., & Hunter, L. (2008). Intrinsic evaluation of text mining tools may not predict performance on realistic tasks. In *Pacific Symposium on Biocomputing, 13*, 640-651). PMID: 18229722 Retrieved from http://psb.stanford.edu/psb-online/proceedings/psb08/

Crémilleux, B., Soulet, A., Klema, J., Hébert, C., & Gandrillon, O. (in press). Discovering Knowledge from Local Patterns in SAGE data. In P. Berka, J. Rauch, & D. A. Zighed, (Eds.), *Data Mining and Medical Knowledge Management: Cases and Applications.* Hershey, PA: IGI Global publications to appear 2008.

Crémilleux, B., & Soulet, A. (2008). Discovering Knowledge from Local Patterns with Global Constraints. In O. Gervasi, *et al.* (Eds) *8th International Conference on Computational Science and Applications ICCSA'08,* (pp. 1242-1257). Springer, LNCS 5073.

Datta, R., Joshi, D., Li, J., & Wang, J. Z. (2008). Image retrieval: Ideas, influences, and trends of the new age. *ACM Computing Surveys, 40*(2), 5, 1-60. doi: http://doi. acm.org/10.1145/1348246.1348248

De Beaugrande, R. A. (1991). *Linguistic theory: The discourse of fundamental works.* London, New York: Longman. [electronic book http://www.beaugrande.com]

de Bruijn, B., & Martin, J. (2002). Getting to the (c)ore of knowledge: Mining biomedical literature. *International Journal of Medical Informatics, 67*, 7-18. PII: S1386-5056(02)0005 0-3

Déjean & Giguet (2008) pdf2xml URL: http://sourceforge.net/projects/pdf2xml

del Lungo, G., & Tognini Bonelli, E. (Eds.). (2006). *Evaluation in academic discourse.* Amsterdam, Herdon: John Benjamins.

Ding, J., Berleant, D., Nettleton, D, & Wurtele, E. (2002). Mining MEDLINE: Abstracts, Sentences, or Phrases? In *Pacific Symposium on Biocomputing PSB 2002* (pp. 326-337). Retrieved from http://helix-web.stanford.edu/psb02/ding.pdf

Feldman, R., Regev, Y., Hurvitz, E., & Finkelstein-Landau, M. (2003). Mining the biomedical literature using semantic analysis and natural language processing techniques. *Biosilico, 1(2),* 69-80. PII: S1478-5282(03)02314-6

Fleischman, S. (2003). Language and medicine. In D. Schiffrin, D. Tannen & H. Hamilton (Eds.), *The Handbook of Discourse Analysis.* Oxford: Blackwell, 470-502.

Fløttum, K., & Rastier, F. (Eds.) (2002). *Academic discourse, multidisciplinary approaches.* Oslo: Novus forlag.

Fløttum, K. (Ed.) (2007). *Language and Discipline Perspectives on Academic Discourse.* Newcastle: Cambridge Scholars Publication.

Fluck, J., Zimmermann, M., Kurapkat, G., & Hofmann, M. (2005). Information extraction technologies for the life science industry. *Drug Discovery Today, 2(3),* 217-224. doi: 10.1016/j.ddtec.2005.08.013

Friedman C., Kra P., Rzhetsky A. (2002). Two biomedical sublanguages: a description based on the theories of Zellig Harris. *Journal of Biomedical Informatics 35(4),* 222-235. doi: 10.1016/j.ddtec.2005.08.013

Grishman R., Huttunen S., Yangarber R. (2002). Information Extraction for Enhanced Access to Disease Outbreak Reports. *Journal of Biomedical Informatics 35 (4),* 236-246. doi:10.1016/S1532-0464(03)00013-3

Hakenberg, J., Rutsch, J., & Leser, U. (2005). Tuning text classification for hereditary diseases with section weighting. In *First International Symposium on Semantic Mining in Biomedicine (SMBM)* (34-37). Retrieved June 2008 from http://www.informatik.hu-berlin.de/forschung/gebiete/wbi/research/publications

Halliday, M.A.K. (1994). *An introduction to functional grammar.* London: Edward Arnold.

Harris, Z. (1982). *A grammar of English on mathematical principles.* New York: Wiley.

Harris, Z., Gottfried, M., Ryckman, T., Mattick, P., Daladier, A., Harris, T. N., *et al.* (1989). *The form of information in science: Analysis of an immunology sublanguage.* Dordrecht: Kluwer Academic.

Harris, Z. (2002). The structure of science information. *Journal of Biomedical Informatics 35(4),* 215-221. doi: 10.1016/S1532-0464(03)00011-X

Hirschman, L., Yeh, A. Blaschke C, & Valencia A. (2005). "Overview of BioCreAtIvE: critical assessment of information extraction for biology" *BMC Bioinformatics* (6 S1). doi:10.1186/1471-2105-6-S1-S1

Hockett, C. F. (1958). *A course in modern linguistics.* New York: MacMillan.

Holmes, J. H., & Peek, N. (2007). Intelligent data analysis in biomedicine. *Journal of Biomedical Informatics, 40(6),* 605-609. doi:10.1016/j.jbi.2007.10.001

Hunter, L., & Bretonnel Cohen, K. (2006). Biomedical language processing: What's beyond Pubmed? *Molecular Cell* (21), 589-594. doi:10.1016/j.molcel.2006.02.012

Hyland, K. (2005). *Metadiscourse.* London, New York: Continuum Publishing Group.

Jelier, R., Schuemie, M., Eijk, C. V. E., Weeber, M., Mulligen, E. V., Schijvenaars, B., *et al.* (2003). Searching for geneRIFs: Concept-based query expansion and Bayes classification. TREC 2003 work notes.

Kando, N. (1992). *Structure of research articles.* (SIG Notes 92-FI-25). Tokyo: Information Processing Society Japan.

Kando, N. (1999). Text structure analysis as a tool to make retrieved documents usable. In *4th International Workshop on Information Retrieval with Asian Languages*, Taipei, Taiwan. Retrieved May 2008 from http://research.nii.ac.jp/~kando/

Krallinger M., & Valencia, A. (2005) Text-mining and information-retrieval services for molecular biology. *Genome Biology* 2005, 6:224. doi:10.1186/gb-2005-6-7-224

Leroy, G., Eryilmaz, E., & Laroya, B. T. (2006). Health information text characteristics. In *AMIA 2006 Symposium* (pp. 479–483). American Medical Informatics Association.

Lisacek, F., Chichester, C., Kaplan, A.. & Sandor, A. (2005). Discovering Paradigm Shift Patterns in Biomedical Abstracts: Application to Neurodegenerative Diseases. In *First International Symposium on Semantic Mining in Biomedicine (SMBM)*, Hinxton, UK.

Lovis, C. (1998). Trends and pitfalls with nomenclatures and classifications in medicine. *International Journal of Medical Informatics* (52), 141-148. PII S1386-5056(98)00133-6

Lucas N., Crémilleux B., Turmel L. (2003) Signalling well-written academic articles in an English corpus by text mining techniques. In Archer D., Rayson P., Wilson A., McEnery T. (Eds) *Corpus Linguistics*. (pp. 465-474). Lancaster: University Centre for Corpus Research on Language, Lancaster University.

Lucas N., Crémilleux B. (2004) Fouille de textes hiérarchisée, appliquée à la détection de fautes. *Document numérique* 8 (3), 107-133.

Mizuta, Y., Korhonen, A., Mullen, T., & Collier, N. (2006). Zone analysis in biology articles as a basis for information extraction. *International Journal of Medical Informatics* (75), 468-487. doi:10.1016/j.ijmedinf.2005.06.013

National Library of Medicine Entrez PubMed website url : http://www.ncbi.nlm.nih.gov/entrez/query.fcgi?DB=pubmed

Netzel, R., Perez-Iratxeta, C., Bork P., & Andrade, M. A. (2003). The way we write. Country-specific variations of the English language in the biomedical literature. *EMBO reports* 4 (5), 446-451. doi:10.1038/sj.embor.embor833

Nwogu, K. N. (1997). "The medical research paper: structure and functions" *English for Specific Purposes* 16 (2), 119-138.

Parsons, G. (1990). *Cohesion and coherence: Scientific texts. A comparative study.* Nottingham, England: Department of English Studies, University of Nottingham.

Perrin, P., & Petry, F. (1999). An information-theoretic based model for large-scale contextual text processing. *Information Sciences* (116), 229-252. PII: S0020-0255(98) 1 0090-7

Perrin, P., & Petry, F. (2003). Extraction and representation of contextual information for knowledge discovery in texts. *Information Sciences* (151), 125-152. doi:10.1016/S0020-0255(02)00400-0

Rebholz-Schumann, D., Kirsh, H., & Couto, F. (2005). Facts from texts — is text mining ready to deliver? *PLoS Biology*, 3(2), e65. doi: 10.1371/journal.pbio.0030065

Regev, Y., Finkelstein-Landau, M., & Feldman, R. (2003). Rule-based extraction of experimental evidence in the biomedical domain – the KDD cup 2002 (task 1). *SIGKDD explorations*, 4(2), 90-91.

Rzhetsky, A., Iossifov, I., Koike, T., Krauthammer, M., Kra, P., Morris, M., *et al.* (2004). Geneways: A system for extracting, analyzing, visualizing and integrating molecular pathway data. *Journal of Biomedical Informatics* (37), 43-53.

Ritchie, A., Robertson, S., & Teufel, S. (2007). Creating a test collection: Relevance judgements of cited and non-cited papers. Paper presented at *RIAO*, Pittsburgh, Pennsylvania, USA.

Roberts, P. M. (2006). Mining literature for systems biology. *Briefings in Bioinformatics*, 7(4), 399-406.

Rowley-Jolivet, Elizabeth (2007). "A Genre Study of *If* in Medical Discourse" In K. Fløttum (Ed.) *Language and discipline perspectives on academic discourse* (pp. 176-201). Cambridge: Cambridge Scholars.

Salager-Meyer, F. (1994). Hedges and textual communicative function in medical English written discourse. *English for Specific Purposes, 13*(2), 149-170.

Schiffrin, D., Tannen, D., & Hamilton, H. (Eds.). (2003). *The handbook of discourse analysis* (2nd ed.). Oxford: Blackwell.

Shah, P., Perez-Iratxeta, C., Bork, P., & Andrade, M. (2003). Information extraction from full text scientific articles: Where are the keywords? *BMC Bioinformatics, 4(20).* http://www.biomedcentral.com/1471-2105/4/20

Shatkay, H., & Feldman, R. (2003). Mining the biomedical literature in the genomic era: an overview. *Journal of Computational Biology 10*(6), 821-855.

Shatkay, H., & Craven, M. (2007). *Biomedical text mining.* Cambridge, Massachussets, USA: MIT Press.

Schilder, Frank (2002). Robust discourse parsing via discourse markers, topicality and position *Natural Language Engineering 8*(2/3), 235-255.

Schuemie, M. J., Weeber, M., Schjivenaars, B. J. A., van Mulligen, E. M., van der Eijk, C. C., Jelier, R., et al. (2004). Distribution of information in biomedical abstracts and full-text publications. *Bioinformatics, 20*(16), 2597-2604.

Skelton, J. R. (1994). Analysis of the structure of original research papers: An aid to writing original papers for publication. *British Journal of General Practitioners* (44), 455-459.

Soulet, A., Crémilleux, B. (2005). An Efficient Framework for Mining Flexible Constraints. In T.B. Ho, D. Cheung, and H. Liu (Eds.) *PAKDD 2005* (pp. 661–671), Springer LNCS 3518.

Spyropoulos, C. D., & Karkaletsis, V. (2005). Information extraction and summarization from medical documents. *Artificial Intelligence in Medicine* (33), 107-110.

Swales, J. (1990). *Genre analysis: English in academic and research settings.* Cambridge: Cambridge University Press.

Teufel, S. (1999). *Argumentative zoning.* Doctoral dissertation, University of Edinburgh Edinburgh. Retrieved June 2008 from http://www.cl.cam.ac.uk/~sht25/az.html

Teufel, S., & Moens, M. (2002). Summarizing scientific articles: Experiments with relevance and rhetorical status. *Computational Linguistics, 28*(4), 409-445.

Vold, E. T. (2006). Epistemic modality markers in research articles. A cross-linguistic and cross-disciplinary study. *International Journal of Applied Linguistics, 16*(1), 61-87.

Webber, B. (1988). Tense as discourse anaphor. *Computational Linguistics, 14*(2), 61-72.

Wilbur, J., Rzhetsky, A., & Shatkay, H. (2006). New directions in biomedical text annotation: Definitions, guidelines and corpus construction. *BMC Bioinformatics, 7(356).* doi:10.1186/1471-2105-7-356

Wren, J. D. (2005). Open access and openly accessible: A study of scientific publications shared via the internet. *BMJ.* doi 10.1136/bmj.38422.611736.E0

Yangarber R., Jokipii L. (2005). Redundancy-based Correction of Automatically Extracted Facts. In *Human Language Technology Conference/ Conference on Empirical Methods in Natural Language Processing HLT/EMNLP-2005* (pp. 57-64) .Morriston, N.J.: Association for Computational Linguistics. doi: http://dx.doi.org/10.3115/1220575.1220583

Zerida, N., Lucas, N., & Crémilleux, B. (2006). Combining linguistic and structural descriptors for mining biomedical literature. In *ACM Symposium on Document Engineering* (pp. 62-64). New York: ACM. doi: doi.acm.org/10.1145/1284420.1284469

Zerida, N., Lucas, N., & Crémilleux, B. (2007). Exclusion-inclusion based text categorization of biomedical articles. In *ACM Symposium on Document engineering* (pp. 202-204). New York: ACM. doi: http://doi.acm.org/10.1145/1284420.1284469

Zipf, G. K. (1939). *The Psycho-biology of Language.* Boston: Houghton Mifflin.

Chapter XIII
A Neural Network Approach Implementing Non-Linear Relevance Feedback to Improve the Performance of Medical Information Retrieval Systems

Dimosthenis Kyriazis
National Technical University of Athens, Greece

Anastasios Doulamis
National Technical University of Athens, Greece

Theodora Varvarigou
National Technical University of Athens, Greece

ABSTRACT

In this chapter, a non-linear relevance feedback mechanism is proposed for increasing the performance and the reliability of information (medical content) retrieval systems. In greater detail, the user who searches for information is considered to be part of the retrieval process in an interactive framework, who evaluates the results provided by the system so that the user automatically updates its performance based on the users' feedback. In order to achieve the latter, we propose an adaptively trained neural network (NN) architecture that is able to implement the non- linear feedback. The term "adaptively" refers to the functionality of the neural network to update its weights based on the user's content selection and optimize its performance.

INTRODUCTION

The rapid progress in publishing articles and the huge amount of data being stored, accessed and transmitted in the biological and medical domain has led to the advent of applications that perform Natural Language Processing (NLP) in order to enable researchers, doctors and other actors in the aforementioned domain to search and retrieve the relevant content. In this context, the traditional approaches of searching, retrieving and organizing the medical data, using only text annotation, cannot describe the medical content with high efficiency. For this reason, several content-based retrieval mechanisms and approaches have been proposed, some of which work by extracting high level semantic features of the content.

Despite, however, the fact that semantic segmentation has attracted much attention recently, other features that describe the content such as keywords or categories are usually used for implementing content-based retrieval algorithms. To reduce the limitations emerged by using low-level descriptors and simultaneously to increase the performance of content-based algorithms, the human can be considered as a part of the retrieval process, in an interactive framework. This means that initially the user evaluates the results, provided by the system and then the system adapts its performance according to the user's demands. In this framework, a feedback is established from the user to the system based on the most relevant articles, which is usually called relevance feedback. Such an approach, apart from eliminating the gap between high-level and low-level features, it also reduces the problems related to the subjectivity of humans, which often interpret the same medical content in a different way.

To address the content interpretation and classification, new adaptive and interactive management schemes should be introduced, which are capable of updating the system response with respect to the current user's information needs and preferences. One way to achieve adaptability of the system response to the users' needs is to modify the similarity measure used for ranking data. In this way, retrieval, organization and transmission of the information are updated in accordance with the humans' perception of the content through a dynamic real time learning strategy based on the users' interaction.

One of the interactive learning techniques is *relevance feedback* (originated from text-based information retrieval systems), which adapts the response of a system according to the relevant information feedback to it so that the adjusted response is a better approximation to the user's information needs. Usually, relevant information is

Figure 1. Design of the relevance feedback mechanism for medical content retrieval systems

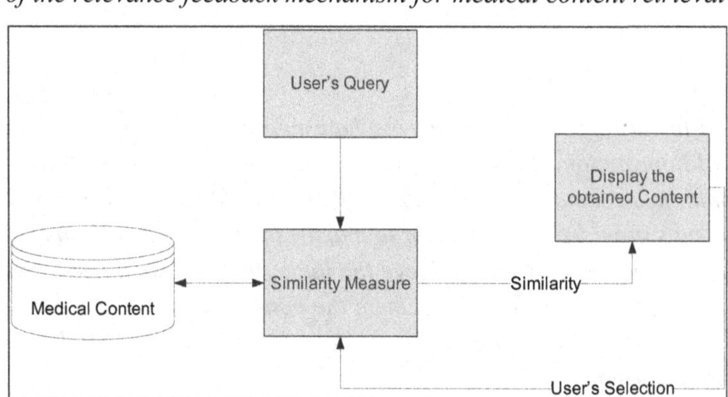

provided by the user in an *interactive framework*, who evaluates the results according to his/her demands and preferences. Relevance feedback has been widely used in text-based information retrieval systems (J. Rocchio, 1971). Although it is not restricted to description environments where similarity measures are used, in databases where similarity-based queries are applied (Y. Ishikawa, 1998), relevance feedback refers to the mechanism which updates the similarity measure with respect to the relevant/irrelevant information, as indicated by the user. Relevance feedback confronts the subjectivity of humans in perceiving medical content and also eliminates the gap between high-level semantics and low-level features, which are often used for content description and modeling (Y. Rui, 1998). The following figure (Figure 1) presents a block diagram of a relevance feedback scheme.

To perform the relevance feedback mechanism a degree of importance should be assigned to each content descriptor, i.e., a different weighed factor to each element of the feature characterizing the medical content. After the first retrieval, the user assigns a degree of appropriateness for each article, which actual indicates the similarity degree of the respective article to the query. The weights are dynamically adapted based on the users' feedback, who selects the most appropriate articles among those retrieved by the system. Furthermore, we propose an enhancement to the relevance feedback mechanism by introducing nonlinearities in the parametric distance. This is implemented by an adaptively trained neural network classifier, the weights of which are adjusted according to the users' feedback. In this case, the network weights define the degree of importance for each descriptor, while the network output indicates the similarity of the examined article to the query one. The network weights are updated each time a new users' selection takes place so that they are closer to the user's selection while simultaneously results in a minimal degradation of the previously learned data.

Concluding, our approach proposes the use of a non-linear relevance feedback mechanism in content-based retrieval systems. To implement this mechanism we use a neural network that is able to dynamically adapt its performance by taking into account both the current knowledge and the previous one. As a result, after the user's feedback, the network output, is optimized since it also takes into account the user's selection. There has to be mentioned, that the proposed relevance feedback mechanism works efficiently independently from the content, which means that it is applicable not only to textual content but to images and video as well. This mechanism can be seen as an additional layer on the retrieval algorithms in medical databases and other sources of content, which improves the overall system performance in terms of the data that are finally obtained by the user.

The remainder of this chapter is structured as follows. The background section presents related work in the field of non-linear relevance feedback as a way to improve systems' performance. The research topic and the focus of our work, is describe thereafter. We present the problem of generalized non-linear relevance feedback and we propose a recursive algorithm for updating the similarity measure to the current users' information needs and preferences. Finally, "Future Trends" section includes a discussion on future research and potentials for the current study, while the chapter is summarized in the "Conclusion" section.

BACKGROUND

As already mentioned, one of the interactive learning techniques is *relevance feedback*, which adapts the response of a system according to the relevant information feedback to it so that the adjusted response is a better approximation to the user's information needs. In this context, recently relevance feedback algorithms have been extended from text-based information retrieval to content-based image retrieval systems. The area of image retrieval is even more complex due to the nature of the content: it is much harder to characterize and make queries on images than on textual information. Given that our approach can be applied to any information retrieval system we briefly present work in this area focusing on the more complex side: the one of the image retrieval in order to show that our approach advances this specific field of research in the most "complex" case. In (I. Cox, 1996), a probabilistic framework was reported based on a Bayesian formulation scheme. In (Y. Rui, 1998), a relevance feedback algorithm is introduced using as metric the weighted Euclidean distance and a heuristic scheme is adopted to perform the weight updating. However, this approach is a heuristic method and as mentioned in the conclusions of this chapter, there is a need for an optimal learning strategy. The first approaches towards this direction have been reported in (Y. Avrithis, 1998; A. D. Doulamis, 1999; Y. Ishikawa, 1998). In particular, in (Y. Avrithis, 1998; A. D. Doulamis, 1999) the weighted Euclidean distance is used as in (Y. Rui, 1998) and the weight updating strategy is performed by minimizing the response of the Euclidean distance metric over all selected samples. Instead, in (Y. Ishikawa, 1998), the generalized Euclidean distance is adopted as similarity metric to take into account the interconnection of different feature elements with each other. Feature element interconnection is also examined in (Y. Choi, 2000). However, the works of (Y. Avrithis, 1998; A. D. Doulamis, 1999) yield unstable performance in case of negative examples, while "smooth" the system response when many positive relevant images are selected. In addition, the work of (Y. Ishikawa, 1998) involves the inversion of the covariance matrix of the selected samples. It is clear, however, that the covariance matrix is not invertible if the number of selected samples is smaller than the size of image feature vectors, which is a common case in real situations. To confront this difficulty, the authors of (Y. Ishikawa, 1998) propose a solution based on the pseudo-inverse of the covariance matrix. Although, however, in theory, such an approach eliminates the singularity problems, in practice, the retrieval performance is not so satisfactory (Y. Rui, 2000). To reduce the aforementioned difficulties, a "hierarchical model" has been proposed in (Y. Rui, 2000) for decomposing the feature vectors into vectors of smaller size. In addition, the algorithm introduces a dynamic switch for performing the weight updating so as to decrease the effect of singularity. A different approach is presented in (Xiang Sean Zhou, 2001), where the relevance feedback problem is addressed using discriminant analysis. In particular, the algorithm proposes Biased discriminant analysis to face the symmetry between positive and negative examples under small training samples, enhanced by a kernel version to facilitate non-linearities. The method non-linearly transforms the feature vector space to adapt the system response to the current users' needs and preferences. However, only the vector norm is exploited in the proposed transformation, while a constant similarity measure is assumed, i.e., the Euclidean distance.

Other relevance feedback algorithms use the cross-correlation measure for similarity. Cross-correlation is a normalized measure, which expresses how similar/dissimilar two feature vectors are. A correlation-based relevance feedback scheme has been reported in (N. Doulamis, 2001), while a recursive learning strategy has been presented in (N. Doulamis, 2001; N. Doulamis 2001) to address the case of multiple feedback iterations. In these methods, the weights (model parameters) express the degree of relevance of the query feature vector to the vector of the selected samples. Again, the aforementioned approaches consider a constant type of similarity measure, e.g., the correlation criterion, regulating only the importance of extracted descriptors to the similarity metric, instead of the similarity type itself.

On the contrary, in this chapter, the problem of relevance feedback is addressed *in the most generic form* by optimally updating the similarity measure type to the current users' information needs and preferences. In this case, instead of adjusting the degree of importance of each descriptor, the similarity measure itself is estimated through an on-line efficient and recursive learning strategy. Therefore, no restrictions on the type of the similarity are imposed, in contrast to the aforementioned approaches, where only a specific type of similarity measure is considered, such as the Euclidean distance (Y. Avrithis, 1998 - Y. Rui, 2000) or the Cross-Correlation criterion (N. Doulamis, 2001 - N. Doulamis 2001). Initially, the similarity measure is assumed to be of any non-linear function type. In the following, the similarity is modeled as a non-linear parametric relation of known functional components (E. Kreyszig, 1989; G. Cybenko, 1989) using concepts derived from functional analysis. More specifically, it has been shown that any non-linear continuous function can be approximated with any degree of accuracy by considering functional components of non-constant, bounded and monotone increasing squashing functions. The contribution of each component to the similarity measure is estimated based on a set of selected relevant / irrelevant samples interactively provided by the user to express the current information needs. As a result, at each feedback iteration, the type of similarity measure is estimated resulting in a *generalized non-linear relevance feedback scheme.*

The contribution of each functional component to the similarity measure is *recursively* estimated through an efficient on-line learning strategy. In particular, the adaptation is performed so that a) the current selected content as expressed by a set of relevant/irrelevant samples is trusted as much as possible, while simultaneously b) a minimal modification of the already estimated similarity measure is encountered. For the satisfaction of the aforementioned conditions, a small modification of the model coefficients is assumed to be sufficient. Then, the first condition is simplified by applying a first order Taylor series expansion to the functional components, which results in a set of linear constraints of the current selected relevant/irrelevant samples. For the second condition, the sensitivity of the error between the system response and the actual degree of relevance, as provided by the user over an indicative learning set, is used. The algorithm results in a constraint minimization problem for the estimation of the coefficients of the functional components and therefore of the type of similarity measure, which approximates as much as possible the current users' information needs and preferences.

IMPROVING THE PERFORMANCE OF MEDICAL INFORMATION RETRIEVAL SYSTEMS

Based on the above, in this section we will briefly present the proposed architectural approach that includes an Artificial Neural Network (ANN) and the relevance feedback mechanism, the combination of which improves the performance of any medical information retrieval system. In general, an ANN is an information processing paradigm that is inspired by the way biological nervous systems, such as the brain, process information. The key element of this paradigm is the novel structure of the information processing system. It is composed of a large number of highly interconnected processing elements (neurones) working in unison to solve specific problems. ANNs, like people, learn by example.

Following the proposed architecture, we will describe the focus of our work which is the ANN's functions and the modeling of the similarity measures through the ANN in order to enable the latter to adjust its weights based on the feedback provided by the user.

Proposed Architectural Approach

The core component of the proposed architectural approach is an Artificial Neural Network used to model the similarity measure of a query for ranking the retrieved data. The aforementioned ANN is adaptable - meaning that the weight factors in its functions are adapted based on the relevance assigned by the user over all selected data. The selected data are the outcome of any content retrieval mechanism in a database / source with medical information. The information regarding the relevance of the results to the user's query is parsed into the ANN from the implemented relevance feedback mechanism as presented in the following figure (Figure 2).

The process is initiated by the content retrieval system each time a user searches for medical content. Based on his / her search, the content retrieval system replies by providing a set of results. Afterwards these results are evaluated by the user who provides feedback on them to the ANN. The ANN "learns" from this process and updates the weights of its functions in order to provide better results in the next iteration. The key point in this process is how the weights are updated based on the user's feedback.

In the following paragraphs we will present an innovative approach that allows the weights update of the ANN's functions in order to include the user's feedback and improve the performance of content retrieval systems in future queries.

Similarity Measures

Regarding the ANN, one way to achieve adaptability of the system response to the users' needs is to modify the *similarity measure* used for ranking data. In this way, retrieval, organization and transmission of the information is updated in accordance with the humans' perception of the content through a dynamic real time learning strategy based on the users' interaction.

Let us assume in the following a *query by example* type of operation for content-based retrieval. This means that the user provides queries in the form of requests for content, which are analyzed similarly to the samples of the database. Thus, for each query by example, a feature vector is constructed to describe the query content. In the following, a similarity measure is applied to find a set of data that best match the query content. The most commonly used similarity measure for data retrieval is the Euclidean distance, where in its generalized form is defined as (*Generalized Euclidean Distance*) (Y. Ishikawa, 1998; Y. Rui, 2000)

$$d(\mathbf{f}_q,\mathbf{f}_i) = (\mathbf{f}_q - \mathbf{f}_i)^T \cdot \mathbf{W} \cdot (\mathbf{f}_q - \mathbf{f}_i) \quad (1)$$

Figure 2. Architectural approach

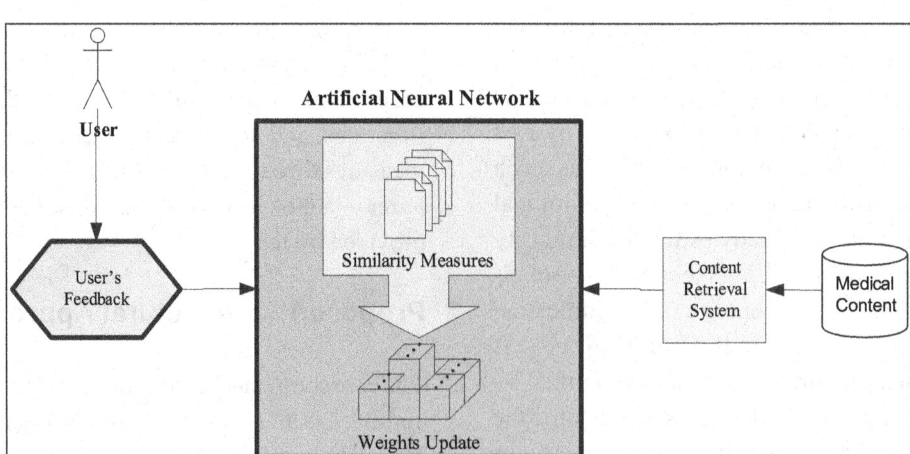

In equation (1), vector $\mathbf{f}_q$ refers to the feature vector of the query, while $\mathbf{f}_i$ to the feature vector of the ith sample in the database. Vectors $\mathbf{f}_q$ and $\mathbf{f}_i$ are estimated as described previously. The $\mathbf{W}$ is a real symmetric matrix, which contains the weights that regulate the degree of importance of the feature elements to the similarity measure. In case that no interconnection among different feature elements is permitted, matrix $\mathbf{W}$ becomes diagonal and the resulted similarity measure is called *Weighted Euclidean Distance*. The weighted Euclidean distance has been adopted in several relevance feedback schemes, such as the works of (Y. Rui, 1998; Y. Avrithis, 1998; A. D. Doulamis, 1999). On the contrary, in (Y. Ishikawa, 1998; Y. Rui, 2000), the generalized Euclidean distance has been involved.

Another interesting similarity measure adopted in the literature for relevance feedback is the cross-correlation criterion, which indicates how similar two feature vectors are and thus provides a measure for their content similarity (N. Doulamis, 2001- N. Doulamis, 2001). Furthermore, correlation remains unchanged with respect to feature vector scaling and translation. For example, adding or multiplying a constant value to all elements of a feature vector affects the Euclidean distance but not the correlation. One way for parametrizing the correlation-based similarity is (N. Doulamis, 2001)

$$\rho_{\mathbf{w}}(\mathbf{f}_q,\mathbf{f}_i)=\frac{\sum_{k=1}^{P} w_k \cdot f_{q,k}\cdot f_{i,k}}{\sqrt{\sum_{k=1}^{P} w_k^2 \cdot f_{q,k}^2}\cdot\sqrt{\sum_{k=1}^{P} f_{i,k}^2}} \quad (2)$$

where $f_{q,k}$ and $f_{i,k}$ are the kth element of vectors $\mathbf{f}_q$ and $\mathbf{f}_i$ respectively. The variable P in (2) indicates the size of feature vector, while parameters w_k the relevance of the kth element of the query feature vector to the selected ones. An optimal learning strategy for estimating the weights w_k has been presented in (N. Doulamis, 2001; N. Doulamis, 2001) along with a recursive weight updating scheme for multiple feedback iterations.

In many relevance feedback approaches the similarity measure used is of constant type. In these scenarios, only regulation of the weighted factors w_k is permitted, which express the degree of importance of each descriptor to the similarity measure. Instead, a more powerful and efficient approach is to implement an on-line learning strategy, which assumes *any generic non-linear similarity measure* with the capability of adapting its type to the current users' information needs and preferences. In this case, instead of regulating the importance of each descriptor to the similarity measure, at each feedback iteration, the type of similarity measure is dynamically estimated, resulting in a *generic non-linear relevance feedback scheme.* In particular, the similarity measure, say $d(\cdot)$, is modeled as a continuous function $g(\cdot)$ of the difference between the query feature vector $\mathbf{f}_q$ and the feature vector $\mathbf{f}_i$ of the ith sample in the database.

$$d(\mathbf{f}_q,\mathbf{f}_i)=g(\mathbf{f}_q-\mathbf{f}_i) \quad (3)$$

Equation (3) models any non-linear similarity measure of the query feature vector $\mathbf{f}_q$ and the ith sample in the database $\mathbf{f}_i$ so that the current user's information needs and preferences are satisfied as much as possible. The above equation is modeled through the proposed ANN.

However in equation (3), the feature vectors $\mathbf{f}_q$ and $\mathbf{f}_i$ are involved, which affect the retrieval results. It is clear that the more efficient a feature vector describes the content, the higher the retrieval performance is. In this chapter, we concentrate on the estimation of the most appropriate similarity measure $g(\cdot)$, which satisfies the user information needs and preferences as much as possible for a *given feature vector representation.*

Generalized Non-Linear Relevance Feedback

The main difficulty in implementing equation (3) is that function $g(\cdot)$ is actually unknown. For this reason, initially modeling of the unknown function $g(\cdot)$ is required in a parametric form. Modeling permits the estimation of similarity measure based on a set of relevant/irrelevant selected data.

Similarity Measure Type Modeling

Concepts derived from functional analysis are adopted in this chapter for modeling and parametrizing the unknown function $g(\cdot)$ (E. Kreyszig, 1989; G. Cybenko, 1989). Particularly, it can be proved that any continuous non-linear function can be expressed as a parametric relation of known functional components $\Phi_l(\cdot)$ within any degree of accuracy (E. Kreyszig, 1989). In this case, we have that

$$d(\mathbf{f}_q,\mathbf{f}_i)=g(\mathbf{f}_q-\mathbf{f}_i)\approx\sum_{l=1}^{L}v_l\cdot\Phi_l\left(\sum_{k=1}^{P}w_{k,l}(f_{q,k}-f_{i,k})\right) \tag{4}$$

where number L expresses the approximation order of function $g(\cdot)$. In equation (4), v_l and $w_{k,l}$ correspond to model parameters, while $\Phi_l(\cdot)$ corresponds to functional components. It is clear that the approximation precision increases, as the order L increases. Equation (4) is the equation used in the proposed ANN.

The most familiar class of functional components $\Phi_l(\cdot)$ is the sigmoid functions, which are equal to

$$\Phi_l(x)=1/(1-\exp(-a\cdot x)) \tag{5}$$

where a is a constant which regulates the curve steepness. It should be mentioned that the parameters v_l, $w_{k,l}$ of (4) *are not related* to the weighted factors (degree of importance) of the descriptors, which are used in the current relevance feedback approaches, such the ones in (Y. Rui, 1998; I. Cox, 1996 - N. Doulamis 2001). On the contrary, they express the coefficients (model parameters) on which function $g(\cdot)$ is expanded to the respective functional components.

From equation (4), it seems that $P\times L$ parameters are required to approximate any continuous similarity measure of order L. The number of parameters can be reduced by imposing constraints on v_l and $w_{k,l}$, which, however, restrict the type of similarity measure of (4). Particularly, let us assume that the same parameters are assigned to all functional components $\Phi_l(\cdot)$. This means that $w_{k,l}=w_{k,q}\ \forall l,q$ and therefore $w_{k,l}=w_k$ since they depend only on the feature vector index and not on the index of the functional components. If we further assume that the functional components are linear, we conclude that

$$d(\mathbf{f}_q,\mathbf{f}_i)=\left(\sum_{l=1}^{L}v_l\right)\cdot\sum_{k=1}^{P}w_k(f_{q,k}-f_{i,k}) \tag{6}$$

which simulates the weighted Euclidean distance with free parameters the P variables w_k. In this case, the parameters v_l *do* not affect the performance of the similarity measure since they just multiply the overall similarity.

Another interesting case results from the assumption that squared functional components $\Phi_l(\cdot)$ are considered, i.e., $\Phi_l(x)=x^2$. In this case, we have that

$$d(\mathbf{f}_q,\mathbf{f}_i)=\sum_{l=1}^{L}v_l\cdot\left(\sum_{k=1}^{P}w_k(f_{q,k}-f_{i,k})\right)^2=\left(\sum_{l=1}^{L}v_l\right)\cdot\sum_{m=1}^{P}\sum_{k=1}^{P}w_k\cdot w_m(f_{q,k}-f_{i,k})\cdot(f_{q,m}-f_{i,m}) \tag{7}$$

Other types of similarity measures are obtained by imposing constraints either on the parameters v_l and $w_{k,l}$ or on the type of the functional components $\Phi_l(\cdot)$. Imposing constraints on v_l, $w_{k,l}$ and

$\Phi_l(\cdot)$ (and thus restricting the type of similarity measure that (4) models), we reduce the number of free parameters, and therefore the relevance feedback computational complexity. However, the most generic case is derived by setting no constraints on (4), which models any continuous non-linear function. All the other types of similarity measures can be considered as special cases of the generic one. In section 4, a recursive algorithm for estimating the free parameters is proposed for the general case. The same methodology can be applied for the special cases too, taking, however, into consideration the constraints.

Similarity Measure Type Estimation

Using, equation (4), it is clear that estimation of similarity measure is equivalent to the estimation of coefficients v_l, $w_{k,l}$. In particular, let us denote as $S^{(r)}$ a set, which contains selected relevant/ irrelevant samples at the r feedback iteration of the algorithm. The set $S^{(r)}$ has the form

$$S^{(r)} = \{\cdots,(\mathbf{f}_q - \mathbf{f}_i, R_i),\cdots\} = \{\cdots,(\mathbf{e}_i, R_i),\cdots\} \tag{8}$$

where $\mathbf{f}_q$ refers to the query feature vector, $\mathbf{f}_i$ to the feature vector of the ith selected sample and R_i to the respective degree of relevance. Negative values of R_i express irrelevant content, whereas positive values of R_i relevant content. Let us denote as $v_l(r + 1)$, $w_{k,l}(r + 1)$ the model parameters at the $(r+1)$ feedback iteration. These coefficients are estimated so that, the similarity measure, after the rth feedback iteration, equals the degree of relevance assigned by the user over all selected data,

$$d^{(r+1)}(\mathbf{f}_q,\mathbf{f}_i) = g^{(r+1)}(\mathbf{f}_q - \mathbf{f}_i) = \sum_{l=1}^{L} v_l(r+1)\cdot \Phi_l\left(\sum_{k=1}^{P} w_{k,l}(r+1)\cdot(f_{q,k} - f_{i,k})\right) \approx R_i,$$

$$\text{with } i \in S^{(r)} \tag{9}$$

where $d^{(r+1)}(\cdot)$ expresses the non-linear similarity measure at the $(r+1)$th feedback iteration of the algorithm.

Usually, the number of samples of set $S^{(r)}$ at the rth feedback iteration is much smaller than the number of coefficients v_l, $w_{k,l}$ that should be estimated. For example, a typical number for the coefficients is around 640 (L=10 and P=64), whereas the number of selected samples at a given feedback iteration is usually less than 10. Therefore, equation (9) is not sufficient to uniquely identify the parameters v_l, $w_{k,l}$. To achieve uniqueness in the solution, an additional requirement is imposed, which takes into consideration the variation of the similarity measure. In particular, among all possible solutions, the one that satisfies (9) and simultaneously causes a minimal modification of the already estimated similarity measure is selected as the most appropriate.

Let us denote as S a set, which contains relevant / irrelevant samples with respect to several queries. The set S is used for the initial estimation of the similarity measure based on a least squared minimization algorithm as described in section 5. At each feedback iteration, the set S is augmented by adding new selected relevant/ irrelevant samples. In order to retain a constant size of S, for computational efficient purposes, the older samples are removed from S as new samples added. Then, the requirement of the minimal modification of the already estimated similarity measure is expressed as

$$\text{minimize } B(r) = \left\| E^{(r+1)} - E^{(r)} \right\|_2 \tag{10}$$

where

$$E^{(r)} = \frac{1}{2} \cdot \sum_{i \in S} \{g^{(r)}(\mathbf{f}_q - \mathbf{f}_i) - R_i\}^2$$

corresponds to the error of the similarity measure over all data of S at the rth feedback iteration.

As a result, the model parameters of the similarity measure are estimated by the following constraint minimization problem

$$\text{minimize } B(r) = \left\| E^{(r+1)} - E^{(r)} \right\|_2 \quad (11a)$$

subject to

$$d^{(r+1)}(\mathbf{f}_q, \mathbf{f}_i) = g^{(r+1)}(\mathbf{f}_q - \mathbf{f}_i) = \sum_{l=1}^{L} v_l(r+1) \cdot$$

$$\Phi_l\left(\sum_{k=1}^{P} w_{k,l}(r+1) \cdot (f_{q,k} - f_{i,k}) \right) \approx R_i ,$$

$$\text{with } (f_{q,k} - f_{i,k}) \in S^{(r)} \quad (11b)$$

The constraint term of equation (11b) indicates that, the proposed on-line learning strategy modifies the similarity measure so that, after the adaptation, the users' information needs are satisfied as much as possible. On the contrary, the term of (11a) expresses that the adaptation is accomplished with a minimal modification of the already estimated similarity measure.

Recursive Similarity Measure Adaptation

In this subsection, a recursive algorithm is presented to perform the constraint minimization of (11). Therefore, the scheme yields to a *Recursive Generalized Non-Linear Relevance Feedback* algorithm for information retrieval.

Let us consider that all coefficients $v_l(r)$, $w_{k,l}(r)$ are included in a vector, say $\mathbf{w}(r)$, i.e.,

$$\mathbf{w}(r) = [\cdots w_{k,l}(r) \cdots v_l(r) \cdots]^T \quad (12)$$

Vector $\mathbf{w}(r)$ is decomposed into

$$\mathbf{w}(r) = [vec\{\mathbf{W}(r)\}^T \, \mathbf{v}(r)^T]^T \quad (13)$$

where vector $\mathbf{v}(r)$ and matrix $\mathbf{W}(r)$ are related with the coefficients $v_l(r)$, $w_{k,l}(r)$ as

$$\mathbf{W}(r) = [\mathbf{w}_1(r) \cdots \mathbf{w}_L(r)] \text{ and}$$

$$\mathbf{v}(r) = [v_1(r) \cdots v_L(r)]^T \quad (14)$$

where

$$\mathbf{w}_l(r) = [w_{1,l}(r) \cdots w_{P,l}(r)]^T$$

and P the feature vector size. Operator $vec\{\cdot\}$ returns a vector formed by stacking up all columns of the respective matrix.

Let us now assume, that the model parameters at the $(r+1)$th feedback iteration, i.e., the $\mathbf{w}(r+1)$, are related to the model parameters $\mathbf{w}(r)$ at the rth iteration as

$$\mathbf{w}(r+1) = \mathbf{w}(r) + \Delta\mathbf{w} \quad (15)$$

where $\Delta\mathbf{w}$ refers to a small increment of the model coefficients. Equation (15) indicates that a small modification of the coefficients is adequate to satisfy the current user's information needs, expressed by (11b).

Adaptation to the Current Selected Relevant/Irrelevant Samples

In the following, we deal with the analysis of equation (11b), i.e., the constraint of the minimization. In particular, based on equation (15), linearization of the functional components $\Phi_l(\cdot)$ is permitted using a first order Taylor series expansion. Then, equation (11b) can be decomposed in a system of linear equations, as indicated by the following theorem

Based on the fact that the constraint expressed by equation (11b) under the assumption of (15) is decomposed to a system of linear equations of the form $\mathbf{c}(r) = \mathbf{A}(r) \cdot \Delta\mathbf{w}$, where vector $\mathbf{c}(r)$ and matrix $\mathbf{A}(r)$ depends only on the model parameters of the previous rth feedback iteration, vector $\mathbf{c}(r)$ expresses the difference between the desired degree of relevance R_i, assigned by the user, and the one provided by the system before the feedback iteration, i.e., using the parameters $\mathbf{w}(r)$.

In particular, vector $\mathbf{c}(r)$ is given as

$\mathbf{c}(r) = [...c^{(r)}(\mathbf{e}_i)...]T$, for all $\mathbf{e}_i \in S^{(r)}$ with

$$c^{(r)}(\mathbf{e}_i) = g^{(r+1)}(\mathbf{e}_i) - g^{(r)}(\mathbf{e}_i) = R_i - g^{(r)}(\mathbf{e}_i) \quad (16)$$

where $\mathbf{e}_i = \mathbf{f}_q - \mathbf{f}_i$

Furthermore, matrix $\mathbf{A}(r)$ is given as

$$\mathbf{A}^T(r) = [...\mathbf{a}^{(r)}(\mathbf{e}_i)...], \text{ for all } \mathbf{e}_i \in S^{(r)} \quad (17)$$

where the columns $\mathbf{a}^{(r)}(\mathbf{e}_i)$ are given as

$$\mathbf{a}^{(r)}(\mathbf{e}_i) = [\text{vec}\{\mathbf{e}_i \cdot (\mathbf{g}^{(r)})^T\}^T \, \mathbf{u}(r)^T]^T \quad (18)$$

where

$$\mathbf{u}(r) = \boldsymbol{\varphi}(\mathbf{W}^T(r) \cdot \mathbf{e}_i) \quad (19)$$

with $\boldsymbol{\varphi}(\cdot) = [\Phi_1(\cdot)...\Phi_L(\cdot)]^T$ a vector containing the functional components $\Phi_l(\cdot)$ [see equation (5)]. Vector $\mathbf{g}(r)$ is given as follows

$$\mathbf{g}(r) = \mathbf{D}(r) \cdot \mathbf{v}(r) \quad (20)$$

with matrix $\mathbf{D}(r)$ expresses the derivatives of the elements of vector $\mathbf{u}(r)$, i.e.,

$$\mathbf{D}(r) = diag\{\delta_1(r),...,\delta_L(r)\} \quad (21)$$

In (21) $diag\{\cdot\}$ refers to a diagonal matrix.

Since in our case the functional components $\Phi_l(\cdot)$ are the sigmoid, the

$$\delta_i(r) = u_i(r) \cdot [1 - u_i(r)] \quad (22)$$

Based on the previous equations, it can be seen that, vector $\mathbf{c}(r)$ and matrix $\mathbf{A}(r)$ are *only* related with the coefficients $v(r)$ and $w_{k,l}(r)$ of the rth feedback iteration.

Minimal Modification of the Similarity Measure

The term of equation (11a), which expresses the minimal modification of the already estimated similarity measure is decomposed under the assumption of equation (15) as follows

The effect of the small weight perturbation to the term of (11a) is provided by minimizing a squared convex function of the form

$$\frac{1}{2}\Delta\mathbf{w}^T \cdot \mathbf{J}^T(r) \cdot \mathbf{J}(r) \cdot \Delta\mathbf{w},$$

where matrix $\mathbf{J}(r)$ is the Jacobian matrix of the error

$$E_i^{(r)} = \frac{1}{2} \cdot (g^{(r)}(\mathbf{f}_q - \mathbf{f}_i) - R_i)$$

over all samples of set S.

The Jacobian matrix $\mathbf{J}(r)$ is given as

$$\mathbf{J} = \begin{bmatrix} \vdots & \vdots & \vdots & \vdots & \vdots \\ \cdots & \frac{\partial E_i}{\partial w_{k,l}} & \cdots & \frac{\partial E_i}{\partial v_l} & \cdots \\ \vdots & \vdots & \vdots & \vdots & \vdots \end{bmatrix} \quad (23)$$

with the derivatives

$$\frac{\partial E_i^{(r)}}{\partial w_{k,l}} \text{ and } \frac{\partial E_i^{(r)}}{\partial v_l}$$

being expressed by the following equations

$$\frac{\partial E_i^{(r)}}{\partial w_{k,l}} = -t_i(r) \cdot v_k(r) \cdot \delta_l(r) \cdot e_{i,l} \quad \text{and}$$

$$\frac{\partial E_i^{(r)}}{\partial v_l} = -t_i(r) \cdot u_l(r) \tag{24}$$

with $t_i(r) = (g^{(r)}(\mathbf{f}_q - \mathbf{f}_i) - R_i)$ and $e_{i,l}$ the lth element of vector $\mathbf{e}_i = \mathbf{f}_q - \mathbf{f}_i$.

Based on the above, the recursive estimation of the model parameters for each feedback iteration is accomplished by calculating the small perturbation of the model coefficients $\Delta\mathbf{w}$ through the following constraint minimization problem

$$\text{Minimize } B(r) = \frac{1}{2} \cdot \Delta\mathbf{w}^T \cdot \mathbf{J}^T(r) \cdot \mathbf{J}(r) \cdot \Delta\mathbf{w} \tag{25a}$$

$$\text{Subject to } \mathbf{c}(r) = \mathbf{A}(r) \cdot \Delta\mathbf{w} \tag{25b}$$

The main steps of the proposed generalized recursive non-linear relevance feedback scheme are the following:

1. Assume that the rth feedback iteration has been completed and the type of the similarity measure has been estimated as expressed by the parameters $\mathbf{v}(r)$ and $\mathbf{W}(r)$. Then, the model parameters for the $(r+1)$ iteration are updated with the following steps.
2. Estimate vector $\mathbf{c}(r)$ using (16) and matrix $\mathbf{A}(r)$ using (17 and 18).
3. Estimate matrix $\mathbf{J}(r)$ as in (23,24).
4. Apply the reduced gradient method for calculating the small increment of the model parameters $\Delta\mathbf{w}$ (this method is described in the following paragraphs).
5. Update model coefficients using (15) and the model parameters $\mathbf{v}(r+1)$ and $\mathbf{W}(r+1)$.
6. The new similarity measure is expressed through (4).

The Reduced Gradient Method

Equation (25a) is a convex function since it is of square form (D. J. Luenberger, 1984). Furthermore, (25b) corresponds to linear constraints. As a result, only one minimum exists, which is the global one (D. J. Luenberger, 1984). One solution for minimizing (25) is to use Lagrange multipliers. However, in this case inversion of matrices of large size is involved, which is a process both computationally and memory demanded. For this reason, in this chapter an iterative constraint minimization technique is adopted to perform the constraint minimization of (25). Among other methods, such as the gradient projection (D. J. Luenberger, 1984), the reduced gradient method has been selected due to the fact that it demands less computational complexity, especially in case of few constraints, which is valid in our case.

The reduced gradient method is an iterative process, which starts from a feasible point (solution) and moves in a direction, which decreases the error function of equation (25a), while simultaneously satisfies the constraint defined by the equation (25b). A point is called feasible if it satisfies the constraints of (25b). To commence the algorithm, an initial feasible point $\Delta\mathbf{w}(0)$ is required.

Initialization Phase

In our case, as initial feasible point, $\Delta\mathbf{w}(0)$, the minimal distance from the origins to the constraint hyper-surface $\mathbf{c}(r) - \mathbf{A}(r) \cdot \Delta\mathbf{w} = \mathbf{0}$ is used. Therefore, $\Delta\mathbf{w}(0)$ is given by minimizing the following equation

$$\text{minimize } \|\Delta\mathbf{w}\|_2 \text{ or equivalently } (\Delta\mathbf{w})^T \cdot \Delta\mathbf{w} \tag{26a}$$

$$\text{subject to } \mathbf{c}(r) - \mathbf{A}(r) \cdot \Delta\mathbf{w} = \mathbf{0} \tag{26b}$$

Minimization of the (26a) subject to (26b) is achieved using Lagrange multipliers (D. J. Luenberger, 1984). In this case, the aforementioned minimization problem is written as

$$\Delta\mathbf{w}(0) = \underset{\Delta\mathbf{w}}{\operatorname{argmin}}\Big((\Delta\mathbf{w})^T \cdot \Delta\mathbf{w} + \boldsymbol{\lambda}^T \cdot (\mathbf{c}(r) - \mathbf{A}(r) \cdot \Delta\mathbf{w})\Big) \tag{27}$$

where the elements of vector λ corresponds to the Lagrange multipliers. Differentiating equation (27) with respect $\Delta\mathbf{w}$ and λ and setting the results equal to zero, we obtain

$$\Delta\mathbf{w}(0) = \mathbf{A}^T(r) \cdot (\mathbf{A}(r) \cdot \mathbf{A}^T(r))^{-1} \cdot \mathbf{c}(r) = \mathbf{Q}(r) \cdot \mathbf{c}(r) \tag{28a}$$

$$\text{with } \mathbf{Q}(r) \equiv \mathbf{A}^T(r) \cdot (\mathbf{A}(r) \cdot \mathbf{A}^T(r))^{-1} \tag{28b}$$

It should be mentioned that matrix $\mathbf{A}(r) \cdot \mathbf{A}^T(r)$ is of size $\zeta \times \zeta$, where ζ corresponds to the number of the imposed constraints, i.e., to the number of selected relevant/irrelevant data. This number is usually small, and inversion of matrix $\mathbf{A}(r) \cdot \mathbf{A}^T(r)$ does not demand high computational complexity and memory requirements.

Iteration Phase

At the mth iteration of the algorithm, the feasible point $\Delta\mathbf{w}(m)$ is arbitrarily partitioned into two groups; the first group contains the dependent (basic) variables, while the second the independent variables. Without loss of generality, we select the first elements of vector $\Delta\mathbf{w}(m)$ as dependent variables. Therefore,

$$\Delta\mathbf{w}(m) = [\Delta\mathbf{w}^D(m)^T \;\; \Delta\mathbf{w}^I(m)^T]^T \tag{29}$$

where $\Delta\mathbf{w}^D(m)$ is a vector, which contains the dependent variables, while $\Delta\mathbf{w}^I(m)$ the independent ones.

Using the constraint $\mathbf{c}(r) = \mathbf{A}(r) \cdot \Delta\mathbf{w}$, we can express the dependent vector $\Delta\mathbf{w}^D(m)$ with respect to the independent variables $\Delta\mathbf{w}^I(m)$ as follows

$$\Delta\mathbf{w}^D(m+1) = (\mathbf{A}^D)^{-1} \cdot \Big(\mathbf{c}(r) - (\mathbf{A}^I(r))^T \cdot \Delta\mathbf{w}^I(m+1)\Big) \tag{30}$$

where $\mathbf{A}^D(r)$ is the part of matrix $\mathbf{A}(r)$ which related to the dependent variables while the $\mathbf{A}^I(r)$ to the independent ones. Thus, $\mathbf{A}(r) = [\mathbf{A}^D(r)\ \mathbf{A}^I(r)]$. Matrix $\mathbf{A}^D(r)$ is always squared with size equals to the number of constraints ζ, thus $\mathbf{A}^D(r)$ is of $\zeta \times \zeta$ elements. This means that vector $\mathbf{c}(r)$ is of size $\zeta \times 1$. On the contrary, matrix $\mathbf{A}^I(r)$ is of size $\zeta \times \{L \cdot P - \zeta)$, where $L \cdot P$ corresponds to the number of the model parameters. Thus, vector $\Delta\mathbf{w}^I(m)$ is of size $(L \cdot P - \zeta) \times 1$.

At next iterations, the independent variables are updated towards the direction of the respective gradient,

$$\Delta\mathbf{w}^I(m+1) = \Delta\mathbf{w}^I(m) - \eta(m) \cdot \mathbf{r}(m) \tag{31}$$

In equation (31), scalar $\eta(m)$ regulates the convergence rate of the weight updating, while $\mathbf{r}(m)$ refers to the reduced gradient, which is given as

$$\mathbf{r}^T(m) = \theta^T - \gamma^T \cdot (\mathbf{A}^D(r))^{-1} \cdot \mathbf{A}^I(r) \tag{32}$$

where vectors θ and γ are provided by splitting the gradient of cost function D into the dependent and independent group

$$\nabla B(r) = \mathbf{J}^T(r) \cdot \mathbf{J}(r) \cdot \Delta\mathbf{w}(m) = [\gamma^T \;\; \theta^T]^T \tag{33}$$

The main steps of the reduced gradient method, which is used in our case for estimating the new network weights, are the following:

1. Initialization Phase
   a. Estimate the initial model increment $\Delta\mathbf{w}(0)$ using equation (28)
   b. Set m=0
2. Iteration Phase
   a. Estimate the reduced gradient $\mathbf{r}(m)$ using equation (32) and (33)
   b. Update the increment of the independent variables at the (m+1) iteration using (31)
   c. Estimate the increment of the dependent variables at the (m+1) iteration using (30)
   d. If the error

      $$\left\|\Delta\mathbf{w}(m+1)-\Delta\mathbf{w}(m)\right\|_2 < T,$$

      where T a threshold then stop the iteration else Set m=m+1 and reinitiate the Iteration Phase.

Following the above analysis, it is clear that the proposed functions and the reduced gradient method allows the update on the weights of the ANN's equation (Equation (3)) in order to enable the integration of the relevance feedback (Equation (9)) as provided by the user.

EVALUATION

In this section, we briefly discuss some experimental results to evaluate the efficiency of the proposed generalized non-linear relevance feedback scheme for content-based retrieval from a database that contains medical data.

The aforementioned database was deployed in the National Technical University of Athens, enhanced by medical information obtained from the university's library. This information refers to scientific content: research papers, journals and case studies; the archives are used for conducting the presented experiments. The overall data set consists of around 15,000 data covering a wide variety of medical content. We also used a "parsing" service that searches in the database's content and annotates it in order to produce specific categories of the content (we concluded to 80 categories). As described previously in this book chapter, several data descriptors are extracted and organized - to which the proposed relevance feedback approach is applied. Each data descriptor includes segments properties that are used to describe this segment. These properties are the type of article, the keywords, the publication area, the authors and the publication date. To these segments we applied specific queries - as described in detail in the following paragraphs - to improve the performance of any retrieval system.

Objective Evaluation Criteria for the Retrieval Performance

Usually, the quantitative evaluation of a content-based retrieval system is performed through the *Precision-Recall Curve* measure.

Precision for a query *q [Pr(q)]* is defined as the ratio of the number of retrieved relevant images, say *N(q)* over the number of total retrieved articles, say *M* [36]. On the other hand, recall of a query *q [Re(q)]* is the ratio of the number of retrieved relevant articles *N(q)* over the total number of relevant articles in the database for the respective query, *G(q)* [36].

$$\Pr(q)=\frac{N(q)}{M},\quad \operatorname{Re}(q)=\frac{N(q)}{G(q)} \tag{34}$$

In a real content-based retrieval system, as the number M of articles returned to the user increases, precision decreases, while recall increases. Because of this, instead of using a single value of $\Pr(q)$ or $\operatorname{Re}(q)$, the curve Precision-Recall is adopted.

In equation (34), precision and recall have been estimated for a given query q. However, to evaluate the performance of a content-retrieval system, many queries should be applied and the average value of precision/recall should be estimated. Assuming that Q queries are submitted, the average precision/recall, APr, ARe are defined as

$$\mathrm{APr}=\frac{1}{Q}\sum_{q=1}^{Q}\Pr(q) \qquad \mathrm{ARe}=\frac{1}{Q}\sum_{q=1}^{Q}\mathrm{Re}(q) \qquad (35)$$

The following figure (Figure 3) presents the average precision-recall curve as obtained by submitted around 3,000 randomly selected queries to the database at the fifth feedback iteration. As is expected, the best precision for every recall value is achieved using the proposed generalized non-linear relevance feedback scheme. This is due to the fact that in this case the type of the similarity measure is recursively updated to fit the current

Figure 3. Relevance feedback performance of the proposed generalized non-linear scheme and the methods of [20] and [22] as expressed by the average precision-recall curve at the 5th feedback iteration.

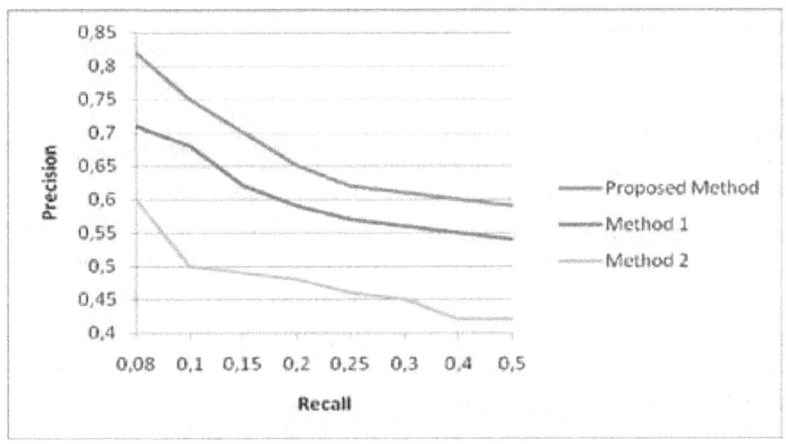

Figure 4. Precision values versus the number of feedback iterations for the investigated relevance feedback schemes and comparisons with the works of [14], [19], [20] and [22].

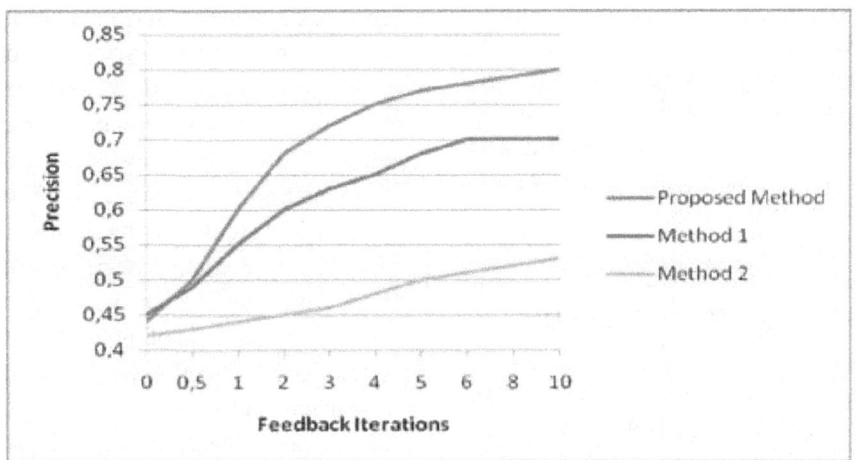

users' information needs. The second best precision performance is noticed for the correlation-based relevance feedback algorithm of Method 1 (N. Doulamis, 2001). This is mainly due to the fact that, in this case, the similarity measure is based on the correlation metric, which provides a better physical representation of the similarity content. In this figure, we have also depicted the performance of the algorithm of (Xiang Sean Zhou, 2001) - Method 2, which presents a slight worse performance compared to the correlation-based approach. It should be mentioned that for all the compared relevance feedback algorithms, the same feature vector representation was used. As a result, the highest retrieval performance obtained by the proposed non-linear relevance feedback scheme is due to the fact that the adopted similarity measure better models the user's information needs and preferences. This means that the proposed scheme estimates the non-linear relationship of the feature vectors used to describe the medical content characteristics and the actual user's information needs in perceiving the content. For this reason, better retrieval results are derived with respect to traditional approaches, where a similarity measure of constant type is used.

The precision values with respect to feedback iterations for recall 10% and 30% are shown in Figure 4 respectively for the aforementioned algorithms. The results have been evaluated on the entire database by submitting around 3,000 randomly selected queries.

In all cases, the precision increases with respect to feedback iterations, with a decreasing, however, improvement ratio, meaning that beyond a certain limit only a slight precision increase is accomplished. It can be seen that the proposed scheme outperforms the compared ones for each one of the feedback iterations.

THE SYSTEM FUTURE TRENDS

Notwithstanding, it is within our future plans to attempt to implement the NN along with the relevance feedback mechanism so as to allow the provision of the functionality that is described in this chapter as a service. As a result, this service could be used as a "filter" service to any information retrieval service providing the most relevant results to the users based on prior searches. The latter is considered of major importance since many approaches have been presented as ways to handle the information retrieval problem in biomedicine. For example, authors of (Min Hong, 2005) present a complete approach for biomedical information retrieval including classification of technical documents, continuous learning on user's interests and requests and provision of an interactive interface to navigate vast information spaces. Moreover, in (Hagit Shatkay, 2005) information retrieval problems focused in the biomedical field are discussed while literature (Y. Kagolovsky, 1998) describes information extraction from medical text resources. The outcome of these approaches can be optimized by a service that comprises both the method for the relevance feedback and the NN modeling described in this chapter.

CONCLUSION

Information retrieval in biomedicine is an important issue but due, however, to the subjective perception of humans as far as the content is concerned, adaptive management algorithms are required to update the system response to actual users' information needs and preferences. Adaptation of content management is achieved through on-line learning strategies, which modify the similarity measure used for ranking visual data.

Providing optimization capabilities to systems that deal with content retrieval - independently both from the content and from the retrieval technique, is a topic of interest in many research areas. To this direction we proposed an architecture that includes an artificial neural network and a relevance feedback scheme. The outcome of the relevance feedback scheme is encompassed into the neural network in order to allow its adaptability to the changes proposed by the user. In order to achieve the latter, the weights on the NN equation need to change in a way to reflect the user's feedback.

One method for on-line learning is *relevance feedback*, an adaptive mechanism, which modifies the response of a system according to the *feedback* about the *relevance* of selected samples so that the system response is adjusted to the current user's information needs. Although relevance feedback is not restricted to description environments where similarity measures are used, in databases where similarity-based queries are applied, relevance feedback refers to the mechanism which updates the similarity measure with respect to the relevant/irrelevant information, as indicated by the user. In this chapter, we address the problem of relevance feedback in the most generic form by updating the type of similarity measure itself, instead of adjusting the degree of importance of the descriptors to the similarity measure. Therefore, *a generalized non-linear relevance feedback scheme* is discussed.

In particular, functional analysis is used to model the non-linear similarity measure, by expressing it as a parametric relation of known monotone increasing functional components. Then, a recursive model parameter updating algorithm is adopted, which adapts the similarity measure type to the current users' information needs and preferences, as expressed by a set of selected relevant/irrelevant data. The adaptation is performed so that a) the current selected data are satisfied as much as possible and b) a minimal modification of the already estimated similarity measure (i.e., existing knowledge) is accomplished. Assuming that a small perturbation of the model parameters is adequate to satisfy the aforementioned conditions, the algorithm results in a constraint minimization problem for estimating the contribution of each functional component to the similarity measure.

The experimental results indicate that the presented *generalized recursive non-linear relevance feedback* scheme yields promising results and the proposed method provides better retrieval ranking due to the fact that no restrictions on the similarity type are imposed, as happens with the previous approaches and therefore better adaptation to the current users' information needs is accomplished. Another advantage of the proposed algorithm is the fact that it can be recursively implemented in case of multiple feedback iterations, in contrast to most of the previous approaches. This results in a computationally efficient algorithm, which further increases the effectiveness of the proposed method. In addition, the algorithm is robust regardless of the number of selected relevant/irrelevant samples, i.e., small selected samples are enough to accurately update the type of similarity measure, in contrast to some of the previously proposed techniques.

REFERENCES

Avrithis, Y., Doulamis, A. D. , Doulamis, N. D., & Kollias, S. D. (1998). An Adaptive Approach to Video Indexing and Retrieval. *Proceedings of the International Workshop on Very Low Bitrate Video Coding (VLBV)*, (pp. 69-72), Urbana IL, October 1998.

Choi, Y., Kim, D., & Krishnapuram, R. (2000). Relevance Feedback for Content-based Image Retrieval using Choquet Integral. *Proceedings of the IEEE International Conference on Multimedia & Expo*, (pp. 1207-1210), New York, August 2000.

Cox, I., Miller, M. L., Omohundro, S. M., & Yianilos, P. N. (1996). Pichunter: Bayesian Relevance Feedback for Image Retrieval. *Proceedings of the International Conference on Pattern Recognition*, *3*, 362-369.

Cybenko, G. (1989). Approximation by Superpositions of a Sigmoidal function. *Mathematics of Control, Signal and Systems, 2*, 303-314.

Doulamis, A. D., Avrithis, Y. S., Doulamis, N. D., & Kollias, S. D. (1999). Interactive Content-Based Retrieval in Video Databases Using Fuzzy Classification and Relevance Feedback. *Proceedings of the IEEE International Conference on Multimedia Computing and Systems (ICMCS), 2,* 954-958, Florence, Italy, June 1999.

Doulamis, N., & Doulamis, A. (2001). A Recursive Optimal Relevance Feedback Scheme for Content Based Image Retrieval," *Proceedings of the IEEE International Conference on Image Processing (ICIP), 2*, 741-744, Thessaloniki, Greece, October 2001.

Doulamis, N., Doulamis, A., & Kollias, S. (2001). Fuzzy Histograms and Optimal Relevance Feedback for Interactive Content-based Image Retrieval. *IEEE Transactions on Image Processing.*

Doulamis, N., Doulamis, A., &. Ntalianis, K. (2001). Optimal Interactive Content-Based Image Retrieval," *Proceedings of the International Conference on Augmented, Virtual Environments and 3D Imaging*, 248-251, Myconos, Greece, May 2001.

Hong, M., Karimpour-Fard, A., Russell, R., & Hunter, L. (2005). Integrated Term Weighting, Visualization, and User Interface Development for Bioinformation Retrieval. *Artificial Intelligence and Simulation, Lecture Notes in Computer Science*, Springer Verlag.

Ishikawa, Y., Subramanya, R., & Faloutsos, C. (1998). Mindreader: Querying Databases through Multiple Examples. *Proceedings of the 24th VLDB conference*, New York, USA.

Kagolovsky, Y., Freese, D., Miller, M., Walrod, T., & Moehr, J. (1998). Towards improved information retrieval from medical sources. *International journal of medical informatics.*

Kreyszig, E. (1989). *Introductory Functional Analysis with Applications.* New York: Wiley & Sons.

Luenberger, D. J. (1984) *Linear and non Linear Programming.* Addison-Wesley.

Rocchio, J. (1971). Relevance Feedback in Information Retrieval. *The SMART Retrieval System: Experiments in Automatic Document Processing,* Prentice Hall.

Rui, Y., Huang, T. S., Ortega, M., & Mehrotra, S. (1998). Relevance Feedback: A Power Tool for Interactive Content-Based Image Retrieval. *IEEE Transactions on Circuits. Systems for Video Technology, 8*(5), 644-655.

Rui, Y., & Huang, T. S. (2000) Optimizing Learning in Image Retrieval. *Proceedings of the IEEE International Conference on Computer Vision and Pattern Recognition*, Jun. 2000.

Salton, G., & McGill, M. J. (1982). *Introduction to Modern Information Retrieval.* New York: McGraw-Hill Book Company.

Shatkay, H. (2005). Information retrieval from biomedical text. *Briefings in Bioinformatics*, Henry Stewart Publications.

Zhou, X . S., & Huang, T. S. (2001). Small Sample Learning during Multimedia Retrieval using BiasMap. *Proceedings of the IEEE Conference on Computer Vision and Pattern Recognition,* Hawaii, December 2001.

Chapter XIV
Extracting Patient Case Profiles with Domain-Specific Semantic Categories

Yitao Zhang
The University of Sydney, Australia

Jon Patrick
The University of Sydney, Australia

ABSTRACT

The fast growing content of online articles of clinical case studies provides a useful source for extracting domain-specific knowledge for improving healthcare systems. However, current studies are more focused on the abstract of a published case study which contains little information about the detailed case profiles of a patient, such as symptoms and signs, and important laboratory test results of the patient from the diagnostic and treatment procedures. This paper proposes a novel category set to cover a wide variety of semantics in the description of clinical case studies which distinguishes each unique patient case. A manually annotated corpus consisting of over 5000 sentences from 75 journal articles of clinical case studies has been created. A sentence classification system which identifies 13 classes of clinically relevant content has been developed. A golden standard for assessing the automatic classifications has been established by manual annotation. A maximum entropy (MaxEnt) classifier is shown to produce better results than a Support Vector Machine (SVM) classifier on the corpus.

INTRODUCTION

The medical diagnosis and treatment of a patient is a complex procedure which requires relevant knowledge and clinical experience of illnesses. In order to distinguish different illnesses that show similar signs and symptoms, or to decide the best available option for treatment of a medical condition, physicians need to have adequate observations of similar patient cases, either from their own previous medical practices, or some external resources, such as the knowledge of more experienced colleagues, and the medical literature on the latest progress in the field.

Clinical case reporting therefore plays an important role in both educating young physicians in the practice of medicine, and sharing clinical experience and exceptional findings among physicians (Jenicek, M., 2001). There are two types of clinical case reports, namely routine patient case reports and clinical case studies. Routine case reports are raw patient records of the diagnostic and treatment procedure and provide information which is necessary for the continuity of patient care, such as progress notes, discharge summaries and pathology reports. Clinical case studies, on the other hand, report rare and abnormal patient cases that are considered as of significant scientific value to the field. They are reported by clinicians, usually in the form of formal journal articles in medical press.

Narrative patient records produced by nurses and physicians everyday in hospitals and clinics, provide first-hand the richest information about the progress of patients. However, the confidentiality of personal records has always been a concern which prevents the research community having access to enough data to develop useful learning systems comparable to human performance. Confidential information includes names of patients and physicians, dates, and geographic clues which are required to be anonymized before any raw patient data can be released to the public. Moreover, the anonymisation task often requires human annotators to manually check every single patient record to satisfy certain laws and ethical guidelines specified by governments. For instance, the 2007 Computational Medicine Challenge had to use human annotators to review all of the 4,055 raw patient records and to remove nearly half of them from the final gold-standard corpus to meet United States HIPAA standards.

With the emergence of publicly available online knowledge bases such as MEDLINE/PubMed and BMC Central, clinicians now have access to a large number of full-text journal articles of clinical case studies. Each case study records a detailed discussion of the patient's abnormal signs and symptoms, or novel conditions which are considered as report-worthy. While all the sensitive privacy information has been carefully removed from the text, a clinical case study still contains rich information about patient case profiles, such as patient demographics, signs and symptoms, laboratory test readings and interpretations, and treatments and subsequent outcomes for patients. This patient profile information is key in answering two fundamental questions dominating the daily practice of physicians: (1) Given the case profile of a patient, what is the best explanation or diagnosis of the condition? (2) Given the specified circumstances of a patient, what is the best treatment available? By exploring clinical case studies with similar patient profiles, physicians can learn, and therefore improve their practices of medicine, from the successes or failures of their peers.

However, the amount of data added into online biomedical databases each year is so large that clinicians cannot keep up to date with the new discoveries and knowledge in the field. For instance, there are 500,000 new journal articles added into the PubMed/MEDLINE database each year (Mitchell, J. A., Aronson, A. R., & Mork, J. G., 2003). An information need therefore arises for building intelligent information retrieval systems which incorporate domain-knowledge to find the right patient cases to support clinical decision making in a timely manner. Most efforts so far in biomedical text-mining have been made to exploit only abstracts of clinical case studies, which is still a small proportion of the fully available text (Cohen, A. M, & Hersh, W. R., 2003). Important clinical information, such as laboratory tests and readings, signs and symptoms of a patient during the diagnosis and treatment, and health profile of a patient, generally missing in the abstract section of a clinical case study. This work therefore turns to full-text articles of clinical case studies for accessing detailed descriptions of diagnoses and treatments of patients. The fingerprint information of each clinical case is exploited to help build an intelligent information retrieval system which is aware of the uniqueness of each individual case in performing tasks such as retrieving similar patient cases.

Since the detailed patient profiles are largely encoded in free-text, Natural Language Processing (NLP) is crucial in extracting the targeted information which provides important clues for differentiating individual patient cases. Most efforts to date using NLP to analyse medical text have focused at a word or phrase level, particularly in identifying appropriate medical concepts in text. Domain-specific ontological resources like Unified Medical Language System (UMLS) and Systematized Nomenclature of Medicine – Clinical Terms (SNOMED CT), which define both medical concept classes and detailed relationships among the concepts, have been used to serve tasks like biomedical entity recognition and entity relation extraction (Cohen, A. M. et al., 2003; Aronson, A. R., 2001). However, a successful mapping between terms in free-text to concepts in a medical ontology only provides an isolated lexical-level interpretation of the text meaning. The understanding of clause or sentence level semantics has largely remained as a challenge for extracting targeted clinical information. For instance, recognising individual concepts of "Isoflavones" and "Hormone replacement therapy" alone in the following sentence does not give people the big picture of the meaning of the sentence.

"Isoflavones are gaining popularity as alternatives to hormone replacement therapy."

A system that works only on the lexical level will return the above sentence as a positive result for enquiries on either "Isoflavones", or "Hormone replacement therapy". However, this example sentence provides only background information about the above two therapies, rather than any useful targeted fact or knowledge which describes the procedures or outcomes of undertaking a treatment for a patient. Therefore, lexical semantics alone does not contain all the necessary information for retrieving the right facts or knowledge according to a requirement determined by clinicians, such as searching for the possible side-effects of a treatment on a specific illness, or causations of a suspicious medical condition on patient.

The syntax of a sentence provides important clues for understanding the full-meaning of the text. Words and phrases in a sentence are organized into a grammatical structure according to their syntactic categories, such as nouns, verbs, and adjectives. The semantics of a sentence can then be represented by the concepts in the text and the relationships among the concepts. Most state-of-the-art statistical parsers are trained and evaluated on newswire text, particularly Wall Street Journal articles of the Penn Tree Bank. Biomedical text, however, shows different characteristics such as a much larger vocabulary involving medical and biological terms, and ungrammatical patterns like missing subjects and verbs as seen in raw clinical records. It is therefore inappropriate to use a parser which is trained on newswire text to understand the meaning of biomedical text. Recent efforts on creating gold-standard syntactically annotated biomedical corpora, notably the GENIA corpus, require that human annotators not only have the knowledge of the grammatical formalism used for annotation, but also a deep understanding of the biomedical domain. The difficulty of assembly a team with enough qualified human annotators, and the slowness of the annotation process has therefore prevented researchers developing useful biomedical corpora comparable to the size of their counterparts in the newswire domain. As a result, statistical parsers tailored to the biomedical domain are hard to train and evaluate. Some systems therefore turn to hand-written domain-specific grammars, or partial parsing to fulfil the syntactic and semantic analysis of clinical narratives.

In order to overcome the clinicians' difficulty of coping with a large amount of data in the clinical domain, this work develops a semantic annotation scheme for patient case studies which serves as an intermediate level of domain description for specific extraction of information. The proposed semantic annotation set helps the unfolding of important scenarios of a patient case study in journal articles, such as the medical procedures undertaken and the diagnostic and treatment processes of a patient. The remainder of this chapter provides a brief introduction of related works in the field. A detailed discussion of the proposed semantic category set follows together with the process of deploying the annotation scheme to create a new clinical case studies corpus from journal articles which report interesting and exceptional patient cases. Possible applications of the new clinical case studies corpus include Information Extraction, Information Retrieval, and Question Answering. As an initial effort, a sentence classification task has been set up to train a system that can automatically identify specific semantic information in the texts.

BACKGROUND

Medical ontologies play an important role in serving tasks like biomedical named-entity recognition, and extraction of relationships among medical concepts. In a manually constructed ontology, equivalent free-text terms are indexed by a single concept identification number, and are organized into an hierarchical structure according to their relationships to other concepts in the ontology.

The Systematized Nomenclature of Medicine (SNOMED CT) is a comprehensive ontology which covers a wide variety of concepts in the healthcare domain. SNOMED CT includes about 360, 000 concepts which are stored in a hierarchical structure connected by over 60 types of relationships. There are 19 top-level concepts in the SNOMED CT hierarchy which represent the highest level of abstraction of elements in the healthcare domain, such as clinical finding, procedure, and body structure (January 2007 release). These 19 top-level concepts subsume all the other concepts in the ontology.

The Unified Medical Language System (UMLS), which was developed by the National Library of Medicine (NLM), is an ongoing project to integrate a wide variety of biomedical vocabularies and terminologies into a single knowledge base to serve the needs for building intelligent medical and health-care management systems (Bodenreider, O., 2004). The UMLS contains three major components, namely, the Metathesaurus, the Semantic Network, and the SPECIALIST lexicon. The UMLS Metathesaurus stores more than one million biomedical concepts which are drawn from over 100 sources in 17 different languages, together with over 12 million relations among the concepts (the 2007 version). Terms referring to the same meaning are clustered into one single concept in the UMLS Metathesaurus. The Semantic Network defines 135 semantic types which categorize all the concepts in the Metathesaurus, together with 54 possible relationships among concepts. Finally, the SPECIALIST Lexicon contains more than 330, 000 common words and biomedical terms in English, together with over 550, 000 variants.

Many systems have been developed to map phrases in biomedical text to concepts in controlled vocabularies or standardized ontologies, notably the UMLS Metathesaurus. The techniques used in the mapping process generally involve string matching, limited syntactic analysis such as part-of-speech (POS) tagging and chunking, and hand-written domain knowledge about the specific genres of biomedical text (Aronson, A. R., 2001;

Brennan, P. F., & Aronson, A. R., 2003; Cooper, G. F., & Miller, R. A., 1998; Friedman, C., Alderson, P. O., Austin, J. H., Cimino, J. J., & Johnson, S. B., 1994; Friedman, C., Shagina, L., Lussier, Y., & Hripcsak, G., 2004; Lussier, Y. A., Shagina, L., & Friedman, C., 2001; Zou, Q., Chu, W. W., Morioka, C., Leazer, G. H., & Kangarloo, H., 2003). MetaMap Transfer (MMTx), for example, uses a five-step algorithm which incorporates knowledge sources like SPECIALIST Lexicon, shallow syntactic analysis of text, and variants generation for terms, to map terms to concepts in the UMLS Metathesaurus (Aronson, A. R., 2001). Users can also specify a sub-domain of the UMLS concept space to restrict the scope of concepts the MMTx system tries to map. MedLEE uses a domain-specific grammar to parse clinical notes (Friedman, C. et al., 1994, 2004. The grammar specifies a frame-based structure of sentences in which concepts, values and modifiers are used to interpret information in clinical notes.

Moreover, applying natural language processing techniques to the clinical domain has recently attracted much attention. To generate better text summarisations, sentence classification methods have been used to first reveal the rhetorical structure of scientific articles, which encodes the argument role of each sentence in a text, such as “introduction”, “method”, “result”, and “conclusion” (McKnight, L., & Srinivasan, P., 2003). Discriminative methods like Support Vector Machines (SVM) have been widely used in the sentence classification task in the biomedical domain (McKnight, L. et al., 2003; Yamamoto, Y., & Takagi, T. A., 2005) Lin et al recently attempted to model the rhetorical structure of MEDLINE abstracts by using a generative model (Yamamoto, Y. et al., 2004).

Hara and Matsumoto used BACT, which is a machine learner that can capture patterns from semi-structured data like parse trees, to classify sentences in MEDLINE abstracts as to whether or not a sentence contains the information extraction targets like “compared treatment”, “endpoint”, and “patient population” (Hara, K., & Matsumoto, Y., 2005). The BACT system is reported as comparable to a SVM learner with tree kernel (Kudo, T., & Matsumoto, Y., 2004).

The literature does not reveal any attempt to identify a clinically appropriate specific set of categories to extract from published texts, nor does it advocate a utilitarian objective for an information extraction process that would motivate its use by clinical practitioners. We propose a specific set of clinical generalized categories suited to clinical practice and then demonstrate the compilation of a training corpus and derive a set of optimal features for automatically extracting sentences which constitute instantiations of the clinical categories.

THE CATEGORY SET

This section proposes a category set aimed at recovering key semantics of clinical case studied in journal articles. The development of this markup scheme is the result of analyzing information needs of clinicians. During the development of this category set, domain experts were constantly consulted for their input and advice.

The categories can be divided into two subgroups, namely the more generic categories representing descriptions of the diagnostic and treatment procedures of clinicians, and the genre-specific categories reflecting the argumentation role of medical research papers. Examples of the tagged sentences are shown in Table 1 and Table 2 respectively.

Justification of the Need for a New Semantic Tag Set

Although standardized medical ontologies cover a wide variety of concepts in biomedical texts, there is still a need to develop fine-grained and application-specific categories for analyzing clinical case studies. This section uses SNOMED CT

Table 1. The categories of diagnostic and treatment procedures with sample phrases

Category name	Frequency	Examples
Sign	955 (18.7%)	"his finger was swollen, tense and tender."
		"electrolytes were normal"
Symptom	145 (2.8%)	"she also complained of right upper quadrant pain, which radiated to her right lower quadrant and upper back."
		"he experienced mild muscle weakness in his lower extremities"
Medical Test	176 (3.4%)	"Her BP was 100/75 mmHg, HR was 110 bpm"
		"respiratory rate was 20 breaths/min"
Diagnostic Test	416 (8.1%)	"Cerebrospinal fluid examination was negative"
		"CT scan with contrast confirmed the vascular nature of the cyst."
Diagnosis	217 (4.2%)	"The diagnosis of Echinococcus granulosus infection was confirmed"
Treatment	460 (9.0%)	"He was placed on triple antibiotics therapy."

Table 2. Categories for genre specific semantics with sample phrases

Category Name	Frequency	Examples
Referral	22 (0.4%)	"The patient was referred to the pediatric surgery department"
Patient Health Profile	166 (3.2%)	"this healthy, well-nourished, normotensive postmenopausal woman"
		"She had a history of symptomatic therapy (non-specific antibiotics)."
Patient Demographics	141 (2.8%)	"A 49 year old woman"
Causation	64 (1.3%)	"due to a malassezia furfur infection on the skin"
		"The rash was thought to be a reaction to the Cephalosporin antibiotic."
Exceptionality	72 (1.4%)	"Our case is the rst male patient reported with SSc and IPH."
		"Situs inversus presenting with acute cholecystitis is very rare."
Case Recommendations	171 (3.3%)	"Conservative treatment should be given unless there are complications."
		"Glucocorticoids should be avoided in diabetic patients."
Exclusion	29 (0.6%)	"She has no history of smoking."
		"There was no current or history of asthma."

as an example to illustrate the problems of using a general-purpose medical knowledge base for extracting targeted information beyond word or phrase level.

The hierarchy in a medical ontology reflects the knowledge of its creators on how the medical concepts should be classified and organized into a unified knowledge base. However, the granularity of concepts in a general-purpose ontology is often found not suitable for a particular health management task. For instance, it is often desirable to distinguish between objective clinical findings observed by physicians and subjective descriptions of symptoms reported by patients. In SNOMED CT, most concepts related to symptoms reported by patients are classified as "finding reported by subject or history provider" which is a child concept of "clinical finding". However, many symptom concepts can also be linked to "clinical finding" through alternative routes which classify them as an objective findings. For example, "symptom of lower limb" is a child of both "finding reported by subject or history provider" and "finding of lower limb". The second concept can be further linked to "finding by site" which is also a child concept of "clinical finding". As a result, a successful mapping of "symptom of lower limb" in text cannot provide information on the coarse-level sense of whether it is a symptom concept or a sign concept.

Meanwhile, concepts of the same semantic type can be distributed into different categories. For example, "pain" and "weakness" are both common subjective descriptions of discomfort and health histories of patients. However, the two concepts belong to different sub-categories of "clinical finding" in SNOMED CT. The concept of "weakness" is a "clinical history and observation findings", while "pain" is a "neurological finding". Interestingly, "no pain", which is a negation of the concept "pain", belongs to "situation with explicit context" which is a sibling of "clinical finding". Therefore, the current granularity of classifying and organizing concepts in a general-purpose medical ontology like SNOMED CT makes it difficult to be adopted into various contexts of health-care management systems.

The Diagnostic and Treatment Procedures

The categories convey a variety of general concepts which occur in descriptions of clinical procedures. These categories are more generic and are not confined to any specific genre of medical text, such as research articles or raw clinical notes. Although the current category set covers a good variety of aspects of the semantics of clinical reports, it does not provide a hierarchy for rhetorical structure of text.

Sign is a signal that indicates the existence or nonexistence of a disease as observed by clinicians during the diagnostic and treatment procedures. Typical signs of a patient include the appearance of the patient, readings or analytical results of laboratory tests, or responses to a medical treatment. Clinical tests which are of particular interest to medical practitioners were given separate categories in this research.

Symptom is also an indication of disorder or disease but is noted by patients rather than by clinicians. For instance, a patient can experience weakness, fatigue, or pain during the illness. In most cases, descriptions of symptoms are expressed as complaints or feelings by patients. However, an interesting exception can be seen in the following sentence:

"He was identified by nursing staff as having knee pain."

In this case a patient with dementia actually lost his ability to feel pain, and his symptom was only noted by clinicians through their observations.

Medical Test is a specific type of sign in which a quantifiable or specific value has been identified by a medical testing procedure, such as by taking a blood pressure or a white blood cell count.

Diagnostic Test gives analytical results for diagnosis purposes as observed by clinicians in a medical testing procedure. It differs from a medical test in that it generally returns no quantifiable value or reading as its result. The expertise of clinicians is required to read and analyse the result of a diagnostic test, such as interpreting an X-ray image.

Diagnosis identifies conditions that are diagnosed by clinicians.

Treatment is the therapy or medication that patients received.

Genre Specific Semantics

The categories described in this section provide genre-specific semantics. These categories tend to occur much more frequently in journal articles of clinical findings than other types of medical text like clinical notes.

Referral specifies another unit or department to which patients are referred for further examination or treatment.

Patient Health Profile identifies characteristics of patient health histories, including social behaviors.

Patient Demographics outline the details and background of a patient.

Causation is a speculation about the cause of a particular abnormal condition, circumstance or case.

Exceptionality states the importance and merits of the reported case.

Case Recommendations mark the advice for clinicians or other readers of the report.

Exclusion rules out a particular causation or phenomenon in a report.

THE CORPUS

The corpus described in this paper is a collection of recent research articles that report clinical findings by medical researchers. To make the data representative of the clinical domain, a wide variety of topics have been covered in the corpus, such as cancers, gene-related diseases, viral and bacterial infections, and sports injuries. The articles were randomly selected and downloaded from BioMed Central[1], which is a freely available online repository of biomedical research papers. During the selection stage, those reports that describe a group of patients were removed. As a result, this corpus is confined to clinical reports on individual patients.

A single annotator (first author) manually tagged all 75 articles in the corpus. Then a second annotator (second author) evaluated all the annotations made by the first annotator. Any disagreement between the two annotators was resolved by discussion between the two annotators. Annotations were done by using Callisto[2], which is a free annotation tool developed by MITRE. The distributions of categories, together with the statistical profile of the corpus are shown in Table 1, Table 2, and Table 3. The category set covers 45.2% of all the sentences in the corpus. The sentences that cannot be properly classified are not assigned any semantic category. Manual inspection of the corpus shows that most sentences not covered by the category set are those that describe background knowledge of the research, or reference the work of other researchers.

Table 3. Descriptive statistics of the corpus

Total articles	75
Total sentences	5,117
Total sentences with at least one category	2,311
Total tokens	112,382
Total tokens with tag	48,267

THE SENTENCE CLASSIFICATION TASK

Many sentences in the corpus contain information that serves more than one function. For instance, the sentence "She was admitted for pneumonectomy with a provisional diagnosis of bronchogenic carcinoma." contains both information of the treatment "pneumonectomy", and the diagnosis "bronchogenic carcinoma".

Among the total of 2,311 sentences with tags, there are 544 (23.5%) sentences assigned more than one category. This overlapping feature of the category assignment makes a single multi-class classifier approach inappropriate for the task. Instead, each category has been given a separate machine-learned classifier capable of assigning a binary "Yes" or "No" label for a sentence according to whether or not the sentence includes the targeted information as defined by the category set. Meanwhile, a supervised-learning approach was adopted in this experiment.

Experiments

Preprocessing

Raw articles were first separated into different sections based on their original formatting information. Then a maximum entropy based sentence splitter was used to detect the boundaries between sentences. Each sentence was tagged for part-of-speech (POS) and chunked using the Genia Tagger (Tsuruoka, Y., Tateishi, Y., Kim, J. D., Ohta, T., McNaught, J., Ananiadou, S., & Tsujii, J., 2005) which is trained on biomedical texts. The POS information was also used as the input for the Bikel parser (Bikel, D. M., 2004) which is trained on newswire text. The system used AGTK[3], an API interface developed for accessing annotation graph compatible file formats, to retrieve human annotations made within Callisto. Figure 1 shows a snapshot of the GUI interface of Callisto for the manual annotation stage of the work.

Classifiers and the Feature Set

Maximum Entropy Modeling (MaxEnt) and Support Vector Machine (SVM) are the two most popular techniques for supervised classification problems. This section briefly discusses the principles of the two methods, together with the feature set and experimental settings.

In a MaxEnt model features are considered as constraints (Berger, A. L., Della Pietra, V. J., & Della Pietra, S. A., 1996). For example, when considering the category "Sign", the system tries to assign either a "YES" or a "NO" label to a sentence based on various features of the instance, such as

$$f_i(y,x) = \begin{cases} 1 \textit{ if } \text{y = YES and has word(x) ='swollen'} \\ 0 \qquad\qquad\qquad \text{otherwise} \end{cases}$$

where y is the outcome class label for the mark-up tag "Sign", and x is the current sentence instance.

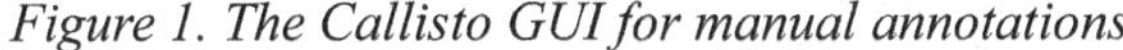

Figure 1. The Callisto GUI for manual annotations

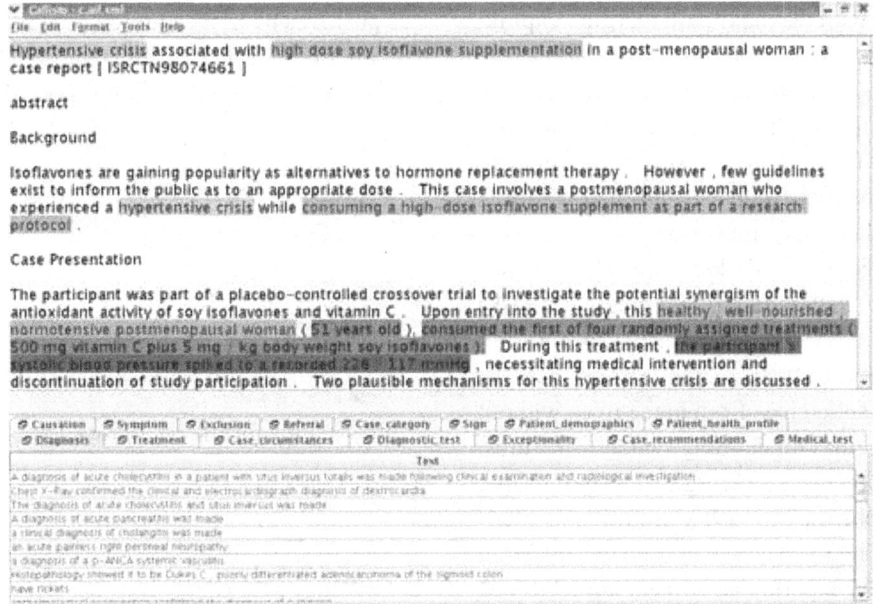

In this example, the feature fires when the current sentence contains the unigram word "swollen". The conditional probability of seeing the class label y given an instance x can be then be defined in terms of its features:

$$P(y\mid x)=\frac{1}{Z(x)}\exp(\sum_i \lambda_i f_i(y,x))$$

where Z(x) is a normalization function, and each feature f_i is associated with a parameter λ_i. An important advantage of MaxEnt modeling is that it can tolerate dependent features within the same feature set. In the experiments, we used a MaxEnt classifier implementation which is developed by Zhang Le[4].

An SVM classifier uses a set of instances $x_i \in R^n$, where R^n is a N dimensional vector space and each x_i is assigned with a binary class label of either -1 or +1, an SVM classifier tries to project input vectors onto a high-dimensional feature space Γ by using a mapping function called a kernel:

$$\Phi : x_i \rightarrow \Gamma$$

It then separates two classes in the high-dimensional feature space Γ by using a linear hyperplane with the maximum margin (Vapnik, V. N., 1995).

The tree kernel proposed by Collins and Duffy (2002) exploits non-flat structure representations and is able to measure the similarity between two parse trees by comparing all their common sub-structures. By combining the tree kernel with other conventional kernels such as linear, polynomial, and radial basis function (RBF) kernels, an SVM classifier is able to not only utilize common flat-structured features, but also exploit syntactic clues from parse trees without any explicit rules for defining syntactic features. In the experiments, a SVM-light package with tree kernel (Joachims, T., 1999; Moschitti, A., 2004) was used. The SVM classifier used two different kernels in the experiment: a linear kernel (SVM t=1), and a combination of the tree kernel and the linear kernel (SVM t=6). The introduction of the tree kernel was an attempt to evaluate the effectiveness of incorporating syntactic features for the task.

The feature set used in the experiment consists of bag-of-words features (unigrams and bigrams) and the document structure information such as the title of the current section. The syntactic features were encoded in parse trees and were therefore only accessed implicitly by the SVM classifier with the tree kernel.

Evaluation

The micro-averaged balanced form of F_1 has been used for evaluating the performance of the sentence classification system. For a semantic category $T_{i,}$ the system tries to assign either a "Yes" or "No" label to each sentence in the corpus according to whether or not the sentence contains the targeted information. As shown in Table 4, TP is the number of correctly predicted positive instances of $T_{i,}$ and FP is the number of wrongly predicted positive instances by the system. For those labeled as not containing information of T_i, FN is the number of instances that are tagged as positives by human annotators, and TN is the number of true negative instances.

The micro-averaged balanced form of F_1 can be calculated as

$$F_1=\frac{2PR}{P+R},$$

where P is the precision rate.

$$P=\frac{\sum TP_i}{\sum TP_i+\sum FP_i},$$

and R stands for the recall rate

$$R=\frac{\sum TP_i}{\sum TP_i+\sum FN_i}.$$

This calculation gives equal importance to each event of a category T_i.

Results

Two machine learning systems (SVM and MaxEnt) were used in the sentence classification experiments. The micro-averaged F_1 results for all the categories are shown in Table 5. Experiments were done using a 4-fold cross validation method. The baseline system S_0 used only bag-of-words (BOW) features (unigrams and bigrams), while S_1 incorporates information from the document structure such as the title of the current section, and the position of the current sentence in the section.

The detailed results for the S_1 MaxEnt system for each clinical category are shown in Table 6. In most cases, categories of diagnostic and treatment procedures have better classification results than those of the categories describing the genre-specific semantics. There is not an entirely linear relationship between sample size and quality of result although a trend is present.

In order to evaluate the sentence classification system in more detail, a close study has been made of the "Sign" category which has the largest frequency in the corpus and is relatively stable according to the inter-annotator agreement. The sentence classification result for the "Sign" category is shown in Table 7. The figures in the table are 10-fold cross validation results. The baseline system reported in Table 7 uniformly assigns a "Yes" label to all sentences as positive "Sign" instances.

The MaxEnt classifier generally outperforms the SVM classifier in every test on the F_1 metric. However, the difference between the two classifiers is not statistically different in some experimental settings based on 10-fold paired t-test results for the significance level of $\alpha = 5\%$. The introduction of the tree kernel in the SVM classifier shows a higher precision rate, which suggests the potential benefits of exploiting syntactic features in the task, and a slight drop in recall rate compared to the MaxEnt system and the SVM system with linear kernel alone. However, the tree kernel suffers the problem of inaccurate input parse trees because of the lack of gold-standard medical tree-banks on which to train a parser. The Bikel parser is trained on newswire text and therefore much less accurate on parsing clinical reports.

The recall rate of SVM classifiers drops when bigrams are added to unigram features, while the MaxEnt classifier shows no significant improvement. Although Niu et.al. reported better performance by incorporating bigram features (Niu, Y., Zhu, X., Li, J., & Hirst, G., 2006) these experiment showed no significant benefits.

Adding title information of the current section into the feature set has given both SVM and MaxEnt classifiers significant improvement in terms of precision and recall. It suggests that the rhetorical role of a sentence, revealed partly by its section title, plays an important role in differentiating the functionality of different text segments. Moreover, this feature can be easily acquired in full journal articles.

Table 4. Contingency table for a Category T_i.

	Gold-standard Yes	Gold-standard No	Total
Predict-Yes	True Positives (TP_i)	False Positives (FP_i)	TP_i+FP_i
Predict-No	False Negatives (FN_i)	True Negatives (TN_i)	TN_i+FN_i
Total	TP_i+FN_i	FP_i+TN_i	$TP_i+FP_i+TN_i+FN_i$

Table 5. Results for all semantic categories (4-fold cross validation)

Features	Classifier	Precision	Recall	F_1
S_0 (BOW)	MaxEnt	65.6	39.4	49.3
	SVM (linear kernel)	42.8	16.7	24.0
	SVM (linear + tree kernel)	81.4	17.1	28.2
S_1 (BOW + Section Title)	MaxEnt	66.4	42.3	**51.7**
	SVM (linear kernel)	66.3	22.9	34.1
	SVM (linear + tree kernel)	79.3	24.2	37.0

Table 6. Sentence classification results for all categories (4-fold cross validation)

Clinical Category	Precision	Recall	F_1	N
Sign	62.4	50.7	56.0	955
Symptom	69.1	44.8	54.4	145
Medical Test	80.7	52.3	63.4	176
Diagnostic Test	65.5	44.7	53.1	416
Diagnosis	65.3	28.6	39.7	217
Treatment	68.9	42.4	52.5	460
Referral	100.0	22.7	37.0	22
Patient Health Profile	47.7	18.8	27.0	166
Patient Demographics	94.1	68.6	79.3	141
Causation	0.0	0.0	0.0	64
Exceptionality	57.1	16.7	25.8	72
Case Recommendations	62.3	29.3	39.8	171
Exclusion	42.9	10.3	16.7	29

Table 7. Sentence classification result for "sign" (10-fold cross validation)

Features	Classifier	Precision	Recall	F_1
	Baseline	18.7	100.0	31.5
Unigram	MaxEnt	58.8	47.7	52.7
	SVM (linear)	36.7	39.3	37.9
	SVM (linear + tree)	70.3	31.7	43.7
Unigram + Bigram	MaxEnt	59.2	48.9	53.6
	SVM (linear)	39.5	27.5	32.4
	SVM (linear + tree)	73.2	27.1	39.6
Unigram + Section Title	MaxEnt	64.5	51.1	**57.0**
	SVM (linear)	56.1	49.3	52.5
	SVM (linear + tree)	71.2	42.2	53.0
Unigram + Bigram + Section Title	MaxEnt	63.5	49.6	55.7
	SVM (linear)	61.6	44.2	51.5
	SVM (linear + tree)	72.9	40.5	52.1

DISCUSSION

The imbalanced class sizes of the target information in the corpus make sentence classification a difficult task. Most classification experiments have an F_1 value well below 60. In this section we review some of the wrongly classified sentences to identify strategies for improving the current information extraction system.

First of all, simple bag-of-words modeling of text is not able to capture the rich and subtle information encoded in the sentences. For example, the sentence "His mother and his brother had a history of deep venous thrombosis and his father died because of pulmonary embolism" was misclassified as a positive instance of "Sign" by both classifiers. This sentence actually mentions the family health history of the patient and therefore includes the ``health profile'' information as decided by human annotators. However, a machine learner with only bag-of-words modeling of text failed to recognize the difference between the switching of person entities from patient to his family members.

Moreover, the manual annotation also introduces some inconsistencies and errors, which will need to be corrected for future annotation. The sentence "Ultrasonographic examination of the mass showed a cystic structure" is classified as "Sign" by the system. However, in manual annotations the sentence is given a "Diagnostic test" tag, and the result of the test is not tagged as "Sign" by human annotator. Although most sentences with "Diagnostic test" or "Medical test" information include "Sign" information too, there are some examples where no description of any sign or symptom occurred with a medical test. This problem can be avoided by introducing more rigid and consistent guidelines on manual annotation.

CONCLUSION

The fast-growing content of online repositories like BioMed Central and MEDLINE provides a useful source for training text-mining systems for the clinical domain. This paper aims to evaluate the possibility of exploiting full journal articles of clinical case studies rather than only abstracts which generally ignore the detailed clinical history of each individual patient. By using simple bag-of-words features and document structure information, machine learned classifiers can easily outperform a naive baseline which uniformly predicts true in the sentence classification task. An overall micro-averaged F_1 value of 51.7 has been reported for 13 semantic categories.

Future work includes annotating more case reports by inviting domain experts to participate in the project. More annotators are needed for evaluating the stability of the tag set on a larger scale. Meanwhile, an active learning approach is considered as an alternative for building a large corpus by learning examples in the manually annotated corpus. There is also a need to add more specialized semantic categories such as "outcomes" of a treatment into the current category set. In order to achieve better performance on the sentence classification task, we plan to incorporate domain knowledge which is partly encoded in biomedical ontologies such as SNOMED CT and UMLS. Successful mapping between free-text to its corresponding clinical concepts should provide more reliable identification and standardisation of features for the system. Moreover, syntactic features need to be evaluated and refined to provide more useful clues about the text.

ACKNOWLEDGMENT

We wish to thank Prof Deborah Saltman for defining the tag categories and Joel Nothman for refining their use on texts. We would also like to thank the support from all members of the Sydney Language Technology Research Group.

REFERENCES

Aronson, A. R. (2001). Effective mapping of biomedical text to the UMLS Metathesaurus: The MetaMap program. *Proc AMIA Symp.,* (pp. 17-21).

Berger, A. L., Della Pietra, V. J., & Della Pietra, S. A. (1996). A maximum entropy approach to natural language processing. *Computational Linguistics, 22*(1), 39-71.

Bikel, D. M. (2004). A distributional analysis of a lexicalized statistical parsing model. *Proceedings of the Conference on Empirical Methods in Natural Language Processing* (pp. 182–9).

Bodenreider, O. (2004). The unified medical language system (UMLS): Integrating biomedical terminology. *Nucleic Acids Research, 32.*

Brennan, P. F., & Aronson, A. R. (2003). Towards linking patients and clinical information: Detecting UMLS concepts in e-mail. *Journal of Biomedical Informatics, 36*(4/5), 334-41.

Cohen, A. M, & Hersh, W. R. (2005). A survey of current work in biomedical text mining. *Briefings in Bioinformatics, 6*(1), 57.

Collins, M., & Duffy, N. (2002). New ranking algorithms for parsing and tagging: Kernels over discrete structures, and the voted perceptron. *Proceedings of the 40th Annual Meeting on Association for Computational Linguistics* (pp. 263-70).

Cooper, G. F., & Miller, R. A. (1998). An experiment comparing lexical and statistical methods for extracting mesh terms from clinical free text. *J Am Med Inform Assoc., 5*(1), 62-75.

Friedman, C., Alderson, P. O., Austin, J. H., Cimino, J. J., & Johnson, S. B. (1994). A general natural-language text processor for clinical radiology. *Journal of the American Medical Informatics Association, 1*(2), 161-74.

Friedman, C., Shagina, L., Lussier, Y., & Hripcsak, G. (2004). Automated encoding of clinical documents based on natural language processing. *Journal of the American Medical Informatics Association, 11*(5), 392.

Hara, K., & Matsumoto, Y. (2005). Information extraction and sentence classification applied to clinical trial medline abstracts. *Proceedings of the 2005 International Joint Conference of InCoB, AASBi and KSB* (pp. 85–90).

Jenicek, M. (2001). Clinical case reporting in evidence-based medicine (2nd edition). Arnold.

Joachims, T. (1999). Making large scale svm learning practical. In B. Scholkopf, C. Burges, & A. Smola (Eds.), *Advances in kernel methods - support vector learning.*

Kudo, T., & Matsumoto, Y. (2004). A boosting algorithm for classification of semi-structured text. *Proc. of EMNLP.,* (pp. 301–8).

Lin, J., Karakos, D., Demner-Fushman, D., & Khudanpur, S. (2006). Generative content models for structural analysis of medical abstracts. *Proceedings of the BioNLP Workshop on Linking Natural Language Processing and Biology at HLT-NAACL.* (pp. 65-72).

Lussier, Y. A., Shagina, L., & Friedman, C. (2001). Automating SNOMED coding using medical language understanding: A feasibility study. *Proc AMIA Symp., 418, 22.*

McKnight, L., & Srinivasan, P. (2003). Categorization of sentence types in medical abstracts. AMIA Annu Symp Proc., (pp. 440-4).

Mitchell, J. A., Aronson, A. R., & Mork, J. G. (2003). Gene indexing: Characterization and analysis of nlm's generifs. *AMIA Annu Symp Proc. 2003,* (pp. 460-4).

Moschitti, A. (2004). A study on convolution kernels for shallow semantic parsing. *Proceedings of ACL-2004.*

Niu, Y., Zhu, X., Li, J., & Hirst, G. (2005). Analysis of polarity information in medical text. *Proceedings of the American Medical Informatics Association 2005 Annual Symposium* (pp. 570–4).

Tsuruoka, Y., Tateishi, Y., Kim, J. D., Ohta, T., McNaught, J., Ananiadou, S., & Tsujii, J. (2005). Developing a robust part-of-speech tagger for biomedical text. *Advances in Informatics - 10th Panhellenic Conference on Informatics* (pp. 382-92).

Vapnik, V. N. (1995). *The nature of statistical learning theory.* Springer.

Yamamoto, Y., & Takagi, T. A. (2005). Sentence classification system for multi biomedical literature summarization. *Proceedings of the 21st International Conference on Data Engineering.*

Zou, Q., Chu, W. W., Morioka, C., Leazer, G. H., & Kangarloo, H. (2003). Indexfinder: A method of extracting key concepts from clinical texts for indexing. *AMIA Annu Symp Proc.,* (pp. 763-7).

ENDNOTES

1 http://www.biomedcentral.com/
2 http://callisto.mitre.org/
3 http://agtk.sourceforge.net/
4 http://homepages.inf.ed.ac.uk/s0450736/

Section IV
NLP Software for IR in Biomedicine

Chapter XV
Identification of Sequence Variants of Genes from Biomedical Literature: The OSIRIS Approach

Laura I. Furlong
Research Unit on Biomedical Informatics (GRIB), IMIM-Hospital del Mar, Universitat Pompeu Fabra, Spain

Ferran Sanz
Research Unit on Biomedical Informatics (GRIB), IMIM-Hospital del Mar, Universitat Pompeu Fabra, Spain

ABSTRACT

SNPs constitute key elements in genetic epidemiology and pharmacogenomics. While data about genetic variation is found at sequence databases, functional and phenotypic information on consequences of the variations resides in literature. Literature mining is mainly hampered by the terminology problem. Thus, automatic systems for the identification of citations of allelic variants of genes in biomedical texts are required. We have reported the development of OSIRIS, aimed at retrieving literature about allelic variants of genes, a system that evolved towards a new version incorporating a new entity recognition module. The new version is based on a terminology of variations and a pattern-based search algorithm for the identification of variation terms and their disambiguation to dbSNP identifiers. OSIRISv1.2 can be used to link literature references to dbSNP database entries with high accuracy, and is suitable for collecting current knowledge on gene sequence variations for supporting the functional annotation of variation databases.

INTRODUCTION

In the last years the focus of biological research has shifted from individual genes and proteins towards the study of entire biological systems. The advent of high-throughput experimentation has led to the generation of large data sets, which is reflected in the constant growth of dedicated repositories such as sequence databases and literature collections. Currently, MEDLINE indexes more than 17 million articles in the biomedical sciences, and it's increasing at a rate of more than 10 % each year (Ananiadou et al., 2006). In this scenario, text mining tools are becoming essential for biomedical researchers to manage the literature collection, and to extract, integrate and exploit the knowledge stored therein. Mining textual data can aid in formulating novel hypothesis by combining information from multiple articles and from biological databases, such as genome sequence databases, microarray expression studies, and protein-protein interaction databases (Jensen et al., 2006) (Ananiadou & McNaught, 2006). These kind of approaches are being applied in different scenarios: the prediction of the function of novel genes, functional annotation of molecules, discovering protein-protein interactions, interpreting microarray experiments and association of genes and phenotypes (for a review see (Ananiadou et al., 2006; Jensen et al., 2006)).

The basis of any text mining system is the proper identification of the entities mentioned in the text, also known as Named Entity Recognition (NER). Genes, proteins, drugs, diseases, tissues and biological functions are examples of entities of interest in the biomedical domain. It has been recognised that naming of these biological entities is inconsistent and imprecise, and in consequence tools that automatically extract the terms that refer to the entities are required to obtain an unambiguous identification of such entities (Park & Kim, 2006). In addition to the identification of a term that refer to, for instance, a protein in a text, it is very advantageous to map this term to its corresponding entry in biological databases. This process, also known as normalization, is very relevant from a biomedical perspective, because it provides the correct biological context to the term identified in the text.

NER has been an intense subject of research in the last years in the biology domain, specially for the identification of terms pertaining to genes and proteins (Jensen et al., 2006). Contrasting, few initiatives have been directed to the task of identification of Single Nucleotide Polymorphisms (SNPs) from the literature. Among other types of small sequence variants, SNPs represent the most frequent type of variation between individuals (0.1 % of variation in a diploid genome (Levy et al., 2007)). This observation, in addition to their widespread distribution in the genome and their low mutation rate, have positioned the SNPs as the most used genetic markers. SNPs are currently being used in candidate gene association studies, genome wide association studies and in pharmacogenomics. In this context they represent promising tools for finding the genetic determinants of complex diseases and for explaining the inter individual variability of drug responses.

From the point of view of NER, SNPs and other types of sequence variants represent a challenging task. Figure 1 illustrates the terminology problem for sequence variants of genes. The text fragments show different terms that can be used to refer to SNPs. It is important to note that the examples shown refer to a single SNP, for which different expressions are used, even in the same abstract. The same SNP can be referred to by its nucleotide representation as well as by its amino acid representation (in such cases where the SNP produces a change at the level of protein sequence). Even in each of these cases, different expressions can be used, and although there is a nomenclature standard for sequence variations (den Dunnen & Antonarakis, 2001) it is not widely used by the authors. The first approach related with NER for sequence variants was MuteXt, which was focused on collecting single point mutations for two protein families: nuclear hormone receptors and G-protein coupled receptors (Horn et al., 2004). A related approach has been implemented in MEMA (Rebholz-Schuhmann et al., 2004), in which regular expressions were used to extract variation-gene pairs from MEDLINE abstracts. The Vtag tagger (McDonald et al., 2004), based on Conditional Random Fields, was developed

Figure 1. Examples of different terms used to refer to sequence variants of genes in MEDLINE abstracts. The examples shown represent text passages extracted from different MEDLINE abstract, that refer to the same dbSNP entry (rs 1799983) mapped to the NOS3 (highlighted terms).

Article PMID: 11017941
In controls, individuals with the **E298D** mutation in exon 7 (136.1 micromol/L) showed significantly higher (P = 0.001) median plasma NOx than those without this mutation (64.5 micromol/L).

Article PMID: 10205226
Allele frequencies of **298Asp** were concordant across the panels: 8.4% in hypertensive subjects, 8.
The relevance of the **Glu298Asp** polymorphism to hypertension in this population was tested in 2 ways.

Article PMID: 10231340
Ten polymorphisms were detected: three in the 5' flanking sequence at positions -1474, -924 and -788, two in coding sequences 774C --> T (silent) and **G894 --> T** (**Glu-298 --> Asp**) and five in introns 2, 11, 12, 22 and 23.

for the identification of several types of sequence variations related to cancer in the literature. Although all these systems represent interesting examples of approaches for the identification of variations, most of them are focused only in protein point mutations (Caporaso et al., 2007; Erdogmus & Sezerman, 2007; Kanagasabai et al., 2007), specific protein families (Horn et al., 2004) or specific diseases (Erdogmus & Sezerman, 2007; McDonald et al., 2004). Very few approaches consider other types of variation like synonymous SNPs or variations located in gene regions other than exons, despite these variations could have functional consequences. Moreover, none of the mentioned approaches tackle the problem of the normalization of the variation terms so far identified. An exception of this is the Mutation Grab approach, which maps the point mutations to the protein using sequence information and the graph bigram approach (Lee et al., 2007). Nevertheless, it does not provide dbSNP identifiers for the point mutations found in the text.

Our goal was to develop a generic approach for NER of sequence variants that satisfied the following criteria: 1) to cover any type of short range sequence variation (SNPS, short insertions, deletions, etc), 2) to cover variations that affect not only the sequence at the protein level but also at the nucleotide level (SNPs in non-coding regions of genes like introns, in intergenic regions, etc), 3) to have a generic method applicable to all the genes, and not restricted to a gene or protein family, and 4) to map the variation mentions to its database identifier (normalization). This is what we call the OSIRIS approach. The first implementation, OSIRISv1.1 (Bonis et al., 2006), was an information retrieval system that integrated different data sources and incorporated tools for terminology generation with the aim of retrieving literature about the allelic variants of a gene using the PubMed search engine (http://www.ncbi.nlm.nih.gov/entrez/query.fcgi?db=PubMed). Although the use of OSIRISv1.1 helped the researchers in the tedious task of searching literature for sequence variants of genes, there was room for improvement. For instance, the first implementation of OSIRIS used the PubMed search engine, and did not include a NER system for the identification and tagging of the terms within the text. This and other features described below were incorporated in the new version of OSIRIS (herein referred to as OSIRISv1.2). A key aspect was to develop a NER system for identification and normalization of any kind of short range sequence variants of human genes. The new implementation of OSIRIS incorporates its own NER module and is built on top of a local mirror of MEDLINE collection and HgenetInfoDB. HgenetInfoDB is a database that integrates data on human entries from the NCBI Gene database (http://www.ncbi.nlm.nih.gov/entrez/query.fcgi?db=gene) and dbSNP (http://www.ncbi.nlm.nih.gov/SNP/). The NER module is based on the new OSIRISv1.2 search algorithm, which uses a pattern matching based search strategy and a dictionary of sequence variant terminology for the identification of terms denoting SNPs and other sequence variants and their mapping to dbSNP identifiers. The use of

Figure 2. Normalization. The process of mapping the variation mention found in the text to its corresponding database identifier is defined as normalization. For variations, the reference repository for sequence variation dbSNP is used. Normalization allows disambiguation of variation entities found in text and thus provide its unique identification, and places the variation mention in a biological context. Several layers of information can be obtained by mapping different databases that contain information of the variation and the gene and protein to which it is mapped to.

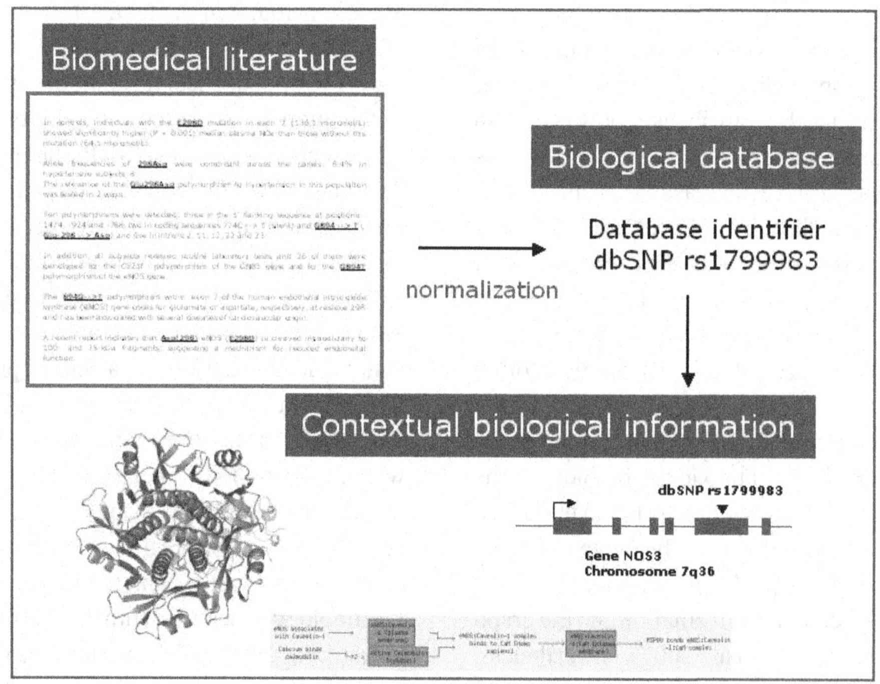

OSIRISv1.2 on MEDLINE abstracts generates a corpus of annotated literature linked to sequence database identifiers (NCBI Gene and dbSNP). OSIRISv1.2 can be used for collecting literature about the allelic variants of genes, which then can be mined for the extraction of interesting associations, for instance of SNPs with disease phenotypes.

DEFINITIONS

We use the term variation to refer to any kind of short range change in the nucleotide sequence of the genome. SNPs are the most studied type of sequence variation, but we can also consider as member of this class short insertions or deletions, named variations as Alu sequences, and other types of variations collected in the dbSNP database (Sherry et al., 1999). These variations can be mapped to the exonic regions of genes, and produce a change at the protein level, or within introns, untranslated regions or between genes. Some variations may alter protein function, such as non synonymous SNPs, or alter other processes related with the regulation of gene expression. Others may have no functional effect, such as synonymous SNPs at the protein level. However, although synonymous SNPs do not alter the protein sequence, are currently being regarded as potentially functional in light of recent reports that document their involvement in other processes such as regulation of mRNA processing or protein folding (Kimchi-Sarfaty et al., 2007). More information on sequence variation can be found elsewhere (Brookes, 1999; Burton et al., 2005; Shastry, 2007). From the point of view of our NER system, a variation entity is defined by the combination of tokens that specify the location of the variation in the sequence and the original and altered alleles. It is important to note that this information can be represented as nucleotide sequence or amino acid sequence. For instance, in Figure 1 the term E298D represents the following: E is the original allele of the variation in the protein (residue E in one letter code or Glu in three letter code for Glutamic acid) while D is the altered residue (residue D or Asp or Aspartic acid) and the variation occurs at position 298 of the protein sequence. The same variation could be referred as using the nucleotide representation G894T: in this case the G original allele stands for a guanine residue in the gene sequence at position 894 of the mRNA that changes to a thymine residue. In this example a first source of ambiguity in SNP notation is found. How can we know that the G894T term refers to a change in the protein or in the nucleotide sequence? Both possibilities are plausible without any additional information: contextual information extracted from the text or biological information from the sequence. Our strategy focuses in the latter source of information as we believe it constitutes the more reliable approach to disambiguate these cases.

IMPLEMENTATION

The OSIRIS approach is built on the basis of a dictionary of terms for the sequence variants of genes. The terminology was compiled from data from dbSNP, using a term expansion approach according to a set of patterns manually developed after inspecting the literature for collecting natural language expressions frequently used to refer to sequence variants. For each variant, the collection of amino acid terminology is built by 286 terms and the nucleotide terminology is composed by 114 terms. Some examples of terms are shown in Table 1. By using the dictionary, it is possible to link the term found in the text with the dbSNP database identifier. This is the so called process of normalization illustrated in Figure 2. Normalization allows the unambiguous identification of the variation, and allows resolving uncertainties in SNP identity as the one mentioned above. Moreover, several layers of information can be added to the information found in the text, in this

Table 1. Terminology for sequence variants. Some examples of the terminology used by the system are shown.

Amino acid terminology	Nucleotide terminology
Q610R	A-161G
R610Q	G-161A
Gln610Arg	G(-161)A
Arg610Gln	-161 A-G
Gln (610) Arg	-161 G-A
Arg (610) Gln	-161 (A-G)
610 Gln>Arg	A(-161)G
610 Arg>Gln	-161 (G-A)

Figure 3. OSIRISv1.2 system workflow. The system is based in a local mirror of MEDLINE database and HgenetInfoDB, which integrates information for human Gene and dbSNP databases from the NCBI. The starting point of the system is a gene, for which a set of articles is annotated by using a gene NER tool and stored in the TextMiningDB (1) . The gene-specific corpus is accessed by OSIRIS (2) to obtain the MEDLINE citations annotated to a NCBI Gene entry. The corresponding MEDLINE abstracts are retrieved from a local repository (3). In addition, sequence data for each gene and its sequence variants are retrieved from HgenetInfoDB, and this information is used to generate the SNP terminology (4). The next step of OSIRISv1.2 is the search for occurrences of the sequence variant terms in each gene-specific corpus by processing the MEDLINE abstracts. This information (SNP-specific corpus) is returned to the TextMiningDB database (5). For simplicity we use in this figure the term SNP to refer to all variations present in the database (SNPs and other types of sequence variants).

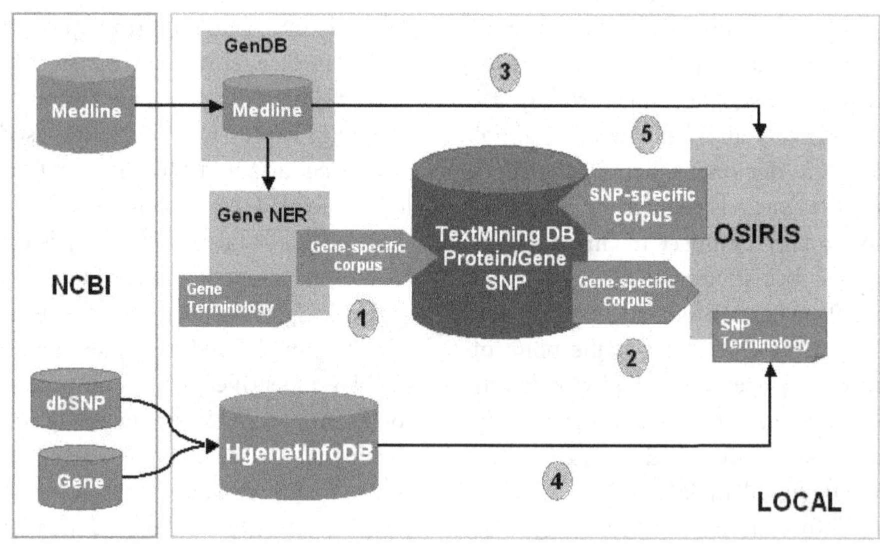

case the mention of a sequence variation. For instance, the gene to which the sequence is mapped to can be obtained, with the precise location in the genome and in the chromosome. Information on the effect of the variation at the protein level, or the participation of the gene or protein in a biological pathway or signalling network can be obtained as well. All these pieces of information are stored in different biological databases and can be integrated with the information found in plain text by means of the normalization process.

The first implementation of the system consisted in an information retrieval tool based on the PubMed search engine and specific queries using the terminology (Bonis et al., 2006). For the OSIRISv1.2 implementation, we sought to develop our own NER system able to find and mark the variation mentions in the texts. To accomplish this, we developed a simple search algorithm that scans the Medline abstracts at the sentence level looking for the terms present in the terminology. This approach improves the recognition of variations from text in terms of recall and precision, allows the mapping to database identifiers, and constitutes a first step towards a system for mining genotype-phenotype relationships.

OSIRISV1.2 SYSTEM WORKFLOW

A schematic view of the workflow of the system is shown in Figure 3. The starting point of OSIRISv1.2 is a gene, for whom a set of abstracts annotated to that gene is obtained. MEDLINE abstracts annotated with NCBI Gene identifiers by a gene NER tool (Hanisch et al., 2005) are stored in the TextMiningDB database and accessed by OSIRISv1.2 to obtain the corpus of MEDLINE citations annotated to a NCBI Gene entry. The corresponding MEDLINE abstracts are retrieved from a local repository and stored for later processing. In addition, sequence data for each gene and its sequence variants are retrieved from HgenetInfoDB. HgenetInfoDB contains information on human genes from the NCBI Gene database and their sequence variants (SNPs, indels, etc.) from the NCBI dbSNP. Using the information obtained from HgenetInfoDB, OSIRISv1.2 generates a dictionary of terms for each variant representing the more frequently used terminology for the variant. The next step of OSIRISv1.2 is the search for occurrences of the sequence variant terms in each gene-specific corpus by processing the MEDLINE abstracts. The search is performed using pattern matching of the terms from the terminology to text passages. This procedure allows the identification of the term that refers to a variant and the assignment of a dbSNP identifier to that term (normalization). By assignment of a dbSNP identifier to a variation, its linkage to the gene to which the variation is mapped is established. Finally, the information extracted from text is stored in the TextMiningDB database (Figure 3).

Once the set of citations that refer to a variations are identified, information extraction tasks can be applied on this set of documents in order to extract relevant information, for instance related phenotypes associated to a SNP. Alternatively, annotations performed by experts in each document, as is the case of the Medical Subject Heading (MeSH) terms (http://www.nlm.nih.gov/mesh/), can be obtained from the document set. MeSH terms are assigned to each MEDLINE abstract by experts in the field who read the full text article, and choose the most representative terms from the MeSH controlled vocabulary to describe the contents of the article. The MeSH terms from the Disease category were chosen to describe the set of articles associated to a dbSNP entry by OSIRISv1.2. The Disease category is formed by 23 sub-categories covering human diseases, with the exception of the C22 branch ('Animal Diseases') which was excluded from the analysis. The branch F03 representing Mental Disorders was added in order to add coverage for psychiatric diseases not included in the above mentioned 23 categories.

Terms from the Disease category of the MeSH hierarchy were extracted from the set of abstracts previously associated to each dbSNP entry by OSIRISv1.2. Then, a weight was assigned to each MeSH term as a measure of the relevance of the term in describing the set of articles associated to each variation. The weights were computed for the set of documents annotated to a variation by OSIRISv1.2, according to the TFxIDF scoring system, frequently used in text mining applications (Shatkay & Feldman, 2003). The use of MeSH terms provides a phenotypic description in the disease area for the allelic variations of genes extracted from the literature, and provides an easy way to retrieve the variations that are associated to a certain disease.

EVALUATION

The performance of OSIRISv1.2 was assessed on a manually annotated corpus developed as described previously (Furlong et al., 2008). During the evaluation, both processes of identification of the terms that refer to variations and disambiguation of the terms to database identifiers (normalization) were assessed.

A comparison of the performance of all the current methodologies is shown in Table 2. Both versions of OSIRIS were evaluated on the corpus developed in our group. Regarding the other approaches, although the results of the evaluations carried out in each case are not directly comparable (different corpora and evaluation criteria were used), it serves as a rough comparison with these selected methods. The evaluation for OSIRISv1.2 showed satisfactory results for both precision and recall. The low recall of OSIRISv1.1 could be explained by the inability of the query expansion approach used by the system to recover all the variation specific terms. The recall was increased in the OSIRISv1.2 implementation by improvement of both the recognition of gene and variation terms. Regarding the other approaches, published results indicate that the MEMA system (Rebholz-Schuhmann et al., 2004) achieved a 75 % recall and 98 % precision for the recovery of mutations from texts. MEMA uses regular expressions for finding mutations-gene pairs, but it does not provide mapping to dbSNP entries. In this system, the association of a mutation with a gene is done by co-occurrence of both terms in a sentence. Contrasting, OSIRISv1.2 uses co-occurrence and a sequence based approach which provides a higher accuracy. The Vtag approach (McDonald et al., 2004), based on a probabilistic model to identify mutation terms, achieves a high recall level, but without providing mapping to

Table 2. Comparison of the performance of NER methods for sequence variants. OSIRISv1.1 and OSIRISv1.2 were evaluated on the corpus described in (Furlong et al., 2008). Performance of other methods correspond to published data for each development and different benchmarks, thus precluding a strict comparison. The results can only be considered for a rough comparison of the state of the art.

Method	Precision	Recall	F-score
OSIRISv1.1	0.97	0.3	0.46
OSIRISv1.2	0.99	0.82	0.89
Vtag	0.85	0.79	0.82
MuteXt	0.87	0.57	0.67
MEMA	0.98	0.75	0.85
MutationFinder	0.98	0.81	0.88

sequence database entries. MutationMiner had a similar performance than OSIRISv1.2, however this system only consider non synonymous SNPs at protein level and do not disambiguate the terms to database identifiers (Caporaso et al., 2007).The strategy used by OSIRISv1.2 provides a way to achieve recognition and mapping of variation terms to dbSNP identifiers with high precision and recall, which are very important features for database annotation purposes and mining information from text. The same strategy for normalization of variation terms to dbSNP identifiers has been implemented in combination with a machine learning approach with promising results (Klinger et al., 2007).

APPLICATION

To illustrate the utility of the approach, OSIRISv1.2 was used to compile a collection of literature references for the allelic variants of genes related with two complex human diseases: breast cancer and intracranial aneurysm and subarachnoid haemorrhage. The results are described in (Furlong et al., 2008) and can be queried through a web interface (http://ibi.imim.es/OSIRISv1.2.html). OSIRISv1.2 is able to collect results for any kind of variation present in reference repositories such as dbSNP. As can be seen in Table 3, for two selected genes among the ones that have been studied in relation to intracranial aneurysm (NOS3 and SERPINE1) the system found documents that mention SNPs located in different gene locations. In a similar way than other approaches, the system is able to find references to SNPs in coding regions of genes: the ones that most probably have an impact in the protein sequence (coding non synonymous SNPs). However, the approach is not limited to SNPs affecting the protein sequence, as the example of non synonymous coding SNPs, and is able to find citations of synonymous or silent SNPs, or SNPs located in other regions of genes, as such as 5' and 3' surrounding regions of genes, that may harbour important regulatory elements. In the small number of examples shown, it can be appreciated that the citations that mention these SNPs are annotated with MeSH disease terms, suggesting that these SNPs may have a functional relationship with the disease phenotype.

CONCLUSIONS AND PERSPECTIVES

We have presented the OSIRIS approach as a system for collecting the current knowledge about the allelic variants of genes from the literature. The evaluation of the system on a manually annotated corpus showed satisfactory results on both precision (99 %) and recall (89 %) for the recognition of variation terms and disambiguation to dbSNP identifiers. The approach here presented has the ability to identify any kind of short range variation independently of its genomic location or the gene to which is mapped to. In addition, it can resolve most cases of ambiguity in SNP identification by means of its normalization process.

To demonstrate the usefulness of the approach, OSIRISv1.2 was applied for the development of a database of literature references associated with allelic variants of genes related with human diseases. The approach illustrates the strategy for linking genetic variants of genes present in sequence databases, such as dbSNP, with disease terms of a controlled vocabulary through the literature. This is a general approach that could be used for developing databases focused in specific diseases of interest, or for mining functional consequences of sequence variants of genes from the literature. Several interesting pieces of information regarding related phenotypes and functional effects of variations can be easily obtained from the literature using OSIRISv1.2 (Furlong et al., 2008).

OSIRISv1.2 is focused in identifying the terms from text that represent variations from reference sequence repositories such as dbSNP. We

Table 3. Example of OSIRISv1.2 results for some SNPs mapped to genes NOS3 and SERPINE1. The identifiers for Gene Id and SNP Id represent NCBI identifiers. The MeSH Disease terms have been extracted from the set of documents annotated to each variation by OSIRISv1.2.

Gene Id	Gene Symbol	Description	SNP Id	Change	Location	MeSH Disease Terms
4846	NOS3	nitric oxide synthase 3	1549758	D258D	coding (synonymous change)	alpha 1-Antitrypsin Deficiency
						Emphysema
						Diabetic Retinopathy
						Diabetes Mellitus, Type 1
						Myocardial Infarction
			1799983	E298D	coding (non synonymous change)	Hypertension
						Coronary Arteriosclerosis
						Coronary Disease
						Cardiovascular Diseases
						Myocardial Infarction
						Pre-Eclampsia
						Carotid Artery Diseases
5054	SERPINE1	serpin peptidase inhibitor 1 or nexin or plasminogen activator inhibitor type 1	6092	T15A	coding (non synonymous change)	Metabolic Syndrome X
						Obesity
						Diabetic Angiopathies
						Diabetic Nephropathies
						Coronary Arteriosclerosis
						Hemorrhage
						Diabetes Mellitus, Type 1
						Myocardial Infarction
						Coronary Disease
			2227631	-914 A/G	in 5' region of gene	Metabolic Syndrome X
						Brain Ischemia
						Myocardial Infarction
						Coronary Disease
			7242	10993 G/T	in 3' UTR region of gene	Metabolic Syndrome X
						Myocardial Infarction

anticipate that a suitable application of OSIRISv1.2 would be for supporting the functional annotation of dbSNP entries. This is a relevant issue since the unravelling of the biological consequences of sequence variants remains a challenging task. The elucidation of the functional impact of predisposing SNP alleles identified by genome wide association studies has important implications in terms of understanding the underlying biology of complex diseases and identifying putative therapeutic targets. This is still a challenging task due to the scarcity of functionally annotated SNP data. In the field of pharmacogenomics, the identification of variations in drug metabolising enzymes is capital and we foresee a promising application in these field as well.

ACKNOWLEDGMENT

This work was generated in the framework of the @neurIST and the ALERT projects co-financed by the European Commission through the contracts no. IST-027703 and ICT-215847, respectively. The Research Unit on Biomedical Informatics (GRIB) is a node of the Spanish National Institute of Bioinformatics (INB). It is also member of the COMBIOMED network.

REFERENCES

Ananiadou, S., Kell, D. B., & Tsujii, J. (2006). Text mining and its potential applications in systems biology. *Trends Biotechnol, 24*(12), 571-579.

Ananiadou, S., & McNaught, J. (2006). *Text mining for biology and biomedicine*. Boston: Artech House.

Bonis, J., Furlong, L. I., & Sanz, F. (2006). OSIRIS: a tool for retrieving literature about sequence variants. *Bioinformatics, 22*(20), 2567-2569.

Brookes, A. J. (1999). The essence of SNPs. *Gene, 234*(2), 177-186.

Burton, P. R., Tobin, M. D., & Hopper, J. L. (2005). Key concepts in genetic epidemiology. *Lancet, 366*(9489), 941-951.

Caporaso, J. G., Baumgartner, W. A., Jr., Randolph, D. A., Cohen, K. B., & Hunter, L. (2007). MutationFinder: a high-performance system for extracting point mutation mentions from text. *Bioinformatics, 23*(14), 1862-1865.

den Dunnen, J. T., & Antonarakis, S. E. (2001). Nomenclature for the description of human sequence variations. *Hum Genet, 109*(1), 121-124.

Erdogmus, M., & Sezerman, O. U. (2007). Application of automatic mutation-gene pair extraction to diseases. *J Bioinform Comput Biol, 5*(6), 1261-1275.

Furlong, L. I., Dach, H., Hofmann-Apitius, M., & Sanz, F. (2008). OSIRISv1.2: a named entity recognition system for sequence variants of genes in biomedical literature. *BMC Bioinformatics, 9*(1), 84.

Hanisch, D., Fundel, K., Mevissen, H. T., Zimmer, R., & Fluck, J. (2005). ProMiner: rule-based protein and gene entity recognition. *BMC Bioinformatics, 6 Suppl 1*, S14.

Horn, F., Lau, A. L., & Cohen, F. E. (2004). Automated extraction of mutation data from the literature: application of MuteXt to G protein-coupled receptors and nuclear hormone receptors. *Bioinformatics, 20*(4), 557-568.

Jensen, L. J., Saric, J., & Bork, P. (2006). Literature mining for the biologist: from information retrieval to biological discovery. *Nat Rev Genet, 7*(2), 119-129.

Kanagasabai, R., Choo, K. H., Ranganathan, S., & Baker, C. J. (2007). A workflow for mutation extraction and structure annotation. *J Bioinform Comput Biol, 5*(6), 1319-1337.

Kimchi-Sarfaty, C., Oh, J. M., Kim, I. W., Sauna, Z. E., Calcagno, A. M., Ambudkar, S. V., et al. (2007). A "silent" polymorphism in the MDR1 gene changes substrate specificity. *Science, 315*(5811), 525-528.

Klinger, R., Friedrich, C. M., Mevissen, H. T., Fluck, J., Hofmann-Apitius, M., Furlong, L. I., et al. (2007). Identifying gene-specific variations in biomedical text. *J Bioinform Comput Biol, 5*(6), 1277-1296.

Lee, L. C., Horn, F., & Cohen, F. E. (2007). Automatic extraction of protein point mutations using a graph bigram association. *PLoS Comput Biol, 3*(2), e16.

Levy, S., Sutton, G., Ng, P. C., Feuk, L., Halpern, A. L., Walenz, B. P., et al. (2007). The diploid genome sequence of an individual human. *PLoS Biol, 5*(10), e254.

McDonald, R. T., Winters, R. S., Mandel, M., Jin, Y., White, P. S., & Pereira, F. (2004). An entity tagger for recognizing acquired genomic variations in cancer literature. *Bioinformatics, 20*(17), 3249-3251.

Park, J. C., & Kim, J.-j. (2006). Named Entity Recognition. In S. Ananiadou & J. McNaught (Eds.), *Text Mining for Biology and Biomedicine.* (pp. 121-142). London: Artech House Books.

Rebholz-Schuhmann, D., Marcel, S., Albert, S., Tolle, R., Casari, G., & Kirsch, H. (2004). Automatic extraction of mutations from Medline and cross-validation with OMIM. *Nucleic Acids Res, 32*(1), 135-142.

Shastry, B. S. (2007). SNPs in disease gene mapping, medicinal drug development and evolution. *J Hum Genet, 52*(11), 871-880.

Shatkay, H., & Feldman, R. (2003). Mining the biomedical literature in the genomic era: an overview. *J Comput Biol, 10*(6), 821-855.

Sherry, S. T., Ward, M., & Sirotkin, K. (1999). dbSNP-database for single nucleotide polymorphisms and other classes of minor genetic variation. *Genome Res, 9*(8), 677-679.

Chapter XVI
Verification of Uncurated Protein Annotations

Francisco M. Couto
Universidade de Lisboa, Portugal

Mário J. Silva
Universidade de Lisboa, Portugal

Vivian Lee
European Bioinformatics Institute, UK

Emily Dimmer
European Bioinformatics Institute, UK

Evelyn Camon
European Bioinformatics Institute, UK

Rolf Apweiler
European Bioinformatics Institute, UK

Harald Kirsch
European Bioinformatics Institute, UK

Dietrich Rebholz-Schuhmann
European Bioinformatics Institute, UK

ABSTRACT

Molecular Biology research projects produced vast amounts of data, part of which has been preserved in a variety of public databases. However, a large portion of the data contains a significant number of errors and therefore requires careful verification by curators, a painful and costly task, before being reliable enough to derive valid conclusions from it. On the other hand, research in biomedical information retrieval and information extraction are nowadays delivering Text Mining solutions that can support curators to improve the efficiency of their work to deliver better data resources. Over the past decades, automatic text processing systems have successfully exploited biomedical scientific literature to reduce the researchers' efforts to keep up to date, but many of these systems still rely on domain knowledge that is integrated manually leading to unnecessary overheads and restrictions in its use. A more efficient approach would acquire the domain knowledge automatically from publicly available biological sources, such as BioOntologies, rather than using manually inserted domain knowledge. An example of this approach is GOAnnotator, a tool that assists the verification of uncurated protein annotations. It provided correct evidence text at 93% precision to the curators and thus achieved promising results. GOAnnotator was implemented as a web tool that is freely available at http://xldb.di.fc.ul.pt/rebil/tools/goa/.

INTRODUCTION

A large portion of publicly available data provided in biomedical databases is still incomplete and incoherent (Devos and Valencia, 2001). This means that most of the data has to be handled with care and further validated by curators before we can use it to automatically draw valid conclusions from it. However, biomedical curators are overwhelmed by the amount of information that is published every day and are unable to verify all the data available. As a consequence, curators have verified only a small fraction of the available data. Moreover, this fraction tends to be even smaller given that the rate of data being produced is higher than the rate of data that curators are able to verify.

In this scenario, tools that could make the curators' task more efficient are much required. Biomedical information retrieval and extraction solutions are well established to provide support to curators by reducing the amount of information they have to seek manually. Such tools automatically identify evidence from the text that substantiates the data that curators need to verify. The evidence can, for example, be pieces of text published in BioLiterature (a shorter designation for the biological and biomedical scientific literature) describing experimental results supporting the data. As part of this process, it is not mandatory that the tools deliver high accuracy to be effective, since it is the task of the curators to verify the evidence given by the tool to ensure data quality. The main advantage of integrated text mining solutions lies in the fact that curators save time by filtering the retrieved evidence texts in comparison to scanning the full amount of available information. If the IT solution in addition provides the data in conjunction with the evidence supporting the data and if the solutions enable the curators to decide on their relevance and accuracy, it would surely make the task of curators more effective and efficient.

A real working scenario is given in the GOA (GO Annotation) project. The main objective of GOA is to provide high-quality GO (Gene Ontology) annotations to proteins that are kept in the UniProt Knowledgebase (Apweiler et al., 2004; Camon et al., 2004; GO-Consortium, 2004). Manual GO annotation produces high-quality and detailed GO term assignments (i.e. high granularity), but tends to be slow. As a result, currently less than 3% of UniProtKb has been confirmed by manual curation. For better coverage, the GOA team integrates uncurated GO annotations deduced from automatic mappings between UniProtKb and other manually curated databases (e.g. Enzyme Commission numbers or InterPro domains). Although these assignments have high accuracy, the GOA curators still have to verify them by extracting experimental results from peer-reviewed papers, which is time-consuming. This motivated the development of GOAnnotator, a tool for assisting the GO annotation of UniProtKb entries by linking the GO terms present in the uncurated annotations with evidence text automatically extracted from the documents linked to UniProtKb entries.

The remainder of this chapter starts by giving an overview on relevant research in biomedical information retrieval and extraction and exposing which contribution GOAnnotator brings to the current state-of-the-art. Afterwards, the chapter describes the main concepts of GOAnnotator and discusses its outcome and its main limitations, as well as proposals how the limitations can be solved in the future. Subsequently, the chapter provides insight into how approaches like GOAnnotator can change the way curators verify their data in the future, making the delivered data more complete and more reliable. For achieving this, the chapter will describe the issues that need to be addressed leading into valuable future research opportunities. The chapter ends by giving an overview of what was discussed and by presenting the concluding remarks.

BACKGROUND

A large amount of the information discovered in Molecular Biology has been mainly published in BioLiterature. However, analysing and identifying information in a large collection of unstructured texts is a painful and hard task, even to an expert.

BioLiterature

The notion of BioLiterature includes any type of scientific text related to Molecular Biology. The text is mainly available in the following formats:

1. **Statement:** a stretch of text that describes the protein similar to comment or description field of a database entry (e.g., in UniProtKb).
2. **Abstract:** a short summary of a scientific document.
3. **Full-text:** the full-text of a scientific document including scattered text such as figure labels and footnotes.

Statements contain more syntactic and semantic errors than abstracts, since they are not peer-reviewed, but they are directly linked to the facts stored in the databases. The main advantage of using statements or abstracts is the brief and succinct format on which the information is expressed. However, usually this brief description is insufficient to draw a solid conclusion, since the authors have to skip some important details given the text size constraint. These details can only be found in the full-text of a document, which contains a complete description of the results obtained. For example, important details are sometimes only present in figure labels.

The full-text document contains the complete information for the presented research. Unfortunately, full-text documents are not yet readily available, since up to now publishers' licensing agreements restrict access to most of the full-text content. In addition, the formats and structures of the full-text document tend to vary according to the needs of the journal in where the document has been published leading to unnecessary complications in processing the documents. Furthermore, processing of full-text documents in comparison to document summaries also increases the complexity for text-mining solutions, leading to the result that the availability of more information is not necessarily all-beneficial to text-mining tools. Some of the information may even induce the production of novel errors, for example, the value of a fact reported in the Results section has to be interpreted differently in comparison to a fact that has been reported in the Related Work section. Therefore, the use of full-text will also create several problems regarding the quality of information extracted (Shah et al., 2004).

Access to BioLiterature is mainly achieved through the PubMed Web portal, which in 2008 delivered more than 17 million[1] references to biomedical documents dating from the 1950s (Wheeler et al., 2003). It is the main task of PubMed to make it easier for the general public to find scientific results in the BioLiterature. The users can search for citations by author name, journal title or keywords. PubMed also includes links to full-text documents and other related resources. More than 96% of the citations available through PubMed are from MEDLINE, a large repository of citations to the BioLiterature indexed with NLM's controlled vocabulary, the Medical Subject Headings (MeSH). Besides the bibliographic citations, PubMed also provides the abstracts of most documents, especially of the newer ones. The articles from 1950 through 1965 are in OLDMEDLINE, which contains approximately 1.7 million citations (Demsey et al., 2003). These old citations do not contain the abstract and certain fields may contain outdated or erroneous data.

MEDLINE was designed to deal with printed documents, but nowadays many journals provide the electronic version of their documents. Moreover, some of them became Open Access Publications, which means that their documents are freely available and can be processed and displayed without any restrictions. These documents have been exploited by tools, such as Google Scholar[2], Scirus[3] or EBSCO[4], which can be used to search and locate scientific documents. One of the major free digital archives of life sciences full-text documents is PMC (PubMed Central), which aims at preserving and maintaining access to this new generation of electronic documents. Presently, PMC includes over 1.3 million documents. The availability of full-text documents offers new opportunities for research to text-mining tool providers, who were up to now often restricted to analysing only the abstracts of scientific documents.

Text Mining

An approach to improve the access to the knowledge published in BioLiterature is to use Text Mining, which aims at automatically retrieving and extracting knowledge from natural language text (Hearst, 1999). The application of text-mining tools to BioLiterature started just a few years ago (Andrade and Bork, 2000). Since then, the interest in the topic has been steadily increasing, motivated by the vast amount of documents that curators have to read to update biological databases, or simply to help researchers keep up with progress in a specific area (Couto and Silva, 2006). Thus, Bioinformatics tools are increasingly using Text Mining to collect more information about the concepts they analyse. Text-mining tools have mainly been used to identify:

1. **Entities**, such as genes, proteins and cellular components;
2. **Relationships**, such as protein localisation or protein interactions;
3. **Events**, such as experimental methods used to discover protein interactions.

One of the most important applications of text-mining tools is the automatic annotation of genes and proteins. A gene or protein annotation consists of a pair composed by the gene or protein and a description of its biological role. The biological role is often a concept from a BioOntology, which organises and describes biological concepts and their relationships. Using a BioOntology to annotate genes or proteins avoids ambiguous statements that are domain specific and context dependent. The best-known example is the gene ontology (GO) that is a well-established structured vocabulary that has been successfully designed and applied for gene annotation of different species (GO-Consortium, 2004). To understand the activity of a gene or protein, it is also important to know the biological entities that interact with it. Thus, the annotation of a gene or protein also involves identifying interacting chemical substances, drugs, genes and proteins.

Very early on the text-mining system AbXtract was developed to identify keywords from MEDLINE abstracts and to score their relevance for a protein family (Andrade and Valencia, 1998). Other systems have been developed in recent years to identify GO terms from the text: MeKE identified potential GO terms based on sequence alignment (Chiang and Yu, 2003) and BioIE uses syntactic dependencies to select GO terms from the text (Kim and Park, 2004). Furthermore, other approaches use IT solutions where GO terminology is applied as a dictionary (Koike et al., 2005; Müller et al., 2004; Pérez et al., 2004; Rebholz-Schuhmann et al., 2007; Jaeger et al., 2008). However, none of these systems have been integrated into the GOA curation process. Moreover, only Perez et al. make use of the hierarchical structure of GO to measure the distance between two terms based on the number of edges that separate them (path length). However, incorrect annotations can be caused by neglecting the semantics of the hierarchical structure of GO causes. For example, if a large number of GO terms from the leaves or the deep levels in GO are assigned then the system tends to generate over-predictions, and if general GO terms from the top levels of the hierarchy are produced then the annotations tend to be useless.

The performance of state-of-the-art text-mining tools for automatic annotation of genes or proteins is still not acceptable by curators, since gene or protein annotation is more subjective and requires more expertise than simply finding relevant documents and recognising biological entities in texts. To improve their performance, state-of-the-art text-mining tools use domain knowledge manually inserted by curators (Yeh et al., 2003). This knowledge consists of rules inferred from patterns identified in the text, or on predefined sets of previously annotated texts. The integration of domain knowledge improves overall the precision of predictions, but it cannot be easily extended to work on other domains and demands an extra effort to keep the knowledge updated as BioLiterature evolves.

The selection of pieces of text that mention a GO term was assessed as part of the first BioCreAtIvE competition (Hirschman et al., 2005). This competition enabled the assessment of different text mining approaches and their ability to assist curators. The system with the best precision predicted 41 annotations, but 27 were not correct, which lead to a 35% precision (14 out of 41) (Chiang and Yu, 2004). The main problem is that the terms denoting GO concepts were never designed to support text-mining solutions. Terms in the vocabulary are ambiguous and could not be easily deciphered by automatic processing and sometimes even by humans (Camon et al., 2005). Without improvements to the precision, such automatic extractions are unhelpful to curators. This reflects the importance of designing more efficient tools to aid in the curation effort.

GOAnnotator uses publicly available biological data sources as domain knowledge for improving the retrieval and extraction tasks requiring minimal human intervention, since it avoids the complexities of creating rules and patterns covering all possible cases or creating training sets that are too specific to be extended to new domains (Shatkay and Feldman, 2003). Apart from avoiding direct human intervention, automatically collected domain knowledge is usually more extensive than manually generated domain knowledge and does not become outdated as easily, if the originating public databases can be automatically tracked for updates as they evolve. The most important data resource used by GOAnnotator is GO.

GENE ONTOLOGY (GO)

The GO project is one of the long-lasting and successful resource building efforts in Molecular Biology constructing a BioOntology of broad scope and wide applicability (Bada et al., 2004). GO provides a structured controlled vocabulary denoting the diversity of biological roles of genes and proteins in a species-independent way (GO-Consortium, 2004). GO comprised 24,397 distinct terms in September 2007. Since the activity or function of a protein can be defined at different levels, GO is composed of three different aspects: *molecular function, biological process* and *cellular component*. Each protein has elementary molecular functions that normally are independent of the environment, such as catalytic or binding activities. Sets of proteins interact and are involved in cellular processes, such as metabolism, signal transduction or RNA processing. Proteins can act in different cellular localisations, such as the nucleus or membrane.

GO organises the concepts as a DAG (Directed Acyclic Graph), one for each aspect. Each node of the graph represents a concept, and the edges represent the links between concepts (see example in Figure 1). Links can represent two relationship types: *is-a* and *part-of*. The content of GO is still evolving dynamically: its content changes every month with the publication of a new release. Any user can request modifications to GO, which is maintained by a group of curators who add, remove and change terms and their relationships in response to modification requests. This prevents GO from becoming outdated and from providing incorrect information.

GOAnnotator

GOAnnotator is a tool for assisting the GO annotation of UniProtKb entries by linking the GO terms present in the uncurated annotations with evidence text automatically extracted from the documents

Figure 1. Sub-graph of GO

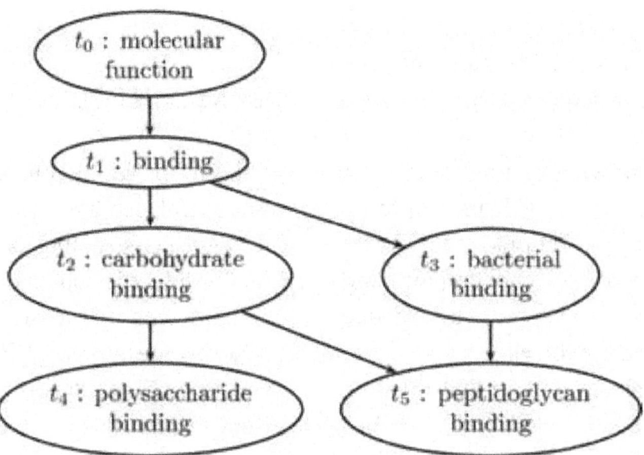

Figure 2. List of documents related with a given protein. The list is sorted by the most similar term extracted from each document. The curator can use the Extract option to see the extracted terms together with the evidence text. By default GOAnnotator uses only the abstract, but the curator can use the AddText option to replace or insert text.

PubMedId	Title	MostSimilarTermExtracted	Scope	Authors	Year	Extract	AddText
11594756(FullText)	Distinct phosphoinositide binding specificity of the GAP1 family proteins: characterization of the pleckstrin homology domains of MRASAL and KIAA0538.	100% GTPase activator activity (f)	GeneRIF	3	2001	Pre-Processed	Text
11448776(FullText)	CAPRI regulates Ca(2+)-dependent inactivation of the Ras-MAPK pathway.	100% GTPase activator activity (f)	SEQUENCE FROM N.A.	3	2001	Pre-Processed	Text
9628581(FullText)	Prediction of the coding sequences of unidentified human genes. IX. The complete sequences of 100 new cDNA clones from brain which can code for large proteins in vitro.	28% cell communication (p)	SEQUENCE FROM N.A.	7	1998	Pre-Processed	Text
14702039(FullText)	Complete sequencing and characterization of 21,243 full-length human cDNAs.	-	GeneRIF	154	2004	Pre-Processed	Text
12853948(FullText)	The DNA sequence of human chromosome 7.	-	SEQUENCE FROM N.A.	107	2003	Pre-Processed	Text

linked to UniProtKb entries. Initially, the curator provides a UniProtKb accession number to GOAnnotator. GOAnnotator follows the bibliographic links found in the UniProtKb database and retrieves the documents. Additional documents are retrieved from the GeneRIF database or curators can add any other text (Mitchell et al., 2003). GOAnnotator prioritizes the documents according to the extracted GO terms from the text and their similarity to the GO terms present in the protein uncurated annotations (see Figure 2).

Any extracted GO term is an indication for the topic of the document, which is also taken from the UniProtKb entry. The curator uses the topic as a hint to potential GO annotation.

The extraction of GO terms is based on FiGO, a method used for the BioCreAtIvE competition (Couto et al., 2005). FiGO receives a piece of text and returns the GO terms that were detected in the given text. To each selected GO term, FiGO assigns a confidence value that represents the terms' likelihood of being mentioned in the text. The confidence value is the ratio of two parameters. The first parameter is called local evidence context and is used to measure the likelihood that words in the text are part of a given GO term. The second parameter is a correction parameter, which increases the confidence value when the words detected in the text are infrequent in GO. In BioCreAtIvE, FiGO predicted 673 annotations but 615 were not correct, which lead to a 8.6% precision (58 of 673). The low performance is the result of the finding that GO terms are not explicitly used in the literature to annotate proteins. As a consequence, contextual information has to be taken into consideration to extract the correct annotations. It is advantageous to this process if additional domain knowledge can be integrated. For instance, experiments performed as part of the KDD2002 Cup challenge (bio-text task) have shown that the statistical text classification systems generate low performance if they refrain from integrating domain knowledge into their reasoning (Yeh et al., 2003). A more effective approach has been used by GOAnnotator. Here the necessary domain knowledge has been acquired from publicly available resources and significantly improves the precision to the annotation process for yet uncurated resources.

GO terms are considered to be similar if they are in the same lineage or if they share a common parent in the GO hierarchy. To calculate a similarity value between two GO terms, we decided to implement a semantic similarity measure. Research on Information Theory proposed many semantic similarity measures. Some of them calculate maximum likelihood estimates for each concept using the corpora, and then calculate the similarity between probability distributions. Semantic similarity measures take into consideration a combination of parameters linked to the structure of an ontology as well as information content based on statistical data from corpora (Rada et al., 1989). The information content of a concept is inversely proportional to its frequency in the corpora. Concepts that are frequent in the corpora have low information content. In case of GO the corpora used to derive the statistical information is the annotations provided by GO, i.e. the information content of a GO term is calculated based on the number of proteins annotated to it. For example, GO terms annotated to most of the proteins normally provide little semantic information.

Many semantic similarity measures applied to ontologies have been developed. We implemented a measure based on the ratio between the information content of the most informative common ancestor and the information content of both concepts (Lin, 1998). Recent studies have explored on the effectiveness of semantic similarity measures over the GO (Couto et al., 2006; Lord et al., 2003; Gaudan et al., 2008). The results have shown that GO similarity is correlated with sequence and family similarity, i.e., they demonstrated the feasibility of using semantic similarity measures in a biological setting.

GOAnnotator displays a table for each uncurated annotation with the GO terms that were extracted from a document and were similar to the GO term present in the uncurated annotation (see Figure 3). The sentences from which the GO terms were extracted are also displayed. Words that have contributed to the extraction of the GO terms are highlighted. GOAnnotator gives the curators the opportunity to manipulate the confidence and similarity thresholds to modify the number of predictions.

RESULTS

The GOA team curated 66 proteins out of a list of 1,953 uncurated UniProtKb/SwissProt proteins that GOAnnotator analysed. This 66 proteins were selected by applying a similarity threshold of 40% and a confidence threshold of 50%. In other words, GOAnnotator identified evidence texts with at least 40% similarity and 50% confidence to selected GO terms for all these 66 proteins. These proteins had 80 uncurated annotations that GOAnnotator analysed, providing 89 similar annotations and the respective evidence text from 118 MEDLINE abstracts. The 80 uncurated annotations included 78 terms from different domains of GO (see Table 1).

After curating the 89 evidence texts, GOA curators found that 83 were valid to substantiate 77 distinct uncurated annotations (see Table 2), i.e. 93% precision.

Table 3 shows that 78% (65 out of 83) of the correct evidence texts confirmed the uncurated annotations, i.e. the extracted annotation and the uncurated annotation contained the same GO identifier. In cases where the evidence text was correct, it did not always contain exactly any of the known variations of the extracted GO term. In the other cases the extracted GO term was similar: in 15 cases the extracted GO term was in the same lineage of the GO term in the uncurated annotation; in 3 cases the extracted GO

Figure 3. Identified and proposed GO terms. For every selected uncurated database resource, GOAnnotator identifies and proposes GO terms extracted from the selected document and displays the sentence that contains the evidence for the GO term. If the curator accepts the evidence as a correct annotation then he can use the Add option to store the annotation together with the document reference, the evidence codes and any comments in the database.

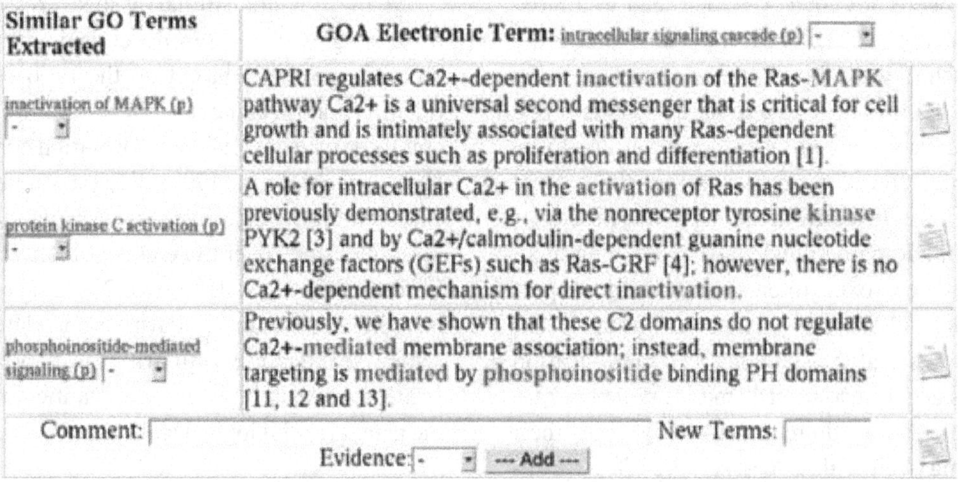

Similar GO Terms Extracted	GOA Electronic Term: intracellular signaling cascade (p) -	
inactivation of MAPK (p) -	CAPRI regulates Ca2+-dependent inactivation of the Ras-MAPK pathway Ca2+ is a universal second messenger that is critical for cell growth and is intimately associated with many Ras-dependent cellular processes such as proliferation and differentiation [1].	
protein kinase C activation (p) -	A role for intracellular Ca2+ in the activation of Ras has been previously demonstrated, e.g., via the nonreceptor tyrosine kinase PYK2 [3] and by Ca2+/calmodulin-dependent guanine nucleotide exchange factors (GEFs) such as Ras-GRF [4]; however, there is no Ca2+-dependent mechanism for direct inactivation.	
phosphoinositide-mediated signaling (p) -	Previously, we have shown that these C2 domains do not regulate Ca2+-mediated membrane association; instead, membrane targeting is mediated by phosphoinositide binding PH domains [11, 12 and 13].	
Comment:	New Terms: Evidence: - --- Add ---	

Table 1. Distribution of the GO terms from the selected uncurated annotations through the different aspects of GO

GO Aspect	GO Terms
molecular function	54
biological process	18
cellular component	6
total	78

Table 2. Evaluation of the evidence text substantiating uncurated annotations provided by the GOAnnotator

Evidence Evaluation	Extracted Annotations
correct	83
incorrect	6
total	89

term was in a different lineage, but both terms were similar (share a parent). In general, we can expect GOAnnotator to confirm the uncurated annotation using the findings from the scientific literature, but it is also obvious that GOAnnotator can propose new GO terms.

Examples

GOAnnotator provided correct evidence for the uncurated annotation of the protein "Human Complement factor B precursor" (P00751) with the term "complement activation, alternative pathway" (GO:0006957). The evidence is the following sentence from the document with the PubMed identifier 8225386: "The human complement factor B is a centrally important component of the alternative pathway activation of the complement system."

GOAnnotator provided a correct evidence for the uncurated annotation of the protein "U4/U6 small nuclear ribonucleoprotein Prp3" (O43395) with the term "nuclear mRNA splicing, via spliceosome" (GO:0000398). From the evidence the tool extracted the child term "regulation of nuclear mRNA splicing, via spliceosome" (GO:0048024). The evidence is the following sentence from the document with the PubMed identifier 9328476: "Nuclear RNA splicing occurs in an RNA-protein complex, termed the spliceosome." However, this sentence does not provide enough evidence on its own, the curator had to analyze other parts of the document to draw a conclusion.

GOAnnotator provided a correct evidence for the uncurated annotation of the protein "Agmatinase" (Q9BSE5) with the term "agmatinase activity" (GO:0008783). From the evidence the tool extracted the term "arginase activity" (GO:0004053) that shares a common parent. The evidence was provided by the following sentence from the document with the PubMed identifier 11804860: "Residues required for binding of Mn(2+) at the active site in bacterial agmatinase and other members of the arginase superfamily are fully conserved in human agmatinase." However, the annotation only received a NAS (Non-traceable author statement) evidence code, as the sentence does not provide direct experimental evidence of arginase activity. Papers containing direct experimental evidence for the function/subcellular location of a protein are more valuable to GO curators.

GOAnnotator provided a correct evidence for the uncurated annotation of the protein "3'-5' exonuclease ERI1" (Q8IV48) with the term "exonuclease activity" (GO:0004527). The evidence is the following sentence from the document with the PubMed identifier 14536070: "Using RNA affinity purification, we identified a second protein, designated 3'hExo, which contains a SAP and a 3' exonuclease domain and binds the same sequence." However, the term "exonuclease activity" is too high level, and a more precise annotation should be "3'-5' exonuclease activity" (GO:0008408).

Table 3. Comparison between the extracted GO terms with correct evidence text and the GO terms from the uncurated annotations

GO Terms	Extracted Annotations
exact	65
same lineage	15
different lineage	3
total	83

Discussion

Researchers need more than facts, they need the source from which the facts derive (Rebholz-Schuhmann et al., 2005). GOAnnotator provides not only facts but also their evidence, since it links existing annotations to scientific literature. GOAnnotator uses text-mining methods to extract GO terms from scientific papers and provides this information together with a GO term from an uncurated annotation. In general, we can expect GOAnnotator to confirm the uncurated annotation using the findings from the scientific literature, but it is obvious as well that GOAnnotator can propose new GO terms. In both cases, the curator profits from the integration of both approaches into a single interface. By comparing both results, the curator gets convenient support to take a decision for a curation item based on the evidence from the different data resources.

GOAnnotator provided correct evidence text at 93% precision, and in 78% of these cases the GO term present in the uncurated annotation was confirmed. These results were obtained for a small subset of the total number of uncurated annotations, but it represents already a significant set for curators. Notice that manual GO annotation covers less than 3% of UniProtKb. Over time, proteins tend to be annotated with more accurate uncurated terms and bibliography. Thus, the percentage of uncurated proteins satisfying the 40% similarity and 50% confidence thresholds will grow, and therefore make GOAnnotator even more effective.

Sometimes, the displayed sentence from the abstract of a document did not contain enough information for the curators to evaluate an evidence text with sufficient confidence. Apart from the association between a protein and a GO term, the curator needs additional information, such as the type of experiments performed and the species from which the protein originates. Unfortunately, quite often this information is only available in the full text of the scientific publication. GOAnnotator can automatically retrieve the abstracts, but in the case of the full text the curator has to copy and paste the text into the GOAnnotator interface, which only works for a limited number of documents. BioRAT solves this problem by retrieving full text documents from the Internet (Corney et al., 2004). In addition, the list of documents cited in the UniProtKb database was not sufficient for the curation process. In most cases, the curators found additional sources of information in PubMed. In the future, GOAnnotator should be able to automatically query PubMed using the protein's names to provide a more complete list of documents.

GOAnnotator ensures high accuracy, since all GO terms that did not have similar GO terms in the uncurated annotations were rejected. Using this 40% similarity threshold may filter out meaningful potential annotations that are not similar to known curated annotations. However, without this restriction the results returned by the text mining method would contain too much noise to be of any use to curators, as it was demonstrated in the BioCreAtIvE competition. GOAnnotator meets the GOA team's need for tools with high precision in preference to those with high recall, and explains the strong restriction for the similarity of two GO terms: only those that were from the same lineage or had a shared parent were accepted. Thus, GOAnnotator not only predicted the exact uncurated annotation but also more specific GO annotations, which was of strong interest to the curators. MeKE selected a significant number of general terms from the GO hierarchy (Chiang and Yu, 2003). Others distinguished between gene and family names to deal with general terms (Koike et al., 2005). GOAnnotator takes advantage of uncurated annotations to avoid general terms by extracting only similar terms, i.e. popular proteins tend to be annotated to specific terms and therefore GOAnnotator will also extract specific annotations to them.

The applied text-mining method FiGO was designed for recognizing terms and not for extracting annotations, i.e. sometimes the GO term is correctly extracted but is irrelevant to the actual protein of interest. The method also generated mispredictions in the instances where all the words of a GO term appeared in disparate locations of a sentence or in an unfortunate order. Improvements can result from the incorporation of better syntactical analysis into the identification of GO terms similar to the techniques used by BioIE (Kim and Park, 2004). For example, a reduction of the window size of FiGO or the identification of noun phrases can further increase precision. In the future, GOAnnotator can also use other type of text-mining methods that prove to be more efficient for extracting annotations.

FUTURE TRENDS

Recent publications on the improvements by using information retrieval and extraction tools are promising and encourage the research community to make an effort to improve their quality and expand their scope. However, the performance of most tools is still highly dependent on domain knowledge provided through experts. Integration of the expert knowledge is time-consuming and imposes limitations whenever services have to be extended to other domains with different user requirements. On the other side, the domain of molecular biology draws profits from publicly available databases containing a significant amount of information. In our opinion, better use of such domain knowledge and automatic integration of the data from these biological information resources will be the key to develop more efficient tools and will thus contribute to their wider acceptance among curators in the biological domain. Apart from avoiding direct human intervention, automatic collection of domain relevant information is usually more comprehensive than any manually generated representation of domain knowledge and does not become outdated, since public databases can be automatically tracked for updates as they evolve.

Domain knowledge is only available thanks to the research community efforts in developing accurate and valuable data resources and by making them publicly available. These data resources are continually being updated with more information. However, they are still too incomplete, too inconsistent and/or too morpho-syntactically inflexible to efficiently be used by automatic tools. For example, GO started by adding generic terms and simple relationships to provide a complete coverage of the Molecular Biology domain. Thus, the main limitation of GO is the lack of specific terms that, for example, represent precise biochemical reactions like EC numbers. However, as different research communities understand the importance of adding their domain knowledge to GO, it will expand its coverage and improve its interoperability with other data sources. While BioOntologies are traditionally used mainly for annotation purposes, their ultimate goal should be to accurately represent the domain knowledge so as to allow automated reasoning and support knowledge extraction. The establishment of guiding principles, as in OBO, to guide the development of new BioOntologies is a step in this direction, by promoting formality, enforcing orthogonality, and proposing a common syntax that facilitates mapping between BioOntologies. This not only improves the quality of individual BioOntologies, but also enables a more effective use of them by information retrieval and extraction tools.

CONCLUSION

This chapter introduced the biomedical information retrieval and extraction research topics and how their solutions can help curators to improve the effectiveness and efficiency of their tasks. It gives an overview on three important aspects of these research topics: BioLiterature, Text Mining and BioOntologies.

It has presented GOAnnotator, a system that automatically identifies evidence text in literature for GO annotation of UniProtKb/SwissProt proteins. GOAnnotator provided evidence text at high precision (93%, 66 sample proteins) taking advantage of existing uncurated annotations and the GO hierarchy. GOAnnotator assists the curation process by allowing fast verification of uncurated annotations from evidence texts, which can also be the source for novel annotations. This document discusses the results obtained by GOAnnotator pointing out its main limitations. This document ends by providing insight into the issues that need to be addressed in this research area and represent good future research opportunities.

The approach developed here constitutes a small and relatively early contribution to the advance of biomedical information retrieval and extraction topics, but the main idea presented here seems promising and the results encourage further study. Still, despite all the limitations presented here, many relevant biological discoveries in the future will certainly result from an efficient exploitation of the existing and newly generated data by tools like GOAnnotator.

ACKNOWLEDGMENT

This work was supported by the Marie Curie Training Sites scheme of the European Commission's Quality of Life Programme (Contract no. QLRI-1999-50595) and by FCT through the Multiannual Funding Programme.

REFERENCES

Andrade, M., & Bork, P. (2000). Automated extraction of information in Molecular Biology. *FEBS Letters*, *476*, 12–17.

Andrade, M., & Valencia, A. (1998). Automatic extraction of keywords from scientific text: Application to the knowledge domain of protein families. *Bioinformatics*, *14*(7), 600–607.

Apweiler, R., Bairoch, A., Wu, C., Barker, W., Boeckmann, B., Ferro, S., Gasteiger, E., Huang, H., Lopez, R., Magrane, M., Martin, M., Natale, D., O'Donovan, C., Redaschi, N., & Yeh, L. (2004). UniProt: the universal protein knowledgebase. *Nucleic Acids Research*, *32*(Database issue), D115–D119.

Bada, M., Stevens, R., Goble, C., Gil, Y., Ashburner, M., Blake, J., Cherry, J., Harris, M., & Lewis, S. (2004). A short study on the success of the gene ontology. *Journal of Web Semantics*, *1*(1), 235–240.

Camon, E., Barrell, D., Dimmer, E., Lee, V., Magrane, M., Maslen, J., Binns, D., & Apweiler, R. (2005). An evaluation of GO annotation retrieval for BioCreAtIvE and GOA. *BMC Bioinformatics*, *6*(Suppl 1), S17.

Camon, E., Magrane, M., Barrell, D., Lee, V., Dimmer, E., Maslen, J., Binns, D., Harte, N., Lopez, R., & Apweiler, R. (2004). The Gene Ontology Annotations (GOA) database: sharing knowledge in UniProt with Gene Ontology. *Nucleic Acids Research*, *32*, 262–266.

Chiang, J., & Yu, H. (2003). MeKE: discovering the functions of gene products from biomedical literature via sentence alignment. *Bioinformatics*, *19*(11), 1417–1422.

Chiang, J., & Yu, H. (2004). Extracting functional annotations of proteins based on hybrid text mining approaches. In *Proc. of the BioCreAtIvE Challenge Evaluation Workshop*.

Corney, D., Buxton, B., Langdon, W., & Jones, D. (2004). BioRAT: Extracting biological information from full-length papers. *Bioinformatics*, 20(17), 3206–3213.

Couto, F., & Silva, M. (2006). Mining the BioLiterature: towards automatic annotation of genes and proteins. In *Advanced Data Mining Techonologies in Bioinformatics*, Idea Group Inc.

Couto, F., Silva, M., & Coutinho, P. (2005). Finding genomic ontology terms in text using evidence content. *BMC Bioinformatics*, *6*(S1), S21.

Couto, F., Silva, M., & Coutinho, P. (2006). Measuring semantic similarity between gene ontology terms. *DKE - Data and Knowledge Engineering, Elsevier Science (in press).*

Demsey, A., Nahin, A., & Braunsberg, S. V. (2003). Oldmedline citations join pubmed. *NLM Technical Bulletin*, *334*(e2).

Devos, D., & Valencia, A. (2001). Intrinsic errors in genome annotation. *Trends Genetics*, *17*(8), 429–431.

Gaudan, S., Jimeno, A., Lee, V., & Rebholz-Schuhmann, D. (2008) Combining evidence, specificity and proximity towards the normalization of Gene Ontology terms in text. *EURASIP JBSB* (accepted).

GO-Consortium (2004). The Gene Ontology (GO) database and informatics resource. *Nucleic Acids Research*, *32*(Database issue), D258–D261.

Hearst, M. (1999). Untangling text data mining. In *Proc. of the 37th Annual Meeting of the Association for Computational Linguistics.*

Hirschman, L., Yeh, A., Blaschke, C., & Valencia, A. (2005). Overview of BioCreAtIvE: critical assessment of information extraction for biology. *BMC Bioinformatics*, *6*(Suppl 1), S1.

Jaeger, S., Gaudan, S., Leser, U., & Rebholz-Schuhmann, D. (2008). Integrating Protein-Protein Interactions and Text Mining for Protein Function Prediction. *Data Integration in The Life Sciences (DILS 2008)*, Evry June 25-27 2008 (accepted for publication in BMC Bioinformatics).

Kim, J., & Park, J. (2004). BioIE: retargetable information extraction and ontological annotation of biological interactions from literature. *Journal of Bioinformatics and Computational Biology*, *2*(3), 551–568.

Koike, A., Niwa, Y., & Takagi, T. (2005). Automatic extraction of gene/protein biological functions from biomedical text. *Bioinformatics*, *21*(7), 1227–1236.

Lin, D. (1998). An information-theoretic definition of similarity. In *Proc. of the 15th International Conference on Machine Learning.*

Lord, P., Stevens, R., Brass, A., & Goble, C. (2003). Investigating semantic similarity measures across the Gene Ontology: the relationship between sequence and annotation. *Bioinformatics*, *19*(10), 1275–1283.

Mitchell, J., Aronson, A., Mork, J., Folk, L., Humphrey, S., & Ward, J. (2003). Gene indexing: characterization and analysis of NLM's GeneRIFs. In *Proc. of the AMIA 2003 Annual Symposium.*

Müller, H., Kenny, E., & Sternberg, P. (2004). Textpresso: an ontology-based information retrieval and extraction system for biological literature. *PLOS Biology*, *2*(11), E309.

Pérez, A., Perez-Iratxeta, C., Bork, P., Thode, G., & Andrade, M. (2004). Gene annotation from scientific literature using mappings between keyword systems. *Bioinformatics*, *20*(13), 2084–2091.

Rada, R., Mili, H., Bicknell, E., & Blettner, M. (1989). Development and application of a metric on semantic nets. *IEEE Transactions on Systems*, *19*(1), 17–30.

Rebholz-Schuhmann, D., Kirsch, H., & Couto, F. (2005). Facts from text - is text mining ready to deliver? *PLoS Biology*, *3*(2), e65.

Rebholz-Schuhmann, D., Kirsch, H., Gaudan, M. A. S., Rynbeek, M., & Stoehr, P. (2007). EBIMed - text crunching to gather facts for proteins from Medline. *Bioinformatics*, *23*(2) e237–44.

Shah, P., Perez-Iratxeta, C., Bork, P., & Andrade, M. (2004). Information extraction from full text scientific articles: Where are the keywords? *BMC Bioinformatics*, *4*(20).

Shatkay, H., & Feldman, R. (2003). Mining the biomedical literature in the genomic era: An overview. *Journal of Computational Biology*, *10*(6), 821–855.

Wheeler, D., Church, D., Federhen, S., Lash, A., Madden, T., Pontius, J., Schuler, G., Schriml, L., Sequeira, E., Tatusova, T., & Wagner, L. (2003). Database resources of the national center for biotechnology. *Nucleic Acids Research*, *31*(1), 28–33.

Yeh, A., Hirschman, L., & Morgan, A. (2003). Evaluation of text data mining for database curation: Lessons learned from the KDD challenge cup. *Bioinformatics*, *19*(1), i331–i339.

ENDNOTES

1 http://www.nlm.nih.gov/bsd/licensee/baselinestats.html

2 http://scholar.google.com/

3 http://www.scirus.com/

4 http://www.epnet.com/

Chapter XVII
A Software Tool for Biomedical Information Extraction (And Beyond)

Burr Settles
University of Wisconsin-Madison, USA

ABSTRACT

ABNER (A Biomedical Named Entity Recognizer) is an open-source software tool for text mining in the molecular biology literature. It processes unstructured biomedical documents in order to discover and annotate mentions of genes, proteins, cell types, and other entities of interest. This task, known as named entity recognition (NER), is an important first step for many larger information management goals in biomedicine, namely extraction of biochemical relationships, document classification, information retrieval, and the like. To accomplish this task, ABNER uses state-of-the-art machine learning models for sequence labeling called conditional random fields (CRFs). The software distribution comes bundled with two models that are pre-trained on standard evaluation corpora. ABNER can run as a stand-alone application with a graphical user interface, or be accessed as a Java API allowing it to be re-trained with new labeled corpora and incorporated into other, higher-level applications. This chapter describes the software and its features, presents an overview of the underlying technology, and provides a discussion of some of the more advanced natural language processing systems for which ABNER has been used as a component. ABNER is open-source and freely available from http://pages.cs.wisc.edu/~bsettles/abner/

INTRODUCTION

Efforts to organize the wealth of biomedical knowledge in the primary literature have resulted in hundreds of databases and other resources (Bateman, 2008), providing scientists with access to structured biological information. However, with nearly half a million new research articles added to PubMed annually (Soteriades & Falagas, 2005), the sheer volume of publications and complexity of the knowledge to be extracted is beyond the means of most manual database curation efforts. As a result, many of these resources struggle to remain current. Automated *information extraction* (IE), or at least automated assistance for such extraction tasks, seems a natural way to overcome these information management bottlenecks.

Named entity recognition (NER) is a subtask of IE, focused on finding mentions of various *entities* that belong to semantic classes of interest. In the biomedical domain, entities of interest are usually references to genes, proteins, cell types, and the like. Accurate NER systems are an important first step for many larger information management goals, such as automatic extraction of biologically relevant relationships (e.g., protein-protein interactions or sub-cellular location of gene products), biomedical document classification and retrieval, and ultimately the automatic maintenance of biomedical databases.

In order to facilitate and encourage research in the area of biomedical NER, several "bake-off" style competitions have been organized, in particular the NLPBA shared task (Kim et al., 2004) and the BioCreative challenge (Yeh et al., 2005). For these events, several research teams rapidly design, build, and submit results for machine learning systems using benchmark annotated text collections. The challenges showcase a variety of approaches to the problem, and provide a wealth of insights into what sorts of models and features are most effective. However, few of the resulting systems have been made publicly available for researchers working in related areas of natural language processing (NLP) in biomedicine.

Figure 1. A screenshot of ABNER's graphical user interface

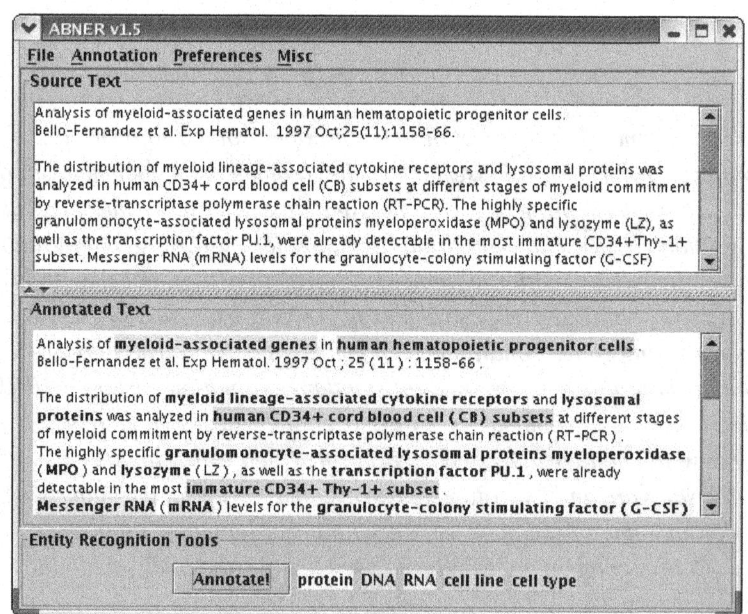

I first released ABNER (Settles, 2005) in July 2004 as a demonstrational graphical user interface (GUI) for the system I developed as part of the NLPBA shared task challenge (Settles, 2004). In March 2005, a revised, open-source version of the software was released with some performance improvements and a new Java application programming interface (API). The goal is to encourage others to write custom interfaces to the core NER software, allowing it to be integrated into other, more sophisticated biomedical information management systems. ABNER also supports training new models on corpora labeled for different knowledge domains (e.g., particular organisms, since gene naming conventions vary from species to species).

Figure 1 shows a screenshot of the intuitive GUI when ABNER is run as a stand-alone application. Text can be typed in manually or loaded from a file (top window), and then automatically tagged for multiple entities in real time (bottom window). Each entity type is highlighted with a unique color for easy visual reference, and tagged documents can be saved in a variety of annotated file formats. The application also has options for processing plain text documents on the file system in batch mode offline.

ABNER has built-in functionality for tokenization and sentence segmentation, which are fairly robust to line breaks and biomedical abbreviations (users can choose to bypass these features in favor of their own text preprocessing as well). The bundled ABNER application is implemented in Java and is therefore platform-independent, and has been tested on Linux, Solaris, Mac OS X, and Windows.

The basic ABNER distribution includes two built-in entity-tagging models trained on the NLPBA (Kim et al., 2004) and BioCreative (Yeh et al., 2005) corpora. The first is a modified version of the GENIA corpus (Kim et al., 2003), containing five entity types labeled for 18,546 training sentences and 3,856 evaluation sentences. The latter corpus contains only one entity type that subsumes both genes and gene products (proteins, RNA, etc.) labeled for 7,500 training sentences and 2,500 evaluation sentences. Evaluation of NER systems is typically done in terms of recall $R = tp/(tp+fn)$, precision $P = tp/(tp+fp)$, and the harmonic mean as a summary statistic, $F_1 = (2 \times R \times P)/(R+P)$, where tp means true positives, fn means false negatives, and fp means false positives. Table 1 presents results for the two built-in models, trained and evaluated on the designated train/evaluation splits for these corpora.

ABNER's accuracy is still roughly state-of-the-art. To my knowledge, only two systems with published results have outperformed ABNER on the NLPBA corpus (Zhou & Su, 2004; Friedrich et al., 2006), and neither is freely available. Comparisons to published results on the BioCreative corpus are more difficult to interpret, as the figures

Table 1. Evaluation results for ABNER's two built-in tagging models

Corpus	Recall	Precision	F1
NLPBA (all entities)	0.720	0.691	0.705
protein	0.778	0.681	0.726
DNA	0.631	0.672	0.651
RNA	0.619	0.613	0.616
cell line	0.582	0.539	0.560
cell type	0.656	0.798	0.720
BioCreative (gene)	0.659	0.745	0.699

in Table 1 reflect only perfectly accurate entity predictions (i.e., exact word-boundary matches), and official BioCreative evaluation gives some "partial credit" to incomplete entity extractions (Yeh et al., 2005). When adjusted for this, ABNER is competitive with the leading systems on this corpus as well, and is again the only freely available open-source system among them.

Third-party research also indicates that ABNER is among the most accurate publicly available NER tools for biomedical text. Kabiljo et al. (2007) performed a comparative analysis of three systems: ABNER (using the BioCreative model), GAPSCORE (Chang et al., 2004), and NLProt (Mika & Rost, 2004) on a new benchmark corpus called ProSpecTome, which is a subset of NLPBA re-annotated with more stringent labeling conventions. They found ABNER to be the most accurate on this new corpus by a significant margin. Lam et al. (2006) also conducted an informal comparison of ABNER (using the NLPBA model) to PowerBioNE (Zhou et al., 2004) when deciding which to use as a component in their automated database maintenance system, and found ABNER to be consistently the best. Furthermore, most other systems are only available as web services or platform-specific compiled binaries, whereas ABNER is designed to be portable, flexible, and integrated into third-party biomedical NLP applications.

BACKGROUND AND TECHNOLOGY

The NER problem can be thought of as a *sequence-labeling task*: each word is a *token* in a sequence to be assigned a *label* (which corresponds to an entity class of interest). Once upon a time *hidden Markov models* (HMMs), which are statistical finite-state machines (Rabiner, 1989), were the machine learning method of choice for sequence labeling, such as part-of-speech tagging. However, more complex problems like NER tend to require larger, more sophisticated sets of features (e.g., words, prefixes or suffixes, capitalization patterns, neighboring words within a certain window of distance, etc.) which are certainly not independent, and can present difficulties for generative models like HMMs if the dependencies are not modeled explicitly. As a result, some researchers opt to use simple discriminative classifiers (which are more robust to such independence violations) to label each word separately, in lieu of graphical sequence models altogether (Kudoh & Matsumoto, 2000; Kazama et al., 2002).

However, *conditional random fields* (CRFs) have emerged as a sort of "best-of-both-worlds" solution (Lafferty et al., 2001). CRFs are undirected statistical graphical models (a special case of which is a linear chain, corresponding to a statistical finite-state machine), but they are also conditionally trained in a way that overcomes feature independence and other shortcomings of HMMs. After being shown effective for other NLP sequence labeling tasks like part-of-speech tagging (Lafferty et al., 2001), phrase chunking (Sha & Pereira, 2003), and named entity recognition for newswire text (McCallum & Li, 2003), they naturally became a popular candidate for solving the biomedical NER problem as well (Settles, 2004; McDonald & Pereira, 2004; Settles, 2005; Friedrich et al., 2006).

Let $\mathbf{x} = \langle x_1, x_2, \ldots, x_T \rangle$ be a sequence of observed words (i.e., a sentence) of length T, and let $\mathbf{y} = \langle y_1, y_2, \ldots, y_T \rangle$ be a sequence of labels that are assigned to the words in the input sequence $\mathbf{x}$. Figure 2(a) illustrates an example sentence and how it might be labeled. The labels in $\mathbf{y}$ represent the entities of interest (e.g., DNA, cell type, other), which also correspond to states in a statistical finite state machine, such as the one in Figure 2(b). A first-order linear-chain CRF defines the conditional probability of a label sequence $\mathbf{y}$ given an input sequence $\mathbf{x}$ to be:

$$P(\mathbf{y} \mid \mathbf{x}) = \frac{1}{Z(\mathbf{x})} \exp\left(\sum_{t=1}^{T} \sum_{k=1}^{K} \theta_k f_k(y_{t-1}, y_t, \mathbf{x}, t) \right),$$

Figure 2. Example CRF graphs for (a) a labeled input sequence, and (b) the structure of a corresponding finite-state machine.

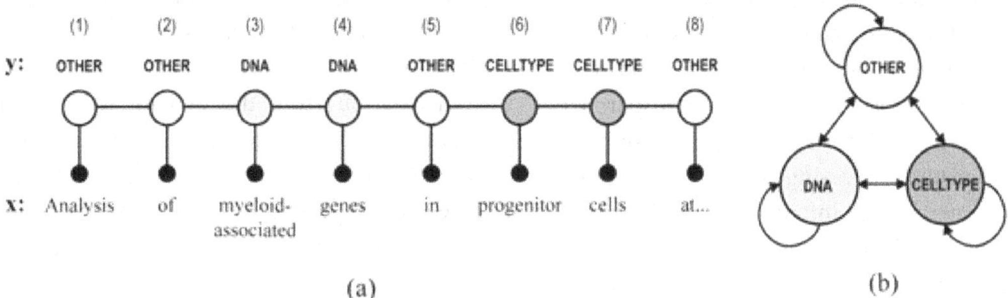

where $Z(\mathbf{x})$ is a normalization factor over all possible label sequences, f_k is one of K binary functions describing a features that characterize position t in sequence $\mathbf{x}$, and θ_k is the weight for that feature. For example, f_k might be the feature WORD=*myeloid-associated* and have value 1 at position t=3 in the sequence from Figure 2(a). Other features that are set to 1 for this position might be HASDASH, SUFFIX=*ated*, and NEXTWORD=*genes*. The weight θ_k for each feature should be positive for a feature correlated with the target label, negative for a feature that is anti-correlated, and near zero for a relatively uninformative feature. One can think of CRFs as a sequence-based generalization of maximum entropy (also known in the literature as multinomial logistic regression) classifiers (Nigam et al., 1999). In order to learn these weights properly, we can use gradient ascent to maximize the conditional log likelihood of N labeled sequences in a training set $D = \{\langle \mathbf{x}, \mathbf{y}\rangle_{(1)}, \ldots, \langle \mathbf{x}, \mathbf{y}\rangle_{(N)}\}$:

$$LL(D) = \sum_{n=1}^{N} \log\left(P(\mathbf{y}_{(n)} \mid \mathbf{x}_{(n)})\right) - \sum_{k=1}^{K} \frac{\theta_k^2}{2\sigma^2},$$

where the second term is simply a Gaussian prior over feature weights to help to prevent over-fitting due to sparsity in D. If the training sequences are fully labeled, the objective function $LL(D)$ is convex and the model is guaranteed to converge to an optimal set of feature weights. New sequences can then be labeled using an inference algorithm such as Viterbi. For more information on CRFs, their typical training procedures, and their relationship with other graphical models, see Sutton & McCallum (2006) for a good introduction.

ABNER uses a first-order CRF with a default feature set comprised of orthographic and contextual features, mostly based on regular expressions, prefixes or suffixes, and neighboring tokens. The full feature set is viewable (and editable) in the ABNER distribution source code. Some research indicates that additional features like part-of-speech tags and lexicon (dictionary) membership can improve accuracy, however ABNER does not have native support for such features at this time. My own research indicates that the gains of such features for ABNER are only slight, and pose several software engineering challenges at the expense of its currently robust, portable, and fast performance.

ABNER is written entirely in Java using graphical window objects from the Swing library. The CRF models are implemented with the MALLET toolkit (http://mallet.cs.umass.edu), which uses a quasi-Newton method called L-BFGS (Nocedal & Wright, 1999) to learn the optimal feature weights efficiently. ABNER conducts its built-in tokenization using a deterministic finite-state lexical scanner built with JLex (http://www.cs.princeton.edu/~appel/modern/java/JLex/).

BEYOND NAMED ENTITIES

As stated earlier, accurate NER systems are an important first step for many larger information management goals. This section briefly discusses some more recent work by other researchers who are using ABNER as a component in larger biomedical text processing systems. These applications generally fall into three main categories: higher-level information extraction, document categorization and information retrieval, and the automatic maintenance or curation of biological databases.

Higher-Level Information Extraction

NER is a basic subtask of information extraction (IE), focused only on finding *entity* mentions in text. Naturally, the next step in IE is identifying the *relationships* among such entities directly from text. For example, in mining the biomedical literature this can mean extracting protein-protein interactions or identifying the sub-cellular localization of gene products.

Madkour et al. (2007) developed an extraction system for protein-protein interactions that employs ABNER in the protein identification phase. After proteins are annotated, the articles are mined using an unsupervised mutual reinforcement algorithm to rank textual patterns indicating an interaction relationship. They report an F_1 score of 0.55 on a corpus of MEDLINE abstracts, which appears to be near the current state-of-the-art for this formulation of the problem. To facilitate further progress in the area of extracting protein-protein interactions, a few variants of the task were proposed as part of the BioCreative2 challenge, and ABNER was also chosen as an NER component in at least four of the competing approaches (Abi-Haidar et al., 2007; Figueroa & Neumann, 2007; Gonzalez et al., 2007; Huang et al., 2007). Results from this evaluation are somewhat mixed, however, and substantially lower than those reported by Madkour et al.

Bethard et al., (2008) propose another interesting IE task that involves extracting semantic role arguments for protein transport predicates. Consider the following sentence: "IRS-3 expression blocked glucose/IGF-1 induced IRS-2 translocation from the cytosol to the plasma membrane." They developed a system that attempts to automatically extract relational predicate records like TRANSLOCATION(*IRS-2*, *cytosol*, *plasma membrane*) from such passages of the biomedical literature. The extracted predicate name represents the type of protein transport, and the arguments correspond to the target protein and the sub-cellular source and destination locations of the transport action, respectively. The authors employ ABNER's protein predictions as part of the predicate extraction system, resulting in an F_1 score of 0.792 (compared to 0.841 if protein mentions are already perfectly known).

Document Categorization and Information Retrieval

Most information retrieval (IR) systems aim to retrieve documents that are relevant to the user's particular information needs. Recently, however, interest has grown in developing systems that combine IR (particularly in the biomedical domain) with text categorization and information extraction, attempting to answer user questions or put them in context, while providing supplementary information and linking to the original sources (Hersh et al., 2007).

Several researchers who work on these more sophisticated IR systems have found that utilizing named entity predictions can improve their accuracy. For example, Tari et al. (2007) employ ABNER to process query topics in a Q&A-style document retrieval system. The extracted entities are then matched against synonym lists in gene databases as part of a query-expansion step to improve recall. Another task, part of the Text Retrieval Conference (TREC) 2005 genomics track, involves filtering a set of documents for those which are appropriate for manual curation in four different biological databases. Several systems developed to solve this task (Yang et al., 2006; Yu et al., 2006; Li et al., 2007) use ABNER's entity predictions to enhance the feature set in this classification problem. Similarly, ABNER is used effectively by IR systems designed to filter passages of text for mentions of protein-protein interactions (Abi-Haidar et al., 2007; Figueroa & Neumann, 2007; Huang et al., 2007).

Automatic Maintenance of Biological Databases

Biological researchers often rely on specialist databases to maintain an in-depth repository of domain knowledge. For example, a database may only catalog information on a single, organism-specific genome, or functionally classified toxins and other chemicals. However, as indicated in the introduction, the rate of growth for new information to be mined from the primary literature or filtered from larger, general-purpose databases each year far eclipses the ability of curators to keep things up-to-date manually, even with a focused and specialized scope of interest.

Lam et al. (2006) present a novel system to address some of these issues, combining ABNER with a protein sequence motif extractor to automatically update special-interest databases. Entities are extracted from the textual fields of target database records (e.g., titles and abstracts or reference articles), and motifs are likewise extracted from the protein sequence fields (i.e., the actual amino acid sequences). The entity keywords and sequence motifs are then combined to generate queries for more general-purpose databases in the public domain, such as GenBank or SwissProt. The idea is to filter the records from these broader interest databases and automatically extract the records that are relevant to the special-interest resources at hand. Their experiments in automatically maintaining a snake venom database achieve an F_1 score of 0.80 using both ABNER keywords and sequence motifs (as opposed to 0.045 and 0.41, respectively, using either one in isolation).

Cakmak & Ozsoyoglu (2007) present another system that uses ABNER to extract gene mentions from the literature, and infer new function annotations from the Gene Ontology (GO Consortium, 2004) that may have been overlooked. The GO is a standardized vocabulary for molecular function of gene products used in most model organism genome databases. The resulting GO annotations can be appended to the extracted genes' database records automatically. They report F_1 scores of 0.66, 0.66, and 0.64 for the Biological Process, Molecular Function, and Cellular Component sub-ontologies, respectively.

CONCLUSION

ABNER is an efficient, accurate, cross-platform software tool for finding named entities in biomedical text. It has been demonstrated to perform at or near the state-of-the-art on multiple benchmark corpora, and remains one of the few high-accuracy NER systems available freely and under an open-source license at the time of this writing. It also ships with its own API, allowing users to re-train the underlying machine learning system for specific tasks, or to integrate it into larger, more sophisticated information management systems. So far, ABNER has been used as a vital component in several such systems, including applications for higher-level information extraction, document classification and retrieval, and the automatic maintenance of biological databases.

ACKNOWLEDGMENT

I would like to thank Mark Craven for his guidance and support of this project. Research related to the software was supported by NLM grant 5T15LM007359 and NIH grant R01-LM07050.

REFERENCES

Abi-Haidar, A., Kaur, J., Maguitman, A., Radivojac, P., Retchsteiner, A., Verspoor, K., Wang, Z., & Rocha, L. (2007). Uncovering protein-protein interactions in the bibliome. In *Proceedings of the BioCreative2 Workshop*, (pp. 247–255).

Bateman, A. (2008). Editorial. *Nucleic Acids Research*, 33(Database issue), D1.

Bethard, S., Lu, Z., Martin, J., & Hunter, L. (2008). Semantic role labeling for protein transport predicates. *BMC Bioinformatics, 9*, 277.

Cakmak, A. & Ozsoyoglu, G. (2007). Annotating genes using textual patterns. In *Proceedings of the Pacific Symposium on Biocomputing (PSB), 12*, 221–232. World Scientific Press.

Chang, J. T., Schutze, H., & Altman, R. B. (2004). GAPSCORE: finding gene and protein names one word at a time. *Bioinformatics, 20*(2), 216-225.

Figueroa, A., & Neumann, G. (2007). Identifying protein-protein interactions in biomedical publications. In *Proceedings of the BioCreative2 Workshop*, 217-225. GO

Consortium (2004). The Gene Ontology (GO) database and informatics resource. *Nucleic Acids Research*, 32, D258-D261.

Friedrich, C., Revillion, T., Hofmann, M., & Fluck, J. (2006). Biomedical and chemical named entity recognition with conditional random fields: The advantage of dictionary features. In *Proceedings of the International Symposium on Semantic Mining in Biomedicine (SMBM)*, (pp. 85-89).

Gonzalez, G., Tari, L., Gitter, A., Leaman, R., Nikkila, S., Wendt, R., Zeigler, A., & Baral, C. (2007). Integrating knowledge extracted from biomedical literature: Normalization and evidence statements for interactions. In *Proceedings of the BioCreative2 Workshop*, (pp. 227-235).

Hersh, W., Cohen, A., Roberts, P., & Rekapalli, H. (2007). TREC 2006 genomics track overview. In *Proceedings of the Text Retrieval Conference (TREC).*

Huang, A., Ding, S., Wang, H., & Zhu, X. (2007). Mining physical protein-protein interactions from literature. In *Proceedings of the BioCreative2 Workshop.*

Kabiljo, R., Stoycheva, D., & Shepard, A. (2007). ProSpecTome: A new tagged corpus for protein named entity recognition. In *Proceedings of the ISMB BioLINK*, 24-27. Oxford University Press.

Kazama, J., Makino, T., Ohta, Y., & Tsujii, J. (2002). Tuning support vector machines for biomedical named entity recognition. In *Proceedings of the ACL Workshop on NLP in the Biomedical Domain*, 1-8.

Kim, J., Ohta, T., Teteisi, Y., & Tsujii, J. (2003). GENIA corpus - a semantically annotated corpus for bio-textmining. *Bioinformatics, 19*(Suppl. 1), I180-I182.

Kim, J., Ohta, T., Tsuruoka, Y., Tateisi, Y., & Collier, N. (2004). Introduction to the bio-entity recognition task at JNLPBA. In *Proceedings of the International Joint Workshop on Natural Language Processing in Biomedicine and its Applications (NLPBA)*, 70–75.

Kudoh, T., & Matsumoto, Y. (2000). Use of support vector learning for chunk identification. In *Proceedings of the Conference on Natural Language Learning (CoNLL)*, 142-144.

Lafferty, J., McCallum, A., & Pereira, F. (2001). Conditional random fields: Probabilistic models for segmenting and labeling sequence data. In *Proceedings of the International Conference on Machine Learning (ICML)*, (pp. 282–289). Morgan Kaufmann.

Lam, K., Koh, J., Veeravalli, B., & Brusic, V. (2006). Incremental maintenance of biological databases using association rule mining. In *Lecture Notes in Computer Science*, 140–150. Springer-Verlag.

Li, Y., Lin, H., & Yang, Z. (2007). Two approaches for biomedical text classification. In Proceedings of the *International Conference Bioinformatics and Biomedical Engineering (ICBBE)*, (pp. 310–313). IEEE Press.

Madkour, A., Darwish, K., Hassan, H., Hassan, A., & Emam, O. (2007). BioNoculars: Extracting protein-protein interatctions from biomedical text. In *BioNLP 2007: Biological, translational, and clinical language processing*, (pp. 89–96). ACM Press.

McCallum, A., & Li, W. (2003). Early results for named entity recognition with conditional random fields, feature induction and web-enhanced lexicons. In *Proceedings of the Conference on Natural Language Learning (CoNLL)*, (pp. 188–191).

McDonald, R., & Pereira, F. (2004). Identifying gene and protein mentions in text using conditional random fields. In *Proceedings of the BioCreative Workshop.*

Mika, S., & Rost, B. (2004). Protein names precisely peeled off free text. *Bioinformatics*, *20*(Suppl. 1), I241-I247.

Nigam, K., Lafferty, J., & McCallum, A. (1999). Using maximum entropy for text classification. In *Proceedings of the IJCAI Workshop on Information Filtering*, (pp. 61-67).

Nocedal, J., & Wright, S. J. (1999). *Numerical Optimization*. Springer.

Rabiner, L. R. (1989). A tutorial on hidden Markov models and selected applications in speech recognition. *Proceedings of the IEEE*, *77*(2), 257–286.

Settles, B. (2004). Biomedical named entity recognition using conditional random fields and rich feature sets. In *Proceedings of the International Joint Workshop on Natural Language Processing in Biomedicine and its Applications (NLPBA)*, (pp. 104–107).

Settles, B. (2005). ABNER: an open source tool for automatically tagging genes, proteins, and other entity names in text. *Bioinformatics*, *21*(14), 3191–3192.

Sha, F., & Pereira, F. (2003). Shallow parsing with conditional random fields. In *Proceedings of the Human Language Technology and North American Association for Computational Linguistics Conference (HLT-NAACL)*, 213–220. ACL Press.

Soteriades, E. S., & Falagas, M. E. (2005). Comparison of amount of biomedical research originating from the European Union and the United States. *British Medical Journal*, *331*, 192-194.

Sutton, C., & McCallum, A. (2006). An introduction to conditional random fields for relational learning. In L. Getoor & B. Taskar (Eds.), *Introduction to Statistical Relational Learning.* MIT Press.

Tari, L., Gonzalez, G., Leaman, R., Nikkila, S., Wendt, R., & Baral, C. (2007). ASU at TREC 2006 genomics track. In *Proceedings of the Text Retrieval Conference (TREC).*

Yang, Z., Lin, H., Li, Y., Liu, B., & Lu, Y. (2006). TREC 2005 genomics track experiments at DUTAI. In *Proceedings of the Text Retrieval Conference (TREC).*

Yeh, A., Morgan, A., Colosimo, M., & Hirschman, L. (2005). BioCreative task 1a: Gene mention finding evaluation. *BMC Bioinformatics*, *6*(Suppl. 1), S2.

Yu, L., Ahmed, S., Gonzalez, G., Logsdon, B., Nakamura, M., Nikkila, S., Shah, K., Tari, L., Wendt, R., Ziegler, A., & Baral, C. (2006). Genomic information retrieval through selective extraction and tagging by the ASU-BoiAI group.

In *Proceedings of the Text Retrieval Conference (TREC)*.

Zhou, G., Zhang, J., Su, J., Shen, D., & Tan, C. L. (2004). Recognizing names in biomedical texts: A machine learning approach. *Bioinformatics*, *20*(7), 1178-1190.

Zhou, G., & Su, J. (2004). Exploring deep knowledge resources in biomedical name recognition. In *Proceedings of the International Joint Workshop on Natural Language Processing in Biomedicine and its Applications (NLPBA)*, (pp. 96-99).

Chapter XVIII
Problems-Solving Map Extraction with Collective Intelligence Analysis and Language Engineering

Asanee Kawtrakul
Kasetsart University, Thailand & Ministry of Science and Technology, Thailand

Chaveevarn Pechsiri
Dhurakij Pundij University, Thailand

Sachit Rajbhandari
Kasetsart University, Thailand

Frederic Andres
National Institute of Informatics, Japan

ABSTRACT

Valuable knowledge has been distributed in heterogeneous formats on many different Web sites and other sources over the Internet. However, finding the needed information is a complex task since there is a lack of semantic relations and organization between them. This chapter presents a problem-solving map framework for extracting and integrating knowledge from unstructured documents on the Internet by exploiting the semantic links between problems, methods for solving them and the people who could solve them. This challenging area of research needs both complex natural language processing, including deep semantic relation interpretation, and the participation of end-users for annotating the answers scattered on the Web. The framework is evaluated by generating problem solving maps for rice and human diseases.

INTRODUCTION

Accumulation ofknowledge and Collective Intelligence on certain topics is crucial for building a Knowledge Society. Best practices or experience on focus areas can be found and shared through writing research reports, visiting blogs, and even participating in Wikipedia. Anyway, Information on new events should be extracted from newspapers and news sites for updating, monitoring or tracking the important events. However, these sources of valuable knowledge are scattered over many different sources, and they come in many different formats. Moreover, desired information/knowledge is more difficult to access from scattered sources since search engines return ranked retrieval lists that offer little or no information on the semantic relationships among scattered information, and even when such information is found, it is often redundant or in excess volume since there is no content filtering or correct answer indicated. Accordingly, as we move beyond the concept of simple information retrieval and simple database queries, automatic content aggregation, question answering, and knowledge visualization become more important.

Moreover, to make smart access to a "one-stop service", semantic-based knowledge aggregating and organizing are needed for shortening the time it takes to grasp the knowledge. PMM map (Problem--Methods of problem solving--huMan map), a smart visual browser, is then developed. Since the web consists to a large extent of unstructured or semi-structured natural language text, generating PMM map needs language engineering techniques such as named entity recognition, discourse relation recognition for specific information and knowledge extraction. However, PMM map generation also needs collaborative intelligence to create the community knowledge pool and contribute to both annotate problem-solving solutions scattered on the web and verify the ones that extracted by the Q&A system.

This chapter focuses on problem solving map extraction using 'know-why' and 'know-how' analyser as a means of indicating specific answers to queries on topics *"cause-and-effect* "such as disease and symptoms, " *problem-and -how-to-do* " such as disease prevention or control, and biomedicine preparation. Section 2 describes the background and related works. Section 3 gives the conceptual framework for PMM map generation. Section 4 describes the problems that need language engineering to solve and gives a brief of specific knowledge annotation. Section 5 summaries the experiments related to the language processing.

BACKGROUND AND RELATED WORKS

The lessons learned from solving past problems (e.g. how to protect oneself from a disease, how to control the plant disease) and gaining valuable information from previous experience (e.g. disease diagnosis) and the history of disease recurrences (e.g. disease outbreaks) are invaluable for guaranteeing food safety and human health. To reduce the time that users take to learn from such information, a salient information space with semantic link should be developed.

Problem-solving is an intelligent behavior (Kennedy J., et al., 2001) where the goal is to find a solution which satisfies certain criteria. It requires abductive reasoning whereby we apply deductive reasoning in combination with natural language processing. In classical applications as well as in expert systems, abductive inference (Shohei K., et al., 2003) is a complex problem (creation and maintenance) as it is simulated by deductive procedures or rules. On the other hand, qualitative reasoning concerns modeling and inference techniques where continuous phenomena are discretized into a finite number of qualitative categories. In this chapter, language engineering is described as a tool for extracting knowledge represented in unstructured format. The extracted knowledge will be a finite number of specific answers to queries on topics *"cause-and-effect* "such as disease and symptoms., *"problem-and -how-to-do"* such disease prevention or control, and biomedicine preparation.

Although we have attempted to use the Semantic Web to bridge content semantically, our framework is also related to BioCaster (Collier,N., et al.,2007). ProMED-PLUS (Yangarber R., et al., 2005), a system for automatic "fact" extraction from plain-text reports about outbreaks of infectious epidemics around the world, and MiTAP (Damianos L., et al., 2004), a prototype SARS detecting, monitoring and analyzing system of infectious disease outbreaks that uses across-language Information Retrieval and works automatically on easy-to-use news servers. The system, called PMM map, is composed of many steps for supporting specific event extraction (what-when-where), such as disease outbreak events, and object-attributes extraction, such as pest-characteristics.

Topic Maps ISO Standard 13250 and their data model provide several advantages (interoperability and composition) for organizing knowledge. Thus, we utilize the topic maps framework to manage the set of topics, associations, and occurrences (Kawtrakul, et al., 2007b). However, to produce the PMM map, we need to exploit the semantic links between problems, methods for solving them and the people who could solve them. This challenging area of research needs both complex natural language processing, including discourse relation interpretation such as cause-effect and problem-solving procedure, and the participation of end-users for annotating the answers scattered on the web.

According to Jana Trnková and Wolfgang Theilmann (2004), there are four kinds of knowledge: (1) orientation knowledge (know-what) including the information what the topic is about, (2) reference knowledge (know-where) referring to the location to find additional or new information that can become know-what, (3) explanation knowledge (know-why) about why something is the way it is and (4) action knowledge (know-how) referring to how to do or to accomplish something.

In order to provide 'know-what' : the oriented knowledge including the information what the topic is about, and 'know-where' , referring to the location to find additional or new information that can become know-what, our model (Kawtrakul, et al., 2007a)formulates the relation extraction problem as a classification problem, and it is motivated by the work of J. Suzuki et al. (2003) on the HDAG kernel to solve classification problems in natural language processing. The use of classification methods in information extraction is not new. Intuitively, we can view the information extraction problem as a problem of classifying a fragment of text into a predefined category, which results in a simple information extraction system such as a system for extracting information from job advertisements (Zavrel J., et al., 2000) and business cards (Kushmerick N., et al. , 2001). However, those techniques require an assumption that there should be only one set of information in each document; the proposed model does not suffer from this constraint.

This chapter focuses on 'know-why', an explanation knowledge about why something is the way it is; such as the cause-and-effect of biomedicine usage, the cause-and-effect of disease outbreaks, and 'know-how', referring to how to do or to accomplish something., such as disease prevention or control, biomedicine preparation, and disease treatment.

PMM MAP GENERATION SCENARIO

The PMM Map generation brings together information from different sources and structures scattered over the web. An ontology-based integration approach is used instead of simple data storage; it provides higher degree of abstraction, extensibility and reusability. We have developed a sample ontology representing the concepts/topics with specific properties as knowledge (see Fig.1) and relationships, such as treatment, expertise, to integrate this knowledge. Note that the problem (P) is related to disease, the methods (M) are from biomedicine, and the human problem solvers (M) are experts in the fields of biomedicine and disease. The problem such as Plant disease refers to the symptoms or characteristics needed for diagnosis and for specific applications such as for early warning through a mobile SMS service by using outbreak period. The problem solver such as disease expert refers to a person or group of persons who have knowledge about the problem. We also used the concept of know-who (Thamvijit D., et al., 2005) to extract information from research documents related to the problems of interest. In order to generate PMM map, at first stage, language engineering techniques such as named entity recognition, discourse relation recognition are needed for information and knowledge extraction. Name entities consist of Person names, Disease names, Herbal names, Location or Organization names and time expressions.

With PMM map generation framework, "one-stop services" for specific domain can be created to serve user in many categories. Example of categories in rice domain is shown in Figure 2

Knowledge resources, shown in Figure 2, come from different websites and other sources over the internet, i.e., (A,B,E)[2] ,(C)[3], (D) newspaper website , (F)[4],(I)[5],(J)[6],(K)[7], and (L)[8]. For more specific scenarios as the follows:

Problem1: Let say <farmers> living in <location1> have some problems in their agri-

Figure 1. Knowledge integration between problem, solution, and solver

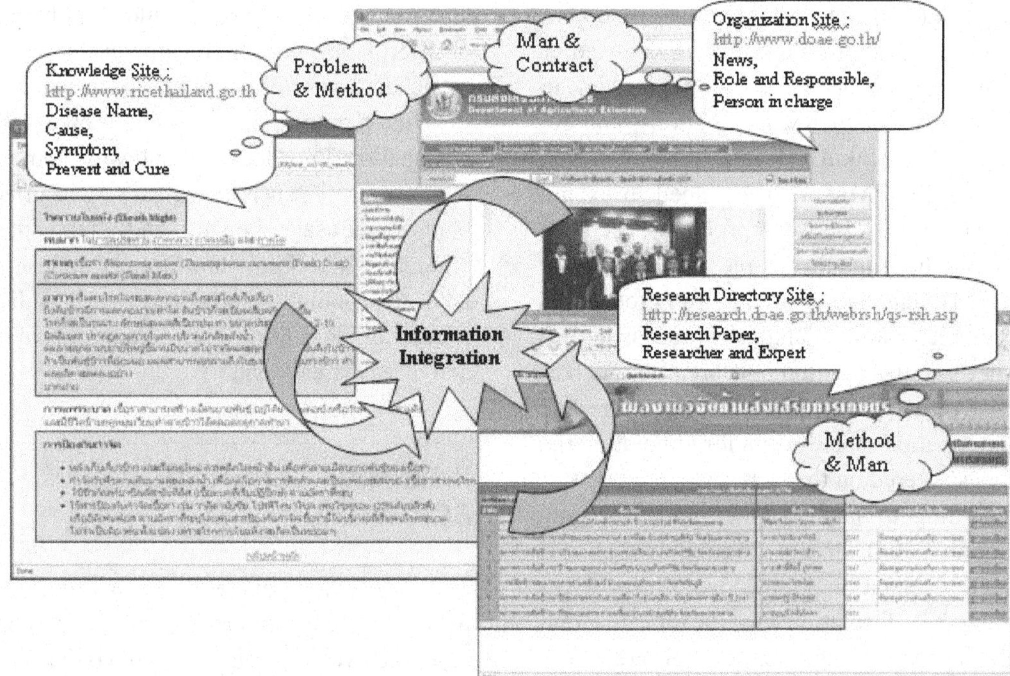

Figure 2. An example of Rice Related Information for providing one-stop service

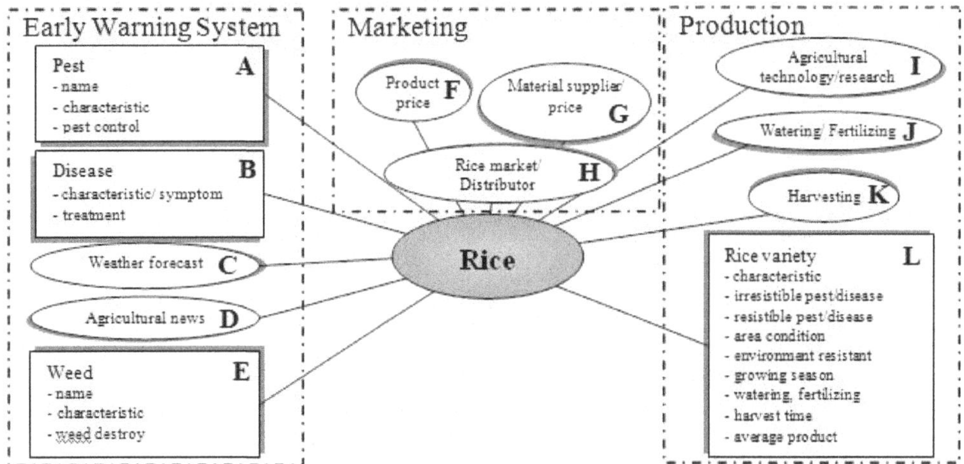

cultural products with <symptoml> and <symptom2>.

Solutionl: <symptoml> and <symptom2> are the symptoms of <diseasel> and this disease is found in <locationl>. Based on the symptoms, we can recognize the disease of those agricultural products. <expertl> and <expert2> are the experts on <diseasel>. Both of them recommend following <treatementl>. <treatmentl> uses <medicinel> and <medicine2> and have 3 steps of usage <stepl>, <step2> and <step3>.

Problem2: Let say <diseasel> {Name, Description, Time, Type} have time properties as Jan-Apr. During these months, automatic warning system can send SMS information about <diseasel> to the farmers living in <locationl>. The message contains <symptomsl> and <symptoms2> to diagnose the disease and follow <treatmentl> using <medicinel>.

Regarding to the above problems, semantic-based knowledge aggregating and organizing the problem and its solution on the basis of the PMM model are shown as Figures 3 and 4, respectively, for providing knowledge service as a "one-stop service".

To create the PMM Map, information is collected from the scenario by following the collective intelligence procedure illustrated in Figure 5. The cycle drawn with the solid line corresponds to a local PMM process involving a single user. The dotted cycle corresponds to a collaborative PMM process involving several users.

Local PMM Process

Local PMM process is a personalized knowledge acquisition. Starting from the PMM definition based on Knowledge portal Model (Kawtrakul A., et al., 2007a), it enables to determine the following knowledge inputs about know-why, and know-how. Human action such as answer indication annotates the knowledge input to be used by the know-why and know-how analyzer component. Then the knowledge results, such as Symptom-Disease, and the process of Disease Prevention or Control, the process of Biomedicine Preparation, the process of Disease Treatment, are extracted and verified by the Problem-Solving Comparison process.

Figure 3. Visual representation of problem and solution

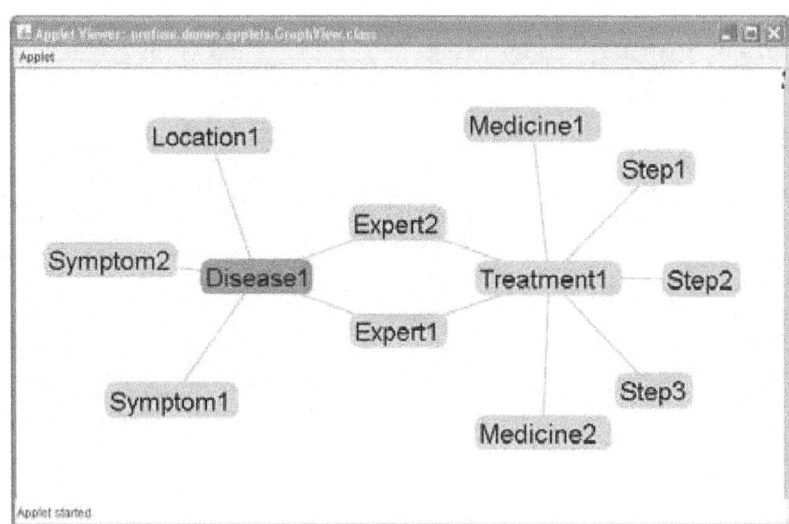

Figure 4. Visual representation of location based Disease Warning

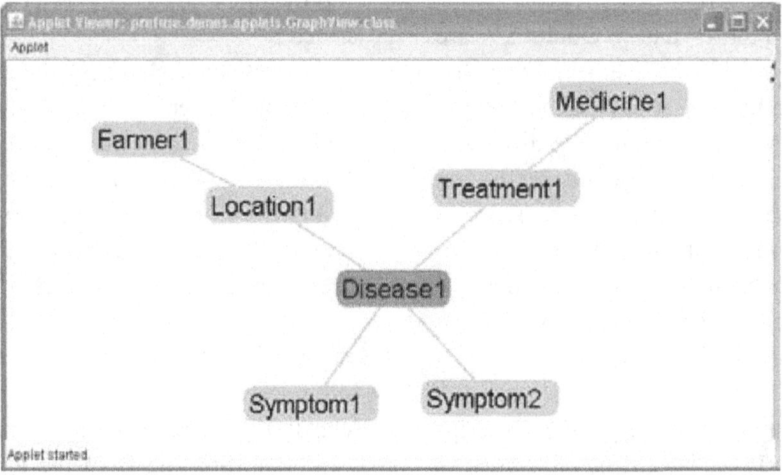

Collaborative PMM Process

Starting from the PMM definition, the collaborative answer indicator annotates the input with know-how and know-why information. The collaborative PMM analyzer produces the knowledge results which will be evaluated by the collaborative PMM verification component.

PMM ANALYZER WITH LANGUAGE ENGINEERING

To provide PMM map as a tool for Knowledge-oriented problem solving, unifying Knowledge Engineering with Language Engineering and Information and Communication Technologies is necessary. The model of Knowledge Engineer-

Figure 5. Collective intelligence PMM process architecture

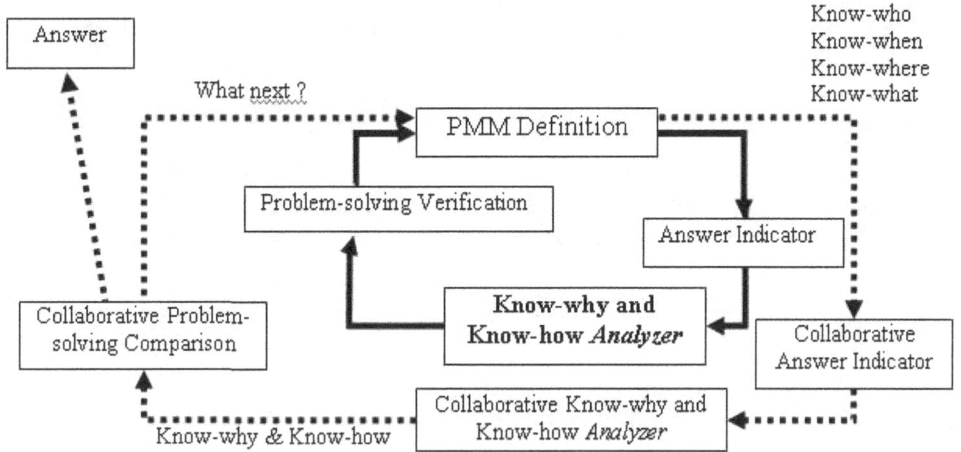

ing and ICT is generic but based on Language Engineering techniques, the language model is specific to a language.

To extract Disease-Symptoms or Pest-Attributes for later diagnosis, Information Extraction technique has been applied. Extracting information in the usual way yields a set of related entities in the format of slot and filler, but information in Thai text indicating locations, plant's condition, time expressions, etc., cannot be limited to a set of related entities because of the problem of zero anaphora (Kawtrakul A. and Yingsaeree C., 2005). Moreover, the name entity classification (e.g., Plant Name, Pest's name) must be robust (Biezunski M., et al., 2002). To deal with semantic-based knowledge aggregating and organizing, especially, in a domain like agriculture, food, or health, we exploit collective intelligence (Segaran T., 2007) for pre-indicating the query-answer pair and for post-verifying the extracted answer ,i.e., cause-effect and how-to-do.

Name Entity Recognition for Problem Definition and Human Expert Information Extraction

The Message Understanding Conference (MUC) framework defines Name Entities (NEs) as names of persons, organizations, and locations, temporal information (date and time), and numerical expressions (monetary values and percentages). To deal with a domain like agriculture, food, or health, we have to extend the NE (Chanlekha H. and Kawtrakul A., 2004) accordingly to fit the new domain. Here, we suggest enriching the list of NEs with the following terms from the domain of agriculture: plant/biomedical name, animal name, disease name, chemical name, and pathogen name. While there are many difficulties in common between NEs in the domain of Agriculture NEs (ANEs) and NEs, there are still some difficult problems specific to the task of ANE extraction.

ANE extraction is hampered by the characteristics peculiar to the Thai language: 1) unlike Western languages, no orthographic information, such as uppercase letters are used, neither can we rely on character types, such as Kanji, or Katakana, as used in Japanese to signal a NE. 2) there is no space or any special character signaling word boundaries. 3) Many NEs in Thai do not have a specific structure. Besides these difficulties, ANE extraction faces problems intrinsically linked to the characteristics of the terms of the agricultural domain:

1. Plant names, animal names, and disease names are usually compound words with a sentence- or NP-like structure. This leads to a lot of ambiguities during the NE extraction process. (see Example 1).
   In Example 1, sentences (a) and (b) are grammatically correct in Thai if we consider only the local context. However, if we take the global context into account, i.e. other occurrences of the same name, we see that only (b) is correct.
2. ANEs usually occur without any explicit clue word. Hence, their extraction depends greatly on the context and the ANE itself. See Example 2.
3. Category Ambiguity: Some words can belong to different NEs classes depending on their surrounding contexts (see Example 3).

Example 1.

a) "**จะพบ**/ We will find ***ด้วงงวง***/ *Pin-Hole Borer* ANIMAL **กัดใบมะม่วง**/ cut mango leaves **จำนวนมาก**/ a lot"
b) "**จะพบ**/ We will find [**ด้วงงวงกัดใบมะม่วง**]/[mango leaf cutting weevil]ANIMAL **จำนวนมาก**/ a lot"

Example 2.

"**ความเป็นพิษของ**/Toxicity of ***ลำโพง***/*Thorn apple* PLANT-NAME:
ทุกส่วนล้วนมีคุณสมบัติเป็นพิษ/ Every part has toxic property",
The word "**ลำโพง**" could be a plant name ("Thorn apple") or a common word ("loudspeaker"). This problem cannot be solved by using simple heuristics. Clearly, more information than POS or syntactic information is needed.

Example 3.

[**ฟักทอง**]/[pumpkin's]PLANT **พันธ์**/varieties, [**ดำ**]/[Dum,]PLANT-NAME **เมื่อแก่**/when the fruit ripes, **เปลือกจะขรุขระเป็นปุ่มปม**/ the skin is rugged, **คล้ายผิว**/which looks like the skin of a [**คางคก**]/[toad]ANIMAL **บางทีก็เรียกพันธ์**/ sometimes call this variety [**คางคก**]/[Kangkok]PLANT-NAME

In the above example, "**คางคก**/toad" could be either the name of a plant or common noun type ANIMAL. It all depends on the context. Furthermore, in Thai, the starting word of an NE is usually considered to be a head word(common noun), and used as NE category. However, it can yield an incorrect NE category , e.g., being animal name instead of being disease name. For example "**ไส้เดือนฝอยรากปม**/Root-knot Nematode" could be the name of Rice Disease . However, "**ไส้เดือนฝอย**/nematode" here is a phyla of animal.

Collaborative Analysis and Annotation for Knowledge Extraction

The use of natural language processing can extend the realm of semi-automatic knowledge acquisition and management. Bookmarks normally are hyperlinks for communities on the web to see who is doing what and what people find interesting . However, such social bookmarks are not adequate for extracting knowledge on providing services. Annotation is also necessary for important information tagging such as the solution to the problem, traditional disease protections, and clinical guidelines for disease diagnosis.

1. **Annotation schema**
   In this chapter, the actual symbolic representations used in the knowledge sources or corpus classify discourse annotations into two sets: causality tags for know-why extraction and procedural tags for know-how extraction.
2. **Causality tags**
   We define tags to learn the verb-pair rules for extracting the inter-causal Elementary Discourse Unit (EDU:where EDU is defined as a simple sentence or a clause, Carlson et al., 2003) that forms a causative unit and its effective information unit. These tags are used to learn cause-effect relations between causative events and effective events from the annotated EDU corpus. Such a relation can be expressed as a combination of a causative verb (v1) and the effective verb or result verb (v2) in verb pairs from different EDUs or as a lexical pair from a lexico-syntactic pattern within one EDU(Pechsiri, C. and Kawtrakul, A.,2007). Each verb in the pair has to be manually annotated with the causative verb concepts derived from Wordnet[1] . To determine the verb-pair rules, each verb concept is learned by Naïve Bayes Classification and Support Vector Machine Model for result comparison.
3. **Procedural tags**
   Collecting knowledge for a question answering system that replies to "how-to" questions involves unifying the question with a goal and providing the user with the instructions associated with that goal. Procedural texts provide instructions to reach this goal. They include documents such as formal recommendations, directions for use/control/protection/prevention, and advice.
   The procedural texts have the following structure: titles, which express a goal to reach; instructions, which express the actions to perform; actions, which are separated by two means: typographic and punctuation marks, for example; bullet, paragraph indent, etc. and linguistic marks that express temporality. e.g., แล้วจึง/laew jung: then],[ขณะ/kana: while] prerequisites; and warnings. Saint-Dizier P., et al (2007) designed the annotation tag types including prerequisite, instruction, recommendation, and warning, to the procedural text for text analysis in the question-answering system.
4. **Annotation process**
   We classify the annotation types into three independent layers; morphological, syntactic and discourse layer. Each layer has specific purpose of observation. A semi-automatic tool is provided to annotate linguistic information. This tool allows users to browse information in three independent layers. The Figure 6 shows the annotation process. Our corpus was automatically word segmented and POS tagged including Name Entity (Chanlekha H. and Kawtrakul A., 2004), and word-formation recognition (Pengphon N., et al., 2002) to solve the boundary of Thai Name Entity and noun phrase. After that, EDU segmentation (Chareonsuk J., et al.,

2005) is then dealt with, to generate EDUs for discourse annotation by using a general-purpose text editor or word processor.

Explanation and Procedural Knowledge Analysis for Problem-Solving Method Extraction

There are several problems in extracting explanation knowledge such as know-why and procedural knowledge such as know-how from textual data on web pages, especially ones dealing with herbal insecticides and herbal medicines.

Know-Why Extraction

There are several views of know-why that can assist us in diagnosing problems. In this chapter, we consider only the disease-effect view. There are two main problems affecting know-why: causality identification and causality boundary determination.

- **Causality identification for the disease-effect view**: According to (Pechsiri, C. and Kawtrakul, A., 2007), the causality is expressed in the form of an inter-causal-EDU which consists of multiple EDUs in both a causative unit and an effect unit and the cue phrase is used for a causality identification and boundary determination. The cue phrase consists of a discourse-marker set and a word-expression set as follows (for the inter-causal EDU) (see Example 4). However, we still have the problems of ambiguity and implicit cue phrase elements.
- **Cue phrase ambiguity:** The discourse marker cue in example a) is a cause-effect expression while in b) it is a condition (see Example 5).
- **Implicit cue phrase:** It is not necessarily the case that the causality expression always contains a cue phrase (see Example 6) where the [..] symbol mean ellipsis.
- **Boundary determination between causative unit and effective unit:** For the disease-effect view, we can generally determine these boundaries by using discourse markers, such as' และ/and', 'และ/or', and 'ก็/then', as delimiters. Here, we address only the boundary with an implicit delimiter.
- **Implicit boundary delimiter:** As stated in the causality identification definition, causal expressions do not always contain cue phrases. This raises the problem of identifying causative antecedents and effective consequence boundaries, especially when each boundary unit contains more than one EDU, as shown in Figure 7.

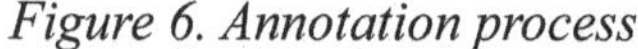

Figure 6. Annotation process

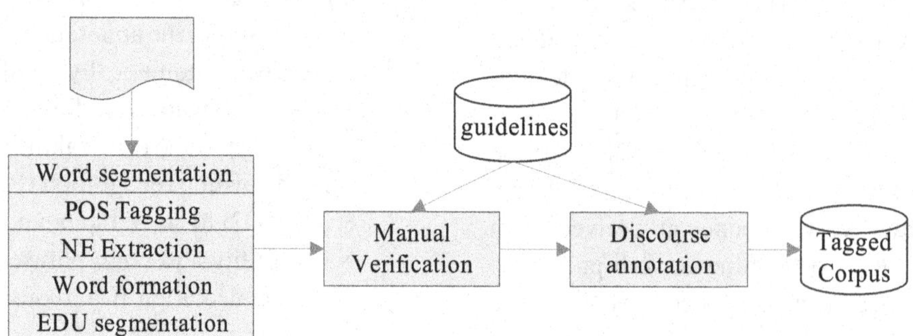

Example 4.

cue phrase set = discourse-marker set Union word-expression set
discourse-marker set = single-marker set Union pair-marker set
single-marker set = {'**เพราะ**/because', '**เนื่องจาก**/since', '**และ**/and', '**หรือ**/or',…}
pair-marker set = {'**ถ้า..แล้ว**/if..then', '**ถ้า..จะ**/if..will', '**เมื่อ..จะ**/when..will',…}
word-expression set = {'**ทำให้**/make', '**เป็นเหตุให้**/cause that', '**เป็นผลจาก**/

Example 5.

a) EDU1: '**ถ้าข้าวถกเชื้อราเข้าทำลาย** '('If rice plants are destroyed by fungi.')
EDU2: '**เมล็ดจะลีบหมด**' ('the seeds will be thin.')
b) EDU1: **ถ้าเป็นรุนแรง** (If (the epidemic) is serious)
EDU2: **จะทำให้ตายได้** (it will have died)

Example 6.

c) EDU1:'**ข้าวเป็นโรคใบหงิก**('Oryza get stunt disease.')
EDU2:'[**ทำให้**]**ต้นจะแคระแกรน**'('[it causes that] the plant to become stunted.')

Example 7.

EDU1 **น้ำเลี้ยงจากใบข้าว** (Aphid sucks sap from a rice plant)
EDU2 **ใบจะบิดโค้งงอ** (Leaf will twist [and] curl.)
EDU3 **ขอบใบจะมีอาการปลายใบแห้ง** (The rim of leaf will have the symptom of dried leaf)

EDU1 **เพลี้ยจักจั่นดูดกิน**

This problem can be solved by using verb-pair rules along with Centering Theory (Grosz, B., Joshi, A., and Weinstein, S., 1995) and cue phrase (see Example 7).

In case of disease-treatment/disease-control view: The problem of causality identification also involves the word level and the sentence level. For the word level, the medicinal name entity may express in the form of a sentence like name entity or an EDU- like name entity which explains the medicinal action as the causative action of medicine, and medical characteristic. The problem of this level is how to identify the causative name entity. See Example 8.

Figure 7. Possible boundaries of causative antecedent and effective consequence

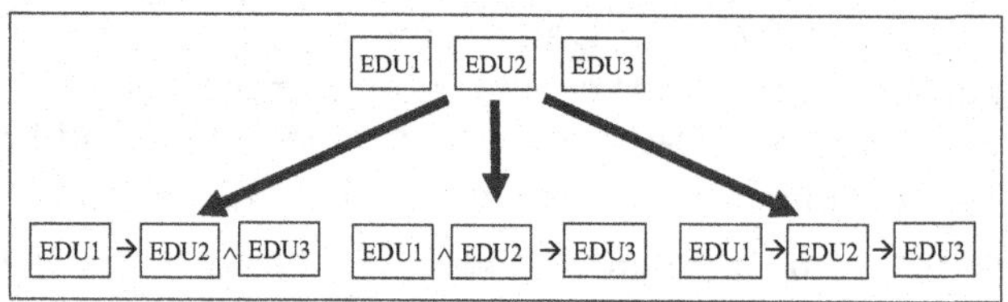

Example 8.

a) "ใบโหระพา/A basil leave ใช้เป็น/is used as ยา/medicine ขับ/releases ลม/gas" where ยา/medicine ขับ/releases ลม/gas (means a medicine releasing gas) is an EDU-like name entity with the causative action, 'release'.
b) "แก่นกระแจะ/ Nicolson stem ใช้ทำ/is used for making ยา/medicine ดอง/soaks in เหล้า/liquor"
where ยา/medicine ดอง/soaks in เหล้า/liquor (means a medicine preserved in liquor) is an EDU-like name entity with the characteristic of medicine being preserved in the alcohol.

Example 9.

Causality
EDU1 "ใบกระเพรา/A basil leave ใช้เป็น/is used as ยา/medicine ขับ/releases ลม/gas"
(=A basil leaf is used as a medicine releasing gas.)
EDU2 "[The basil leaf] แก้/stop คลื่นไส้/being nauseate."
(=It causes that the basil leaf stops being nausea.)

Non-causality
EDU1 "ใบกระเพรา/A basil leave ใช้เป็น/is used as ยา/medicine ขับ/releases ลม/gas"
(=A basil leaf is used as a medicine releasing gas.)
EDU2 "[the basil leave]รักษา/relieves แผล/ulcerใน/inกระเพาะอาหาร/stomach."
(=The basil leaf relives ulcer in a stomach.)

For the sentence level, the EDU containing an EDU-like name entity with the causative action may be followed by an effect EDU(s) to form the cause-effect or causality relation between the EDU like name entity and that following EDU(s). See Example 9.

And in case of Boundary determination for disease-treatment/disease-control view: Some cause-effect relations from the herbal web sites are expressed in the form of the EDU containing an EDU like name entity with the causative action followed by some effect EDUs without any cue of ending effect boundary, e.g. "และ/and". See Example 10.

Mostly, Causality extraction is based on multiple EDUs. However, most of causality

Example 10.

EDU1 "**ใบกระเพรา**/A basil leave **ใช้เป็น**/is used as **ยา**/medicine **ขับ**/releases**ลม**/gas"
(=A basil leaf is used as a medicine releasing gas.)

EDU2 "[The basil leaf] **แก้**/stop **ปวดท้อง**/stomachache."
(=It causes that the basil leaf stops paining abdomen.)

EDU3 "[**And** the basil leaf]**แก้**/stop **คลื่นไส้**/being nauseate."
(=And the basil leaf stops being nausea.)

expressions are realized in two main forms: an inter-causal EDU and an intra-causal EDU. The inter-causal EDU is defined above as a causality expression of more than one simple EDU and intra-causal EDU as a causality expression occurring within one EDU. Moreover, there are 20% of inter-causal EDU and 7% of intra-causal EDU from the annotated-causality corpora are found. Then, Causality extraction focuses only on the inter-causal EDU. To extract a causative unit and its effective information unit in the form of the inter-causal EDU, these tags are defined for verb-pair rules learning for extracting the inter-causal EDU. Table 1 shows causality tag schema.

The cause-effect schema is used for annotating in an EDU corpus for machine learning in cause-effect relation between causative events and effective events. These relation can be expressed by a combination of the causative verb (vc) and the effective verb or result verb (ve) in the verb pairs from different EDUs or by a lexical pair from a lexico syntactic pattern within one EDU (in case of intra-causality)

Know-How Extraction

Procedural texts can indeed be a simple, ordered list of instructions to reach a goal, but they can also be less linear, outlining different ways to realize something, with arguments, advices, conditions, hypothesis, and preferences. The organization of a procedural text is in general made visible by means of linguistic and typographic marks. However, there are problems remained to be solved.

Therefore, by the observation, there are many problems in procedural extraction process according to procedural text ambiguities and it, sometimes, mixes style of procedural text with and without markers or clues and also the complex intertwining of lexical, syntactic, semantic and pragmatic factors. See Figure 8.

As shown in the Figure 8, it is noticeable that the process number 1 to 6 is not procedure but the procedure is shown in only 7 and 8. Moreover, the complete procedure is reviewed in unstructured part. In the procedural structure, it also has explanation as in "5% while the rice is in booting stage" and condition as "before harvesting for one week by randomly taking 100 ears of paddy in each sub-plot". These kinds of text structure cause the ambiguity in Thai language since the structures were described by sentences or clauses that make the difficulty of procedural text annotation process.

- **Instruction identification for Herbal Medicine Preparation:** The problem is how to identify the herbal medicine instruction or how-to preparation without any starting-preparation cue, e.g. "**ดังต่อไปนี้**/as in the following" "**ดังนี้**/as follows" "**โดย**/by", etc. Example 11 shows the instruction EDUs with and without instruction cue word.
- **Determination of procedural knowledge boundary:** The problem is how to identify the ending of herbal medicine preparation without any hint cue (see Example 12), where the ending preparation is EDU2.

Table 1. Annotation schema for causality extraction

Tag type	Description
Cause-Boundary tag <C id=*num* type=*cause/noncause*> EDU1 EDU2 … EDUn </C>	-To annotate the starting point of the **cause** unit by "<C id=*num* type=*cause/noncause*>" tag (where the attribute **id** is a cause number and the attribute **type** is type of EDUs in this boundary) -ending boundary with" </C>" tag
Effect-Boundary tag <R id=*num* type=*effect/noneffect*> EDU1 EDU2 … EDUn </R>	-To annotate the starting point of the **effect** unit by "<R id=*num* type=*effect/noneffect*>" tag (where the attribute **id** is a effect number corresponding to the cause **id** and the attribute **type** is type of EDUs in this **effect** unit) -ending boundary with" </R>" tag
Embedded cause tag inside the result EDU <EmC id=*num* type=*cause/noncause*> … </EmC>	-To annotate the embedded cause by "<EmC id=*num* type=*cause/noncause*>" tag (where the attribute **id** is a cause number and the attribute **type** is type of the EDU that is embedded into the result EDU -ending boundary with "</EmC>" tag
Effect-Boundary tag of the effect EDU containing an embedded-cause EDU <EmR id=*num* type=*effect/noneffect*> EDU1 EDU2.....EDUn </EmR>	-To annotate the starting point of the **effect** unit by "<EmR id=*num* type=*effect/noneffect*>" tag (where the attribute **id** is an effect number corresponding to the cause **id** and the attribute **type** is type of EDUs in this **effect** unit) -ending boundary with "</EmR>" tag
<np1 concept='.....'> noun-phrase </np1>	To annotate the concept of an agent. This concept will be useful for selecting word sense of verb to be causative.
<VC concept='....'>verb</VC>	To annotate the concept of verb for solving the word form variety
<np2 concept='.....'> noun-phrase </np2>	To annotate the concept of a patient. This concept will be useful for selecting word sense of verb to be causative.
<VE concept='....'>verb</VE>	To annotate the concept of verb for solving the word form variety

Figure 8. Example of ambiguity and mixed style procedural corpus

… To test the efficiency of Discoloration Disease with two isolates, there is a comparative testing methodology by using water spraying with the procedure as the following,

1. Disease B. subtilis No.4
2. Disease B. subtilis No.9
3. Disease B. subtilis No.33
4. Disease B. subtilis No.4 + B. subtilis No.9
5. Disease B. subtilis No.4 + B. subtilis No.33
6. Disease B. subtilis No.9 + B. subtilis No.33
7. Spray with the propiconazol 25% E.C
8. Spray with water

instruction

For the procedure for spraying Discoloration Disease chemical, uses the antagonistic bacterium two times with suggestion scale; 5% while the rice is in booting stage, evaluates the severe of Discoloration Disease in each plot before harvesting for one week by randomly taking 100 ears of paddy in each sub-plot. After that, takes the seed to count for disease attacked rice gain and non disease attacked rice gain for calculating of suppressing disease rice grain discoloration percentage including the evaluating of rice product with 14 % moisture in each plot. Then take the result to analyze with the statistical process.

Example 11.

Using Explicit Cue:
EDU1 "สกัด/Extract น้ำมัน/oil จาก/from ใบตะไคร้หอม/lemon grass leaves ด้วย/with วิธีง่ายๆ /the simple method ดังนี้/as follows"
EDU2 "นึ่ง/steam ใบตะไคร้/lemon grass leaves" ......

Using Implicit Cue:
EDU1 "นอกจากนี้/Furthermore[, we] ใช้/use ใบสดและรากทองพันชั่ง/Kurz leaves and roots โขลก ละเอียด/to mash finely"
EDU2 "แช่ /soak เหล้าโรง/in the liquor 1 สัปดาห์/ for 1 week" ....

Example 12.

implicit cue:
EDU1 "นอกจากนี้/Furthermore[, we] ใช้/use ใบสดและรากทองพันชั่ง/Kurz leaves and roots โขลก ละเอียด/to mash finely"
EDU2 "แช่ /soak เหล้าโรง/in the liquor 1 / for 1 week สัปดาห์"
EDU3 "เอา/take น้ำเหล้า/liquor ทา/to apply"
EDU4 "แก้/inhibit กลากเกลื้อน/chloasma"

Example 13.

modal marker ต้อง [tong] (must), advice marker ควร [kuan] (should) and temporal marker such as และ[lae] (and), แล้ว [laew] (then), แล้วก็[laew ko] (and then), แล้วจึง[laew jung] (and.... then) , ต่อมา[tor ma](after that), ถัดมา[tat ma] (from then on), ต่อจากนั้น[tor jak nan] (next), หลังจาก[lung jak] (after), หลังจากนั้น[lung jak nun] (after that). Additionally, some elements such as number, bullet, pictures, etc. are used.

To solve the problems mentioned above, morphological processing is mainly used to recognize word boundary instead of recognizing lexicon form like English and EDU Segmentation have to be applied for finding the boundary of text unit as sentence or clause. The markers for instruction are a slightly different,i.e.,

1. Typographic especially, new paragraph delimit titles, instruction zones, prerequisites and warnings
2. Verb in imperative form is utilized as in English. However Thai have no voice form as active or passive voice as in English.
3. various classes of markers (see Example 13).

Currently, we also use the following annotation types for indicating procedural instructions in the corpus. The annotated corpus , then, will be used for extracting regular expressions for further recognizing know-how automatically.

- Title: <title> … </title>
- Instruction: <instruction> … </instruction>
- Advice: <advice> … </advice>
- Warning: <warning> … </warning>
- Condition: <condition > … </condition >
- Elaboration: <elaboration> … </elaboration>
- Prerequisite: <prerequisite> … </prerequisite>

EXPERIMENTAL RESULTS AND CONCLUSION

NE Recognition Experiment with Various Feature Types

We did the experiment on various feature types to see their impact on the performance of the extraction system when adding some new features. In this evaluation, we considered context ranges from w-2 to w2 with bigrams and trigrams. The evaluations are 10-fold cross-validation. The results are shown in Table 2.

We can see from Table 2 that the Global features and Document-style-dependent features contribute a lot to the system's performance except for disease and pathogen name. **Note:** Local features here mean lexie/word's information such as Orthography, being a word in a dictionary. Global features here mean string matching with the other words in the corpus, being a word in the title/section/sub-section.

Knowledge Extraction Experiment

How to solve know-why extraction problems for the disease-effect view: A Naïve Bayes classifier is needed to start the causality recognition process. A Naïve Bayes classifier is implemented in Weka, which is for inter-causal EDU learning with causative and effective verbs and their concepts. The EDUs are classified as class 1 (cause-effect EDUs) and class 0 (non cause-effect EDUs). The precision and recall of causality extraction (Pechsiri et. al., 2007) are 86% and 70%, respectively, with a boundary accuracy of 94%.

$$\begin{aligned} EDUclass &= \arg\max_{class \in Class} P(class \mid v_c, v_e) \\ &= \arg\max_{class \in Class} P(v_c \mid class)\, P(v_e \mid class)\, P(class) \end{aligned}$$

$$v_c \in V_c \text{ where } V_c \text{ is a CausativeVerb set}$$

$$v_e \in V_e \text{ where } V_e \text{ is an EffectiveVerb set}$$

How to solve know-why extraction problems for disease-treatment/disease-control view: These problems can be solved by using Naïve Bayes to learn three verbs with concepts from the following EDUs. The first EDU is from the EDU containing an EDU like name entity and the verb in this EDU is called "supporting causative verb, v_s". The second EDU is from the EDU like name entity which contains a causative verb, v_c. The last EDU is from the EDU following the EDU containing the EDU like name entity, and this last EDU contains an effect verb, v_e. All these verbs are shown as the features in the following equation , where EDUs class is determined by

Table 2. Performance of the system with different features

Features	Plant	Animal	Chemical	Disease	Pathogen
Local feature	88.07	87.12	78.27	91.55*	85.47*
Local feature + Global feature	88.51	88.92*	79.43	91.30	85.44
Local feature + Global feature + Document-style-dependent feature	89.07*	87.46	80.26*	90.48	85.27

class1 (cause-effect EDUs) and class0 (non cause-effect EDUs) with the extraction result of 88% as precision, 69% as recall, and with a boundary accuracy of 85%.

$$\begin{aligned} EDUclass &= \underset{class \in Class}{\arg\max}\ P(class \mid v_s, v_c v_e pair) \\ &= \underset{class \in Class}{\arg\max}\ P(v_s \mid class) P(v_c v_e pair \mid class) P(class) \end{aligned}$$

$$v_s \in V_s \text{ where } V_s \text{ is a Supporting Causative Verb set}$$

$$v_c v_e pair \in V_{cepair} \text{ where } V_{cepair} \text{ is a Cause-Effect Verb Pair set}$$

How to solve know-how extraction problem: Currently, "know-how" extraction uses the regular expression to identify the procedural knowledge and the boundary of procedural, which created from the typographic markers, linguistic markers and position markers.

CONCLUSION

This chapter gives an overview of our on-going research on collaborative knowledge annotation based on 'know-why' and 'know-how' analyzer for specific answer indications (e.g. cause-and-effect of biomedicine usage, disease prevention or control, and biomedicine preparation). We introduced the conceptual collaborative framework for PMM map generation. Then we explained the problems of Thai language processing. With PMM model, knowledge service could be provided more efficiently with the smart browser.

ACKNOWLEDGMENT

The work described in this chapter was supported by a grant from the National Electronics and Computer Technology Center (NECTEC) No. NT-B-22-14-12-46-06 for the project, "A Development of Information and Knowledge Extraction from Unstructured Thai Documents". We would like to thank the National Institute of Informatics for supporting the visiting of Frederic Andres to work with our project team. We, also, would like to thank Mukda Suktarachan, Patcharee Varasai for their support in corpus preparation. Last but not least, we would like to give a special thanks to Patrick Saint-Dizier for his invaluable discussion related to know-how and also thank Therawat Tooumnauy and Patthrawan Rattanamanee for their support in data testing and paper formatting.

REFERENCES

Biezunski, M., Bryan, M., & Newcomb S. (2002). *ISO/IEC 13250, Topic Maps (Second Edition)* In proceeding of ISO/IEC JTC1/SC34. Retrieved on May 22, 2002.Available at: *http://www1.y12.doe.gov/capabilities/sgml/sc34/document/0322.htm*

Carlson L., Marcu D., & Okurowski M. E. (2003). *Build a discourse-tagged corpus in the framework of Rhetorical structure theory.* In Current and new direction in discourse and dialogue, Springer, (pp. 85-122).

Chanlekha, H., & Kawtrakul, A. (2004). Thai Named Entity Extraction by incorporating Maximum Entropy Model with Simple Heuristic Information. *In proceeding of IJCNLP' 2004*, Hainan Island, China.

Chareonsuk J., Sukvakree T., & Kawtrakul A. (2005). Elementary Discourse Unit Segmentation for Thai using Discourse Cue and Syntactic Information. *In proceeding of NCSEC2005.*

Damianos, L., Bayer, S., Chisholm, M. A., Henderson, J., Hirschman, L., Morgan, W., Ubaldino, M., & Zarrella, J. (2004). *MiTAP for SARS detection.* In proceeding of the Conference on Human Language Technology, (pp. 241–244). Boston, USA.

Grosz, B., Joshi, A., & Weinstein, S. (1995). Centering: A Framework for Modeling the Local Coherence of Discourse. *Computational Linguistics, 21*(2), 203–225.

Kawtrakul, A., Permpool, T., Yingsaeree, C., & Andres, F. (2007a). *A Framework of NLP based Information Tracking and Related Knowledge Organizing with Topic Maps* In proceeding of NLDB2007, LNCS No. 4592, Springer-Verlag, pp. 272-283, ISBN 978-3-540-73350-8, June 27-29, 2007, CNAM, Paris, France.

Kawtrakul, A., Yingsaeree, C., & Andres, F. (2007b). Semantic Tracking in Peer-to-Peer Topic Maps Management. *In proceeding of LNCS*, (pp. 54-69), October 17-19, 2007.

Kawtrakul, A., & Yingsaeree, C. (2005). A Unified Framework for Automatic Metadata Extraction from Electronic Document. *In proceeding of The International Advanced Digital Library Conference.* Nagoya, Japan.

Kennedy, J. F., Eberhart, R., & Shi, Y. (2001). Swarm Intelligence. In proceeding of Morgan Kaufmann Publishers Inc. San Francisco, CA.

Kushmerick N., Johnston E., & McGuinness S. (2001). Information extraction by text classification. *In Proceedings of IJCAI-2001 Workshop on Adaptive Text Extraction and Mining.*

Pengphon N., Kawtrakul A., & Suktarachan M. (2002). Word Formation Approach to Noun Phrase Analysis for Thai. *In proceeding of The 5th Symposium on Natural Language Processing.*

Pechsiri C., Kawtrakul A., & Piriyakul R. (2005). Mining Causality Knowledge From Thai Textual Data. *In proceeding of The 6th Symposium on Natural Language Processing, SNLP'2005*, Chiang Rai, Thailand.

Pechsiri, C., & Kawtrakul, A. (2007). Mining Causality from Texts for Question Answering System. *In proceeding of IEICE on Transactions on Information and Systems, 90*-D, No 10.

Saint-Dizier, P., Delpech, E., Kawtrakul, A., Suktarachan, M., & Varasai, P. (2007). Annotating the Facets of Procedural Texts. *In proceeding of the 7th International Symposium on Natural Language Processing (SNLP),* Pattaya, Chonburi, Thailand, December 13-15, 2007. (p. 143).

Segaran T. *(2007). Programming Collective Intelligence Building Smart Web 2.0 Applications.* O'Reilly Media, ISBN, 0-59652932-5, 2007, (p. 360).

Shohei, K., Hirohisa, S., & Hidenori, I. (2003). PARCAR: A Parallel Cost-based Abductive Reasoning System. *In proceeding of Transactions of Information Processing Society of Japan, 41*(3), 668-676.

Thamvijit, D., Chanlekha, H., Sirigayon, C., Permpool, P., & Kawtrakul, A. (2005). Person Information Extraction from the Web. *In proceeding of the 6th Symposium on Natural Language Processing 2005 (SNLP 2005),* Chiang Rai, Thailand, Dec 13-15, 2005.

Yangarber, R., Jokipii, L., Rauramo, A., & Huttunen, S. (2005). Information Extraction from Epidemiological Reports. *In Proceedings of HLT/EMNLP-2005.* Canada.

Zavrel, J., Berck, P., & Lavrijssen, W. (2000). Information extraction by text classification: Corpus mining for features. *In proceedings of the workshop Information Extraction Meets Corpus Linguistics.* Athens, Greece.

ENDNOTES

1. http://wordnet.princeton.edu/
2. www.doa.go.th/php/homepage/homepage.htm
3. www.dit.go.th, www.oae.go.th, www.tmd.go.th, www.oae.go.th/mis/predict
4. www.dit.go.th, www.riceexporters.or.th/price.htm
5. www.doa.go.th/apsrdo/index.html, www.soilwafer.com, www.doa.go.th/AedWeb/main.htm
6. www.doa.go.th, www.doae.go.th

[7] www.doa.go.th/pprdo/index.htm, www.phtnet.org

[8] www.doa.go.th/rri, www.doae.go.th

Chapter XIX
Seekbio:
Retrieval of Spatial Relations for System Biology

Christophe Jouis
Université Paris III – Sorbonne, France, & LIP6 (Laboratoire d'Informatique de Paris VI – Université Pierre et Marie Curie), ACASA team, France

Magali Roux-Rouquié
LIP6 (Laboratoire d'Informatique de Paris VI – Université Pierre et Marie Curie), ACASA team, France

Jean-Gabriel Ganascia
LIP6 (Laboratoire d'Informatique de Paris VI – Université Pierre et Marie Curie), ACASA team, France

ABSTRACT

Identical molecules could play different roles depending of the relations they may have with different partners embedded in different processes, at different time and/or localization. To address such intricate networks that account for the complexity of living systems, systems biology is an emerging field that aims at understanding such dynamic interactions from the knowledge of their components and the relations between these components. Among main issues in system biology, knowledge on entities spatial relations is of importance to assess the topology of biological networks. In this perspective, mining data and texts could afford specific clues. To address this issue we examine the use of contextual exploration method to develop extraction rules that can retrieve information on relations between biological entities in scientific literature. We propose the system Seekbio that could be plugged at Pubmed output as an interface between results of PubMed query and articles selection following spatial relationships requests.

INTRODUCTION

For decades, it was thought that more an organism was complex, more the number of genes they contain had to be high. At the completion of the Human Genome Project, it was found that living systems were having approximately the same number of genes coding for proteins (about 20,000) and these assessments resulted in biology's big bang undergoing a paradigmatic change to address biological complexity. Accordingly, the universe of biologists was changing and the challenge of unravelling complexity of living organisms was stipulated on the spatio-temporal variety of the biological components and their relations. Countless examples show that identical molecules could play different roles depending of the relations they may have with different partners embedded in different processes, at different time and/or localization; let mention, muscle differentiation that is orchestrated by the differential localization of a molecular species (Misca et al., 2001) or molecular gradients that regulate the developing eye polarity (Strutt, 1999). To address such intricate networks that account for the complexity of living systems, systems biology is an emerging field that aims at understanding such dynamic interactions from the knowledge of their components and the relations between these components. Among main issues in systems biology, knowledge on entities spatial relations is of importance to assess the topology of biological networks; in this perspective, mining data and texts could afford specific clues. To address this issue, we examine the use of contextual exploration method (Jouis, 1993; Jouis, 2007) to develop extraction rules that can retrieve information on relations between biological entities in scientific literature. To achieve this, we propose SEEK*bio* tool. Among further uses, SEEK*bio* could be plugged at Pubmed (Srinivasan, P., 2001) output as an interface between results of PubMed query and articles selection following spatial relationships requests. These spatial relationships requests would consist of terms graph of the original query and location relations put by the user in the SEEK*bio* graphs editor. The built graph would act as a filter to select relevant articles from a spatial point of view (see figure 1). Enabling this strategy should return selected documents in which relations arguments could be added automatically.

RELATED WORKS

Two different approaches to extracting relationships from biological texts are used (Ananiadou, S., Kell, D. B. & J. Tsujii., 2006).

Co-occurrence

The simplest approach is to identify entities that co-occur within abstracts or sentences in texts. Most of techniques make use of a score based on the apparition frequency of terms to establish and classify terms relationships (Donaldson, I et al., 2003), (Cooper, J.W. & Kershenbaum, A., 2005), (Stapley, B. J. & Benoit, G., 2000). If a couple of terms is regularly repeated, the terms are supposed to have relations although the type of relation is not precised (Wren, J. D. & Garner, H. R., 2004). Learning techniques such as artificial neural networks (ANNs), support vector machines (SVMs), hidden Markov models (HMMs), and naïve Bayes classifiers (NB) are used to detect such relations. They have been adapted for spatial information retrieval in biology. For example, the sub-cellular location of proteins was predicted from text using support vectors machines (Stapley, B. J. et al. 2002).

Otherwise, Protein location was predicted using sequence homology and retrieved information on known or predicted functions, interacting partners, additional sequence motifs, source organism, etc. This approach used a Naïve Bayes classifier to make a prediction about the place where a protein should be located, using only the protein sequence as its input and search against

Figure 1. Utilisation of SEEKbio for collecting all relevant information through Pubmed applied to Medline. As a first step, the user makes a query in the form of a Boolean expression of terms. In step (2), the request is submitted to Pubmed via Medline database. Quite often, the user gets out of a hundred references. This result is not exploitable. So, in a third step, the user specifies his request in the form of a graph in the system SEEKbio. This graph represents a hierarchy of spatial terms of the original request. The graph serves as a filter. With the contextual exploration rules, SEEKbio detects texts in which appear the spatial relationships expressed by the graph. Finally, in Step 4, we get a few abstracts which verify the conditions expressed by the spatial hierarchy.

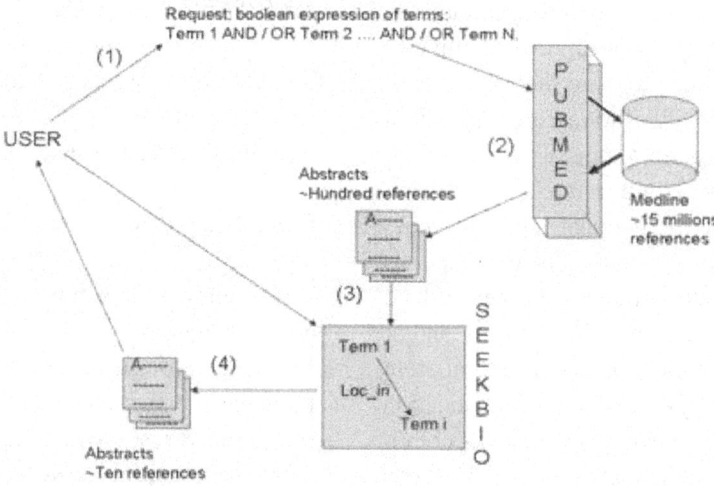

databases to assemble the necessary information (Lu, D. et al, 2004).

Although very powerful, these methods do not allow to infer the type of a relationship (Jensen, L. J., Saric. J. & Bork, P., 2006).

Natural-Language Processing

With natural-language processing, grammar and extraction rules have to be developed (Jensen, L. J., Saric. J., & Bork, P., 2006). Shortly, a syntactic tree is built for each sentence and a rule set is used to extract relationships on the basis of both this syntactic tree and the semantic labels that are used for tagging the entities of interest. Several program exist for tokenization and part-of-speech tagging of English texts, most of which are easily adapted to biomedical texts by retraining them on a manually tagged corpus such as GENIA[a] or PennBioIE[b] (Finkel, J. et al., 2005). Recently, mereological analysis of spatial representations was reported (Donnelly, M., 2005; Donnelly, M., 2004; Donnelly, M, 2006) that used the formal theory of parthood and relations –such as overlap (having a common part) and discreteness (having no common part) –defined in terms of parthood. There are already several works on the spatial reasoning which is a central component of biomedical research and practice.

CONTEXTUAL EXPLORATION METHODOLOGY AND SEEK-CLIPS

Most of natural language processing systems are based on language parsers (syntactic analysis) intended to build a syntactic tree structure essential step for semantic interpretation. The tree is a three-phase one: morphological analysis based on morphological rules, a dictionary of general language and domain-specific terms (lexical analysis) and a grammar (syntactic analysis).

A complete analysis of each sentence is required. It is also necessary to make decisions about correct syntactic rules to be applied if the sentence is ambiguous. Moreover, sentences should be grammatically correct, a requirement imposed by this type of analysis, what is not often where in PUBMED summaries.

SEEK-CLIPS (Jouis, 1993; Jouis, 2007) is an independent module because it neither necessarily requires a general language dictionary nor does it need a preliminary semantic representation of the field nor a parser. In this manner, SEEK-CLIPS permits an "economical" textual analysis. It uses contextual exploration rules. These rules are in fact linguistic markers which convey a linguistic knowledge. Besides, this approach does not need a complete analysis of the text: it simply simulates a reader's strategy whose knowledge of the field is rather limited. Generally, text contextual exploration strategy consists in taking into consideration only the linguistic markers in a text. These elements are considered as relevant identificators. There is, therefore, no need for a complete sentence analysis. For a rapid analysis of a great number of texts, contextual exploration aims at building semantic representations that are not so polished but sufficient (concerning the objectives to be reached) by being satisfied with an approximate syntactical analysis. Contextual exploration detects some markers in the analyzed sentences which stand as key-markers in order to establish relations among concepts.

SEEK-CLIPS design was based exclusively on the language knowledge of the text reader. The method that was developed did not used any specific terms (or arguments) but only "delimiters" between terms such as connectors, grammatical words and symbols of punctuation that delimitate the context. In our hands, exploring a phrase consists in "context exploration". As generally accepted, arguments are "full words" as opposed to "empty words". Under contextual exploration, the "empty words" are seen as containing meaning to connect the entities in the field and independent of a particular area. SEEK-CLIPS provides interactive assistance for information extraction searching in textual data the relations between objects in the field: static relations, and especially the spatial relationships.

Furthermore, SEEK-CLIPS could be used for automatic processing of texts to build ontologies by:

1. defining semantic value sets (SVS), and then by
2. building systems that could identify these semantic values in texts.

These systems take the form of knowledge-based systems and consist of declarative rules. These rules express for the observer (the linguist), decision-making skills of a reader who has to interpret a text.

Rules are as follows: IF <conditions> THEN <conclusions>.

- <conditions> reflect the presence or absence of some linguistic indicators in the context.
- <conclusions> allow gradually building semantic representations.

For instance, we have the contextual exploration rule:

Rule Loc-in1
IF we observe an occurrence of the list $VerbLoc
Followed by (not necessarily immediately) an occurrence of the list $PrepLocIn
Followed by (not necessarily immediately) an occurrence of the list $NounLoc
THEN Intend: Location-in

Where the lists are as below:

$PrepLocIn = to / in / inside / in the middle / halfway /midway / into / within / at the heart /...
$VerbLoc = Locate / localize / place / put / position / situate / set / observe / express / be localized / take place / confine / position /...
$NounLoc = region / area / section / zone / locality /...etc.

The rule Loc-in1 apply the following subtext:

In deuterostomes, B1-type Soxs are asymmetricallylocalized to the future animal/ectodermal region where they act to suppress mesendodermal, and favor neuroectodermal differentiation, while vegetally localized F-type Soxs are involved in mesendodermal differentiation. (PMID: 17608734)

FROM SEEK-CLIPS TO SEEK*BIO*: THE *PLACE AND MOVEMENT* CASE STUDY

Principles for Rules Design Using the SNAP/SPAN BFO Ontology

Using SEEK-CLIPS for identifying *place* and *movement* (also named as *location*) relationships in scientific biological and medicine literature requires establishing the linguistic markers accounting for location; these are general terms that include (1) prepositions of place and movement: *in, inside, to, into*, etc., (PrepLoc) (2) verbs and phrasal verbs: *to locate, to situate, to localize*, etc., (VerbLoc) (3) place nouns: *region, area, zone*, etc., (NounLoc). Nevertheless, general terms are not enough sufficient to infer correct topological relations because domain-specific vocabulary is largely used in scientific literature. The main challenge is to delineate rules and markers lists

Figure 2. Location hierarchies in SEEKbio

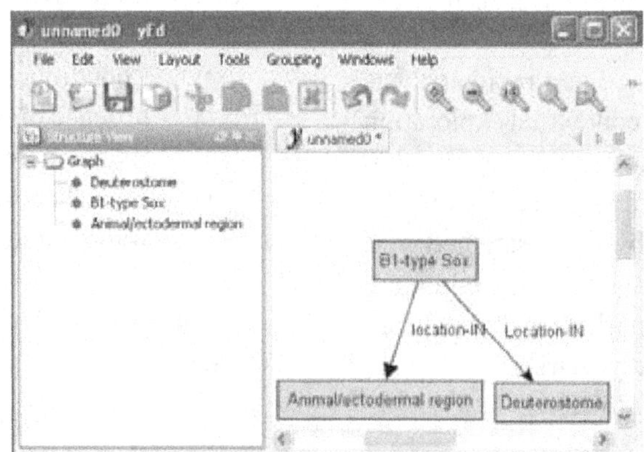

that will identify the relevant relation(s) among the huge complexity of scientific phraseology. To address this issue, let's take as example, relatively simple and short sentences that use makers from place and movement lists; there are mainly of the form:

1. Parthenogenesis *occurs in* insects and microbes.
2. DNA synthesis *occurs in* both chromosome *regions*.
3. A unique protein that only *occurs in* sperm.
4. ABCB1 protein *occurs at* E12.5.
5. This protein *occurs at* a developmental stage.

In this series, sentences use domain-specific vocabulary (*parthenogenesis*, *insects*, *microbe*, *DNA synthesis*, *chromosome*, *protein*, *sperm*, *ABCB1 protein*, *E12.5*, *developmental stage*), and markers of place consisting in prepositions: *in*, *at*; verb: *to occur*, *occurs*; and nouns: *region*, *regions*.

Domain-specific vocabulary can be easily arranged in anatomic and physiologic terms.

- Anatomy (*sensu largo*) is used to refer to anatomical *structures* which contain a certain ordered aggregate of material objects and physical spaces filled with substances that define a collection of regions. All parts of anatomical structures are *located* in the corresponding wholes and among location relations, a second type is that of *containment*. With this respect, in the example above, *insects*, *microbe*, *chromosome*, *protein*, *sperm*, *ABCB1 protein* belongs to anatomic terms.
- Physiology (again, *sensu largo*) deals with *processes* and *functioning* that is the realization of functions and is a process too. Biological processes have a beginning and an end and occur in time and space; *parthenogenesis*, *DNA synthesis*, *E12.5*, *developmental stage*, are biological processes.

This central dichotomy between structure and processes concerns two distinct modes of existence in time and corresponds to a dual view of a given domain. This was the foundation of the Basic Formal Ontology (BFO) (Grenon, P. and Smith, B., 2003) that consists in two orthogonal ontologies, a SNAP ontology made of entities that exist in full at any time (*insects*, *microbe*, *chromosome*, *protein*, *sperm*, *ABCB1 protein* are SNAP entities) and a SPAN ontology made of entities that that have temporal parts and develop in time (as it is the case for *parthenogenesis*, *DNA synthesis*, *E12.5*, *developmental stage*).

The classes of SNAP and SPAN entities are strictly disjoint from each other because SNAP and SPAN entities enjoy distinct temporal modes of being; what does it happen when the two views are bringing together (as it is the case in the example above)?

According to (B. Smith, 2004), the parts and aggregates of SNAP entities are themselves in every case SNAP entities; the parts and aggregates of SPAN entities are likewise themselves SPAN entities; no SNAP entity is ever a part of any SPAN entity and vice versa. Nevertheless, BFO recognizes a number of relations between SNAP and SPAN. Only, relations used in this study are listed below:

- *Relations with Signatures <SNAP , SNAP> and <SPAN, SPAN>;*
  The *place* and *movement* relations may occur only in …; spatiotemporal location is a relation between a processual entity and the spatiotemporal region at which it takes place;
- *Relations with Signature <SNAP, SPAN>: realization* is a relation between SNAP dependent entities and processes;

- *Relations with Signature <SPAN, SNAP>*: *participation* is the most general form of relation between a processual and a substantial entity.

Among the examples given above, only sentence (3) accounts for correct mapping of relation type to *location*; it states that "a special protein is located inside the sperm cell". Otherwise, sentences (1) and (2), on the one hand, and (4) and (5), on the other hand, deal with *realization* and *participation* relations, respectively. Such clear-cut assignment of relation type takes benefits of specific-vocabularies relevant to physiology (*sensu largo*) that deals with functions and processes: *parthenogenesis, DNA synthesis, E12.5, developmental stage* and anatomy (again, *sensu largo*) that deals with structures:

Based on SNAP/SPAN ontologies and relations ontologies (RO), we designed the general frame of rules as below:

In the case of SNAP entities:

IF *(SNAP* or *NounLoc)(VerbLoc* or *PrepLoc)(SNAP* or *NounLoc)*
THEN Intend: *Location*

Several alternatives could instantiated this general frame, depending of the marker list types. For example, the *PrepLoc* set would include a *PrepLocIn* list (*in, at, inside*, etc.), a *PrepLocOn* list (*on, upon, over*, etc.); accordingly, rule activation would intend the specific location type: *Loc-in* and *Loc-on*, respectively.

In the case of SPAN entities:

IF *(SPAN) (VerbLoc* or *PrepLoc)(SPAN)*
THEN Intend: *Location*

In this case, there is no use of *NounLoc* list markers as they consist in entities that endure over time (*region, area, zone*, etc.) and we mentioned above (cf. RO) that no SPAN entity is ever a part (or located in) of any SNAP entity and vice versa.

Principles for Markers Design in the Context of OBO Foundry

In the context of OBO foundry (Smith, B, et al, 2007), biological and medical ontologies were categorized according to BFO entities (SNAP and SPAN) on the one hand, and biological granularity, on the other hand. Main ontologies and the corresponding URL are presented below (Table 1). Using the OBO foundry classification ensures easy and secure marker lists design and instantiation; lists could be fill-in automatically and very refined sub-lists could be further created according to the ontology under consideration (for example, a marker list dedicated RNA molecules based on Rna0).

For the purpose of this study, marker lists were designed and filled by hand, with terms collected from the careful reading of selected abstracts. Nevertheless, these terms were checked for their presence in any of the ontologies mentioned above, with special attention to Gene Ontology (GO).

Corpus Selection and Analysis

As our purpose was to identify location relationships in biological literature, we focused in the field of "developmental biology" know to take special attention to molecule and cell location and movement.

A text corpus was selected from PubMed using the following query equation on September 25th, 2007:

<< Development Drosophila Location >>

A set of 221 occurrences were found. From this list, the 50 more recent abstracts were download and 513 full sentences (text between two full

Table 1. Ontologies of the OBO Foundry arranged according to the BFO (SNAP/SPAN) entities

BFO entity / Granularity	SNAP				SPAN
	Substance		Property		
Organ and organism	**NCBI taxonomy: http://www.ncbi.nlm.nih.gov/Taxonomy**	**FMA:fma.biostr.washington.edu CARO:http://www.bioontology.org/wiki/index.php/CARO:Main_Page**	**FMP: PubMedID15360830 CPRO: http://www.cpro.ubc.ca**	**PaTO: obo.sourceforge.net/cgi-bin/ detail.cgi?attribute_and_value**	GO:www.geneontology.org (Organ Processes)
Cell and cell component	**CL:obo.sourceforge.net/cgi-bin/detail.cgi?cell**	**FMA:fma.biostr.washington.edu GO: www.geneontology.org (Cellular Components)**	**GO: www.geneontology.org (Cellular Function)**		GO:www.geneontology.org (Cellular Processes)
Molecule	ChEBI: ebi.ac.uk/chebi PrO: http://pir.georgetown.edu/pro/ RnaO: http://roc.bgsu.edu/ SO: song.sf.net		GO: www.geneontology.org (Molecular Function)		GO:www.geneontology.org (Molecular Processes)

List of abbreviations: CARO: Common Anatomy Reference Ontology , ChEBI: Chemical Entities of Biological Interest , FMA: Foundational Model of Anatomy, FMP: Foundational Model of Physiology:, CPRO: Clinical Pharmacology Research Organization (University of British Columbia), GO: Gene Ontology (cellular components, molecular functions, biological processes), PaTO: Phenotypic Quality Ontology , PrO: Protein Ontology, RnaO: RNA Ontology, SO: Sequence Ontology

stop) were identified; in addition, 17 artefactual sentences were discarded.

Careful reading of these abstracts allows the writing of rules and 4 tests were necessary to achieve a working set of rules. The first run allows designing n/m rules. The effects of new changes and additional rules were checked in the following tests.

A set of 38 rules was designed and a part of the complete set of rules is given in table 2. The first column presents some of the marker list and the rule structure is detailed in the following columns.

For example, rule 1 states:

IF $VerbLoc $PrepLocIn ($NounLoc + $NounSnapBio)
THEN Intend Loc-in

The positions in the rule was presented as the following in the table

$VerbLoc 1
$PrepLocIn 2
$NounLoc 3
$NounSnapBio 3
($NounSnapBio + $NounLoc) 3+3

Similarly, let's consider rule 4:

IF ($NounSnapBio or $NounLoc) $VerbLoc ($NounSnapBio or $NounLoc)
THEN Intend Loc-in

The positions in the rule was corresponding as follows in the table

$NounSnapBio 1
$NounLoc 1
$VerbLoc 2
$NounSnapBio 3
$NounLoc 3
($NounSnapBio or $NounLoc) 1 or 1
3 or 3
(terms into brackets in the rule were specified as "or" choice in the table).

A set of 10 rules of 38 are presented below (Table 2)

VALIDATION

Validation was performed by looking at recall (ρ) and precision (π) that are two common measures for assessing a text categoriser:

- Recall states how good is the system at finding the relevant document for a specific task; and formally can be written as the ratio of true-positives and the sum of true-positives and false-negatives

$$\rho = \frac{\mathtt{true\_positives}}{\mathtt{true\_positives} + \mathtt{false\_negatives}}$$

- Precision measures the quality of selected data and formally can be written as the ratio

Table 2. Structure of the rules in SEEKbio

Marker lists	Rule 1	Rule 2	Rule 3	Rule 4	Rule 5	Rule 6	Rule 7	Rule 8	Rule 9	Rule 22
$ConjFr										
$ConjLoc										
$Gene										
$IsExpressed										
$NounLoc	3		1 / 3	1 / 3						
$NounSnapBio	3	1	1 / 3	1 / 3	1 / 3	4	1, 4	1 / 5		
$NounSpanBio		3				1 /3	2	2 /4	1 / 4	1 / 3
$PrepLocAfter										
$PrepLocEx										
$PrepLocFr										
$PrepLoc	2	2	2		2		3	3	3	
$PrepLocOn										
$PrepLocOrg										
$PrepLocTarget										
$PrepLocTi										2
$VerbBe										
$VerbCaus										
$VerbFr										
$VerbInit									2	
$VerbLoc	1			2		2				1
$VerbMov										
"+"						3 + 4	1 + 2	1 + 2 / 4 + 5		
"or"	3 or 3		1 or 1 / 3 or 3	1 or 1 / 3 or 3						1 or 1
	Loc-in	Participle	Loc-in	Loc-in	Realize	Realize	Realize	Realize	Loc-in	Loc-st

of true-positives and the sum of true-positives and false-negatives:

$$\pi = \frac{\texttt{true\_positives}}{\texttt{true\_positives} + \texttt{false\_positives}}$$

This validation was performed using a new corpus selected from PubMed. To make sure that enough location relations would be identified for our validation purpose, the query equation was similar (although more precise) to the first series unless the animal species was changed (mouse instead drosophila).

<< "Embryonic development" mouse location >>

This was performed on February 19th, 2008 and a set of 71 occurrences were found from which the 50 more recent abstracts were download.

The 13th first abstracts consist in 178 sentences (any text between two full points) of which 145 correspond to full sentences and the 23 left were artefactual material. These 145 full sentences were checked for rule activation. Among them, we found the following relations: loc_in: 87; Loc_St: 14; Loc_After: 1; Loc_Fr: 3,; Loc_On: 3; Loc_Origin: 3; Realize: 16 and Participle: 20. The sum of these relations was stated as the True_positive and equals to 146. In addition, 8 false_positive and 6 false_negative were found (see below, for discussion).

Accordingly, recall (ρ) and precision (π) were found equal to 0.96 and 0.95, respectively.

FUTURE TRENDS

False positives result, mostly, from the fact that a sentence can have one or more clauses that come either before or after the main clause and begin with a conjunction (when, if, because, etc.) or is made of two sentences that are separated by a coma.

For example, in SEEK*bio* analysis of the following sentence:

One dataset contained genes that are expressed solely in a single developmental stage; the second was made of genes expressed at different developmental stages

The following rules were found:

Loc-in (19-1)
Participle (participle)

Actually, the Participle (participle 1-1) rule was activated two times: once for :

genes ... expressed ... in ...stage

and second,in the following sentence:

genes expressed at ...stages

In addition, a Location-in (19-1) rule was activated of which signature was <*SPAN, SPAN*> according to the sequence:

stage... at... stages

This sequence was made possible because the ";" between the two sentences was not taken into account in SEEK*bio* accounting for false positive.

Otherwise, false negatives were mostly due to the absence of the relevant marker, for example, quail, in the following example, that would allow activating the rule Location-in (1-2):

Further analysis by immunochemistry showed that the location of qbrn-1 protein was consistent with that of the transcripts in the developing quail.

Further improvements in SEEK*bio* would allow to take into consideration the present continuous (*is occurring in*), the simple past tense

(*It occurred in*) and the present perfect (*has occurred in*), when the verb *to occur* is listed in the VerbLoc list.

In addition, the present progressive (is undergoing) is actually not distinguished of the–ing and the –ed forms (participles) used as adjectives; these make rules difficult to apply and can result if false positive and negative forms. More work is required to answer this issue.

REFERENCES

Ananiadou, S. Kell, D. B., & Tsujii, J. (2006). Text mining and its potential applications in systems biology. *TRENDS in Biotechnology, 24*(12), 571-579.

Cooper, J. W., & Kershenbaum, A. (2005). Discovery of protein-protein interactions using a combination of linguistic, statistical and graphical information. *BMC Bioinformatics, 6*, 143.

Donaldson, I et al. (2003). PreBIND and Textomy–mining the biomedical literature for protein-protein interactions using a support vector machine. *BMC Bioinformatics, 4*, 11.

Donnelly, M., Bittner, T., & Rosse, C. (2006).A Formal Theory for Spatial Representation and Reasoning in Biomedical Ontologies. *Artificial Intelligence in Medicine, 36*(1), 1 – 27.

Donnelly, M., Bittner, T., & Rosse, C. . (2005) A formal theory for spatial representation and reasoning in biomedical ontologies. *Artif Intell Med., 21*, 16249077.

Donnelly, M. (2004). On parts and holes: the spatial structure of human body. In M. Fieschi, E. Coiera, & Y. J. Li (Eds.), *Proceedings of the 11th World Congress on Medical Informatics*. IOS Press, Amsterdam.

Finkel, J. et al. (2005). Exploring the boundaries: gene and protein identification in Biomedial text. *BMC Bioinformatics, 6*, S5.

Grenon, P., & Smith, B. (2003). SNAP and SPAN: Towards Geospatial Dynamics. *Spatial Cognition and Computation, 4*(1), 69-104.

Jensen, L. J., Saric, J., & Bork, P. (2006). Literature mining for the biologist: from information retrieval to biological discovery. *Nature Reviews Genetics, 7*, 119-129.

Jouis C. (2007). SEEK-CLIPS : construction d'ontologies en utilisant l'exploration contextuelle. Extraction semi-automatique des relations puis des concepts à partir de textes, *OntoTexte 2007 («Ontologies et Textes»)*, Sophia Antipolis, 10 oct. 2007, France, 5-8.

Jouis, C., (1993). *Contributions à la conceptualisation et à la modélisation des connaissances à partir d'une analyse linguistique de textes. Réalisation d'un prototype : le système SEEK*, PhD dissertation, Ecole des Hautes Etudes en Sciences Sociales (EHESS), Paris France.

Lu, D., Szafron, R., Greiner, P., Lu, D.S., Wishart, B. Poulin, J., Anvik, C., Macdonell, & Eisner, R.(2004). Predicting Subcellular Localization of Proteins using Machine-Learned Classifiers, *Bioinformatics, 20*(4), 547-556.

Miska, E.A., Langley, E., Wolf, D., Karlsson, C., Pines, J., & Kouzarides, T. (2001). Differential localization of HDAC4 orchestrates muscle differentiation. *Nucleic Acids Res, 29*(16), 3439–3447.

Smith, B., & Grenon, P. (2004). The Cornucopia of Formal-Ontological Relations. *Dialectica,* 58(3), 279—296.

Smith, B. et al. (2007). The OBO Foundry: coordinated evolution of ontologies to support biomedical data integration. *Nature Biotechnology, 25*, 1251 – 1255.

Srinivasan, P. (2001). MeSHmap: a text mining tool for MEDLINE. *Proceedings of AMIA Sym*, (pp. 642-646).

Stapley, B. J. et al. (2002). Predicting the sub-cellular location of proteins from text using support vectors machines. *Pacific Symposium on Biocomputing, 7*, 734-385.

Stapley, B. J., & Benoit, G. (2000). Biobibliometrics: information retrieval and visualization from co-occurrence of gene names in Medline abstracts. *Pacific Symposium on Biocomputing, 5*, 529-540.

Strutt, H., & Strutt, D. (1999). Polarity determination in the Drosophila eye. *Curr Opin Genet Dev, 9*, 442-446.

Wren, J. D., & Garner, H. R. (2004). Shared relationships analysis: ranking set cohesion and commonalities within a literature-derived relationships network. *Bioinformatics, 20*, 191-198.

ENDNOTES

[a] http://www-tsujii.is.s.u-tokyo.ac.jp/GENIA

[b] http://bioie.ldc.upenn.edu

Section V

Conclusion and Perspectives

Chapter XX
Analysing Clinical Notes for Translation Research:
Back to the Future

Jon Patrick
The University of Sydney, Australia

Pooyan Asgari
The University of Sydney, Australia

ABSTRACT

There have been few studies of large corpora of narrative notes collected from the health clinicians working at the point of care. This chapter describes the principle issues in analysing a corpus of 44 million words of clinical notes drawn from the Intensive Care Service of a Sydney hospital. The study identifies many of the processing difficulties in dealing with written materials that have a high degree of informality, written in circumstances where the authors are under significant time pressures, and containing a large technical lexicon, in contrast to formally published material. Recommendations on the processing tasks needed to turn such materials into a more usable form are provided. The chapter argues that these problems require a return to issues of 30 years ago that have been mostly solved for computational linguists but need to be revisited for this entirely new genre of materials. In returning to the past and studying the contents of these materials in retrospective studies we can plan to go forward to a future that provides technologies that better support clinicians. They need to produce both lexically and grammatically higher quality texts that can then be leveraged successfully for advanced translational research thereby bolstering its momentum.

INTRODUCTION

This volume gives a picture of the current progress in using Natural Language Processing to provide better access to written materials that are on the whole published under formal assessments and processes. Such materials are more amenable to different NLP tasks than the genre of content produced by clinicians working at the point of care with very sick and dying patients. The point-of-care texts are distinctly different in two important ways - *weaker adherence to grammatical structure*, and *the complexity and veracity of lexical form*. A further difference is in the objectives of the processing tasks themselves. The papers of this volume have defined the necessary task as that of information retrieval in and of itself. Processing clinical notes has a much larger number of objectives which makes it both more complex but also provides a greater number of opportunities to be creative and contribute to enhancements to the field of health care. Translational research, or more colloquially known as "bench to bed" research, is looming to be by far the most important field for improving our health care. This is the process of linking together the research performed in the laboratory to the processes and treatments conducted at the bedside. Much of this work is seen as personalized medicine that will produce drugs targeted at an individual's personal genome, however research into this ideal healthcare is highly restricted without technology that enables linking of the patient records created at the point-of-care with the models of drug-genome interaction built in the laboratory. NLP is a most important bridge between these two end points in the search for better healthcare. Without effective and accurate processing of the point-of-care records to provide evidence of the effectiveness of drugs and the course of diseases in patients under drug treatment there can be no development of evidence based drug treatment, and translational research will progress more slowly than it would otherwise.

This paper presents some of the models we have developed for representing the different processing needs of clinical staff and describes the lessons we have learned from problems encountered in analysing a large corpus of 44 million words of clinical notes.

BACKGROUND

The task of performing natural language processing over clinical notes goes back to 1983 Chi, E. C., Sager, N., Tick, L. J., & Lyman, M. S.; Gabrieli, E. R., Speth, D. J. , 1986) with the work Chi, Sager, Tick and Lyman, and it is only gradually increased in activity to this date. However, in 2008 with have had the first conference specifically targeted at the "Text and Data Mining of Clinical Documents" with a conference organized by the Turku Centre for Computer Science, in Finland (Karsten, H., Back, B., Salakoski, T., Salanterä, S., & Suominen, H., 2008). Much of the work prior to the 1990s has been superceded by later shifts in processing power and new ideas on the software development for this task. The review of the literature in this paper is restricted to later topics that are particularly relevant to automated processing of the language of clinical notes.

In 2001, Taira and Soderland published their approach to information extraction from clinical notes in the radiology domain. They proposed a general structure for such applications which was later used by many other research groups (Huang, Y., Lowe, H., Klein, D., & Cucina, R., 2005; Arnold, C. W., Bui, A. A. T., Morioka, C., El-Saden, S., & Kangarloo, H., 2007; Thomas, B. J., Ouellette, H., Halpern, E. F., & Rosenthal, D. I., 2005; Sinha, U., & Kangarloo, H., 2002). Their proposal had five steps of processing for a complete data retrieval system: *Structural analyzer, Lexical analyzer, Parser, Semantic interpreter and Frame constructor.* They performed an evaluation on this structuring and reported obstacles in: deep understanding of the domain, ability to deal with ungrammatical writing styles, shorthand and telegraphic writings, finding solutions for assumed knowledge between the writer and reader, and handling a large vocabulary. Following their work, different studies have expanded their proposed system to other clinical domains or addressed the reported issues (Sun, J. Y., & Sun, Y., 2006) and in some cases reported new obstacles.

Our discussion of a structure for a medical information extraction system has some parts in common with Taira and Soderland. Moreover, we describe the commonalities in efforts which have been made to address existing issues in the life cycle and the operational objectives of an information extraction system. Table 1 shows a summary of this survey.

Lexical & Phrasal Issues

In clinical notes there is a high complexity to orthography not found in other prose materials such as press reports and formal publications. Some of these domain specific issues are:

1. A large number of mistakes especially for long words.
2. Special abbreviations for entities such as chemical names.
3. Specialist shorthand for idiosyncratic cultural items
4. LOTE (Language other than English) staff using different phonological transformations
5. Keyboard competency
6. Specialty complex terms with variable greco-latin roots
7. Neologisms
8. Verbalization of named entities, especially drug names
9. Productive morphology combined with neologisms
10. Staff access and use of correct materials

In the past decade, researchers have tried to address some of the above issues in many dif-

Table 1. Summary of survey of the literature on processing clinical note

<table>
<tr><th>NLP Topics</th><th>Major Issues</th><th colspan="2">Proposed Solutions</th></tr>
<tr><td rowspan="9">Lexical
&
Phrasal</td><td>Orthography, Keyboard competency & Spell Checking</td><td colspan="2">Regular expression and UMLS based dictionaries</td></tr>
<tr><td>Verbalization of named-entities
& Drug names</td><td colspan="2">No Clear Answer</td></tr>
<tr><td>Abbreviations & Shorthand</td><td colspan="2">Regular expressions and disambiguation algorithms</td></tr>
<tr><td>LOTE issues: Phonological Transformation</td><td colspan="2">No Clear Solution</td></tr>
<tr><td>Neologisms & productive morphology</td><td colspan="2">No Clear Solution</td></tr>
<tr><td rowspan="4">Issue with Multi-word expressions & Capturing Phrases</td><td colspan="2">Complex parser and external knowledge source</td></tr>
<tr><td colspan="2">compositional mapping</td></tr>
<tr><td colspan="2">Part of speech tagging</td></tr>
<tr><td colspan="2">statistical natural language parser</td></tr>
<tr><td rowspan="10">Semantics</td><td>Word sense disambiguation</td><td colspan="2">Variety of algorithms</td></tr>
<tr><td rowspan="4">Mapping issue among Terminologies, Thesauri, Ontologies & classifications (TTOCs)</td><td colspan="2">Frames</td></tr>
<tr><td colspan="2">semantic definitions</td></tr>
<tr><td colspan="2">Diagrams</td></tr>
<tr><td colspan="2">combination oflexical, logical & morphological</td></tr>
<tr><td rowspan="2">Negation</td><td colspan="2">regular expression matching</td></tr>
<tr><td colspan="2">grammatical parsing</td></tr>
<tr><td rowspan="3">Concept Recognition</td><td>Statistical</td><td>Rule based</td></tr>
<tr><td colspan="2">Lexical</td></tr>
<tr><td colspan="2">Hybrid</td></tr>
</table>

ferent ways. A short summary of these efforts follows.

Lexical Verification

NLP is used to perform a variety of low level tasks in information retrieval systems such as term identification. Ananiadou et al in 1994, Frantzi and others in 1998 and Savova et al in 2003 reported different approaches in term identification (Savova, G., Harris, M. R., Johnson, T., Pakhomov, S.V., &. Chute, C. G., 2003; Ananiadou, S., 1994; Frantzi, K., Ananiadou, S., & Tsujii, J., 1998). All reported the affect of orthographic variations in their results. In 2002, Ruch described an IR system which was able to cope with textual misspellings. He demonstrated the extent to which dealing with spelling issues can improve the performance of an IR system (Ruch, P., 2002).

In 2007, Tolentino, Matters, Walop, Law, and Tong described a prototype spell checker which used UMLS and WordNet as primary and secondary domain specific dictionaries, and regular expressions as a look up method. The result was satisfactory except they reported relatively slow processing and low performance.

Lexical verification in clinical notes deals with different types of data for which some researchers suggested different approaches. In 2005 Zhou and Han introduced a new approach in extracting three groups of data from clinical notes: *numeric values, medical terms and categorical values.* Their approach considered three different approaches for these three different groups of data. It was extended in 2006 and they reported satisfactory results (Zhou, X., Han, H., Chankai, I., Prestrud, A., & Brooks, A., 2006).

Abbreviation Identification

Pustejovsky et al. (2001) described a solution for identifying abbreviations based on regular expressions and syntactic information which lead to an increase in the accuracy of identification of noun phrase boundaries. Chang et al (2001) described an algorithm that uses linear regression, Park and Byrd (2001) and Yu et al. (2002) introduced some rule-based algorithms for extraction of abbreviations. Schwartz in 2003 described a very simple but effective algorithm for identifying abbreviations in the biomedical domain. Systems have also been developed to map abbreviations to full forms such as AbbRE (abbreviation recognition and extraction) by Yu et al (2002). There does not seem to be any comprehensive or specific studies on mnemonics in clinical contexts.

Phrasal Level

Dealing with multi-word expressions (MWE) and phrases has been a principal focus of researchers in recent years. Multi-word expressions have been traditionally recognised though standard terminologies. However non-standardized MWEs (e.g. weights and measures, administrative entities) are major issues in phrase processing.

Identification of NPs in both simple and complex forms is one of the challenges in this field where achieving a high precision is the main goal (Yu et al., 2002). In past work MetaMap (Aronson, A. R., 2001), MedLee (Friedman, C., Alderson, P. O., Austin, J. H., et al., 1994) use phrase identification as one of their important steps. MedLee has a Component for Phrase-regularization which regularizes the output forms of phrases that are not contiguous. Moreover MedLee uses a compositional mapping approach which is the combination of central finding (mapped term e.g. enlarged) with its attributes (e.g. severe) or body location modifier (e.g. heart) compared to a concept dictionary and if there are new matches with more accuracy then the combination of words they would be captured as a phrase.

Part of speech tagging for phrase identification also has been used since 1994 when Sager et al. reported a preliminary investigation on mapping clinical terms to SNOMED III (Sager, N., Lyman, M., Nhan, N. T., et al., 2004).

In 2005, Huang et al addressed this issue by using a statistical natural language parser trained on a nonmedical domain in conjunction with using a UMLS Specialist Lexicon. Their results were promising when their custom-designed system achieved almost similar performance figures for both medical and general domains (Huang, Y., Lowe, H., Klein, D., & Cucina, R., 2005).

Semantic Level

Concept Recognition

There are a number of different approaches in concept matching. Between 1990 and 1994, a project at the University of Pittsburgh (Lowe, H. J., Buchanan, B. G., Cooper, G. F., & Vries, J. K., 2005; Miller, R. A., Gieszczykiewicz, F. M., Vries, J. K., & Cooper, G. F.· 1992· Kanter, S. L., Miller, R. A., Tan, M., & Schwartz, J.· 1994) compared two available methods in concept matching - lexical and statistical - evaluated and combine them. The results of their efforts were two different systems: PostDoc (lexical) and Pindex (statistical). Each program takes free text as input from a patient's electronic medical record, and as output it returns a list of suggested MeSH terms. Cooper and Miller (Cooper, G. F., & Miller, R. A., 1998) followed the Pittsburgh's Project in 1998 and performed evaluation on both statistical, lexical and the hybrid methods.

Lexical analysis is one of these approaches. The lexical approach is computationally fast and useful for real-time applications (Huang, Y., Lowe, H., Klein, D., & Cucina, R., 2005); however, this approach may not provide optimal results without combination with other methods (Zou, Q., Chu, W. W., Morioka, C., et al., 2003). An example of this combination is Purcell et al.'s study. In 1995 Purcell and Shortliffe reported their experience in considering context in concept matching where they used concepts encoded in headings of clinical documents to elevate the accuracy (Purcell, G. P., & Shortliffe, E. H., 1995). Following their study, Berrios combined Purcell's technique together with a vector space model and a statistical method to match text content to a set of query types (Huang, Y., Lowe, H., Klein, D., & Cucina, R., 2005; Berrios, D. C., 2000). In 2003 *IndexFinder* was developed by Zou et al. to add syntactic and semantic filtering to improve performance on top of lexical mapping (Huang, Y. et al., 2005; Zou, Q., et al., 2003). Before this point some important research had been done with researchers focused on applying more sophisticated NLP techniques to improve concept recognition accuracy. Friedmen (1994) by using phrase identification tried to improve the concept matching.

In 2001, Nedkarni et al. performed a feasibility study on using UMLS in a computational strategy to identify concepts in medical narrative text. They concluded that the level of noise in the UMLS database impacted on the accuracy of their system and considerable filtering needed to be performed to define a UMLS subset that is suitable for concept matching. In 2007 *Osornio et al·* developed a local interface for SNOMED CT to let users design their own concept subsets or to modify the database to make it more amenable to their concept matching needs.

In 2006, Elkin et al· evaluated the Content Coverage of SNOMED in representing a clinical problem list. They reported encouraging results but they reported improvements to synonymy and adding missing modifiers would lead to a better coverage of SNOMED and address some common problems. Later In 2007, Patrick et al. proposed a system to translate free text clinical notes into SNOMED CT as a web service. They installed their system in an intensive care unit (ICU) to be tested and evaluated in a real scenario. They reported restricting the concept mapping to noun phrase chunks can rule out many false positives and also increase the speed of processing. They also reported on issues like many pre-coordinated terms and qualifications cross noun phrase boundaries.

MedLEE (Friedman, C., et al., 2003) a system developed by Friedman et al. to encode clinical texts, is a well known example of a concept matching through structure detection. Along with MedLEE there are a few other applications (Taira, R. K., & Soderland, S. G., 1999; Taira, R. K., Soderland, S. G., & Jakobovits, R. M., 2001; Christensen, L., Haug, P. J., & Fiszman, M., 2002) which encode modifiers together with core concepts in noun phrases (NPs). The MedLee authors and others in 2005 have extended this approach to other clinical domains and reported encouraging results however they reported that there were many different fields open for improvement and research (Hripcsak, G., Kuperman, G. J., & Friedman, C., 1998; Hripcsak, G., Austin, J. H., Alderson, P. O., & Friedman, C., 2002; Friedman, C. 2000).

MetaMap (Aronson, A. R., 2001) is another concept matching method by structure detection which identifies UMLS concepts in text and returns them in a ranked list in a five step process. Step 1: parsing text for syntactic tagging and then indicating the most important parts of a phrase. Step 2: extracting all possible variants of a phrase and scoring them, Step 3: retrieve all concepts from UMLS which has at least one listed variant. Step 4: evaluate the candidates based on their score. Step 5: combine best candidates to generate the closest concept in UMLS.

Word Sense Disambiguation (WSD)

Although word sense disambiguation is a general field in which a great deal of work has been done, it is still a major field of study and open to research in clinical domain. Ruch et al. (2001) reported that clinical notes compared to unrestricted or general texts is much less ambiguous, however Weeber et al. (2001) reported that the world's largest medical thesaurus (UMLS), has more than 7,000 ambiguous strings that map to more than one concept in a thesaurus.

Nadkarni et al. (2001) reported that a complete automatic concept indexing in medical notes may not be achieved without addressing ambiguity issue in free text. A good example of the efforts in this area is Aronson (2001) study. In 2001, Aronson reported that addressing ambiguity issues is important for enhancing the performance of MetaMap, a mapping program for UMLS concepts. Later in 2001, Weeber and Aronson with an intention to evaluate different available algorithms for WSD, developed a manually sense-tagged test collection of data (Weeber, M., Mork, J., & Aronson, A., 2001) suitable for this purpose. This test collection became a good resource for different researchers to evaluate their algorithms against a standard corpus like the study which has been done by Liu et al. (2002).

Most of the available approaches to word sense disambiguation use or combine different machine learning techniques and refer to characteristics of the ambiguity and its surrounding words relying on a collection of examples Schuemie, M. J., Kors, J. A., & Mons, B., 2005; Leroy, G., &. Rindflesch, T. C., 2003; Resnik, P., & Yarowsky, D., 2000; Dorow, B., & Widdows, D., 2003). In 2005 by Schuemie et al. performed a comprehensive study about WSD in biomedical domain in recent years. They classified the current available approaches into a 5 major branches namely, WSD using:

1. Established knowledge.
2. Bilingual corpora.
3. Supervised learning.
4. Feature vectors.
5. Unsupervised learning.

They concluded that the lack of adequate test sets is probably the most important obstacle to the development and evaluation of effective WSD methods in this field.

Negation

One of most extensive studies on negation was published by Mutalik et al. in 2001. They reported Negation of most concepts in medical narratives can be reliably detected by a simple strategy depending on several factors, the most important being the accuracy of concept matching. Later in the same year, Chapman et al. conducted a study about negation recognition algorithms and they concluded that to be robust a negation algorithm triggered by the negation phrases should apply syntactic and lexical knowledge.

In 2005, Elkin et al improved the Chapman and Mutalik findings by comparing the accuracy of an automated mechanism for assignment of negation to clinical concepts with human assigned negation. They performed a failure analysis to identify the causes of poorly identified negation. Based on their findings, they introduced a new strategy of association of the negative concept to other concept(s) to increase the accuracy.

While most of the negation identification approaches rely on either regular expression matching (Chapman, W. W., Bridewell, W., Hanbury, P., Cooper, G. F., & Buchanan, B., 2001) or grammatical parsing (Huang, Y., & Lowe, H. J., 2005). In 2007 **Huang** and his group introduced a new hybrid method combining regular expression matching with grammatical parsing. They reported the grammatical parser enabled them to detect negated concepts more accurately at a distance from the negation phrase.

It seems, negation identification in clinical notes cannot be done effectively without addressing special requirements of these types of text such as multiple negations and indirect negations are important sub-types of negation.

Mapping between Terminologies, Thesauri, Ontologies & Classifications (TTOCs)

There are a variety of lexical resources available for processing clinical texts. Bodenreider [(2006)] completed a study of many of them and concluded there are difficulties in differentiating between terminologies, thesauri, ontologies and classifications (TTOCs). Each however can be used solely as a lexical resource without considering its structural organisation. Nevertheless, a major issue in natural language processing is a lack of a truly comprehensive clinical vocabulary (Sun, J. Y., & Sun, Y., 2006). Several algorithms have been proposed to automate translation across the variety of TTOCs. Frames (Rocha, R. A., Rocha, B. H. S. C., & Huff, S. M., 1993), semantic definitions (Dolin, R. H., Huff, S. M., Rocha, R. A., Spackman, K. A., & Campbell, K. E., 1998) adopting diagrams [11], and a mix of lexical, logical and morphological methods (Rocha, R. A., & Huff, S. M., 1994) are examples of these algorithms.

In 2004 a comprehensive study was published by Sun (2004) about different techniques and approaches to finding a mapping between two different medical terminologies. He introduced an application, MEDIATE, which adopted semantic networks as an intermediary representation of the databases then an automated mapping algorithm can locate equivalent concepts in different TTOCs. The algorithms take advantage of the conceptual "context" implemented within a semantic network to populate a list of candidate concepts (Sun, Y., 2004). Later in 2006 he extended his work and introduced the LINC tool and listed some new obstacles that confront the data mapping efforts. (Sun, J. Y., & Sun, Y., 2006) This remains an unsolved problem with most practical solutions resorting to some degree of manual processing.

A MODEL OF NLP SERVICES FOR CLINICAL WORK

There are two classes of written materials relevant to studies of clinical narratives. The first class is published content for example, case studies, medical knowledge and clinical protocols/pathways, and standardized care plans. These have correct English prose, shifting contexts, and scientific background knowledge from many aspects of medicine: diseases, procedures, chemistry, pharmaceuticals, family history, and current care plans.

The good prose strategy allows for the use of many of the traditional methods of NLP analysis.

The second class of materials is progress notes or clinical notes from the point-of-care. They are collected in acute care as ward notes and are very different (putting handwriting problems aside) in that they are written rapidly, have rapid shifts in context, extensive abbreviations, significant faulty and improvised orthography and grammar. Sources of some errors are LOTE background and poor typing skills. They make significant assumptions about context and in the limit are written in the highest order of assumptions about a priori knowledge being solely for the benefit and understanding of the writer without consideration of another reader.

Content analysis of published materials is about supporting IR to deliver general medical knowledge to the practitioner. Ward notes are multi-pronged and directed at supporting the attending physicians and their team for a much broader range of activities. We define physicians as needing to serve four roles in their working environment:

1. Point-of-care clinician
2. Researcher
3. Administrator
4. Auditor

In each of these roles the experienced physician has to constantly serve the modes of both the professional and the teacher. The use of progress notes and therefore the types of processing that they require varies between these roles.

The *point-of-care clinician* requires access to the narrative of the notes to determine their next act of care, hence the processing system needs to produce an extract of the current state of the patient and the issues that need to be addressed immediately about their ongoing care whether that is a short term decision as in the Emergency Department or the Intensive Care Unit, or for the longer term at the point of discharge from a hospital. The processing needs are essentially information extraction of particular items such as current diagnoses, care plans, current pathology results (taken from a narrative report) etc. These needs have a high requirement for precision of retrieval as errors of "fact" can lead to disastrous consequences, were as errors of omission are less likely to have such effect and more likely to lead to user discontent of the system.

The *researcher physician* has a somewhat different demand in that they are most interested in aggregation over sets of patient records in the process of performing analytics. Under these circumstances some errors in retrieval are likely to be tolerable as the conclusions one draws from aggregation are likely to be understood to have their own error behaviors. However as the research process is seeking associations between variables the nature of retrieval is intrinsically about the association of one phenomenon with another. This problem can be defined if one so wishes as two or more independent information extraction tasks, however it is likely to be more valuable and possibly more reliable to perform retrieval exploiting a supposed relationship between two variables of interest. For example a study of fractures and hips, would lead to a strategy to extract references to either collocated or anaphoric cross-references to hips and fractures with processing to assess their grammatical relationships (the x-ray showed a 20mm mass just above the hip which became fractured in a later fall") rather than a hunt for "fractured hip" and its string variants. This role and the language processing functions to be provided for it are fundamental to translational research both for retrospective studies and prospective studies.

The *administrator physician* has similar functions to that of the researcher physician in that they require aggregation of content across collections of patients. The difference is that the target variables will come from issues about usage and management of clinical resources.

The fourth role is that of *auditor physician*, that is, a person who audits the processes in the clinical unit to ensure they are maximized for patient safety as well as throughput. The auditor needs processing systems to support analysis of both single patient records and aggregation. When investigating an individual case the auditor will need tools to make ad hoc queries about a single case and at the same time seek to understand the performance of the unit over collections of cases to establish if single cases are out of the norm.

Understanding the roles of clinicians and their needs enables targeting the design and development of language technology to attend to those needs and so deliver productivity and patient safety gains in the workplace.

In summary, the processing requirements are to perform information retrieval on single records to find the precise location in the record for a precise piece of information. For example a staff member attending a patient might want to ask a specific question *"what medications were ordered by this morning ward rounds staff"* which most closely matches an information extraction or Q&A process. Nevertheless another question could be *"what is this patient's care plan and how far have we progressed with?"* This question requires extracting a set of information that has some intrinsic coherence which may well not be all in the one place, in particular the record of actions in executing the care plan will be distributed over pages of notes recorded across the whole time period the patient has been in hospital.

The role of the researcher physician has both different and overlapping needs to the point-of-care clinician. The researcher requires aggregation over records as they investigate the behaviors of staff/processes/drugs/procedures over a collection of specially defined patients. They also need to be able to frame their questions in a manner that is linguistically formal but in the terminology of the clinical setting. The language processing needs for this role are formidable as it requires a number of processing sub-systems to be delivered:

1. Support the common language in the clinical setting in use in the user interface.
2. Information extraction from the individual patient records.
3. Co-ordination of record retrieval based on language and non-language variables.
4. Descriptive statistics analytics using the two types of variables concurrently. An example question might be: "*what is the mean hospital bed occupancy of all males over the 5-year age groups of 40-90 with lung cancer?*"
5. Analytical Statistics comparing hypotheses, for example: "*is there a statistically significant difference in the age of admission for women compared to men for an upper respiratory tract cancers treated by chemotherapy compared to radiotherapy?*"

The processing systems required by the roles of administrator and auditing should be catered for by the systems needed for point-of-care clinician and the researchers if they are designed with sufficient generality.

Experienced staff will need to place themselves in all four of these roles, and their modes of practitioner and teacher, many times in the working week. The objective of NLP should be to develop systems to serve these roles and their modes. The following case study of a corpus analysis identifies many of the problems associated with the current quality of clinical documentation and the strategies we have to implement to overcome them, so that the contents can be used for retrospective clinical research. Moreover building new language technologies to eliminate or minimise these problems paves the way to doing prospective studies in situ in the clinical context and thereby support the enhancement and momentum of translational research.

A CORPUS OF NARRATIVE NOTES FROM AN INTENSIVE CARE UNIT

Building practical language processing systems to serve the roles of physicians and hence support the care and safety of patients and as well as the advancement of medical science requires learning from retrospective studies the limitations of already recorded information and then to design and build new technologies to overcome them. This has been achieved in the case of a study of intensive care notes from an Australian hospital.

The corpus of this study was drawn from 6 years of progress notes (2002-2006) consisting of 44,000,000 words written about 12,000 patients. The notes represent the recordings of all disciplines working in the Intensive Care Service of the Royal Prince Alfred Hospital, Sydney Australia, including intensivists, visiting medical officers (medical specialists), nurses and allied health workers (physiotherapists, psychologists, dietitians, etc.). The corpus is to be known as the RPAH-ICU corpus.

Stages of Processing

This paper deals with a range of issues important to processing these materials before they reach the stage of being usable for information extraction, plus some of the issues related to working as collaborators with clinicians pertinent to the privacy of the records.

Anonymisation

While anonymisation is not directly related to information extraction for use in the clinical wards, it is important in obtaining access to these records so that they can be removed off-site to our own installation for extensive analysis. Hence it is a matter that all researchers have to resolve early in their work. The simplest form of anonymisation is achieved by removing the names and address of patients from the header of the record and only use a Medical Record Number (MRN) to identify the record. This step provides surface anonymisation but there may be other personal information in the record that can enable reconstruction of the patient identity. This can happen especially with distinctive information such as rare disorders, rare locations (e.g. the location of a motor car accident), distinctive names of relatives or attending physicians when combined with information such as age and gender of the patient.

Deep anonymisation requires replacement of the names of all third parties in the narrative notes, including hospital staff and relatives, the names of organisations including other hospitals. It is not normally sensible to remove references to age and gender of a patient as this information tends to be important in many aspects of care and so for any future processing tasks, however reference to specific dates of birth should be removed.

An effective method for identifying names of entities not found in suitable gazetteers is to complete a process of lexical verification over the complete corpus and then manually search the list of unknown words for named entities. Whilst this does not guarantee all named entities will be identified it will capture a very large proportion. We have found that the only names we have not been able to recognise are those from languages with which we are unfamiliar. One confounding variable in this process is the names of medical entities which carry the name of a person. This is a problem in two situations: when the word is miss-spelt and when the name is not recorded in the medical lexicon, e.g. Hudson mask.

Lexical Verification

Lexical verification is specifically separated from other lexical processing e.g. tagging, spelling correction, because there is a very significant problem in completing this task with narrative clinical notes. We have identified three phases to lexical verification. The first phase is compiling a set of lexica that can be used for verification.

The second phase is separating out the unknown words and providing putative known words, and the third stage is capturing true words unknown to the current lexica in an automatic way that makes them readily re-usable.

Assembling Lexica

Lexica for medical NLP need to be assembled from a variety of locations. A lexicon of common English words was taken from the MOBY resource. Medical terminology was drawn from the UMLS and also SCT. SCT is not strictly a lexicon but an ontology consisting of a large collection of medical concepts (approx 360,000). In our work we stripped the individual words of each concept to make a lexicon. The concepts were used in a later processing stage. Many more lexical resources can be found on the Internet for single word processing but are not available for high volume batch throughput. The RPAH-ICU corpus was processed through each of these lexica with the results shown in Table 2.

Identifying and Correcting Unknown Words

Medicine has a highly productive use of language that is, it uses the rules of English word formation very regularly to produce new words, especially the combination of semantic fragments to form new clinical words. In our corpus we have discovered approximately 1000 words indicating medical anatomy and procedures that are not present in SNOMED CT, e.g. anteroseptoapicolateral, heparinise.

The former example shows the morphology of the concepts antero-, septo-, apico- and lateral. The later example has a range of forms that show multiple morphologoical transformations, its longest form so far discovered is "reheparinisation", which demonstrates a process of taking a noun neologism, verbalizing it, nominalising the verb and then adding a prefix of repetition. Further cases are new forms of existing abbreviations, which might be treated as spelling errors, entirely new abbreviations, and new/proprietary drug names.

The RPAH-ICU corpus provided 120,780 unknown word types representing about 5% of the alphabetic words (Table 2) although they only constitute 3.6% of the total corpus. Whilst there is some temptation to treat this error rate as tolerable in a very large corpus it is not advisable. On an assumption of an average of 10 words per sentence then this error rate represents one unknown word in every second sentence which would produce a parsing error in 50% of the sentences, without allowing for errors from other sources.

The unknown word list was processed for putative corrections by computing the edit distances

Table 2. Distribution of the known and unknown words in the RPAH-ICU corpus

Token Type	No. of token types	No. of tokens in corpus	Percentage
Alphabetic words	157,866	31,646,421	71.8%
Words in Moby	32,081	28,095,490	63.7%
Words in SNOMED	22,421	29,008,594	65.8%
Words in UMLS (excludes SNOMED words)	25,956	27,893,156	63.3%
Words in SNOMED but not in Moby	5,005	1,985,391	4.5%
Words in either SNOMED or Moby	37,086	30,080,881	68.3%
Words in neither SNOMED nor Moby (Unknown words)	120,780	1,565,540	3.6%

of 1 and 2 edits to known words. The results were divided into three classes: words that had only one candidate correct word (64,152), words that had multiple candidates (27,610), and words that had no candidates (29,018). The verification process involved inserting the words into a spreadsheet with their putative correct forms, manually checking the offered correction and accepting it or providing an alternative word. Checking was done by an experienced English speaker (JP) from personal knowledge and with support from use of dictionaries sources available from the Internet and Google searching. Unidentifiable words were referred to medical colleagues. Ever word type in the single candidate and no candidate classes have been manually corrected in this way. In the multiple candidate class all words down to a frequency of 4 (6312 types) have been manually verified, giving a total of about 100,000 corrected words.

Avenues of research created by having this material will be valuable for future work. Better automatic spell checking at the point of data entry of narrative notes will enhance the quality of the English and make post processing and especially semantic search and concomitant analytics more reliable. Further support at the point and time of data entry can be created and improved, e.g. automatic expansion of acronyms and abbreviations, verification of clinical terminology, auto-completion of difficult terminology for trainees and LOTE speakers.

Two other ICU corpora have been offered to us for similar analyses. This processing will significantly reduce the amount of effort we have to input into preparing these materials and providing analyses. Also we will be able to investigate the differences in lexicon and language usage from different instances of the same communities and thereby recognise the phenomena that are common to all and also triangulate on the level of differences that exist. The continuity of this work both within the community of Intensive Care Services and the potential to expand into other clinical disciplines makes it vitally important to effectively and automatically manage the collection of new language lexica and usage in the course of studying each corpus.

Capturing New Words

Identifying a "correct" form of a word is straight forward despite being very time consuming. However it is most important that the results of this work are captured whilst the work is progressing. Part of the process of manually verifying unknown words provide the opportunity to collect other information to attach to the word. In our case we have added semantic classes to words and descriptions of their morphological components where applicable. The morphology is useful in the future to recognise hyphenated and un-hyphenated version of words even though they have not been seen in the current corpus. The semantic class information we expect to assist us in later tasks of knowledge representation of the patient case, but we have no specific need for it at this stage.

New words need to be provided to subsequent lexical verification processes after they are initially captured. In principle this merely requires adding the word to the current word list used in the processing system. However if the full value of the process of acquiring new words is to be obtained a record needs to be kept of the source of the word and any other classificatory information that is collected at the time of verification, as described above. This approach demands the compilation of the history of the discovery and usage of the lexical item, which self evidently indicates the need to develop a lexical database to record the relevant content. The database should contain all the words identified from the corpus, which by implication includes the misspelt forms so that they can be readily used in later spell checking software. However, the primary function of the lexical database is to record the first source of the word (to the processing system) and then other classical lexicographical information. In a large production processing system the database itself would not be invoked but rather wordlists would be extracted from it for use in "in-memory" processing applications.

Spelling Correction

Automatic and semi-automatic spelling correction at the time of data entry can be based on two alternative premises. The first premise is that the true word can be found by searching a nearby space of letter configurations for the incorrect word – this is the edit distance model and it is effective if the true solution is truly close to the original word. The limitation is created by the fact that computing edit distance alternatives is expensive given real-time response is needed and it generates a large number of alternative answers. The second premise is that a mapping from the erroneous form to the true form is stored in a lexical database with perhaps better than 90% reliability. This approach is most limited when the true word is not stored. The alternative strategy is to build a statistical spell checker based on a supervised machine learner that estimates the type of mistake made by the user and offers alternatives based on the statistical characteristics of typical spelling errors. To develop such an approach requires the accumulation of the data we have collected by manually correcting the RPAH-ICU corpus.

Spell correcting as a post hoc process required for the analysis of a collected corpus requires some variations in these processes.

1. Word substitutions may sometimes be incorrect because the corrected word has not been identified in situ.
2. Some words cannot be corrected and remain "unknown".
3. The consequences of changing the text after the fact can be serious if any mark-up annotation has already been done to the text.

Appropriate planning for the acquisition of new words and their reuse in later processing needs to be carefully engineered. This is an on-going task for poorly composed materials which arises from the continual variation of content that is introduced in a large and busy hospital unit with diverse and ever-changing staff and patient populations.

The objective of the NLP research in this domain should be to draw an ever increasing amount of content from other clinical disciplines, where each new additional corpus will be better served with a continued accumulation of new terminology and new usages of it.

Entity and Concept Recognition

The recognition of medical entities is a vexed and thorny problem for a number of reasons, namely:

1. There are many knowledge resources in existence and a subset has to be chosen to do a particular piece of work, and any selected resources will have their own gaps in the knowledge one needs to give complete coverage for a given corpus.
2. Even with the use of a comprehensive resource like SNOMED CT when gaps are detected there is no ready mechanisms for inserting the nearly discovered content into the original resource.
3. Rich entity resources have concept entities written in linguistically idiosyncratic ways which create their own obstacles to being used for ready recognition in narrative notes. For example the SCT concept of "third degree burn of elbow with loss of limb" can be written in a myriad of other grammatical forms. In another classification it might have the form "burn, 3rd degree". The processing system needs to be able to reduce both the resource text and the narrative text into canonical forms so there is a better chance of matching the narrative with the concept definitional text.

The RPAH-ICU corpus was analysed for concepts using a methodology reported in Patrick et al. (2007) which indexes every SCT concept for its words (excluding stop words) and then reduces the target text to chunks which are in turn canonicalised. Matches with the SCT words are made and the highest ranked matching concept is accepted as the authentic concept representation of that chunk in the narrative notes. Figure 1 shows an example of a block of narrative text, the SCT concepts recognised and the locations they have in the SCT ontology. Apart from 6 true positives there are 4 false negatives: "Cholycystectomy" is "Cholecystectomy" in SCT, a spelling error in "hypogylcaemics", BSL is an unknown abbreviation in SCT, and cardiac failure is an incomplete expression in SCT used in a total of 27 different concepts. Manual inspection of concept identification suggests the error rate on false negatives is between 20-30% without allowing for all forms of orthographic variation. The amount of false of positives has not been estimated yet, as they require extensive manual analysis of the texts.

Terminology Server

An infrastructure for supporting the analysis of text requires an underpinning data repository that stores all the language resources and also supports a variety of processing tasks. Typically NLP projects have used a lexical database for this function however this is not sufficient for clinical NLP. In this field the medical knowledge is invariably stored in more complex knowledge schemata such as TTOCs, from which the terminology server has to deliver all their structure to an application as is necessary. Design issues of terminology servers have not been visited since the late 1990s (Chute, C., Elkin, P. L., Sheretz, D. D., & Tuttle, M. S., 1999) and require a review which we are undertaking. However the practical experience of this research indicates that a terminology server must serve at least the needs of concept identification, data analytics, Inter TTOC mapping, and decision support. It is within the terminology server that medical terminology that is acquired during processing a corpus is not only recorded but placed within a TTOC framework to maximize its potential re-use in knowledge modelling – not just language processing.

Research Objectives

A set of SCT concepts extracted from a large corpus brings the opportunity to inductively infer the most appropriate subset of SCT for Intensive Care services. There are 13,136,022 concept instances making up about 30,000 unique concept types detected in the corpus. Reducing the set of concepts to those of a frequency 100 and more yields the reduced set comprising 2718 codes, which covers 6,177,077 of the 6,428,597 codable item instances or 96.09% of all codable items. The remaining 3.91% of codable items (n=251,520) requires an additional 21,375 SCT codes. Restricting the set to only the top 1000 codes by usage would cover 89.25% of the codable items in the corpus.

Subsequent to computing the SCT subset evidenced in the corpus another stage of computing the minimal superset of the evidenced set and the local sub-trees around them has to be performed. This ensures coverage beyond what has been observed to what might reasonably be observed without allowing the subset to expand too greatly. The subset inferred from this strategy produced about 15,000 concepts and relationships or about 1% of the total SCT database.

The process has a number of advantages over recruiting a panel of experts to define a suitable SCT subset, namely:

1. It constitutes the evidence for the subset in an unchallengeable manner.
2. It is not susceptible the vagaries of human memory and preferences to compose the list.

Figure 1. Example of clinical narrative notes annotated of SCT codes and illustration of their relationships in the SNOMED CT ontological structure

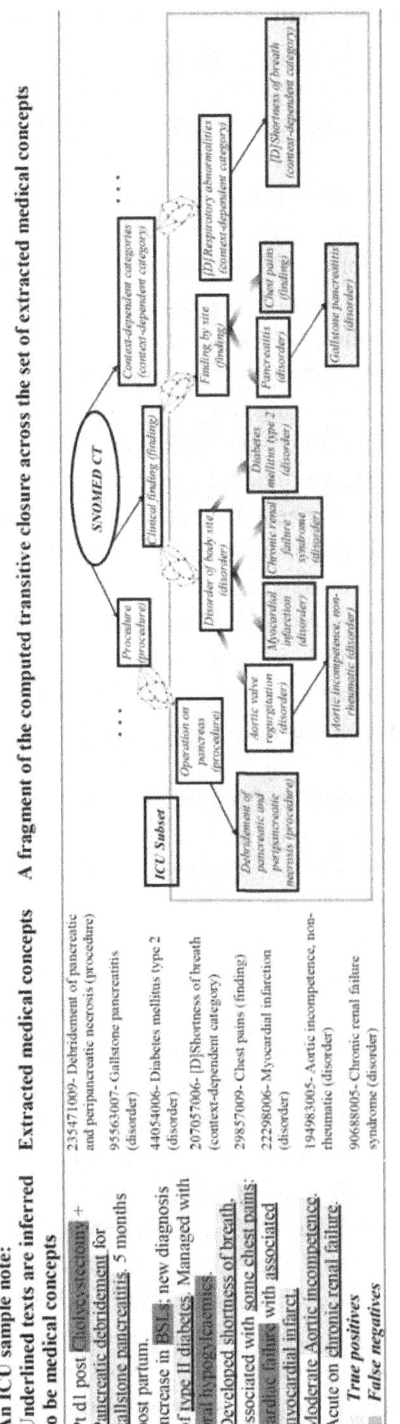

3. It provides a small enough list for the subset to be manually reviewed and modified to create an improvement on "native" SCT.
4. Once the methodology is systematized it provides a strategy reusable for any and all clinical specialties.
5. It should prove to be both a highly economical and efficient method of deriving subsets that are more reliable.
6. It shrinks SCT enough so that description logic engines might perform queries for users in real-time.

PRACTICAL APPLICATIONS OF NLP IN THE HOSPITAL WARD

The use of entity and concept identification can assist in a number of fundamental tasks in the care process. In the two use cases described below (WRIS and CliniDAL) the SCT concept identification enables a semantic index to be created over the narrative notes and thereby provide a mechanism for fast retrieval and categorization of their contents. Much of the activities in processing narrative notes can be viewed as research for academic purposes and contributing to computational linguistics research in its own right. However, it is more valuable and rewarding to affix the research to objectives of providing improved processing for the medical care work of itself. Described below are two projects that require the use of our knowledge and research into the ICU corpus but where that knowledge has been put to use for practical benefit for our medical collaborators.

Ward Rounds Information System

The Ward Rounds Information System (WRIS) is a two part processing system aimed at gaining work productivity in carrying out ward rounds in the ICU (Ryan, A., Patrick, J., & Herkes, R., 2008). In the past the system for performing ward rounds entailed a junior doctor reading many pages of the clinical IS and compiling the most appropriate recent information into a report. This process was error prone, tedious and timely costly taking between 5-10 minutes per patient and needing to be repeated across a 50 bed ward. The first phase of WRIS was to build a complementary system that read the wanted data from the host IS and presented it on a web page. The second phase of the WRIS was for the medical staff to write their clinical notes into the web page and then submit them for conversion to SCT codes. These codes are presented to the staff along with the original text and they are asked to confirm or reject the computed codes. The accepted codes can then be written to the patient record and by being resident there they constitute an index of the record for later retrievals and analytics. The rejected codes form a body of knowledge that can be used to improve the text to SCT encoding process. This technology is now the basis of a wider project to produce a generic strategy for generating Handover reports based on natural language processing.

Clinical Data Analytics Language (CliniDAL)

The CliniDAL is a controlled language for expressing queries to perform retrievals and data analytics on the patient records held in the host clinical information system. It is especially designed to support the use of local clinical dialectal language to express queries, but also it executes those queries over the clinical notes as well as the structured parts of the database. CliniDAL contains a mapping table of every data field in the database relating it to a user interface term, SCT expression (where possible) and the community's clinical sociolect. Furthermore the SCT indices created in the WRIS process are used for retrievals across the clinical notes.

CONCLUSION

All medical imaging and measurement eventually becomes language so NLP is the most important innovation required to advance medical research using the information captured at the coalface of health care – the patient record. Using the patient record retrospectively requires solving serious problems in dealing with linguistically inferior content. Learning how to solve these problems for the retrospective material is fundamental to creating aids for current staff to create future records of a much better linguistic quality and thereby enhance the quality and purposefulness of future language processing systems. There are major problems in giving full coverage to a very broad range of terminologies and concepts needed to be recorded in acute care situations. Better language processing is needed but it is also important that mechanisms ensure knowledge is captured at its time of first recognition and passed back into the processing system for continual reuse. It is an important facet of language processing that any created resource is always reusable and never suffers from depreciation, although the technology that exploits it might.

The narrative of the clinical record constitutes the most important piece of evidence collected in the process of caring for sick and infirmed people. Efforts to relate the outcomes of care processes to their interventions and the medicines will only be achieved on a large scale by harnessing the contents of the patient record, and at the moment, most of the relevant content is locked in the written text. While some valuable content is available from the structured part of the clinical record substantial advances in translational research are dependent on retrieving content locked up in the narrative texts. The technology required to achieve this access has to move through two major phases. Firstly significant studies have to make use of retrospective content to establish the nature of the contents and the best methods for dealing with the processing problems intrinsic to the nature of the data. We have described examples of those problems in this paper with respect to materials from one intensive care service. The second phase is inferring from this knowledge the technologies we have to build to support and shape the behaviours of clinical staff in the future so that firstly they minimise the problems we currently encounter, but also that the technology supports improvement in the way they record the content relevant to not only patient needs at the point of care but also to the larger objectives of translational research. Once such objectives are attained then natural language processing will be able to serve the prospective needs of medical science in very significant ways.

ACKNOWLEDGMENT

We wish to acknowledge the contributions of our partners and collaborators: Dr Robert Herkes and Angela Ryan from the Royal Prince Alfred Hospital, Peter Budd, Yefeng Wang and Yitao Zhang from the University of Sydney, and Prof Alan Rector, Dr. Sebastian Brandt and Jeremy Rogers from the University of Manchester,and Bahram Vazirnezhad, Tehran University of Technology, Iran.

REFERENCES

Ananiadou, S. (1994). A methodology for automatic term recognition. In *Proceedings of COLING*, (pp. 1034—1038).

Arnold, C. W., Bui, A. A. T., Morioka, C., El-Saden, S., & Kangarloo, H. (2007). Informatics in Radiology: A Prototype Web-based Reporting System for Onsite-Offsite Clinician Communication. *RadioGraphics*, *27*(4), 1201 - 1211.

Aronson, A. R. (2001). Effective mapping of biomedical text to the UMLS Metathesaurus: the MetaMap program. *Proc AMIA Symp.*, (pp. 17–21).

Berrios, D. C. (2000). Automated indexing for full text information retrieval. *Proc AMIA Symp.*, (pp. 71–5).

Bodenreider, O. (2006). Lexical, terminological and ontological resources for biological text mining. *Text mining for biology and biomedicine*, (pp. 43-66). Artech House.

Chang, J. T., Schütze, H., & Altman, R. B. (2001). Creating an Online Dictionary of Abbreviations from MEDLINE. *J Am Med Inform Assoc.*

Chapman, W. W., Bridewell, W., Hanbury, P., Cooper, G. F., & Buchanan, B. (2001). Evaluation of negation phrases in narrative clinical reports. In *Proceedings of AMIA Symposium*, (pp. 105—109).

Chi, E. C., Sager, N., Tick, L. J., & Lyman, M. S. (1983). Relational data base modelling of free-text medical narrative. *Med Inform* (London).

Christensen, L., Haug, P. J., & Fiszman, M. (2002). MPLUS: a probabilistic medical language understanding system. *Proc Workshop on Natural Language Processing in the Biomedical Domain* (pp. 29–36). Philadelphia, PA.

Chute, C., Elkin, P. L., Sheretz, D. D., & Tuttle, M. S. (1999). Desiderata for a Clinical Terminology Server. *Proceedings of the AMIA Symposium* (pp. 42-46).

Cohen, A., & Hersh, W. (2005). A survey of current work in biomedical text mining. *Brief Bioinform*, *6*, 57–71.

Cooper, G. F., & Miller, R. A. (1998). An experiment comparing lexical and statistical methods for extracting MeSH terms from clinical free text. *J. Am Med Inform Assoc.*, *5*, 62-75.

Dolin, R. H., Huff, S. M., Rocha, R. A., Spackman, K. A., & Campbell, K. E. (1998). Evaluation of a "lexically assign, logically refine" strategy for semi-automated integration of overlapping terminologies. *J Am Med Inform Assoc.*, *5*, 203–13.

Dorow, B., & Widdows, D. (2003). Discovering corpus-specific word senses. *EACL, Conference Companion* (research notes and demos), (pp. 79–82).

Elkin, P. L., Brown, S. H., Bauer, B. A., Husser, C. S., Carruth, W., Bergstrom, L. R., & Wahner-Roedler, D. L. (2005). A controlled trial of automated classification of negation from clinical notes. *BMC Medical Informatics and Decision Making, 5*, 13 doi:10.1186/1472-6947-5-13.

Elkin, P. L., et al. (2006). Evaluation of the content coverage of SNOMED CT: Ability of SNOMED clinical terms to represent clinical problem lists. *Mayo Clin Proc, 81*(6), 741-8.

Frantzi, K., Ananiadou, S., & Tsujii, J. (1998). The *C*-value/NC-value method of automatic recognition for multi-word terms. In *Proceedings of ECDL Symposium*, (pp. 585—604).

Friedman, C. (2000). A broad-coverage natural language processing system. *Proc AMIA Symp.*, (pp. 270–4).

Friedman, C., Alderson, P. O., Austin, J. H., et al. (1994). A general natural language text processor for clinical radiology. *J Am Med Inform Assoc., 1*, 161–74.

Friedman, C., Shagina, L., Lussier, Y., & Hripcsak, G. (2004). Automated encoding of clinical documents based on natural language processing. *J. Am Med Inform Assoc., 11*(5), 392-402.

Gabrieli, E. R., Speth, D. J. (1986). Automated analysis of the discharge summary,. *J. Clin Comput.*

Hahn, U., Honeck, M., Piotrowski, M., & Schulz, S. (2001). Subword segmentation—leveling out morphological variations for medical document retrieval. *Proc AMIA Symp.*, (pp. 229–33).

Hahn, U., Romacker, M., & Schulz, S. (2002). MedsynDikate—a natural language system for the extraction of medical information from findings reports. *Int J Med inform., 67*, 63–74.

Hearst, M. (1999). Untangling text data mining. In *Proceedings of the 37th Annual Meeting of the Association for Computer Linguistics (*ACL'99), (pp. 3—10).

Hripcsak, G., Austin, J. H., Alderson, P. O., & Friedman, C. (2002). Use of natural language processing to translate clinical information from a database of 889,921 chest radiographic reports. *Radiology, 224*, 157–63.

Hripcsak, G., Friedman, C., Alderson, P. O., DuMouchel, W., Johnson, S. B., & Clayton, P. D. (1995). Unlocking clinical data from narrative reports: a study of natural language processing. *Annals of Internal Medicine, 122*(9), 681-8.

Hripcsak, G., Kuperman, G. J., & Friedman, C. (1998). Extracting findings from narrative reports: software transferability and sources of physician disagreement. *Methods Inf Med., 37*, 1–7.

Huang, Y., & Lowe, H. J. (2007). A novel hybrid approach to automated negation detection in clinical radiology reports. *J. Am Med Inform Assoc., 14*, 304-11.

Huang, Y., & Lowe, H. J. (2005). A grammar based classification of negations in clinical radiology reports. *Proc AMIA Annu Fall Symp*, (pp. 988-92).

Huang, Y., Lowe, H., Klein, D., & Cucina, R. (2005). Improved Identification of Noun Phrases in Clinical Radiology Reports Using a High-Performance Statistical Natural Language Parser Augmented with the UMLS Specialist Lexicon. *J Am Med Inform Assoc, 12*, 275–85.

Humphrey, S. M. (1999). Automatic indexing of documents from journal descriptors: A preliminary investigation. *J Am Soc Inf Sci, 50*(8), 661-674.

Kanter, S. L., Miller, R. A., Tan, M., & Schwartz, J. (1994). Using PostDoc to recognize biomedical concepts in medical school curricular documents. *Bull Med Libr Assoc., 82,* 283 -7.

Karsten, H., Back, B., Salakoski, T., Salanterä, S., & Suominen, H. (Eds.) (2008). *Proceedings of The First Conference on Text and Data Mining of Clinical Documents.* Louhi'08. Turku, Finland.

Lau, L. M., Johnson, K., Monson, K., Lam, S. H., & Huff, S. M. (2002). A method for automated mapping of laboratory results to LOINC. *Proc AMIA Symp.*

Leroy, G., &. Rindflesch, T. C. (2005). Effects of information and machine learning algorithms on word sense disambiguation with small datasets. *Int. J. Med. Inform., 74*, 573–585.

Liu, H., Johnson, S. B., & Friedman, C. (2002). Automatic resolution of ambiguous terms based on machine learning and conceptual relations in the UMLS. *J. Am Med Inform Assoc., 9,* 621–36.

Lopez Osornio, A., Luna, D., Gambarte, M. L., Gomez, A., Reynoso, G., & Gonzalez Bernaldo de Quiros, F. (2007). Creation of a Local Interface Terminology to SNOMED CT [online]. In K. A. Kuhn, J. R. Warren, & T-Y. Leong (Ed.), *Medinfo 2007: Proceedings of the 12th World Congress on Health (Medical) Informatics; Building Sustainable Health Systems* (pp. 765-769). Amsterdam: IOS Press, 2007. Studies in health technology and informatics, ISSN0926-9630.

Lowe, H. J., Buchanan, B. G., Cooper, G. F., & Vries, J. K. (1995). Building a medical multimedia database system to integrate clinical information: an application of high performance computing and communications technology. *Bull Med Libr Assoc., 83,* 57 -64.

Miller, R. A., Gieszczykiewicz, F. M., Vries, J. K., & Cooper, G. F. (1992). Chartline: Providing bibliographic references relevant to patient charts using the UMLS Metathesaurus knowledge sources. *Proc Symp Comput Appl Med Care,* (pp. 86-90).

Mutalik, P. G., Deshpande, A., &Nadkarni, P. M. (2001). Use of general-purpose negation detection to augment concept indexing of medical documents: A quantitative study using the UMLS. *J Am Med Inform Assoc., 8*, 598–609.

Nadkarni, P., Chen, R., & Brandt, C. (2001). UMLS concept indexing for production databases: A feasibility study. *J Am Med Inform Assoc., 8*, 80–91.

Park, Y., & Byrd, R. J. (2001). Hybrid Text Mining for Finding Abbreviations and Their Definitions. *Proceedings of the Conference on Empirical Methods in Natural Language Processing,* (pp. 126- 133). Pittsburgh, PA, June 2001.

Patrick, J., Budd, P., & Wang, Y. (2007). An automated system for Conversion of Clinical notes into SNOMED CT. Health Knowledge & Data Mining Workshop. *Research & Practice in Information Technology, 68*, 195-202.

Prather, J. C., Lobach, D. F., Goodwin, L. K., Hales, J. W., Hage, M. L., & Hammond, W. E. (1997). Medical Data mining: Knowledge discovery in a clinical data warehouse. *AMIA Annual Fall Symposium*, (pp. 101-5).

Purcell, G. P., & Shortliffe, E. H. (1995). Contextual models of clinical publications for enhancing retrieval from full-text databases. *Proc Annu Symp Comput Appl Med Care*, (pp. 851–7).

Pustejovsky, J. et al. (2001). Automation Extraction of Acronym-Meaning Pairs from Medline Databases. *Medinfo, 10*(Pt 1), 371-375.

Pustejovsky, J., Castaño, J., Cochran, B., Kotecki, M., Morrell, M., &. Rumshisky, A. (2001). Extraction and Disambiguation of Acronym-Meaning Pairs in Medline. *unpublished manuscript.*

Resnik, P., & Yarowsky, D. (2000). Distinguishing systems and distinguishing senses: New evaluation tools for words sense disambiguation. *Natural Lang. Eng., 5*(3), 113–133.

Rocha, R. A., & Huff, S. M. (1994). Using diagrams to map controlled medical vocabularies.

Proc Annu Symp Comput Appl Med Care, (pp. 172–6).

Rocha, R. A., Rocha, B. H. S. C., & Huff, S. M. (1993). Automated translation between medical vocabularies using a frame-based interlingua. *Proc Annu Symp Comput Appl Med Care*, (pp. 690–4).

Rosenbloom, S. T., Kiepek, W., Belletti, J., et al. (2004). Generating complex clinical documents using structured entry and reporting. *Medinfo, 11*, 683–687.

Ruch, P. (2002). Using contextual spelling correction to improve retrieval effectiveness in degraded text collections. In *Procedings of the 19th international Conference on Computational Linguistics (COLING) - Volume 1* (Taipei, Taiwan, August 24 - September 01, 2002).

Ruch, P., Baud, R., Geissbuhler, A., &. Rassinoux, A. M. (2001). Comparing general and medical texts for information retrieval based on natural language processing: an inquiry into lexical disambiguation. In *Proceedings of Medinfo Symposium*, (pp. 261—265).

Ryan, A., Patrick, J., & Herkes, R. (2008). Introduction of Enhancement Technologies into the Intensive Care Service, Royal Prince Alfred Hospital, Sydney. *Health Information Management Journal, 37*(1), 39-44.

Sager, N., Lyman, M., Nhan, N. T., et al. (1994). Automatic encoding into SNOMED III: A preliminary investigation. *Proc Annu Symp Comput Appl Med Care*, (pp. 230–4).

Savova, G., Harris, M. R., Johnson, T., Pakhomov, S.V., &. Chute, C. G. (2003). A data-driven approach for extracting "the most specific term" for ontology development. In *Proceedings of the AMIA Symposium*, (pp. 579—583).

Schuemie, M. J., Kors, J. A., & Mons, B. (2005). Word sense disambiguation in the biomedical domain: An overview. *J Comput Biol., 12*, 554-565.

Schwartz, A. S., & Hearst, M. A. (2003). A simple algorithm for identifying abbreviation definitions in biomedical text. In *Proceedings of the 8th Pacific Symposium on Biocomputing* (pp. 451–462).3rd–7th January, Hawaii.

Sinha, U., & Kangarloo, H. (2002). Principal Component Analysis for Content-based Image Retrieval. *RadioGraphics, 22*(5), 1271-1289.

Sun, J. Y., & Sun, Y. (2006). A system for automated lexical mapping. *Am Med Inform Assoc, 13*(3), 334-343.

Sun, Y. (2004). Methods for automated concept mapping between medical databases. *J Biomed Inform, 37*(3), 162-178.

Taira, R. K., & Soderland, S. G. (1999). A statistical natural language processor for medical reports. *Proc AMIA Symp.*, (pp. 970–4).

Taira, R. K., Soderland, S. G., & Jakobovits, R. M. (2001). Automatic structuring of radiology free-text reports. *RadioGraphics, 21*, 237–245.

Taira, R. K., Soderland, S. G., & Jakobovits, R. M. (2001). Automatic structuring of radiology free-text reports. *Radiographics, 21*, 237–45.

Thomas, B. J., Ouellette, H., Halpern, E. F., & Rosenthal, D. I. (2005). Automated Computer-Assisted Categorization of Radiology Reports. *Am. J. Roentgenol., 184*(2), 687-690.

Tolentino, H. D., Matters, M. D., Walop, W., Law, & Tong, W. (2007). *BMC Medical Informatics and Decision Making.*

Weeber, M., Mork, J., & Aronson, A. (2001). Developing a Test Collection for Biomedical Word Sense Disambiguation. *Proc. AMIA Symp.*, (pp. 746-750).

Yu, H., Hripcsak, G., & Friedman, C. (2002). Mapping abbreviations to full forms in biomedical articles. *J Am Med Inform Assoc 2002*; *9*(3), 262-272.

Zhou, X., Han, H., Chankai, I., Prestrud, A., & Brooks, A. (2006). Approaches to text mining for clinical medical records. In *Proc ACM Sympos Applied Computing* (SAC 2006), (pp. 235–239). April 2006. NY: ACM Press.

Zou, Q., Chu, W. W., Morioka, C., et al. (2003). IndexFinder: a method of extracting key concepts from clinical texts for indexing. *Proc AMIA Symp.*, (pp. 763–7).

Compilation of References

Abdalla, R., & Teufel, S. (2006). A bootstrapping approach to unsupervised detection of cue phrase variants. In *21st international Conference on Computational Linguistics Coling06* (pp.921-928). Morriston, N.J.: Association for Computational Linguistics. doi: http://dx.doi.org/10.3115/1220175.1220291

AbdulJaleel, N., & Larkey, L. S. (2003). Statistical transliteration for English-Arabic cross language information retrieval. In *Proceedings of the 12th International Conference on Information and Knowledge Management, CKIM'03*, (pp. 139–146), New Orleans, United-States of America.

Abi-Haidar, A., Kaur, J., Maguitman, A., Radivojac, P., Retchsteiner, A., Verspoor, K., Wang, Z., & Rocha, L. (2007). Uncovering protein-protein interactions in the bibliome. In *Proceedings of the BioCreative2 Workshop*, (pp. 247–255).

Agirre, E., & Edmonds, P. (Eds.). (2006). *Word Sense Disambiguation - Algorithms and Applications*: Springer.

Ahrenberg, L., Andersson, M., & Merkel, M. (2000). *A knowledge-lite approach to word alignment,* (pp. 97–138). In Véronis.

Alexa, M., Kreissig, B., Liepert, M., Reichenberger, K., Rostek, L., Rautmann, K., Scholze-Stubenrecht, W., & Stoye, S. (2002). The Duden Ontology: An Integrated Representation of Lexical and Ontological Information. In K. Simov, N. Guarino, & W. Peters, (Eds.), Proceedings of the OntoLex Workshop at LREC (pp. 1-8). Spain.

Allwein, E. L., Schapire, R. E., & Singer, Y. (2000): Reducing Multiclass to Binary: A Unifying Approach for Margin Classifiers. *In Proceedings of the 17th International Conf. on Machine Learning* (pp. 9-16). San Francisco, CA.: Morgan Kaufmann.

Almeida, F., Bell, M., & Chavez, E. (2003). Controlled health thesaurus for the CDC web redesign project. *AMIA Annu Symp Proc.* (p. 777).

Al-Onaizan, Y., & Knight, K. (2002a). Machine transliteration of names in arabic text. In *Proceedings of ACL Workshop on Computational Approaches to Semitic Languages*, Philadelphia, United-States of America.

Al-Onaizan, Y., & Knight, K. (2002b). Translating named entities using monolingual and bilingual resources. In *Proceedings of the Conference of the Association for Computational Linguistics, ACL'02*, (pp. 400–408), Philadelphia, United-States of America.

Amrani, A., Azé, J., Heitz, T., Kodratoff, Y., & Roche, M. (2004). From the texts to the concepts they contain: a chain of linguistic treatments. In *Proc. TREC'04* (Text REtrieval Conference), National Institute of Standards and Technology, Gaithersburg Maryland USA, (pp. 712-722).

Ananiadou, S. (1994). A methodology for automatic term recognition. In *Proceedings of COLING*, (pp. 1034—1038).

Ananiadou, S. Kell, D. B., & Tsujii, J. (2006). Text mining and its potential applications in systems biology. *TRENDS in Biotechnology, 24*(12), 571-579.

Ananiadou, S., & McNaught, J. (2006). *Text mining for biology and biomedicine.* Boston: Artech House.

Ananiadou, S., & Nenadic, G. (2006). Automatic terminology management in biomedicine. In S. Ananiadou & G. McNaught (Eds.), *Text mining for biology and biomedicine.* Artech House Books.

Ananiadou, S., & Tsujii, J. (Eds.) (2003). *Proceedings of the ACL 2003 Workshop on Natural Language Processing in Biomedicine.* Stroudsburg, PA, USA: Association for Computational Linguistics.

Ananiadou, S., Kell, D. B., & Tsujii, J. (2006). Text mining and its potential applications in systems biology. *Trends Biotechnol, 24*, 571-579.

Ananiadou, S., Procter, R., Rea, B., Sasaki, Y., & Thomas, J. (2007). Supporting Systematic Reviews using Text Mining. *3rd International Conference on e-Social Science,* Ann Arbor.

Andrade, M., & Bork, P. (2000). Automated extraction of information in Molecular Biology. *FEBS Letters, 476*, 12–17.

Andrade, M., & Valencia, A. (1998). Automatic extraction of keywords from scientific text: Application to the knowledge domain of protein families. *Bioinformatics, 14*(7), 600–607.

Andreopoulos, B., Alexopoulou, D., & Schroeder, M. (2007). Word Sense Disambiguation in Biomedical Ontologies with Term Co-occurrence Analysis and Document Clustering. *Int J Data Mining Bioinf,* Special Issue on Biomedical Text Retrieval and Mining.

Apweiler, R., Bairoch, A., & Wu, et al. (2004). UniProt: the Universal Protein knowledgebase. *Nucleic Acids Res,* (32), 115-119.

Apweiler, R., Bairoch, A., Wu, C., Barker, W., Boeckmann, B., Ferro, S., Gasteiger, E., Huang, H., Lopez, R., Magrane, M., Martin, M., Natale, D., O'Donovan, C., Redaschi, N., & Yeh, L. (2004). UniProt: the universal protein knowledgebase. *Nucleic Acids Research, 32*(Database issue), D115–D119.

Arens, Y., Hsu, C. N., & Knoblock, C. A. (1996). Query processing in the SIMS information mediator. In A. Tate (Ed.), *Advanced Planning Technology* (pp. 61-69). Menlo Park, California, USA: AAAI Press.

Argamon, S., Whitelaw, C., Chase, P. J., Hota, S. R., Garg, N., & Levitan, S. (2007). Stylistic text classification using functional lexical features. *Journal of American Society for Information Science & Technology (JASIST), 58*(6), 802-822. doi: doi.org/10.1002/asi.20553

Arnold, C. W., Bui, A. A. T., Morioka, C., El-Saden, S., & Kangarloo, H. (2007). Informatics in Radiology: A Prototype Web-based Reporting System for Onsite-Offsite Clinician Communication. *RadioGraphics, 27*(4), 1201 - 1211.

Aronson, A. (2001). *Effective mapping of biomedical text to the UMLS Metathesaurus: the MetaMap program.* Technical report.

Aronson, A. R. (2001). Effective mapping of biomedical text to the UMLS Metathesaurus: the MetaMap program. *Proc AMIA Symp.*, (pp. 17–21).

Aronson, A. R. (2001). Effective mapping of biomedical text to the UMLS Metathesaurus: the MetaMap program. In S. Bakken (Ed.), *American Medical Informatics Association Symposium* (pp. 17–21). Bethesda, MD, USA: American Medical Informatics Association.

Aronson, A. R. (2006). *MetaMap: Mapping Text to the UMLS Metathesaurus*: National Library of Medicine.

Aronson, A. R., & Rindflesch, T. C. (1997). Query Expansion Using the UMLS Metathesaurus. *Proceedings of the 1997 AMIA Annual Fall Symposium*, (pp. 485-489).

Arvelakis, A., Reczko, M., Stamatakis, A., Symeonidis, A., & Tollis, I. (2005). Using Treemaps to visualize phylogenetic trees. In J. L. Oliveira *et al.* (Eds.), *ISBMDA 2005, LNBI 3745* (pp. 283–293). Springer-Verlag Berlin Heidelber.

Avrithis, Y., Doulamis, A. D. , Doulamis, N. D., & Kollias, S. D. (1998). An Adaptive Approach to Video Indexing and Retrieval. *Proceedings of the International Workshop on Very Low Bitrate Video Coding (VLBV)*, (pp. 69-72), Urbana IL, October 1998.

Bada, M., Stevens, R., Goble, C., Gil, Y., Ashburner, M., Blake, J., Cherry, J., Harris, M., & Lewis, S. (2004). A short study on the success of the gene ontology. *Journal of Web Semantics, 1*(1), 235–240.

Baeza-Yates, R., & Ribeiro-Neto, B. (1999). *Modern Information Retrieval.* Addison Wesley.

Bairoch, A., Boeckmann, B., Ferro, S., & Gasteiger E. (2004). Swiss-Prot: Juggling between evolution and stability Brief. *Bioinform,* (5), 39-55.

Barton, S. (Ed.). (2002). *Clinical Evidence.* London, England: BMJ Publishing Group.

Bateman, A. (2008). Editorial. *Nucleic Acids Research,* 33(Database issue), D1.

Baumgartner, W. A. J., Bretonnel Cohen, K., & Hunter, L. (2008). An open-source framework for large-scale, flexible evaluation of biomedical text mining systems. *Journal of Biomedical Discovery and Collaboration, 3*(1). doi:10.1186/1747-5333-3-1

Berger, A. L., Della Pietra, V. J., & Della Pietra, S. A. (1996). A maximum entropy approach to natural language processing. *Computational Linguistics, 22*(1), 39-71.

Berger, A., Caruana, R., Cohn, D., Freitag, D., & Mittal, V. (2000). Bridging the lexical chasm: statistical approaches to answer-finding. In N. J. Belkin, P. Ingwersen, & M. Leong (Eds.), *23rd International Conference on Research and Development in Information Retrieval* (pp. 192–199). New York, NY, USA: Association for Computing Machinery Press.

Berrios, D. C. (2000). Automated indexing for full text information retrieval. *Proc AMIA Symp.*, (pp. 71–5).

Bethard, S., Lu, Z., Martin, J., & Hunter, L. (2005). *Semantic role labeling for protein transport predicates.* Under Review.

Bhogal, J., Macfarlane, A., & Smith, P. (2007). A review of ontology based query expansion. *Information Processing & Management, 43*(4), July 2007, 866-886.

Biezunski, M., Bryan, M., & Newcomb S. (2002). *ISO/IEC 13250, Topic Maps (Second Edition)* In proceeding of ISO/IEC JTC1/SC34. Retrieved on May 22, 2002. Available at: *http://www1.y12.doe.gov/capabilities/sgml/sc34/document/0322.htm*

Bikel, D. M. (2004). A distributional analysis of a lexicalized statistical parsing model. *Proceedings of the Conference on Empirical Methods in Natural Language Processing* (pp. 182–9).

Biomedical Literature Mining Publication (BLIMP) website URL: http://blimp.cs.queensu.ca

Blaschke, C., Andrade, M. A., Ouzounis, C., & Valencia, A. (1999). Automatic extraction of biological information from scientific text: Protein-protein interactions. *Proc Int Conf Intell Syst Mol Biol,* (pp. 60-67).

Blaschke, C., Leon, E., Krallinger, M., & Valencia, A. (2005). Evaluation of Biocreative assessment of task 2. *BMC Bioinformatics, 6*, S16.

Blum, A., & Mitchell, T. (1998). Combining labeled and unlabeled data with co-training. In *Proceedings of the 11th Annual Conference on Computational Learning Theory* (pp. 92–100). New York, NY, USA: Association for Computing Machinery Press.

Bodenreider, O. (2004). The Unified Medical Language System (UMLS): integrating biomedical terminology. *Nucleic Acids Research, 32*, 267-270.

Bodenreider, O. (2006). Lexical, terminological and ontological resources for biological text mining. *Text mining for biology and biomedicine*, (pp. 43-66). Artech House.

Bodenreider, O. (2007). *Personal Communication*. July 5, 2005.

Bodenreider, O., Burgun, A., & Rindflesch, T.C. (2001). Lexically-suggested hyponymic relations among medical terms and their representation in the UMLS. *Proceedings of the TIA Conference*. Nancy, France.

Bonis, J., Furlong, L. I., & Sanz, F. (2006). OSIRIS: a tool for retrieving literature about sequence variants. *Bioinformatics, 22*(20), 2567-2569.

Boser, B. E., Guyon, I., & Vapnik, V. (1992). A training algorithm for optimal margin classifiers. In H. Haussler (Ed.), *The 5th Annual ACM Workshop on Computational Learning Theory* (pp. 144-152). Pittsburgh, PA, USA: ACM.

Brennan, P. F., & Aronson, A. R. (2003). Towards linking patients and clinical information: Detecting UMLS concepts in e-mail. *Journal of Biomedical Informatics, 36*(4/5), 334-41.

Brill, E. (1993). A *corpus-based approach to language learning*. Unpublished doctoral dissertation, University of Pennsylvania, Philadelphia, PA.

Brill, E. (1994). Some Advances in Transformation-Based Part of Speech Tagging. *AAAI, 1*, 722-727.

Brodda, B. (1979). Något om de svenska ordens fonotax och morfotax: Iakttagelse med utgångspunkt från experiment med automatisk morfologisk analys. *PILUS nr 38*. Department of Swedish, Stockholm University. (In Swedish).

Brookes, A. J. (1999). The essence of SNPs. *Gene, 234*(2), 177-186.

Brookes, M. (2001) *Fly - the Unsung Hero of Twentieth Century Science*: Ecco.

Brown, P. F., Cocke, J., Stephen A., Della Pietra, V. J. D. P., Jelinek, F., Lafferty, J. D., Mercer, R. L., & Roossin, P. S. (1990). A statistical approach to machine translation. *Computational Linguistics, 16*(2).

Brown, P. F., Pietra, S. D., Pietra, V. J. D., & Mercer, R. L. (1994). The mathematic of statistical machine translation: Parameter estimation. *Computational Linguistics, 19(2)*, 263-311.

Buchanan, B. G., & Shortliffe, E. H. (1984). Rule-based expert systems: The MYCIN experiments of the Stanford heuristic programming project. *Technical report from the Stanford Center for Biomedical Informatics Research*. (Electronic book) American Association for Artificial Intelligence http://www.aaaipress.org/Classic/Buchanan/buchanan.html.

Buckley, C., Salton, G., Allan, J., & Singhal, A. (1994). Automatic query expansion using SMART: TREC 3. *In Text REtrieval Conference*.

Buitelaar, P., & Sacaleanu, B. (2001). Ranking and selecting synsets by domain relevance. In D. Moldovan, S. Harabagiu, W. Peters, L. Guthrie, & Y. Wilks, (Eds.), *Proceedings of the Workshop on WordNet and other Lexical Resources: Applications, Extensions and Customizations at NAACL*. Pittsburgh, U.S.A.

Buitelaar, P., Cimiano, P., & Magnini, B. (2005). Ontology learning from text: An overview. In P. Buitelaar, P. Cimiano & B. Magnini (Eds.), *Ontology learning from text: Methods, applications and evaluation* (pp. 3-12). IOS Press.

Buitelaar, P., Sintek, M., & Kiesel, M. (2006). A Lexicon Model for Multilingual/Multimedia Ontologies. In Y. Sure & J. Domingue (Eds.), *The Semantic Web: Research and Applications. Proceedings of the 3rd European Semantic Web Conference (ESWC)*. Budva, Montenegro.

Burton, P. R., Tobin, M. D., & Hopper, J. L. (2005). Key concepts in genetic epidemiology. *Lancet, 366*(9489), 941-951.

Cakmak, A. & Ozsoyoglu, G. (2007). Annotating genes using textual patterns. In *Proceedings of the Pacific Symposium on Biocomputing (PSB), 12*, 221–232. World Scientific Press.

Camon, E., Barrell, D., Dimmer, E., Lee, V., Magrane, M., Maslen, J., Binns, D., & Apweiler, R. (2005). An evaluation of GO annotation retrieval for BioCreAtIvE and GOA. *BMC Bioinformatics*, *6*(Suppl 1), S17.

Camon, E., Magrane, M., Barrell, D., Lee, V., Dimmer, E., Maslen, J., Binns, D., Harte, N., Lopez, R., & Apweiler, R. (2004). The Gene Ontology Annotations (GOA) database: sharing knowledge in UniProt with Gene Ontology. *Nucleic Acids Research*, *32*, 262–266.

Camous, F., Blott, S., & Smeaton, A.F. (2007). Ontology-based MEDLINE document classification. In: *Proc BIRD*, 439-452.

Caporaso, G. J., Deshpande, N., Fink, L. J., Bourne, P. E., Bretonnel Cohen, K., & Hunter, L. (2008). Intrinsic evaluation of text mining tools may not predict performance on realistic tasks. In *Pacific Symposium on Biocomputing, 13*, 640-651). PMID: 18229722 Retrieved from http://psb.stanford.edu/psb-online/proceedings/psb08/

Caporaso, J. G., Baumgartner, W. A., Jr., Randolph, D. A., Cohen, K. B., & Hunter, L. (2007). MutationFinder: a high-performance system for extracting point mutation mentions from text. *Bioinformatics, 23*(14), 1862-1865.

Cardie, C., Wiebe, J., Wilson, T., & Litman, D. (2004). Combining low-level and summary representations of opinions for multi-perspective question answering. In L. Greenwald, Z. Dodds, A. Howard, S. Tejada, & J. Weinberg (Eds.), *AAAI Spring Symposium: New Directions in Question Answering* (pp. 20–27). Menlo Park, CA, USA: AAAI Press.

Carlson L., Marcu D., & Okurowski M. E. (2003). *Build a discourse-tagged corpus in the framework of Rhetorical structure theory.* In Current and new direction in discourse and dialogue, Springer, (pp. 85-122).

Carr, L., Hall, W., Bechhofer, S., & Goble, C. (2001). Conceptual linking: ontology-based open hypermedia. *In Proceedings of the 10th international Conference on World Wide Web* (Hong Kong, Hong Kong, May 01 - 05, 2001). WWW '01. ACM, New York, NY, (pp. 334-342).

Castano, S., Antonellis, V. D., & di Vimercati, S. D. C. (2001). Global viewing of heterogeneous data sources. *IEEE Transaction Knowl. Data Eng., 13(2),* 277-297.

Ceausu, A., Stefanescu, D., & Tufis, D. (2006). Acquis communautaire sentence alignment using Support Vector Machines. In L. Marconi (Ed.), *The 5th LREC Conference* (pp. 2134-2137). Paris, France: ELRA.

Chang, C. C., & Lin, C. J. (2001). *LIBSVM — A library for support vector machines.* http://www.csie.ntu.edu.tw/~cjlin/libsvm/.

Chang, J. T., Schütze, H., & Altman, R. B. (2001). Creating an Online Dictionary of Abbreviations from MEDLINE. *J Am Med Inform Assoc.*

Chang, J. T., Schutze, H., & Altman, R. B. (2004). GAPSCORE: finding gene and protein names one word at a time. *Bioinformatics*, *20*(2), 216-225.

Chanlekha, H., & Kawtrakul, A. (2004). Thai Named Entity Extraction by incorporating Maximum Entropy Model with Simple Heuristic Information. *In proceeding of IJCNLP' 2004*, Hainan Island, China.

Chapman, W. W., Bridewell, W., Hanbury, P., Cooper, G. F., & Buchanan, B. (2001). Evaluation of negation phrases in narrative clinical reports. In *Proceedings of AMIA Symposium*, (pp. 105—109).

Chareonsuk J., Sukvakree T., & Kawtrakul A. (2005). Elementary Discourse Unit Segmentation for Thai using Discourse Cue and Syntactic Information. *In proceeding of NCSEC2005.*

Chazard, E., Puech, P., Gregoire, M., & Beuscart, R. (2006). Using Treemaps to represent medical data. *Ubiquity: Technologies for Better Health in Aging Societies - Proceedings of MIE2006*, (pp. 522-527). Maastricht, Holland.

Chen, S. F. (1993). Aligning sentences in bilingual corpora using lexical information. In L. Schubert (Ed.), *The 31st Annual Meeting of the Association for Computational Linguistics* (pp.9-16). Morristown, NJ, USA: Association for Computational Linguistics.

Cheng, G. Y. (2004). A study of clinical questions posed by hospital clinicians. *Journal of the Medical Library Association*, *93*(4), 445–458.

Chi, E. C., Sager, N., Tick, L. J., & Lyman, M. S. (1983). Relational data base modelling of free-text medical narrative. *Med Inform* (London).

Chiang, J. H., Shin, J. W., Liu, H. H., & Chin, C. L. (2006). GeneLibrarian: an effective gene-information summarization and visualization system. *Bioinformatics, 7,* 392.

Chiang, J., & Yu, H. (2003). MeKE: discovering the functions of gene products from biomedical literature via sentence alignment. *Bioinformatics, 19*(11), 1417–1422.

Chiang, J., & Yu, H. (2004). Extracting functional annotations of proteins based on hybrid text mining approaches. In *Proc. of the BioCreAtIvE Challenge Evaluation Workshop.*

Chieu, H. L., & Ng, H. T. (2003). Named entity recognition with a maximum entropy approach. In W. Daelemans & M. Osborne (Eds.), *7th Conference on Computational Natural Language Learning* (pp. 160–163). Stroudsburg, PA, USA: Association for Computational Linguistics.

Choi, Y., Kim, D., & Krishnapuram, R. (2000). Relevance Feedback for Content-based Image Retrieval using Choquet Integral. *Proceedings of the IEEE International Conference on Multimedia & Expo,* (pp. 1207-1210), New York, August 2000.

Christensen, L., Haug, P. J., & Fiszman, M. (2002). MPLUS: a probabilistic medical language understanding system. *Proc Workshop on Natural Language Processing in the Biomedical Domain* (pp. 29–36). Philadelphia, PA.

Chu, W., & Liu, V. (2004). *A knowledge-based approach for scenario-specific content correlation in a medical digital library.*

Chute, C., Elkin, P. L., Sheretz, D. D., & Tuttle, M. S. (1999). Desiderata for a Clinical Terminology Server. *Proceedings of the AMIA Symposium* (pp. 42-46).

Cimiano, P. & Staab, S. (2004). Learning by Googling. *SIGKDD Explorations, 6*(2): 24-34.

Cimino, J. J. (1996). Linking patient information systems to bibliographic resources. *Methods of Information in Medicine, 35*(2), 122–126.

Claveau, V. & Zweigenbaum, P. (2005a). Automatic translation of biomedical terms by supervised transducer inference. *In Proceedings of the 10th Conference on Artificial Intelligence in Medicine, AIME 05, Lecture Notes of Computer Science*, Aberdeen, Scotland, UK. Springer.

Claveau, V., & Zweigenbaum, P. (2005b). Traduction de termes biomédicaux par inférence de transducteurs. In *Actes de la conférence Traitement automatique des langues naturelles, TALN'05*, Dourdan, France.

Clemons, T. E., Edwin L., & Bradley, J. (2000). A nonparametric measure of the overlapping coefficient. *Comput. Stat. Data Anal., 34(1),* 51-61.

Cohen, A. M., & Hersh, W. R. (2005). A survey of current work in biomedical text mining. *Briefings in Bioinformatics, 6*(1), 57-71.

Cohen, K. B., & Hunter, L. (2008). Getting started in text mining. *PLoS Comput Biol, 4,* e20.

Cohen, K. B., Ogren, P. V., Fox, L., & Hunter, L. (2005). Empirical Data on Corpus Design and Usage in Biomedical Natural Language Processing. *AMIA Annu Symp Proc.* (pp. 156–160). Washington, USA.

Collins, M., & Duffy, N. (2002). New ranking algorithms for parsing and tagging: Kernels over discrete structures, and the voted perceptron. *Proceedings of the 40th Annual Meeting on Association for Computational Linguistics* (pp. 263-70).

Collins, M., & Singer, M. (1999). Unsupervised models for named entity classification. In *Proceedings of the 1999 Joint SIGDAT Conference on Empirical Methods in Natural Language Processing and Very Large Corpora* (pp. 189–196). Stroudsburg, PA, USA: Association for Computational Linguistics.

Consortium (2004). The Gene Ontology (GO) database and informatics resource. *Nucleic Acids Research*, 32, D258-D261.

Cooper, G. F., & Miller, R. A. (1998). An experiment comparing lexical and statistical method for extracting MeSH terms from clinical free text. *Journal of Am Med Inform Assoc., 5*, 62–75.

Cooper, J. W., & Kershenbaum, A. (2005). Discovery of protein-protein interactions using a combination of linguistic, statistical and graphical information. *BMC Bioinformatics, 6*, 143.

Corbett P., Batchelor, C., & Teufel S. (2007). Annotation of Chemical Named Entities. *Biological, translational, and clinical language processing,* (pp. 57-64).

Cormen, T., Leiserson, C., & Rivest, R. (1990). *Introduction to Algorithms.* Cambridge, MA, USA: MIT Press.

Corney, D., Buxton, B., Langdon, W., & Jones, D. (2004). BioRAT: Extracting biological information from full-length papers. *Bioinformatics*, 20(17), 3206–3213.

Cortes, C., & Vapnik, V. (1995). Support-vector networks. *Machine Learning, 20(3),* 273-297.

Couto, F., & Silva, M. (2006). Mining the BioLiterature: towards automatic annotation of genes and proteins. In *Advanced Data Mining Techonologies in Bioinformatics*, Idea Group Inc.

Couto, F., Silva, M., & Coutinho, P. (2005). Finding genomic ontology terms in text using evidence content. *BMC Bioinformatics*, *6*(S1), S21.

Couto, F., Silva, M., & Coutinho, P. (2006). Measuring semantic similarity between gene ontology terms. *DKE - Data and Knowledge Engineering, Elsevier Science (in press).*

Cover, T. M., & Hart, P. E. (1967). Nearest neighbor pattern classification. *IEEE Transactions on Information Theory, 13(1)*, 21-27.

Cox, I., Miller, M. L., Omohundro, S. M., & Yianilos, P. N. (1996). Pichunter: Bayesian Relevance Feedback for Image Retrieval. *Proceedings of the International Conference on Pattern Recognition, 3*, 362-369.

Crammer, K., Dredze, M., Ganchev, K., Talukdar, P. P., & Caroll, S. (2007). Automatic code assignment to medical text. *Biological, Translational and Clinical Language processing (BioNLP 2007)* (pp. 129-136). Prague.

Crémilleux, B., & Soulet, A. (2008). Discovering Knowledge from Local Patterns with Global Constraints. In O. Gervasi, *et al.* (Eds) *8th International Conference on Computational Science and Applications ICCSA'08,* (pp. 1242-1257). Springer, LNCS 5073.

Crémilleux, B., Soulet, A., Klema, J., Hébert, C., & Gandrillon, O. (in press). Discovering Knowledge from Local Patterns in SAGE data. In P. Berka, J. Rauch, & D. A. Zighed, (Eds.), *Data Mining and Medical Knowledge Management: Cases and Applications.* Hershey, PA: IGI Global publications to appear 2008.

Cristianini, N., & Shawe-Taylor, J. (2000). *An Introduction to Support Vector Machines.* Cambridge, UK: Cambridge Univ. Press.

Croft, W. B. (2000). Combining approaches to information retrieval. In W. B. Croft (Ed.), *Advances in Information Retrieval: Recent Research from the CIIR* (pp. 1-36). Norwell, MA, USA: Kluwer Academic Publishers.

Cucchiarelli, A., & Velardi, P. (1998). Finding a domain-appropriate sense inventory for semantically tagging a corpus. *Natural Language Engineering, 4*(4), 325–344.

Cucerzan, S., & Yarowsky, D. (1999). Language independent named entity recognition combining morphological and contextual evidence. In *Proceedings of the 1999 Joint SIGDAT Conference on Empirical Methods in Natural Language Processing and Very Large Corpora* (pp. 90–99). Stroudsburg, PA, USA: Association for Computational Linguistics.

Cussens J. (1997). Part-of-speech tagging using Progol. In S. Dzeroski and N. Lavrac, editors. *Proc. of the 7th International Workshop on Inductive Logic Programming, LNCS, 1297,* 93-108.

Cybenko, G. (1989). Approximation by Superpositions of a Sigmoidal function. *Mathematics of Control, Signal and Systems, 2*, 303-314.

Damianos, L., Bayer, S., Chisholm, M. A., Henderson, J., Hirschman, L., Morgan, W., Ubaldino, M., & Zarrella, J. (2004). *MiTAP for SARS detection.* In proceeding of the Conference on Human Language Technology, (pp. 241–244). Boston, USA.

Daraselia, N., Yuryev, A., Egorov, S., Novichkova, S., Nikitin, A., & Mazo, I. (2004). Extracting human protein interactions from MEDLINE using a full-sentence parser. *Bioinformatics, 20*, 604-11.

Darmoni, S. J., Leroy, J. P., Baudic, F., Douyere, M., Piot, J., & Thirion, B. (2000) CISMeF: a structured health resource guide. *Methods of information in medicine, 39(1)*, 30-35.

Dasarathy, B. V. (1991). *Nearest Neighbor (NN) Norms: Nearest Neighbor Pattern Classification Techniques.* New York, USA: IEEE Press.

Datta, R., Joshi, D., Li, J., & Wang, J. Z. (2008). Image retrieval: Ideas, influences, and trends of the new age. *ACM Computing Surveys, 40*(2), 5, 1-60. doi: http://doi.acm.org/10.1145/1348246.1348248

De Beaugrande, R. A. (1991). *Linguistic theory: The discourse of fundamental works.* London, New York: Longman. [electronic book http://www.beaugrande.com]

de Bruijn, B., & Martin, J. (2002). Getting to the (c)ore of knowledge: Mining biomedical literature. *International Journal of Medical Informatics, 67*, 7-18. PII: S1386-5056(02)0005 0-3

De Buenaga Rodríguez, M., Gómez Hidalgo, J. M., & Díaz Agudo, B. (1997). Using WordNet to Complement Training Information in Text Categorization. *Proceedings of RANLP-97. 2nd International Conference on Recent Advances in Natural Language Processing.* Tzigov Chark, Bulgary. 11-13 September 1997.

Déjean & Giguet (2008) pdf2xml URL: http://sourceforge.net/projects/pdf2xml

del Lungo, G., & Tognini Bonelli, E. (Eds.). (2006). *Evaluation in academic discourse.* Amsterdam, Herdon: John Benjamins.

Deléger, L., Namer, F., & Zweigenbaum, P. (2007). Defining medical words: Transposing morphosemantic analysis from french to english. In *Proceedings of MEDINFO 2007*, volume 129 of Studies in Health Technology and Informatics, Amsterdam, Netherlands.

Demsey, A., Nahin, A., & Braunsberg, S. V. (2003). Oldmedline citations join pubmed. *NLM Technical Bulletin, 334*(e2).

den Dunnen, J. T., & Antonarakis, S. E. (2001). Nomenclature for the description of human sequence variations. *Hum Genet, 109*(1), 121-124.

Devos, D., & Valencia, A. (2001). Intrinsic errors in genome annotation. *Trends Genetics, 17*(8), 429–431.

Díaz-Galiano, M. C., García-Cumbreras, M. A., Martín-Valdivia, M. T., Montejo-Ráez, A., & Urea-López, L. A. (2007). SINAI at ImageCLEF 2007. *Workshop of the Cross-Language Evaluation Forum.*

Dice, L. (1945). Measures of the amount of ecologic association between species. *Ecology 26*(3), 297-302.

Diekema, A., Yilmazel, O., Chen, J., Harwell, S., He, L., & Liddy, E. D. (2004). What do you mean? Finding answers to complex questions. In L. Greenwald, Z. Dodds, A. Howard, S. Tejada, and J. Weinberg (Eds.), *AAAI Spring Symposium: New Directions in Question Answering* (pp. 87–93). Menlo Park, CA, USA: AAAI Press.

Ding, J., Berleant, D., Nettleton, D, & Wurtele, E. (2002). Mining MEDLINE: Abstracts, Sentences, or Phrases? In *Pacific Symposium on Biocomputing PSB 2002* (pp. 326-337). Retrieved from http://helix-web.stanford.edu/psb02/ding.pdf

Dioşan, L., Rogozan, A., & Pécuchet, J. P. (2007). Alignement des definitions par un apprentissage SVM avec optimisation des hyper-paramtres. In *Grand Colloque STIC 2007* (pp. 1-6). Paris, France.

Dioşan, L., Rogozan, A., & Pécuchet, J. P. (2008a). Apport des traitements morpho-syntaxiques pour l'alignement des dénitions par SVM. In F. Guillet & B. Trousse (Eds.), *Extraction et gestion des connaissances (EGC'2008), Actes des 8µemes journees Extraction et Gestion des*

Connaissances, Sophia-Antipolis, France, (pp. 201-202). France: Cepadues-Editions.

Dioşan, L., Rogozan, A., & Pécuchet, J. P. (2008b). Automatic alignment of medical *vs.* general terminologies. In *11th European Symposium on Artificial Neural Networks, ESANN 2008,* Bruges, Belge.

Djebbari, A., Karamycheva, S., Howe, E., & Quackenbush, J. (2005). MeSHer: identifying biological concepts in microarray assays based on PubMed references and MeSH terms. *Bioinformatics, 21*(15), 3324-3326. doi:10.1093/bioinformatics/bti503.

Do, H. H., & Rahm, E. (2002). COMA - A system for flexible combination of schema matching approaches. In P. A. Bernstein et al. (Eds.), *International Conference on Very Large Data Bases* (pp. 610-621). Los Altos, CA, USA: Morgan Kaufmann.

Doan, A., Madhavan, J., Domingos, P., & Halevy, A. Y. (2002). Learning to map between Ontologies on the Semantic Web. In D. Lassner (Ed.), *The World-Wide Web Conference* (pp. 662-673). New York, NY, USA: ACM.

Dolin, R. H., Huff, S. M., Rocha, R. A., Spackman, K. A., & Campbell, K. E. (1998). Evaluation of a "lexically assign, logically refine" strategy for semi-automated integration of overlapping terminologies. *J Am Med Inform Assoc., 5,* 203–13.

Donaldson, I et al. (2003). PreBIND and Textomy–mining the biomedical literature for protein-protein interactions using a support vector machine. *BMC Bioinformatics, 4,* 11.

Donaldson, I., Martin, J., de Bruijn, B., Wolting, C., Lay, V., Tuekam, B., Zhang, S., Baskin, B., Bader, G. D., Michalickova, K., Pawson, T., & Hogue, C. W. (2003). PreBIND and Textomy--mining the biomedical literature for protein-protein interactions using a support vector machine. *BMC Bioinformatics, 4*(1), 11.

Donnelly, M. (2004). On parts and holes: the spatial structure of human body. In M. Fieschi, E. Coiera, & Y. J. Li (Eds.), *Proceedings of the 11th World Congress on Medical Informatics.* IOS Press, Amsterdam.

Donnelly, M., Bittner, T., & Rosse, C. (2006).A Formal Theory for Spatial Representation and Reasoning in Biomedical Ontologies. *Artificial Intelligence in Medicine, 36*(1), 1 – 27.

Dorow, B., & Widdows, D. (2003). Discovering corpus-specific word senses. *EACL, Conference Companion* (research notes and demos), (pp. 79–82).

Doulamis, A. D., Avrithis, Y. S., Doulamis, N. D., & Kollias, S. D. (1999). Interactive Content-Based Retrieval in Video Databases Using Fuzzy Classification and Relevance Feedback. *Proceedings of the IEEE International Conference on Multimedia Computing and Systems (ICMCS), 2,* 954-958, Florence, Italy, June 1999.

Doulamis, N., & Doulamis, A. (2001). A Recursive Optimal Relevance Feedback Scheme for Content Based Image Retrieval," *Proceedings of the IEEE International Conference on Image Processing (ICIP), 2,* 741-744, Thessaloniki, Greece, October 2001.

Doulamis, N., Doulamis, A., & Kollias, S. (2001). Fuzzy Histograms and Optimal Relevance Feedback for Interactive Content-based Image Retrieval. *IEEE Transactions on Image Processing.*

Doulamis, N., Doulamis, A., &. Ntalianis, K. (2001). Optimal Interactive Content-Based Image Retrieval," *Proceedings of the International Conference on Augmented, Virtual Environments and 3D Imaging,* 248-251, Myconos, Greece, May 2001.

Douyere, M., Soualmia, L. F., Neveol, A., Rogozan, A., Dahamna, B., Leroy, J. P., Thirion, B., & Darmoni, S. J. (2004). Enhancing the MeSH thesaurus to retrieve French online health resources in a quality-controlled gateway. *Health Info Libr J., 21*(4), 253-61.

Dowty, D. R. (1991). Proto-roles and argument selection. *Language, 67*(3), 547–619.

DUC. (2005). *Document Understanding Conference.* http://duc.nist.gov/duc2005.

Dutoit, D, & Nugues P. (2002). A lexical network and an algorithm to find words from definitions. In F. van

Harmelen (Ed.), *European Conference on Artificial Intelligence, ECAI 2002* (pp. 450-454). Amsterdam: IOS.

Dutoit, D., Nugues, P., & de Torcy, P. (2003). The integral dictionary: A lexical network based on componential semantics. In V. Kumar et al. (Eds.), *Computational Science and Its Applications - ICCSA 2003* (pp. 368-377). Berlin, DE: Springer.

Ebell, M. H. (1999). Information at the point of care: answering clinical questions. *Journal of the American Board of Family Practice, 12*(3), 225–235.

Efthimiadis, E. (1996). Query expansion. Im M. E. Williams (Ed.), *Annual Review of Information Systems and Technologies (ARIST), v31,* 121-187.

Eichmann, D., Ruiz, M. E., & Srinivasan, P. (1998). Cross-language information retrieval with the UMLS metathesaurus. In *Proceedings of the 21st International Conference on Research and Development in Information Retrieval, SIGIR 98,* (pp. 72–80), Melbourne, Australia.

Elkin, P. L., Brown, S. H., Bauer, B. A., Husser, C. S., Carruth, W., Bergstrom, L. R., & Wahner-Roedler, D. L. (2005). A controlled trial of automated classification of negation from clinical notes. *BMC Medical Informatics and Decision Making, 5,* 13 doi:10.1186/1472-6947-5-13.

Elkin, P. L., et al. (2006). Evaluation of the content coverage of SNOMED CT: Ability of SNOMED clinical terms to represent clinical problem lists. *Mayo Clin Proc, 81*(6), 741-8.

Erdogmus, M., & Sezerman, O. U. (2007). Application of automatic mutation-gene pair extraction to diseases. *J Bioinform Comput Biol, 5*(6), 1261-1275.

Erik, F., Sang, T. K., & Meulder, F. D. (2003). Introduction to the CoNLL-2003 shared task: language-independent named entity recognition. *Proceedings of Conference on Computational Natural Language Learning* (pp. 142–147). Stroudsburg, PA, USA: Association for Computational Linguistics.

Erjavec, T., & Dˇzeroski, S. (2004). Machine learning of morphosyntactic structure: Lemmatizing unknown Slovene words. *Applied Artificial Intelligence, 18*(1), 17–41.

Euzenat, J., & Shvaiko, P. (2007). Ontology matching. Berlin, DE: Springer.

Farkas, R. (2008) The strength of co-authorship in gene name disambiguation. *BMC Bioinformatics, 9*(1), 69.

Feldman, R., & Sanger, J. (2006). *The Text Mining handbook: Advanced approaches in analyzing unstructured data.* Cambridge University.

Feldman, R., Regev, Y., Hurvitz, E., & Finkelstein-Landau, M. (2003). Mining the biomedical literature using semantic analysis and natural language processing techniques. *Biosilico, 1(2),* 69-80. PII: S1478-5282(03)02314-6

Fellbaum, C. (1998). *WordNet: an Electronic Lexical Database.* Cambridge, Mass. MIT Press.

Figueroa, A., & Neumann, G. (2007). Identifying protein-protein interactions in biomedical publications. In *Proceedings of the BioCreative2 Workshop,* 217-225. GO

Fillmore, C. J. (1976). Frame semantics and the nature of language. *Annals of the New York Academy of Sciences: Conference on the Origin and Development of Language and Speech, 280,* 20–32.

Finkel, J. et al. (2005). Exploring the boundaries: gene and protein identification in Biomedial text. *BMC Bioinformatics, 6,* S5.

Fleischman, S. (2003). Language and medicine. In D. Schiffrin, D. Tannen & H. Hamilton (Eds.), *The Handbook of Discourse Analysis.* Oxford: Blackwell, 470-502.

Florian, R., & Yarowsky, D. (2002). *Modeling Consensus: Classifier Combination for Word Sense Disambiguation.* Paper presented at the Conference on empirical methods in natural language processing.

Florian, R., Ittycheriah, A., Jing, H., & Zhang, T. (2003). Named entity recognition through classifier combination. In W. Daelemans & M. Osborne (Eds.), *7th Conference on Computational Natural Language Learning* (pp. 168–171). Stroudsburg, PA, USA: Association for Computational Linguistics.

Fløttum, K. (Ed.) (2007). *Language and Discipline Perspectives on Academic Discourse*. Newcastle: Cambridge Scholars Publication.

Fløttum, K., & Rastier, F. (Eds.) (2002). *Academic discourse, multidisciplinary approaches*. Oslo: Novus forlag.

Fluck, J., Zimmermann, M., Kurapkat, G., & Hofmann, M. (2005). Information extraction technologies for the life science industry. *Drug Discovery Today, 2(3),* 217-224. doi: 10.1016/j.ddtec.2005.08.013

Fluhr, C., Bisson, F., & Elkateb, F. (2000). Parallel text alignment using crosslingual information retrieval techniques, chapter 9. In (Véronis, 2000).

Fontaine, L., & Kodratoff, Y. (2002). Comparaison du rôle de la progression thématique et de la texture conceptuelle chez des scientifiques anglophones et francophones s'exprimant en Anglais. *Asp, La revue du GERAS*, n° 37-38, 2002, pp. 59 - 83, Bordeaux, France. [English version available online; The role of thematic and concept texture in scientific text http://www.lri.fr/~yk/fon-kod-eng.pdf].

Fontelo, P., Liu, F., Leon, S., Anne, A., & Ackerman, M. (2007). PICO linguist and BabelMeSH: Development and partial evaluation of evidence-based multilanguage search tools for Medline/Pubmed. *Studies of Health Technology and Informatics, 129.*

Frantzi, K., Ananiadou, S., & Mima, H. (2000). Automatic Recognition of Multi-Word Terms: the C-value/NC-value Method. *International Journal on Digital Libraries, 3,* 115-130.

Frantzi, K., Ananiadou, S., & Tsujii, J. (1998). The *C*-value/NC-value method of automatic recognition for multi-word terms. In *Proceedings of ECDL Symposium*, (pp. 585—604).

Friedman C., Kra P., Rzhetsky A. (2002). Two biomedical sublanguages: a description based on the theories of Zellig Harris. *Journal of Biomedical Informatics 35(4),* 222-235. doi: 10.1016/j.ddtec.2005.08.013

Friedman, C. (2000). A broad-coverage natural language processing system. *Proc AMIA Symp.*, (pp. 270–4).

Friedman, C., Alderson, P. O., Austin, J. H., Cimino, J. J., & Johnson, S. B. (1994). A general natural-language text processor for clinical radiology. *Journal of the American Medical Informatics Association, 1*(2), 161-74.

Friedman, C., Alderson, P. O., Austin, J. H., et al. (1994). A general natural language text processor for clinical radiology. *J Am Med Inform Assoc., 1,* 161–74.

Friedman, C., Kra, P., Yu, H., Krauthammer, M., & Rzhetsky, A. (2001). GENIES: A natural-langauge processing system for the extraction of molecular pathways from journal articles. *Bioinformatics, 17*(Suppl 1), 74-82.

Friedman, C., Shagina, L., Lussier, Y., & Hripcsak, G. (2004). Automated encoding of clinical documents based on natural language processing. *Journal of the American Medical Informatics Association, 11*(5), 392.

Friedrich, C., Revillion, T., Hofmann, M., & Fluck, J. (2006). Biomedical and chemical named entity recognition with conditional random fields: The advantage of dictionary features. In *Proceedings of the International Symposium on Semantic Mining in Biomedicine (SMBM)*, (pp. 85-89).

Fu, G., Jones, C. B., & Abdelmoty, A. I. (2005). *Ontology-Based Spatial Query Expansion in Information Retrieval ODBASE: OTM Confederated International Conferences.*

Fundel, K., & Zimmer, R. (2007) *Human Gene Normalization by an Integrated Approach including Abbreviation Resolution and Disambiguation.* In: *Proc Second BioCreative Challenge Evaluation Workshop*, Madrid, Spain.

Fung, P., & McKeown, K. (1997a). Finding terminology translations from non-parallel corpora. In *Proceedings of the 5th Annual Workshop on Very Large Corpora*, Hong Kong.

Fung, P., & McKeown, K. (1997b). A technical word and term translation aid using noisy parallel corpora across language groups. *Machine Translation, 12*(1/2), 53–87.

Furlong, L. I., Dach, H., Hofmann-Apitius, M., & Sanz, F. (2008). OSIRISv1.2: a named entity recognition system for sequence variants of genes in biomedical literature. *BMC Bioinformatics, 9*(1), 84.

Gabrieli, E. R., Speth, D. J. (1986). Automated analysis of the discharge summary,. *J. Clin Comput.*

Gale, W. A., & Church, K. W. (1991). A program for aligning sentences in bilingual corpora. *ACL, 19*(1), 177-184.

Gale, W. A., Church, K. W., & Yarowsky, D. (1992). *One sense per discourse.* Paper presented at the Workshop on Speech and Natural Language Harriman, New York.

Gale, W., & Church, K. (1991). Identifying word correspondences in parallel texts. In *Proceedings of the 4th DarpaWorkshop on Speech and Natural Language*, (pp. 152–157), Pacific Grove, CA, United-States of America.

Galley, M., & McKeown, K. (2003). *Improving word sense disambiguation in lexical chaining.* Paper presented at the 18th Int. Joint Conference on Artificial Intelligence, Acapulca, Mexico.

Gangemi, A., Navigli, R., & Velardi, P. (2003). The OntoWordNet Project: extension and axiomatization of conceptual relations in WordNet. In *Proceedings of ODBASE 2002.*

Gangemi, A., Pisanelli, D. M., & Steve, G. (1999). An overview of the ONIONS project: Applying ontologies to the integration of medical terminologies. *Data Knowledge Engeneering., 31*(2), 183- 220.

Gaudan, S., Jimeno, A., Lee, V., & Rebholz-Schuhmann, D. (2008) Combining evidence, specificity and proximity towards the normalization of Gene Ontology terms in text. *EURASIP JBSB* (accepted).

Gaudan, S., Kirsch, H., & Rebholz-Schuhmann, D. (2005). Resolving abbreviations to their senses in Medline. *Bioinformatics, 21*(18), 3658-3664.

Gaussier, E. (1999). Unsupervised Learning of Derivational Morphology from Inflectional Corpora. In *Proceedings of Workshop on Unsupervised Methods in Natural Language Learning, 37th Annual Meeting of the Association for Computational Linguistics, ACL 99*, (pp. 24–30), Maryland, United-States of America.

GeneOntology Consortium, T. (2001). Creating the gene ontology resource: design and implementation. *Genome Research, 11*(8), 1425-1433.

Gildea, D., & Jurafsky, D. (2002). Automatic labeling of semantic roles. *Computational Linguistics, 28*(3), 245–288.

GO-Consortium (2004). The Gene Ontology (GO) database and informatics resource. *Nucleic Acids Research, 32*(Database issue), D258–D261.

Goldberg, D. E. (1989). *Genetic Algorithms in Search, Optimization and Machine Learning.* Reading, MA, USA: Addison Wesley.

Gómez-Pérez, A., & Manzano-Macho, D. (2003). *OntoWeb D.1.5 A survey of ontology learning methods and techniques.* The OntoWeb Consortium. Retrieved March 07, 2008, from http://ontoweb.aifb.uni-karlsruhe.de/Members/ruben/Deliverable1.5.

Gonzalez, G., Tari, L., Gitter, A., Leaman, R., Nikkila, S., Wendt, R., Zeigler, A., & Baral, C. (2007). Integrating knowledge extracted from biomedical literature: Normalization and evidence statements for interactions. In *Proceedings of the BioCreative2 Workshop*, (pp. 227-235).

Gonzalo, J., Verdejo, F., Chugur, I., & Cigarrán, J (1998). Indexing with WordNet synsets can improve text retrieval. *Coling-ACL 98*, (pp. 38-44).

Gorman, P., Ash, J., & Wykoff, L. (1994). Can primary care physicians' questions be answered using the medical journal literature? *Bulletin of the Medical Library Association, 82*(2), 140–146.

Grenon, P., & Smith, B. (2003). SNAP and SPAN: Towards Geospatial Dynamics. *Spatial Cognition and Computation, 4*(1), 69-104.

Grishman, R., Huttunen, S., & Yangarber, R. (2002). Information extraction for enhanced access to disease outbreak reports. *Journal of Biomedical Informatics. Special Issue Sublanguage - Zellig Harris Memorial, 35*(4), 236-246.

Grosz, B., Joshi, A., & Weinstein, S. (1995). Centering: A Framework for Modeling the Local Coherence of Discourse. *Computational Linguistics, 21*(2), 203–225.

Gruber, T. (1995). Towards Principles for the Design of Ontologies used for Knowledge Sharing. *International Journal of Human-Computer Studies, 43*, 907-928.

Gruber, T. R. (1993). A translation approach to portable ontology specifications. *Knowledge Acquisition, 5*(2), 199–220.

Hahn, U., Honeck, M., Piotrowski, M., & Schulz, S. (2001). Subword segmentation—leveling out morphological variations for medical document retrieval. *Proc AMIA Symp.*, (pp. 229–33).

Hahn, U., Romacker, M., & Schulz, S. (2002). Medsyn-Dikate—a natural language system for the extraction of medical information from findings reports. *Int J Med inform., 67*, 63–74.

Hakenberg, J., Rutsch, J., & Leser, U. (2005). Tuning text classification for hereditary diseases with section weighting. In *First International Symposium on Semantic Mining in Biomedicine (SMBM)* (34-37). Retrieved June 2008 from http://www.informatik.hu-berlin.de/forschung/gebiete/wbi/research/publications

Hakenberg, J., Schmeier, S., Kowald, A., Klipp, E., & Leser, U. (2004). Finding Kinetic Parameters Using Text Mining. *OMICS: A Journal of Integrative Biology, 8*(2), 131-152. Special issue on Data Mining meets Integrative Biology - a Symbiosis in the Making.

Halliday, M.A.K. (1994). *An introduction to functional grammar.* London: Edward Arnold.

Hanisch, D., Fundel, K., Mevissen, H. T., Zimmer, R., & Fluck, J. (2005). ProMiner: rule-based protein and gene entity recognition. *BMC Bioinformatics, 6 Suppl 1*, S14.

Hara, K., & Matsumoto, Y. (2005). Information extraction and sentence classification applied to clinical trial medline abstracts. *Proceedings of the 2005 International Joint Conference of InCoB, AASBi and KSB* (pp. 85–90).

Harabagiu, S., Maiorano, S., Moschitti, A., & Bejan, C. (2004). Intentions, implicatures and processing of complex questions. In S. Harabagiu and F. Lacatusu (Eds.), *Human Language Technology Conference of the North American Chapter of the Association for Computational Linguistics, Workshop on Pragmatics of Question Answering* (pp. 31–42). Stroudsburg, PA, USA: Association for Computational Linguistics.

Harnad, S., Brody, T., Vallieres, F., Carr, L., Hitchcock, S., Gingras, Y., Oppenheim, C., Stamerjohanns, H., & Hilf, E. (2004). The Access/Impact Problem and the Green and Gold Roads to Open Access. *Serials review, 30.*

Harris, Z. (1982). *A grammar of English on mathematical principles.* New York: Wiley.

Harris, Z. (2002). The structure of science information. *Journal of Biomedical Informatics 35(4),* 215-221. doi: 10.1016/S1532-0464(03)00011-X

Harris, Z., Gottfried, M., Ryckman, T., Mattick, P., Daladier, A., Harris, T. N., *et al.* (1989). *The form of information in science: Analysis of an immunology sublanguage.* Dordrecht: Kluwer Academic.

Hausser, R. (2001). *Foundations of Computational Linguistics: Human-Computer Communication in Natural Language.* Heidelnerg, Berlin, New York: Springer-Verlag.

Hearst, M. (1999). Untangling Text Data Mining. *Proceedings of the 37th Annual Meeting of the Association for Computational Linguistics (ACL 1999)* (pp. 3-10).

Hearst, M. A. (1992). Automatic acquisition of hyponyms from large text corpora. *Proc. of the 14th International*

Conf. on Computational Linguistics, (pp 539-545). Nantes, France.

Hersh, W. R., Price, S., & Donohoe, L. (2000). Assessing thesaurus-based query expansion using the UMLS Metathesaurus. *Proceedings of the 2000 Annual AMIA Fall Symposium*, (pp. 344-348).

Hersh, W., Buckley, C., Leone, T. J., & Hickam, D. (1994). OHSUMED: an interactive retrieval evaluation and new large test collection for research. In Springer-Verlag New York, Inc. *SIGIR '94: Proceedings of the 17th annual international ACM SIGIR conference on Research and development in information retrieval* (pp. 192-201).

Hersh, W., Cohen, A., Roberts, P., & Rekapalli, H. (2007). TREC 2006 genomics track overview. In *Proceedings of the Text Retrieval Conference (TREC).*

Hersh, W., Price, S., & Donohoe, L. (2000). Assessing Thesaurus-Based Query Expansion Using the UMLS Metathesaurus. *In Proceedings of the AMIA Symposium* (pp. 344-348).

Herskovic, J. R., Tanaka, L. Y., Hersh, W., & Bernstam, E. V. (2007). A Day in the Life of PubMed: Analysis of a Typical Day's Query Log. *Journal of American Medical Informatics Association*, *14*, 212–220.

Hickl, A., Lehmann, J., Williams, J., & Harabagiu, S. (2004). Experiments with interactive question answering in complex scenarios. In S. Harabagiu & F. Lacatusu (Eds.), *Human Language Technology Conference of the North American Chapter of the Association for Computational Linguistics, Workshop on Pragmatics of Question Answering* (pp. 60–69). Stroudsburg, PA, USA: Association for Computational Linguistics.

Hirschman, L., Morgan, A. A., & Yeh, A. S. (2003). Rutabaga by any other name: extracting biological names. *Journal of Biomedical Informatics*, *35*, 247-259. Elsevier.

Hirschman, L., Park, J. C., Tsujii, J., & Wong, L. (2002). Accomplishments and challenges in literature data mining for biology. *Bioinformatics, 18,* 1553-1561.

Hirschman, L., Yeh, A. Blaschke C, & Valencia A. (2005). "Overview of BioCreAtIvE: critical assessment of information extraction for biology" *BMC Bioinformatics* (6 S1). doi:10.1186/1471-2105-6-S1-S1

Hirschman, L., Yeh, A., Blaschke, C., & Valencia, A. (2005). Overview of BioCreAtIvE: critical assessment of information extraction for biology. *BMC Bioinformatics*, *6*(Suppl 1), S1.

Hockett, C. F. (1958). *A course in modern linguistics.* New York: MacMillan.

Hofmann, R., & Valencia, A. (2003). Life cycles of successful genes. *Trends in Genetics*, *19*, 79-81.

Holland, J. H. (1975). *Adaptation in Natural and Artificial Systems.* Michigan, USA: University of Michigan Press.

Holmes, J. H., & Peek, N. (2007). Intelligent data analysis in biomedicine. *Journal of Biomedical Informatics, 40(6)*, 605-609. doi:10.1016/j.jbi.2007.10.001

Hong, M., Karimpour-Fard, A., Russell, R., & Hunter, L. (2005). Integrated Term Weighting, Visualization, and User Interface Development for Bioinformation Retrieval. *Artificial Intelligence and Simulation, Lecture Notes in Computer Science*, Springer Verlag.

Horn, F., Lau, A. L., & Cohen, F. E. (2004). Automated extraction of mutation data from the literature: application of MuteXt to G protein-coupled receptors and nuclear hormone receptors. *Bioinformatics, 20*(4), 557-568.

Hripcsak, G., Austin, J. H., Alderson, P. O., & Friedman, C. (2002). Use of natural language processing to translate clinical information from a database of 889,921 chest radiographic reports. *Radiology*, *224*, 157–63.

Hripcsak, G., Friedman, C., Alderson, P. O., DuMouchel, W., Johnson, S. B., & Clayton, P. D. (1995). Unlocking clinical data from narrative reports: a study of natural language processing. *Annals of Internal Medicine*, *122*(9), 681-8.

Hripcsak, G., Kuperman, G. J., & Friedman, C. (1998). Extracting findings from narrative reports: software transferability and sources of physician disagreement. *Methods Inf Med., 37*, 1–7.

Hristovski, D., Friedman, C., Rindflesch, T. C., & Peterlin, B. (2006). Exploiting semantic relations for literature-based discovery. *AMIA Annu Symp Proc.* (pp. 349-353). Washington, DC.

Hu, Z. Z., Mani, I., Hermoso, V., Liu, H., & Wu, C. H. (2004). iProLINK: an integrated protein resource for literature mining. *Comput Biol Chem, 28*, 409-416.

Hu, Z. Z., Narayanaswamy, M., Ravikumar, K. E., Vijay-Shanker, K., & Wu, C. H. (2005). Literature mining and database annotation of protein phosphorylation using a rule-based system. *Bioinformatics, 21*, 2759-65.

Huang, A., Ding, S., Wang, H., & Zhu, X. (2007). Mining physical protein-protein interactions from literature. In *Proceedings of the BioCreative2 Workshop.*

Huang, T. M., Kecman, V., & Kopriva, I. (2006). *Kernel based algorithms for mining huge data sets.* Berlin, Germany: Springer.

Huang, Y., & Lowe, H. J. (2007). A novel hybrid approach to automated negation detection in clinical radiology reports. *J. Am Med Inform Assoc., 14*, 304-11.

Huang, Y., & Lowe, H. J. (2005). A grammar based classification of negations in clinical radiology reports. *Proc AMIA Annu Fall Symp*, (pp. 988-92).

Huang, Y., Lowe, H., Klein, D., & Cucina, R. (2005). Improved Identification of Noun Phrases in Clinical Radiology Reports Using a High-Performance Statistical Natural Language Parser Augmented with the UMLS Specialist Lexicon. *J Am Med Inform Assoc, 12*, 275–85.

Humphrey, S. M. (1999). Automatic indexing of documents from journal descriptors: A preliminary investigation. *J Am Soc Inf Sci, 50*(8), 661-674.

Humphreys, B. L., Lindberg, D. A. B., Schoolman, H. M., & Barnett, G. O. (1998). The Unified Medical Language System: An Informatics Research Collaboration. *Journal of the American Medical Informatics Association (JAMIA), 5*, 1-11.

Hunter, L., & Bretonnel Cohen, K. (2006). Biomedical language processing: What's beyond Pubmed? *Molecular Cell* (21), 589-594. doi:10.1016/j.molcel.2006.02.012

Hyland, K. (2005). *Metadiscourse*. London, New York: Continuum Publishing Group.

Ide, N. C., Loane, R. F., & Demner-Fushman, D. (2007). Essie: A Concept Based Search Engine for Structured Biomedical Text. *Journal of the American Medical Informatics Association, 14*(3), 253-263.

Ide, N., & Veronis, J. (1998). Word Sense Disambiguation: The State of the Art. *Computational Linguistics, 14*(1), 1-40.

Ishikawa, Y., Subramanya, R., & Faloutsos, C. (1998). Mindreader: Querying Databases through Multiple Examples. *Proceedings of the 24th VLDB conference*, New York, USA.

Jaccard, P. (1912). The distribution of the flora in the alpine zone. *New Phytologist, 11(2)*, 37-50.

Jacquemin, C. (2001). *Spotting and discovering terms through natural language processing.* Cambridge, MA, USA: MIT Press.

Jacquemin, C., & Tzoukermann, E. (1999). NLP for term variant extraction: A synergy of morphology, lexicon and syntax. In T. Strzalkowski (Ed.), *Natural Language Information Retrieval* (pp. 25-74). Kluwer: Boston.

Jaeger, S., Gaudan, S., Leser, U., & Rebholz-Schuhmann, D. (2008). Integrating Protein-Protein Interactions and Text Mining for Protein Function Prediction. *Data Integration in The Life Sciences (DILS 2008)*, Evry June 25-27 2008 (accepted for publication in BMC Bioinformatics).

Jelier, R., Schuemie, M., Eijk, C. V. E., Weeber, M., Mulligen, E. V., Schijvenaars, B., *et al.* (2003). Searching for geneRIFs: Concept-based query expansion and Bayes classification. TREC 2003 work notes.

Jenicek, M. (2001). Clinical case reporting in evidence-based medicine (2nd edition). Arnold.

Jensen, L. J., Saric, J., & Bork, P. (2006). Literature mining for the biologist: from information retrieval to biological discovery. *Nature Reviews Genetics, 7*, 119-129.

Jensen, L. J., Saric, J., & Bork, P. (2006). Literature mining for the biologist: from information retrieval to biological discovery. *Nat Rev Genet, 7*(2), 119-129.

Jensen, L., Saric, J., & Bork, P. (2006). Literature mining for the biologist: From information retrieval to biological discovery. *Nature Reviews, Genetics, 7*,119-129.

Jimeno, A., Jimenez-Ruiz, E., Lee, V., Gaudan, S., Berlanga-Llavori, R., & Rebholz-Schuhmann, D. (2008). Assessment of disease named entity recognition on a corpus of annotated sentences. *BMC Bioinformatics* (to appear).

Jimeno, A., Pezik, A., & Rebholz-Schuhmann, D. (2007). Information retrieval and information extraction in TREC Genomics 2007. *In Text REtrieval Conference.*

Jin-Dong, K., Ohta, T., Teteisi, Y., & Tsujii, J. (2003). GENIA corpus - a semantically annotated corpus for bio-textmining. *Bioinformatics, 19*(1), i180-i182. OUP.

Joachims, T. (1997). A probabilistic analysis of the Rocchio algorithm with TFIDF for text categorization. In D. H. Fisher, (Ed.), *Proceedings of ICML-97, 14th International Conference on Machine Learning,* (pp. 143-151), Nashville, US, 1997. Morgan Kaufmann Publishers, San Francisco, US.

Joachims, T. (1998). Text Categorization with Support Vector Machines: Learning with Many Relevant Features. *Proc ECML.*

Joachims, T. (1998). Text categorization with support vector machines: learning with many relevant features. *In Proceedings of ECML-98, 10th European Conference on Machine Learning,* 1398 (pp. 137-142). Berlin, Germany: Springer Verlag, Heidelberg.

Joachims, T. (1999). Making large scale svm learning practical. In B. Scholkopf, C. Burges, & A. Smola (Eds.), *Advances in kernel methods - support vector learning.*

Joachims, T. (1999). Making Large-Scale SVM Learning Practical. In: B. Schoelkopf, C. J. C. Burges, & A. J. Smola (Eds.), *Advances in Kernel Methods - Support Vector Learning*, Cambridge, MA, USA.

Jouis C. (2007). SEEK-CLIPS : construction d'ontologies en utilisant l'exploration contextuelle. Extraction semi-automatique des relations puis des concepts à partir de textes, *OntoTexte 2007 («Ontologies et Textes»),* Sophia Antipolis, 10 oct. 2007, France, 5-8.

Jouis, C., (1993). *Contributions à la conceptualisation et à la modélisation des connaissances à partir d'une analyse linguistique de textes. Réalisation d'un prototype : le système SEEK*, PhD dissertation, Ecole des Hautes Etudes en Sciences Sociales (EHESS), Paris France.

Kabiljo, R., Stoycheva, D., & Shepard, A. (2007). ProSpecTome: A new tagged corpus for protein named entity recognition. In *Proceedings of the ISMB BioLINK*, 24-27. Oxford University Press.

Kagolovsky, Y., Freese, D., Miller, M., Walrod, T., & Moehr, J. (1998). Towards improved information retrieval from medical sources. *International journal of medical informatics.*

Kanagasabai, R., Choo, K. H., Ranganathan, S., & Baker, C. J. (2007). A workflow for mutation extraction and structure annotation. *J Bioinform Comput Biol, 5*(6), 1319-1337.

Kando, N. (1992). *Structure of research articles.* (SIG Notes 92-FI-25). Tokyo: Information Processing Society Japan.

Kando, N. (1999). Text structure analysis as a tool to make retrieved documents usable. In *4th International Workshop on Information Retrieval with Asian Languages*, Taipei, Taiwan. Retrieved May 2008 from http://research.nii.ac.jp/~kando/

Kanter, S. L., Miller, R. A., Tan, M., & Schwartz, J. (1994). Using PostDoc to recognize biomedical concepts in medical school curricular documents. *Bull Med Libr Assoc., 82,* 283 -7.

Karsten, H., Back, B., Salakoski, T., Salanterä, S., & Suominen, H. (Eds.) (2008). *Proceedings of The First*

Conference on Text and Data Mining of Clinical Documents. Louhi'08. Turku, Finland.

Kawtrakul, A., & Yingsaeree, C. (2005). A Unified Framework for Automatic Metadata Extraction from Electronic Document. *In proceeding of The International Advanced Digital Library Conference.* Nagoya, Japan.

Kawtrakul, A., Permpool, T., Yingsaeree, C., & Andres, F. (2007a). *A Framework of NLP based Information Tracking and Related Knowledge Organizing with Topic Maps* In proceeding of NLDB2007, LNCS No. 4592, Springer-Verlag, pp. 272-283, ISBN 978-3-540-73350-8, June 27-29, 2007, CNAM, Paris, France.

Kawtrakul, A., Yingsaeree, C., & Andres, F. (2007b). Semantic Tracking in Peer-to-Peer Topic Maps Management. *In proceeding of LNCS,* (pp. 54-69), October 17-19, 2007.

Kazama, J., Makino, T., Ohta, Y., & Tsujii, J. (2002). Tuning support vector machines for biomedical named entity recognition. In *Proceedings of the ACL Workshop on NLP in the Biomedical Domain,* 1-8.

Kekäläinen, J., & Järvelin, K. (1998). The impact of query structure and query expansion on retrieval performance. *In Proceedings of the 21st annual international ACM SIGIR conference on Research and development in information retrieval,* (pp. 130-137). ACM Press.

Kennedy, J. F., Eberhart, R., & Shi, Y. (2001). Swarm Intelligence. In proceeding of Morgan Kaufmann Publishers Inc. San Francisco, CA.

Kilgariff, A., & Rose, T. (1998). Measures for corpus similarity and homogenity. In *Proceedings of the 3rd Conference on Empirical Methods in Natural Language Processing* (pp. 46-52). Granada, Spain.

Kim, J., & Park, J. (2004). BioIE: retargetable information extraction and ontological annotation of biological interactions from literature. *Journal of Bioinformatics and Computational Biology, 2*(3), 551–568.

Kim, J., Ohta, T., Teteisi, Y., & Tsujii, J. (2003). GENIA corpus - a semantically annotated corpus for bio-textmining. *Bioinformatics, 19*(Suppl. 1), I180-I182.

Kim, J., Ohta, T., Tsuruoka, Y., Tateisi, Y., & Collier, N. (2004). Introduction to the bio-entity recognition task at JNLPBA. In *Proceedings of the International Joint Workshop on Natural Language Processing in Biomedicine and its Applications (NLPBA),* 70–75.

Kimchi-Sarfaty, C., Oh, J. M., Kim, I. W., Sauna, Z. E., Calcagno, A. M., Ambudkar, S. V., et al. (2007). A "silent" polymorphism in the MDR1 gene changes substrate specificity. *Science, 315*(5811), 525-528.

Klein, D., Smarr, J., Nguyen, H., & Manning, C. D. (2003). Named entity recognition with character-level models. In W. Daelemans & M. Osborne (Eds.), *7th Conference on Computational Natural Language Learning* (pp. 180–183). Stroudsburg, PA, USA: Association for Computational Linguistics.

Klinger, R., Friedrich, C. M., Mevissen, H. T., Fluck, J., Hofmann-Apitius, M., Furlong, L. I., et al. (2007). Identifying gene-specific variations in biomedical text. *J Bioinform Comput Biol, 5*(6), 1277-1296.

Knight, K., & Graehl, J. (1998). Machine transliteration. *Computational Linguistics, 24*(4), 599–612.

Koeling, R., & McCarthy, D. (2007). Sussx: WSD using Automatically Acquired Predominant Senses. *In Proceedings of the Fourth International Workshop on Semantic Evaluations* (pp. 314–317). Association for Computational Linguistics.

Kohomban, U. S., & Lee, W. S. (2005). Learning semantic classes for word sense disambiguation. In *Proceedings of the 43rd Annual Meeting of the Association for Computational Linguistics* (pp. 34–41). Stroudsburg, PA, USA: Association for Computational Linguistics.

Koike, A., Kobayashi, Y., & Takagi, T. (2003). Kinase pathway database: an integrated protein-kinase and NLP-based protein-interaction resource. *Genome Res., 13,* 1231-43.

Koike, A., Niwa, Y., & Takagi, T. (2005). Automatic extraction of gene/protein biological functions from biomedical text. *Bioinformatics, 21*(7), 1227–1236.

Kokkinakis, D. (2006). Collection, encoding and linguistic processing of a Swedish medical corpus – The MEDLEX experience. *Proceedings of the 5th Conference on Language Resources and Evalutaion (LREC).* Genoa, Italy.

Kokkinakis, D. (2008). A semantically annotated Swedish medical corpus. *Proceedings of the 6th Conference on Language Resources and Evalutaion (LREC).* Marrakech, Morocco.

Kokkinakis, D., & Dannélls, D. (2006). Recognizing acronyms and their definitions in Swedish medical texts. *Proceedings of the 5th Conference on Language Resources and Evalutaion (LREC).* Genoa, Italy.

Kokkinakis, D., Toporowska Gronostaj, M., & Warmenius, K. (2000). Annotating, disambiguating & automatically extending the coverage of the Swedish SIMPLE lexicon. *Proceedings of the 2nd Language Resources and Evaluation Conference (LREC)*, Athens, Greece.

Kolárik, C., Hofmann-Apitius, M., Zimmermann, M., & Fluck, J. (2007). Identification of new drug classification terms in textual resources. *Bioinformatics, 23*(13), i264-72.

Krallinger M., & Valencia, A. (2005) Text-mining and information-retrieval services for molecular biology. *Genome Biology* 2005, 6:224. doi:10.1186/gb-2005-6-7-224

Krallinger, M., & Valencia, A. (2005). Text mining and information retrieval services for Molecular Biology. *Genome Biology, 6*, 224.

Krallinger, M., & Valencia, A. (2007). Evaluating the Detection and Ranking of Protein Interaction relevant Articles: the BioCreative Challenge Interaction Article Sub-task (IAS). In: *Proc 2nd BioCreative Challenge Evaluation Workshop*, Madrid, Spain, (pp. 29-39).

Krauthammer, M., & Nenadic, G. (2004). Term identification in the biomedical literature. *Journal of Biomedical Informatics. Special issue: Named entity recognition in biomedicine, 37*(6), 512-526.

Kreyszig, E. (1989). *Introductory Functional Analysis with Applications.* New York: Wiley & Sons.

Kudo, T., & Matsumoto, Y. (2004). A boosting algorithm for classification of semi-structured text. *Proc. of EMNLP.,* (pp. 301–8).

Kudoh, T., & Matsumoto, Y. (2000). Use of support vector learning for chunk identification. In *Proceedings of the Conference on Natural Language Learning (CoNLL)*, 142-144.

Kushmerick N., Johnston E., & McGuinness S. (2001). Information extraction by text classification. *In Proceedings of IJCAI-2001 Workshop on Adaptive Text Extraction and Mining.*

Lacoste, C. Chevallet, J. P., Lim, J. H., Wei, X. Raccoceanu, D., Thi Hoang, D. L., Teodorescu, R., & Vuillenemot, N. (2006). IPAL Knowledge-based Medical Image Retrieval in ImageCLEFmed 2006. *Workshop of the Cross-Language Evaluation Forum.*

Lafferty, J., McCallum, A., & Pereira, F. (2001). Conditional random fields: Probabilistic models for segmenting and labeling sequence data. In *Proceedings of the International Conference on Machine Learning (ICML)*, (pp. 282–289). Morgan Kaufmann.

Lam, K., Koh, J., Veeravalli, B., & Brusic, V. (2006). Incremental maintenance of biological databases using association rule mining. In *Lecture Notes in Computer Science*, 140–150. Springer-Verlag.

Lan, M., Tan, C. L., & Low, H. B. (2006). Proposing a New Term Weighting Scheme for Text Classification. In: *Proc 21st AAAI,* (pp. 763-768).

Lan, M., Tan, C. L., & Su, J. (2007). A Term Investigation and Majority Voting for Protein Interaction Article Sub-task (IAS). In: *Proc 2nd BioCreative Challenge Evaluation Workshop*, Madrid, Spain, (pp. 183-185).

Langlais, P., & Carl, M. (2004). General-purpose statistical translation engine and domain specific texts: Would it work? *Terminology, 10*(1), 131–152.

Langlais, P., & Patry, A. (2007). Translating unknown words by analogical learning. In *Proceedings of the 2007 Joint Conference on Empirical Methods in Natural Language Processing and Computational Natural Language Learning (EMNLP-CoNLL)*, Prague, Czech Republic.

Langlais, P., Yvon F., & Zweigenbaum, P. (2007). What analogical learning can do for terminology translation? In *Proceedings of Computational Linguisitics in Netherlands*, CLIN'07, Nijmegen, Netherlands.

Lapata, M., & Keller, F. (2005). Web-based models for natural language processing. *ACM Transactions on Speech and Language Processing, 2*(1), 1-31.

Lau, L. M., Johnson, K., Monson, K., Lam, S. H., & Huff, S. M. (2002). A method for automated mapping of laboratory results to LOINC. *Proc AMIA Symp.*

Lee, L. C., Horn, F., & Cohen, F. E. (2007). Automatic extraction of protein point mutations using a graph bigram association. *PLoS Comput Biol, 3*(2), e16.

Lee, Y. K., & Ng, H. T. (2002). *An empirical evaluation of knowledge sources and learning algorithms for word sense disambiguation.* Paper presented at the Conference on empirical methods in natural language processing.

Leech, G., Rayson, P., & Wilson, A. (2001). *Word Frequencies in Written and Spoken English: based on the British National Corpus*: Longman, London.

Leroy, G., & Rindflesch, T. C. (2004). Using Symbolic Knowledge in the UMLS to Disambiguate Words in Small Datasets with a Naive Bayes Classifier. In: M. Fieschi et al. (Eds), *MEDINFO.* IOS Press.

Leroy, G., &. Rindflesch, T. C. (2005). Effects of information and machine learning algorithms on word sense disambiguation with small datasets. *Int. J. Med. Inform., 74*, 573–585.

Leroy, G., Eryilmaz, E., & Laroya, B. T. (2006). Health information text characteristics. In *AMIA 2006 Symposium* (pp. 479–483). American Medical Informatics Association.

Leser, U., & Hakenberg, J. (2005). What Makes a Gene Name? Named Entity Recognition in the Biomedical Literature. *Briefings in Bioinformatics, 6*(4), 357-369.

Levy, S., Sutton, G., Ng, P. C., Feuk, L., Halpern, A. L., Walenz, B. P., et al. (2007). The diploid genome sequence of an individual human. *PLoS Biol, 5*(10), e254.

Lewis, D. D. (1991). *Evaluating Text Categorization. In Proceedings of Speech and Natural Language Workshop* (pp. 312-318). Morgan Kaufmann (publisher).

Lewis, D. D., Schapire, R. E., Callan, J. P., & Papka, R. (1996). Training algorithms for linear text classifiers. *In Proceedings of SIGIR-96, 19th ACM International Conference on Research and Development in Information Retrieval* (pp. 298-306). New York, US: ACM Press.

Li, W. S., & Clifton, C. (2000). SEMINT: A tool for identifying attribute correspondences in heterogeneous databases using neural networks. *Data Knowledge Engeneering, 33*(1), 49-84.

Li, Y., Lin, H., & Yang, Z. (2007). Two approaches for biomedical text classification. In Proceedings of the *International Conference Bioinformatics and Biomedical Engineering (ICBBE)*, (pp. 310–313). IEEE Press.

Li, Y., Zaragoza, H., Herbrich, R., Shawe-Taylor, J., & Kandola, J. (2002) The Perceptron Algorithm with Uneven Margins. *In Proceedings of the International Conference of Machine Learning (ICML'2002)* (pp. 379-386).

Lin, D. (1994). Principar — an efficient, broad-coverage, principle-based parser. In *Proceedings of the 15th International Conference on Computational Linguistics* (pp. 482–488). Stroudsburg, PA, USA: Association for Computational Linguistics.

Lin, D. (1998). An information-theoretic definition of similarity. In *Proc. of the 15th International Conference on Machine Learning.*

Lin, D. (1998). Automatic retrieval and clustering of similar words. In *Proceedings of the 17th International Conference on Computational Linguistics* (pp. 768–774).

Stroudsburg, PA, USA: Association for Computational Linguistics.

Lin, J., Karakos, D., Demner-Fushman, D., & Khudanpur, S. (2006). Generative content models for structural analysis of medical abstracts. *Proceedings of the BioNLP Workshop on Linking Natural Language Processing and Biology at HLT-NAACL.* (pp. 65-72).

Lindberg, D. A. B., Humphreys, B. L., & McCray, A. T. (1993). The Unified Medical Language System. *Methods of Information in Medicine, 32*, 281-291.

Lisacek, F., Chichester, C., Kaplan, A.. & Sandor, A. (2005). Discovering Paradigm Shift Patterns in Biomedical Abstracts: Application to Neurodegenerative Diseases. In *First International Symposium on Semantic Mining in Biomedicine (SMBM)*, Hinxton, UK.

Liu, H., Aronson, A. R., & Friedman, C. (2002). *A study of abbreviations in MEDLINE abstracts.* Paper presented at the AMIA Symposium.

Liu, H., Hu, Z. Z., & Wu, C. H. (2006a). BioThesaurus: a web-based thesaurus of protein and gene names. *Bioinformatics, 22*, 103-105.

Liu, H., Hu, Z. Z., Torii, M., Wu, C., & Friedman, C. (2006b). Quantitative Assessment of Dictionary-based Protein Named Entity Tagging. *J Am Med Inform Assoc, 13*, 497-507.

Liu, H., Hu, Z., Zhang, J., & Wu, C. (2006). BioThesaurus: a web-based thesaurus of protein and gene names. *Bioinformatics, 22*(1), 103-105.

Liu, H., Johnson, S. B., & Friedman, C. (2002). Automatic resolution of ambiguous terms based on machine learning and conceptual relations in the UMLS. *J. Am Med Inform Assoc., 9,* 621–36.

Liu, Z., & Chu, W. (2005). Knowledge-based query expansion to support scenario-specific retrieval of medical free text. *In SAC '05: Proceedings of the 2005 ACM symposium on Applied computing*, (pp. 1076-1083), New York, NY, USA: ACM Press.

Lopez Osornio, A., Luna, D., Gambarte, M. L., Gomez, A., Reynoso, G., & Gonzalez Bernaldo de Quiros, F. (2007). Creation of a Local Interface Terminology to SNOMED CT [online]. In K. A. Kuhn, J. R. Warren, & T-Y. Leong (Ed.), *Medinfo 2007: Proceedings of the 12th World Congress on Health (Medical) Informatics; Building Sustainable Health Systems* (pp. 765-769). Amsterdam: IOS Press, 2007. Studies in health technology and informatics, ISSN0926-9630.

Lord, P., Stevens, R., Brass, A., & Goble, C. (2003). Investigating semantic similarity measures across the Gene Ontology: the relationship between sequence and annotation. *Bioinformatics, 19*(10), 1275–1283.

Lortal, G., Diosan, L., Pecuchet, J. P., & Rogozan, A. (2007). Du terme au mot: Utilisation de techniques de classification pour l'alignement de terminologies. In *Terminologie et Intelligence Artificielle, TIA2007, Sophia Antipolis, France.*

Lovis, C. (1998). Trends and pitfalls with nomenclatures and classifications in medicine. *International Journal of Medical Informatics* (52), 141-148. PII S1386-5056(98)00133-6

Lowe, H. J., Buchanan, B. G., Cooper, G. F., & Vries, J. K. (1995). Building a medical multimedia database system to integrate clinical information: an application of high performance computing and communications technology. *Bull Med Libr Assoc., 83,* 57 -64.

Lu, D., Szafron, R., Greiner, P., Lu, D.S., Wishart, B. Poulin, J., Anvik, C., Macdonell, & Eisner, R.(2004). Predicting Subcellular Localization of Proteins using Machine-Learned Classifiers, *Bioinformatics, 20*(4), 547-556.

Lucas N., Crémilleux B. (2004) Fouille de textes hiérarchisée, appliquée à la détection de fautes. *Document numérique* 8 (3), 107-133.

Lucas N., Crémilleux B., Turmel L. (2003) Signalling well-written academic articles in an English corpus by text mining techniques. In Archer D., Rayson P., Wilson

A., McEnery T. (Eds) *Corpus Linguistics*. (pp. 465-474). Lancaster: University Centre for Corpus Research on Language, Lancaster University.

Luenberger, D. J. (1984) *Linear and non Linear Programming*. Addison-Wesley.

Lussier, Y. A., Sarkar, I. N., & Cantor, M. (2002). An integrative model for in-silico clinical-genomics discovery science. *Proc AMIA Symp*. (pp. 469-73).

Lussier, Y. A., Shagina, L., & Friedman, C. (2001). Automating SNOMED coding using medical language understanding: A feasibility study. *Proc AMIA Symp., 418, 22.*

Ma., J., Zhao, Y., Ahalt, S., & Eads, D. (2003). *OSU SVM classifier Matlab toolbox*. http://svm.sourceforge.net/docs/3.00/api/.

Madhavan, J., Bernstein, P. A., & Rahm, E. (2001). Generic schema matching with Cupid. In P. M. G. Apers et al. (Eds.), *The 27th International Conference on Very Large Data Bases VLDB '01* (pp. 49-58). Orlando, USA: Morgan Kaufmann.

Madkour, A., Darwish, K., Hassan, H., Hassan, A., & Emam, O. (2007). BioNoculars: Extracting protein-protein interatctions from biomedical text. In *BioNLP 2007: Biological, translational, and clinical language processing*, (pp. 89–96). ACM Press.

Magnini, B., & Cavaglia, G. (2000). Integrating subject field codes into WordNet. *In Proceedings of the International Conference on Language Resources and Evaluation* (pp. 1413–1418).

Magnini, B., Strapparava, C., Pezzulo, G., & Gliozzo, A. (2001). Using domain information for word sense disambiguation. *In Proceeding of Second International Workshop on Evaluating Word Sense Disambiguation Systems* (pp. 111–114).

Mandala, R., Tokunaga, T., & Tanaka, H. (1998). The use of WordNet in information retrieval. In S. Harabagiu, (Ed.), *Use of WordNet in Natural Language Processing Systems: Proceedings of the Conference*, (pp. 31-37). Association for Computational Linguistics, Somerset, New Jersey.

Manning, C., & Schütze, H. (1999). *Foundation of Statistical Natural Language Processing*. Cambridge, MA.

Manning, C., & Schütze, H. (1999). *Foundations of Statistical Natural Language Processing*. Cambridge, Massachusetts: MIT Press.

Markellos, K., Markellou, P., Rigou, M., & Sirmakessis, S. (2004). Web mining: Past, present and future. In S. Sirmakessis (Ed), *Text Mining and Its Applications* (pp. 25-35). Springer.

Markó, K., Stefan Schulz, O. M., & Hahn, U. (2005). Bootstrapping dictionaries for crosslanguage information retrieval. In *Proceedings of the 28th International Conference on Research and Development in Information Retrieval, SIGIR 05*, (pp. 528–535), Salvador, Brasil.

Martín-Valdivia, M. T., Ureña López, L. A., & García Vega, M. (2007). The learning vector quantization algorithm applied to automatic text classification tasks. *Neural Networks, 20*(6), 748-756.

McCallum, A., & Li, W. (2003). Early results for named entity recognition with conditional random fields, feature induction and web-enhanced lexicons. In *Proceedings of the Conference on Natural Language Learning (CoNLL)*, (pp. 188–191).

McCarthy, D., Koeling, R., Weeds, J., & Carroll, J. (2004). Finding predominant senses in untagged text. *In Proceedings of the 42nd Annual Meeting of the Association for Computational Linguistics*, (pp. 280–287).

McCray, A.T., Bodenreider, O., Malley J. D., & Browne (2001). Evaluating UMLS Strings for Natural Language Processing. *AC Proc AMIA Symp*, (pp. 448-52).

McDonald, R. T., Winters, R. S., Mandel, M., Jin, Y., White, P. S., & Pereira, F. (2004). An entity tagger for recognizing acquired genomic variations in cancer literature. *Bioinformatics, 20*(17), 3249-3251.

McDonald, R., & Pereira, F. (2004). Identifying gene and protein mentions in text using conditional random fields. In *Proceedings of the BioCreative Workshop.*

McKnight, L., & Srinivasan, P. (2003). Categorization of sentence types in medical abstracts. AMIA Annu Symp Proc., (pp. 440-4).

McNaught, J., & Black, W. (2006). Information Extraction. In S.Ananiadou & J. McNaught (Eds.), *Text Mining for Biology and Biomedicine.* Artech house.

Meadow, T. C. (1992). *Text Information Retrieval Systems.* San Diego, CA, USA: Academic Press.

MEDLINE/PubMed database. Accessed March XX, 2008: http://www.nlm.nih.gov/pubs/factsheets/medline.html.

Mena, E., Kashyap, V., Sheth, A., & Illarramendi, A. (2000). OBSERVER: An approach for query processing in global information systems based on interoperation across pre-existing ontologies. *Journal on Distributed and Parallel Databases, 8*(2), 223-272.

Mendonça, E. A., Cimino, J. J., Johnson, S. B., & Seol, Y. H. (2001). Accessing heterogeneous sources of evidence to answer clinical questions. *Journal of Biomedical Informatics, 34,* 85–98.

Meystre, S., & Haug, P. J. (2006). Natural language processing to extract medical problems from electronic clinical documents: Performance evaluation. *Journal of Biomedical Informatics, 39,* 589-599.

Mihalcea, R. (2007). Using Wikipedia for Automatic Word Sense Disambiguation. *In Proceedings of the North American Chapter of the Association for Computational Linguistics.* Rochester, U.S.A.

Mika, S., & Rost, B. (2004). Protein names precisely peeled off free text. *Bioinformatics, 20*(Suppl 1), I241-I247.

Mika, S., & Rost, B. (2004). Protein names precisely peeled off free text. *Bioinformatics, 20*(Suppl. 1), I241-I247.

Miller, G. A. (1995). Introduction to WordNet: A lexical database for English. *Communication ACM, 38,* 39-41.

Miller, R. A., Gieszczykiewicz, F. M., Vries, J. K., & Cooper, G. F. (1992). Chartline: Providing bibliographic references relevant to patient charts using the UMLS Metathesaurus knowledge sources. *Proc Symp Comput Appl Med Care,* (pp. 86-90).

Miska, E.A., Langley, E., Wolf, D., Karlsson, C., Pines, J., & Kouzarides, T. (2001). Differential localization of HDAC4 orchestrates muscle differentiation. *Nucleic Acids Res, 29*(16), 3439–3447.

Mitchell, J. A., Aronson, A. R., & Mork, J. G. (2003). Gene indexing: Characterization and analysis of nlm's generifs. *AMIA Annu Symp Proc. 2003,* (pp. 460-4).

Mitchell, J., Aronson, A., Mork, J., Folk, L., Humphrey, S., & Ward, J. (2003). Gene indexing: characterization and analysis of NLM's GeneRIFs. In *Proc. of the AMIA 2003 Annual Symposium.*

Mitchell, T. (1997). *Machine Learning*: McGraw Hill.

Mitkov, R. (2002). *Anaphora resolution (Studies in Language & Linguistics).* Longman.

Mitra, M., Singhal, A., & Buckley, C. (1998). Improving automatic query expansion. *In Research and Development in Information Retrieval,* (pp. 206-214).

Miyao, Y., & Tsujii, J. (2008). Feature Forest Models for Probabilistic HPSG Parsing. *Computational Linguistics, 34,* 35-80.

Miyao, Y., Ohta, T., Masuda, K., Tsuruoka, Y., Yoshida, K., Ninomiya, T., & Tsujii, J. (2006). Semantic Retrieval for the Accurate Identification of Relational Concepts in Massive Textbases. *Annual Meeting- Association for Computational Linguistics, 2,* 1017-1024.

Mizuta, Y., Korhonen, A., Mullen, T., & Collier, N. (2006). Zone analysis in biology articles as a basis for information extraction. *International Journal of Medical Informatics* (75), 468-487. doi:10.1016/j.ijmedinf.2005.06.013

Montejo-Ráez, A., Martín-Valdivia, M. T., & Ureña-López, L. A. (2007). Experiences with the LVQ algorithm in multilabel text categorization. *In Proceedings of the 4th International Workshop on Natural Language Processing and Cognitive Science* (pp. 213-221.), Funchal, Madeira - Portugal.

Moore, R. C. (2002). Fast and accurate sentence alignment of bilingual corpora. In S. D. Richardson (Ed.), *Machine Translation: From Research to Real Users, 5th Conference of the Association for Machine Translation in the Americas* (pp. 135-144). Berlin, DE: Springer-Verlag.

Moreau, F., Claveau, V., & Sebillot, P. (2007). Automatic morphological query expansion using analogy-based machine learning. In G. Amati et al. (Eds.), *Advances in Information Retrieval, 29th European Conference on IR Research, ECIR 2007, Vol. 4425* (pp. 222-233), Berlin, DE: Springer.

Moreau, F., Claveau, V., & Sébillot, P. (2007). Automatic morphological query expansion using analogy-based machine learning. In *Proceedings of the 29th European Conference on Information Retrieval, ECIR 2007*, Roma, Italy.

Morgan, A., Lu, Z., Wang, X., Cohen, A., Fluck, J., Ruch, P., Divoli, A., Fundel, K., Leaman, R., Hakenberg, J., Sun, C., Liu, H-H., Torres, R., Krauthammer, M., Lau, W., Liu, H., Hsu, C-N., Schuemie, M., Cohen, K. B., & Hirschman, L. (2008) Overview of BioCreative II Gene Normalization. *Genome Biology*, Special Issue on BioCreative Challenge Evaluations.

Moschitti, A. (2004). A study on convolution kernels for shallow semantic parsing. *Proceedings of ACL-2004.*

MUC. (2003). Message Understanding Conference. http://www.cs.nyu.edu/cs/faculty/grishman/muc6.html

Müller, H., Deselaers, T., Lehmann, T., Clough, P., & Hersh, W. (2007). Overview of the ImageCLEFmed 2006 medical retrieval and annotation tasks. Evaluation of Multilingual and Multi-modal Information Retrieval. *Workshop of the Cross-Language Evaluation Forum 2006, Springer Lecture Notes in Computer Science* (2007).

Müller, H., Kenny, E., & Sternberg, P. (2004). Textpresso: an ontology-based information retrieval and extraction system for biological literature. *PLOS Biology, 2*(11), E309.

Müller, H., Kenny, E., & Sternberg, P. (2004). Textpresso: an ontology-based information retrieval and extraction system for biological literature. *PLOS Biology, 2*(11), E309.

Mutalik, P. G., Deshpande, A., &Nadkarni, P. M. (2001). Use of general-purpose negation detection to augment concept indexing of medical documents: A quantitative study using the UMLS. *J Am Med Inform Assoc., 8*, 598–609.

Nadkarni, P., Chen, R., & Brandt, C. (2001). UMLS concept indexing for production databases: A feasibility study. *J Am Med Inform Assoc., 8*, 80–91.

Nakov, P., & Hearst, M. (2006). Using verbs to characterize noun-noun relations. *Proc. of the 12th International Conference on AI: Methodology, Systems, Applications.* Bulgaria.

Narayanaswamy, M., Ravikumar, K. E., & Vijay-Shanker, K. (2005). Beyond the clause: Extraction of phosphorylation information from Medline abstracts. *Bioinformatics,* (Suppl 1), i319-i327.

National Library of Medicine Entrez PubMed website url : http://www.ncbi.nlm.nih.gov/entrez/query.fcgi?DB=pubmed

Navigli, R., & Velardi, P. (2003). An Analysis of Ontology-based Query Expansion Strategies. *Workshop on Adaptive Text Extraction and Mining (ATEM 2003), in the 14th European Conference on Machine Learning (ECML 2003),* (pp. 42-49).

Navigli, R., Velardi, P., & Gangemi, A. (2003). Ontology learning and its application to automated terminology translation. *Intelligent Systems, IEEE, 18*(1), 22–31.

Nelson, S. J., Johnston, D., & Humphreys, B. L. (2001). Relationships in medical subject headings. In C. A. Bean & R. Green (Eds.), *Relationships in the Organization of*

Knowledge. New York: Kluwer Academic Publishers (pp. 171-184).

Netzel, R., Perez-Iratxeta, C., Bork P., & Andrade, M. A. (2003). The way we write. Country-specific variations of the English language in the biomedical literature. *EMBO reports* 4 (5), 446-451. doi:10.1038/sj.embor.embor833

Névéol, A., Mary V., Gaudinat, A., Boyer, C., Rogozan, A., & Darmoni, S. (2005). *A benchmark evaluation of the French MeSH indexing systems*. In S. Miksh, J. Hunter, & E. Keravnou (Eds.), *Springer's Lecture Notes in Computer Science, Artificial Intelligence in Medicine. Proc. AIME*. (pp. 251-255).

Névéol, A., Mork, J. G., & Aronson, A. R. (2007). Automatic indexing of specialized documents: Using generic vs. domain-specific document representations. *Biological, Translational and Clinical Language processing (BioNLP 2007)*. (pp. 183-190). Prague.

Ng, H. T., Lim, C. Y., & Foo, S. K. (1999). *A Case Study on Inter-Annotator Agreement for Word Sense Disambiguation*. Paper presented at the ACL SIGLEX Workshop: Standardizing Lexical Resources.

Nigam, K., Lafferty, J., & McCallum, A. (1999). Using maximum entropy for text classification. In *Proceedings of the IJCAI Workshop on Information Filtering*, (pp. 61-67).

Niles, I., & Pease A. (2003). Linking Lexicons and Ontologies: Mapping WordNet to the Suggest Upper Merged Ontology. *In Proceedings of the Conference on Information and Knowledge Engineering*.

Nilsson, K., Hjelm, H., & Oxhammar, H. (2005). SUiS – cross-language ontology-driven information retrieval in a restricted domain. *In Proceedings of the 15th NODALIDA conference*, (pp. 139-145).

Niu, Y. (2007). *Analysis of semantic classes: toward non-factoid question answering*. Unpublished doctoral dissertation, University of Toronto, Toronto, Canada.

Niu, Y., & Hirst, G. (2004). Analysis of semantic classes in medical text for question answering. In D. Mollá & J. L. Vicedo, *42nd Annual Meeting of the Association for Computational Linguistics, Workshop on Question Answering in Restricted Domains* (pp. 54–61). Stroudsburg, PA, USA: Association for Computational Linguistics.

Niu, Y., & Hirst, G. (2007). Identifying cores of semantic classes in unstructured text with a semi-supervised learning approach. In *Proceedings of Recent Advances in Natural Language Processing 2007* (pp. 418–424).

Niu, Y., Hirst, G., McArthur, M., and Rodriguez-Gianolli, P. (2003). Answering clinical questions with role identification. In Ananiadou, S., & Tsujii, J. (Eds.), *41st Annual Meeting of the Association for Computational Linguistics, Workshop on Natural Language Processing in Biomedicine* (pp. 73–80). Stroudsburg, PA, USA: Association for Computational Linguistics.

Niu, Y., Zhu, X., Li, J., & Hirst, G. (2005). Analysis of polarity information in medical text. *Proceedings of the American Medical Informatics Association 2005 Annual Symposium* (pp. 570–4).

Niu, Y., Zhu, X., Li, J., & Hirst, G. (2005). Analysis of polarity information in medical text. In C. P. Friedman (Ed.), *American Medical Informatics Association 2005 Annual Symposium* (pp. 570–574). Bethesda, MD, USA: American Medical Informatics Association.

Niu, Y., Zhu, X.D., & Hirst, G. (2006). Using outcome polarity in sentence extraction for medical question-answering. In Daniel Masys (Ed.), *American Medical Informatics Association 2006 Annual Symposium* (pp. 599–603). Bethesda, MD, USA: American Medical Informatics Association.

Nocedal, J., & Wright, S. J. (1999). *Numerical Optimization*. Springer.

Nwogu, K. N. (1997). "The medical research paper: structure and functions" *English for Specific Purposes* 16 (2), 119-138.

Oakes, M. P. (2005). Using Hearst's rules for the automatic acquisition of hyponyms for mining a Pharmaceutical corpus. *Proc. of the RANLP 2005 Workshop* (pp 63-67). Bulgaria.

Oflazer, K., & Nirenburg, S. (1999). Practical bootstrapping of morphological analyzers. In *Proceedings of EACL Workshop on Computational Natural Language Learning, CONLL 99*, Bergen, Norway.

Pahikkala, T., Ginter, F., Boberg, J., Jarvinen, J., & Salakoski, T. (2005) Contextual weighting for Support Vector Machines in Literature Mining: An Application to Gene versus Protein Name Disambiguation. *BMC Bioinformatics*, *6*, 157.

Pang, B., & Lee, L. (2003). A sentimental education: sentiment analysis using subjectivity smmarizaiton based on minimum cuts. In *Proceedings of the 42th Annual Meeting of the Association for Computational Linguistics* (pp. 271–278). Stroudsburg, PA, USA: Association for Computational Linguistics.

Pang, B., Lee, L., & Vaithyanathan, S. (2002). Thumbs up? sentiment classification using machine learning techniques. In *Proceedings of 2002 Conference on Empirical Methods in Natural Language Processing* (pp. 79–86). PA, USA: Association for Computational Linguistics.

Park, J. C., & Kim, J.-j. (2006). Named Entity Recognition. In S. Ananiadou & J. McNaught (Eds.), *Text Mining for Biology and Biomedicine.* (pp. 121-142). London: Artech House Books.

Park, Y., & Byrd, R. J. (2001). Hybrid Text Mining for Finding Abbreviations and Their Definitions. *Proceedings of the Conference on Empirical Methods in Natural Language Processing,* (pp. 126- 133). Pittsburgh, PA, June 2001.

Parsons, G. (1990). *Cohesion and coherence: Scientific texts. A comparative study.* Nottingham, England: Department of English Studies, University of Nottingham.

Patrick, J., Budd, P., & Wang, Y. (2007). An automated system for Conversion of Clinical notes into SNOMED CT. Health Knowledge & Data Mining Workshop. *Research & Practice in Information Technology, 68,* 195-202.

Pazienza, M., & Stellato, A. (2006). An environment for semi-automatic annotation of ontological knowledge with linguistic content. In Y. Sure & J. Domingue (Eds.), *The Semantic Web: Research and Applications. Proceedings of the 3rd European Semantic Web Conference (ESWC).* Budva, Montenegro.

Pechsiri C., Kawtrakul A., & Piriyakul R. (2005). Mining Causality Knowledge From Thai Textual Data. *In proceeding of The 6th Symposium on Natural Language Processing, SNLP'2005*, Chiang Rai, Thailand.

Pechsiri, C., & Kawtrakul, A. (2007). Mining Causality from Texts for Question Answering System. *In proceeding of IEICE on Transactions on Information and Systems, 90*-D, No 10.

Pengphon N., Kawtrakul A., & Suktarachan M. (2002). Word Formation Approach to Noun Phrase Analysis for Thai. *In proceeding of The 5th Symposium on Natural Language Processing.*

Pérez, A., Perez-Iratxeta, C., Bork, P., Thode, G., & Andrade, M. (2004). Gene annotation from scientific literature using mappings between keyword systems. *Bioinformatics*, *20*(13), 2084–2091.

Perrin, P., & Petry, F. (1999). An information-theoretic based model for large-scale contextual text processing. *Information Sciences* (116), 229-252. PII: S0020-0255(98) 1 0090-7

Perrin, P., & Petry, F. (2003). Extraction and representation of contextual information for knowledge discovery in texts. *Information Sciences* (151), 125-152. doi:10.1016/S0020-0255(02)00400-0

Pezik, P, Jimeno, A., Lee, V., & Rebholz-Schuhmann, D. (2008b). *Static Dictionary Features for Term Polysemy Identification submitted to Workshop Proceedings of 5th International Conference on Language Resources and Evaluation (LREC 2008).*

Pezik, P., Kim, J., & Rebholz-Schuhmann, D. (2008a). MedEvi – a permuted concordancer for the biomedical domain. *In Proceedings of PALC 2008 Conference.*

Plake, C., Schiemann, T., Pankalla, M., Hakenberg, J., & Leser, U. (2006). AliBaba: PubMed as a graph. *Bioinformatics, 22*(19), 2444-2445.

Porter, M. F. (1980). An algorithm for suffix stripping. *Program, 14*(3), 130-137.

Poulter, G. L., Rubin, D. L., Altman, R. B., & Seoighe, C. (2008). MScanner: a classifier for retrieving Medline citations. *BMC Bioinformatics, 9*, 108.

Prather, J. C., Lobach, D. F., Goodwin, L. K., Hales, J. W., Hage, M. L., & Hammond, W. E. (1997). Medical Data mining: Knowledge discovery in a clinical data warehouse. *AMIA Annual Fall Symposium*, (pp. 101-5).

Proux, D., Rechenmann, F., & Julliard, L. (2000). A Pragmatic Information Extraction Strategy for Gathering Data on Genetic Interactions. *Proc Int Conf Intell Syst Mol Biol, 8*, 279-285.

Purcell, G. P., & Shortliffe, E. H. (1995). Contextual models of clinical publications for enhancing retrieval from full-text databases. *Proc Annu Symp Comput Appl Med Care*, (pp. 851–7).

Pustejovsky, J. et al. (2001). Automation Extraction of Acronym-Meaning Pairs from Medline Databases. *Medinfo, 10*(Pt 1), 371-375.

Pustejovsky, J. *et al.* (2001). Automation Extraction of Acronym-Meaning Pairs from MEDLINE Databases. *Medinfo 2001, 10*(Pt 1), 371-375.

Pustejovsky, J., Castaño, J., Cochran, B., Kotecki, M., Morrell, M., &. Rumshisky, A. (2001). Extraction and Disambiguation of Acronym-Meaning Pairs in Medline. *unpublished manuscript.*

Pustejovsky, J., Castaño, J., Zhang, J., Kotecki, M., & Cochran, B. (2002). Robust relational parsing over biomedical literature: Extracting inhibit relations. *Pac Symp Biocomput*, (pp. 362-373).

Qiu, Y., & Frei, H. (1993). Concept-based query expansion. *In Proceedings of SIGIR-93, 16th ACM International Conference on Research and Development in Information Retrieval*, (pp. 160-169), Pittsburgh, US.

Qu, Y., Grefenstette, G., & Evans, D. A. (2003). Automatic transliteration for Japanese-to-English text retrieval. In *Proceedings of the 26th International Conference on Research and Development in information Retrieval, SIGIR 03*, Toronto, Canada.

Quirk, R., Greenbaum, S., Leech, S., & Svartvik, J. (1985). *A comprehensive grammar of the English language.* London: Longman.

Rabiner, L. R. (1989). A tutorial on hidden Markov models and selected applications in speech recognition. *Proceedings of the IEEE, 77*(2), 257–286.

Rada, R., Mili, H., Bicknell, E., & Blettner, M. (1989). Development and application of a metric on semantic nets. *IEEE Transactions on Systems, 19*(1), 17–30.

Ray, S., & Craven, M. (2001). Representing sentence structure in hidden Markov models for information extraction. In B. Nebel (Ed.), *17th International Joint Conferences on Artificial Intelligence* (pp. 1273–1279). San Fransisco, CA, USA: Morgan Kaufmann Publishers Inc.

Rebholz-Schuhmann, D., Arregui, M., Gaudan, S., Kirsch, H., & Jimeno, A. (2008). Text processing through Web services: Calling Whatizit. *Bioinformatics 2008* (to appear).

Rebholz-Schuhmann, D., Kirsch, H., & Couto, F. (2005). Facts from text - is text mining ready to deliver? *PLoS Biology, 3*(2), e65.

Rebholz-Schuhmann, D., Kirsch, H., & Couto, F. (2005). Facts from text - is text mining ready to deliver? *PLoS Biology, 3*(2), e65.

Rebholz-Schuhmann, D., Kirsch, H., & Nenadic, G. (2006). IeXML: towards a framework for interoperability of text processing modules to improve annotation of semantic types in biomedical text. *Proc. of BioLINK, ISMB 2006*, Fortaleza, Brazil.

Rebholz-Schuhmann, D., Kirsch, H., Arregui, M., Gaudan, S., Rynbeek, M., & Stoehr, P. (2007). EBIMed: Text crunching to gather facts for proteins from Medline. *Bioinformatics, 23*(2), e237-44.

Rebholz-Schuhmann, D., Kirsch, H., Gaudan, M. A. S., Rynbeek, M., & Stoehr, P. (2007). EBIMed - text crunching to gather facts for proteins from Medline. *Bioinformatics, 23*(2) e237–44.

Rebholz-Schuhmann, D., Marcel, S., Albert, S., Tolle, R., Casari, G., & Kirsch, H. (2004). Automatic extraction of mutations from Medline and cross-validation with OMIM. *Nucleic Acids Res, 32*(1), 135-142.

Rebholz-Schumann, D., Kirsh, H., & Couto, F. (2005). Facts from texts — is text mining ready to deliver? *PLoS Biology,* 3(2), e65. doi: 10.1371/journal.pbio.0030065

Rechtsteiner, A., & Rocha, L. M. (2004). MeSH key terms for validation and annotation of gene expression clusters. In A. Gramada & E. Bourne (Eds), *Currents in Computational Molecular Biology. Proceedings of the Eight Annual International Conference on Research in Computational Molecular Biology (RECOMB 2004).* (pp 212-213).

Regev, Y., Finkelstein-Landau, M., & Feldman, R. (2003). Rule-based extraction of experimental evidence in the biomedical domain – the KDD cup 2002 (task 1). *SIGKDD explorations*, 4(2), 90-91.

Reiter, N. (2007). *Towards a Linking of FrameNet and SUMO.* Diploma thesis, Saarland University, Saarbrücken, Germany.

Reiter, N., & Buitelaar, P. (2008). Lexical Enrichment of a Human Anatomy Ontology using WordNet. In A. Tanács, D. Csendes, V. Vincze, C. Fellbaum, & P. Vossen, (Eds.), *Proceedings of the 4th Global WordNet Conference* (pp. 375-387). Szeged, Hungary.

Resnik, P., & Yarowsky, D. (2000). Distinguishing systems and distinguishing senses: New evaluation tools for words sense disambiguation. *Natural Lang. Eng., 5*(3), 113–133.

Richardson, W. S., Wilson, M. C., Nishikawa, J., & Hayward, R. S. (1995). The well-built clinical question: a key to evidence-based decisions. *ACP Journal Club, 123*(3), 12–13.

Riloff, E. (1999). Information extraction as a stepping stone toward story understanding. In A. Ram & K. Moorman (Eds.), *Computational Models of Reading and Understanding.* Cambridge, MA, USA: The MIT Press.

Ritchie, A., Robertson, S., & Teufel, S. (2007). Creating a test collection: Relevance judgements of cited and non-cited papers. Paper presented at *RIAO*, Pittsburgh, Pennsylvania, USA.

Roberts, A. (2005). Learning meronyms from biomedical text. In C. Callison-Burch & S. Wan (Eds). *Proceedings of the Student Research Workshop of ACL*, (pp. 49-54). Ann Arbor, Michigan.

Roberts, P. M. (2006). Mining literature for systems biology. *Briefings in Bioinformatics*, 7(4), 399-406.

Robertson, S. E., Walker, S., & Hancock-Beaulieu, M. (1998). Okapi at TREC-7: Automatic Ad Hoc, Filtering, VLC and Interactive. In *Proceedings of the 7th Text Retrieval Conference, TREC-7,* Gaithersburg, United-States of America.

Rocchio, J. (1971). Relevance Feedback in Information Retrieval. *The SMART Retrieval System: Experiments in Automatic Document Processing*, Prentice Hall.

Rocha, R. A., & Huff, S. M. (1994). Using diagrams to map controlled medical vocabularies. *Proc Annu Symp Comput Appl Med Care*, (pp. 172–6).

Rocha, R. A., Rocha, B. H. S. C., & Huff, S. M. (1993). Automated translation between medical vocabularies using a frame-based interlingua. *Proc Annu Symp Comput Appl Med Care*, (pp. 690–4).

Rosario, B., & Hearst, M. A. (2004). Classifying semantic relations in bioscience texts. In *Proceedings of 42nd Annual Meeting of the Association for Computational Linguistics* (pp. 431–438). Stroudsburg, PA, USA: Association for Computational Linguistics.

Rosario, B., Hearst, M. A., & Fillmore, C. (2002). The descent of hierarchy, and selection in relational semantics. *Proceedings of the ACL-02.* Pennsylvania USA.

Rosenbloom, S. T., Kiepek, W., Belletti, J., et al. (2004). Generating complex clinical documents using structured entry and reporting. *Medinfo, 11*, 683–687.

Rosse C., & Mejino J. L. V. Jr (2003). A reference ontology for biomedical informatics: the foundational model of anatomy. *Journal of Biomedical Informatics, 36*(6), 478–500.

Rowley-Jolivet, Elizabeth (2007). "A Genre Study of *If* in Medical Discourse" In K. Fløttum (Ed.) *Language and discipline perspectives on academic discourse* (pp. 176-201). Cambridge: Cambridge Scholars.

Ruch, P. (2002). Using contextual spelling correction to improve retrieval effectiveness in degraded text collections. In *Procedings of the 19th international Conference on Computational Linguistics (COLING) - Volume 1* (Taipei, Taiwan, August 24 - September 01, 2002).

Ruch, P. (2004). Query Translation by Text Categorization. *COLING 2004.*

Ruch, P. (2006). Automatic assignment of biomedical categories: toward a generic approach. *Bioinformatics, 22,* 6(Mar. 2006), 658-664.

Ruch, P., Baud, R., Geissbuhler, A., &. Rassinoux, A. M. (2001). Comparing general and medical texts for information retrieval based on natural language processing: an inquiry into lexical disambiguation. In *Proceedings of Medinfo Symposium*, (pp. 261—265).

Ruch, P., Jimeno, A., Gobeill, J., Tbarhriti, I., & Ehrler, F. (2006). Report on the TREC 2006 Experiment: Genomics Track. *TREC 2006.*

Rui, Y., & Huang, T. S. (2000) Optimizing Learning in Image Retrieval. *Proceedings of the IEEE International Conference on Computer Vision and Pattern Recognition*, Jun. 2000.

Rui, Y., Huang, T. S., Ortega, M., & Mehrotra, S. (1998). Relevance Feedback: A Power Tool for Interactive Content-Based Image Retrieval. *IEEE Transactions on Circuits. Systems for Video Technology, 8*(5), 644-655.

Ryan, A., Patrick, J., & Herkes, R. (2008). Introduction of Enhancement Technologies into the Intensive Care Service, Royal Prince Alfred Hospital, Sydney. *Health Information Management Journal, 37*(1), 39-44.

Rzhetsky, A., Iossifov, I., Koike, T., Krauthammer, M., Kra, P., Morris, M., *et al.* (2004). Geneways: A system for extracting, analyzing, visualizing and integrating molecular pathway data. *Journal of Biomedical Informatics* (37), 43-53.

Sackett, D. L., & Straus, S. E. (1998). Finding and applying evidence during clinical rounds: the "evidence cart". *Journal of the American Medical Association, 280*(15), 1336–1338.

Sackett, D. L., Straus, S. E., Richardson, W. S., Rosenberg, W., & Haynes, R. B. (2000). *Evidence-based medicine: How to practice and teach EBM.* Edinburgh: Harcourt Publishers Limited.

Safar, B., Kefi, H., & Reynaud, C. (2004). OntoRefiner, a user query refinement interface usable for Semantic Web Portals. *In Applications of Semantic Web technologies to web communities, Workshop ECAI.*

Sager, N., Lyman, M., Nhan, N. T., et al. (1994). Automatic encoding into SNOMED III: A preliminary investigation. *Proc Annu Symp Comput Appl Med Care*, (pp. 230–4).

Saint-Dizier, P., Delpech, E., Kawtrakul, A., Suktarachan, M., & Varasai, P. (2007). Annotating the Facets of Procedural Texts. *In proceeding of the 7th International Symposium on Natural Language Processing (SNLP),* Pattaya, Chonburi, Thailand, December 13-15, 2007. (p. 143).

Salager-Meyer, F. (1994). Hedges and textual communicative function in medical English written discourse. *English for Specific Purposes, 13*(2), 149-170.

Salton, G. (1989). *Automatic text processing: the transformation, analysis, and retrieval of information by computer.* Reading, MA, USA: Addison Wesley.

Salton, G., & Buckley, C. (1987). *Term Weighting Approaches in Automatic Text Retrieval.* Technical Report, Cornell University. Ithaca, NY, USA.

Salton, G., & McGill, M. J. (1982). *Introduction to Modern Information Retrieval.* New York: McGraw-Hill Book Company.

Salton, G., Wong, A., & Yang, C. S. (1975). A vector space model for automatic indexing. *Communications of the ACM, 18*(11), 613–620.

Savova, G., Harris, M. R., Johnson, T., Pakhomov, S.V., &. Chute, C. G. (2003). A data-driven approach for extracting "the most specific term" for ontology development. In *Proceedings of the AMIA Symposium,* (pp. 579—583).

Schiffrin, D., Tannen, D., & Hamilton, H. (Eds.). (2003). *The handbook of discourse analysis* (2nd ed.). Oxford: Blackwell.

Schilder, Frank (2002). Robust discourse parsing via discourse markers, topicality and position *Natural Language Engineering 8*(2/3), 235-255.

Schmid, H. (1994). Probabilistic Part-of-Speech Tagging Using Decision Trees. *In Proceedings of the International Conference on New Methods in Language Processing.* Manchester, United Kingdom.

Schuemie, M. J., Kors, J. A., & Mons, B. (2005). Word sense disambiguation in the biomedical domain: An overview. *J Comput Biol., 12*, 554-565.

Schuemie, M. J., Kors, J. A., & Mons, B. (2005). Word Sense Disambiguation in the Biomedical Domain: An Overview. *Journal of Computational Biology, 12*(5), 554-565.

Schuemie, M. J., Weeber, M., Schjivenaars, B. J. A., van Mulligen, E. M., van der Eijk, C. C., Jelier, R., et al. (2004). Distribution of information in biomedical abstracts and full-text publications. *Bioinformatics, 20*(16), 2597-2604.

Schulz, S., Markó, K., Sbrissia, E., Nohama, P., & Hahn, U. (2004). Cognate Mapping - A Heuristic Strategy for the Semi-Supervised Acquisition of a Spanish Lexicon from a Portuguese Seed Lexicon. In *Proceedings of the 20th International Conference on Computational Linguistics, COLING'04*, (pp. 813–819), Geneva, Switzerland.

Schwartz, A. S., & Hearst, M. A. (2003). A simple algorithm for identifying abbreviation definitions in biomedical text. In *Proceedings of the 8th Pacific Symposium on Biocomputing* (pp. 451–462).3rd–7th January, Hawaii.

Schwartz, A., & Hearst, M. (2003). A simple algorithm for identifying abbreviation definitions in biomedical texts. *Proceedings of the Pacific Symposium on Biocomputing (PSB).* Hawaii, USA.

Sebastiani, F. (2002) Machine learning in automated text categorization. *ACM Computing Surveys, 34*(1), 1-47.

Sebastiani, F. (2002). Machine learning in automated text categorization. *ACM Comput. Surv., 34*(1), 1–47.

Segaran T. *(2007). Programming Collective Intelligence Building Smart Web 2.0 Applications.* O'Reilly Media, ISBN, 0-59652932-5, 2007, (p. 360).

Sehgal, A. K., & Srinivasan, P. (2006). Retrieval with Gene Queries. *BMC Bioinformatics* (Research Paper), 7, 220.

Sekimizu, T., Park, H. S., & Tsujii, T. (1998). Identifying the interaction between genes and gene products based on frequently seen verbs in Medline abstracts. *Genome Inform Ser Workshop Genome Inform., 9*, 62-71 11072322.

Sekine, S. (1997). *Apple Pie Parser.* http://nlp.cs.nyu.edu/app/.

Settles, B. (2004). Biomedical named entity recognition using conditional random fields and rich feature sets. In *Proceedings of the International Joint Workshop on Natural Language Processing in Biomedicine and its Applications (NLPBA)*, (pp. 104–107).

Settles, B. (2005). ABNER: an open source tool for automatically tagging genes, proteins, and other entity names in text. *Bioinformatics, 21*(14), 3191–3192.

Sha, F., & Pereira, F. (2003). Shallow parsing with conditional random fields. In *Proceedings of the Human Language Technology and North American Association for Computational Linguistics Conference (HLT-NAACL)*, 213–220. ACL Press.

Shah, P., Perez-Iratxeta, C., Bork, P., & Andrade, M. (2003). Information extraction from full text scientific articles: Where are the keywords? *BMC Bioinformatics, 4(20).* http://www.biomedcentral.com/1471-2105/4/20

Shah, P., Perez-Iratxeta, C., Bork, P., & Andrade, M. (2004). Information extraction from full text scientific articles: Where are the keywords? *BMC Bioinformatics*, *4*(20).

Shastry, B. S. (2007). SNPs in disease gene mapping, medicinal drug development and evolution. *J Hum Genet, 52*(11), 871-880.

Shatkay, H. (2005). Information retrieval from biomedical text. *Briefings in Bioinformatics*, Henry Stewart Publications.

Shatkay, H., & Craven, M. (2007). *Biomedical text mining.* Cambridge, Massachussets, USA: MIT Press.

Shatkay, H., & Feldman, R. (2003). Mining the biomedical literature in the genomic era: An overview. *Journal of Computational Biology, 10*(6), 821–855.

Shatkay, H., & Feldman, R. (2003). Mining the biomedical literature in the genomic era: an overview. *J Comput Biol, 10*(6), 821-855.

Shatkay, H., & Feldman, R. (2003). Mining the biomedical literature in the genomic era: an overview. *Journal of Computational Biology 10*(6), 821-855.

Shatkay, H., & Feldman, R. (2003). Mining the biomedical literature in the genomic era: an overview. *J Comput Biol., 10*(6), 821-55.

Sherry, S. T., Ward, M., & Sirotkin, K. (1999). dbSNP-database for single nucleotide polymorphisms and other classes of minor genetic variation. *Genome Res, 9*(8), 677-679.

Shin, K., Han, S-Y., & Gelbukh, A. (2004). Balancing manual and automatic indexing for retrieval of paper abstracts. *TSD 2004: Text, Speech and Dialogue. Lecture Notes in Computer Science.* (pp. 203-210) Brno.

Shneiderman, B. (2006a). Discovering business intelligence using treemap visualizations. *b-eye. HCIL-2007-20.* Retrieved February 29, from http://www.b-eye-network.com/view/2673.

Shneiderman, B. (2006b). Treemaps for space-constrained visualization of hierarchies. Retrieved March 10, 2008, from http://www.cs.umd.edu/hcil/treemap-history/.

Shohei, K., Hirohisa, S., & Hidenori, I. (2003). PARCAR: A Parallel Cost-based Abductive Reasoning System. *In proceeding of Transactions of Information Processing Society of Japan, 41*(3), 668-676.

Shultz, M. (2006). Mapping of medical acronyms and initialisms to Medical Subject Headings (MeSH) across selected systems. *Journal Med Libr Assoc., 94*(4), 410–414.

Shvaiko, P., & Euzenat, J. (2005). A survey of schema-based matching approaches. *Journal on data semantics, 4*(1), 146-171.

Simon, J., Dos Santos, M., Fielding, J., & Smith, B. (2006). Formal ontology for natural language processing and the integration of biomedical databases. *International Journal of Medical Information, 75*(3-4), 224-231.

Sinha, U., & Kangarloo, H. (2002). Principal Component Analysis for Content-based Image Retrieval. *Radio-Graphics, 22*(5), 1271-1289.

Sirmakessis, S. (2004). *Text Mining and Its Applications: Results of the Nemis Launch.* Springer.

Skelton, J. R. (1994). Analysis of the structure of original research papers: An aid to writing original papers for publication. *British Journal of General Practitioners* (44), 455-459.

Small, S., Strzalkowski, T., Liu, T., Ryan, S., Salkin, R., Shimizu, N., Kantor, P., Kelly, D., Rittman, R., Wacholder, N., & Yamrom, B. (2004). HITIQA: Scenario based question answering. In S. Harabagiu and F. Lacatusu (Eds.), *Human Language Technology Conference of the North American Chapter of the Association for Computational Linguistics, Workshop on Pragmatics of Question Answering* (pp. 52–59). Stroudsburg, PA, USA: Association for Computational Linguistics.

Smith, B. et al. (2007). The OBO Foundry: coordinated evolution of ontologies to support biomedical data integration. *Nature Biotechnology, 25*, 1251 – 1255.

Smith, B., & Grenon, P. (2004). The Cornucopia of Formal-Ontological Relations. *Dialectica,* 58(3), 279—296.

Smith, C. L., Goldsmith, C. A., & Eppig, J. T. (2005). The Mammalian Phenotype Ontology as a tool for annotating, analyzing and comparing phenotypic information. *Genome Biol, 6*(1), R7.

Soricut, R., & Brill, E. (2006). Question answering using the web: Beyond the factoid. *Information Retrieval—Special Issue on Web Information Retrieval, 9*, 191–206.

Soteriades, E. S., & Falagas, M. E. (2005). Comparison of amount of biomedical research originating from the European Union and the United States. *British Medical Journal, 331*, 192-194.

Soulet, A., Crémilleux, B. (2005). An Efficient Framework for Mining Flexible Constraints. In T.B. Ho, D. Cheung, and H. Liu (Eds.) *PAKDD 2005* (pp. 661–671), Springer LNCS 3518.

Spasic, I., Ananiadou, S., McNaught, J., & Kumar, A. (2005). Text mining and ontologies in biomedicine: making sense of raw text. *Brief Bioinform, 6*, 239-251.

Spyropoulos, C. D., & Karkaletsis, V. (2005). Information extraction and summarization from medical documents. *Artificial Intelligence in Medicine* (33), 107-110.

Srinivasan, P. (2001). MeSHmap: a text mining tool for MEDLINE. *Proceedings of AMIA Sym*, (pp. 642-646).

Stapley, B. J. et al. (2002). Predicting the sub-cellular location of proteins from text using support vectors machines. *Pacific Symposium on Biocomputing, 7*, 734-385.

Stapley, B. J., & Benoit, G. (2000). Bio-bibliometrics: information retrieval and visualization from co-occurrences of gene names in Medline abstracts. *Pac Symp Biocomput*, (pp. 529-540).

Stapley, B. J., & Benoit, G. (2000). Biobibliometrics: information retrieval and visualization from co-occurrence of gene names in Medline abstracts. *Pacific Symposium on Biocomputing, 5*, 529-540.

Stephens, M., Palakal, M., Mukhopadhyay, S., Raje, R., & Mostafa, J. (2001). Detecting gene relations from Medline abstracts. *Pac Symp Biocomput*, (pp. 483-495).

Stevens, R., Goble, C. A., & Bechhofer, S. (2000). Ontology-based knowledge representation for bioinformatics. *Brief Bioinformatics 2000, 1*, 398-414.

Stoyanov, V., Cardie, C., & Wiebe, J. (2005). Multi-perspective question answering using the OpQA Corpus. In *Proceedings of Human Language Technology Conference/Conference on Empirical Methods in Natural Language Processing* (pp. 923–930). Stroudsburg, PA, USA: Association for Computational Linguistics.

Straus, S. E., & Sackett, D. L. (1999). Bring evidence to the point of care. *Journal of the American Medical Association, 281*, 1171–1172.

Struble, C. A., & Dharmanolla, C. (2004). Clustering MeSH representations of biomedical literature. *ACL Workshop: Linking Biological Literature, Ontologies, and Databases, BioLINK*. (pp. 41-48). Boston USA.

Strutt, H., & Strutt, D. (1999). Polarity determination in the Drosophila eye. *Curr Opin Genet Dev, 9*, 442-446.

Stubbs, M. (1993). British Traditions in Text Analysis: From Firth to Sinclair. In M. Baker, G. Francis, & E. Tognini-Bonelli (Eds.), *Text and Technology: In honour of John Sinclair* (pp. 1-33). Amserdam: John Benjamins Publishing Company.

Sun, J. Y., & Sun, Y. (2006). A system for automated lexical mapping. *Am Med Inform Assoc, 13*(3), 334-343.

Sun, Y. (2004). Methods for automated concept mapping between medical databases. *J Biomed Inform, 37*(3), 162-178.

Sutton, C., & McCallum, A. (2006). An introduction to conditional random fields for relational learning. In L. Getoor & B. Taskar (Eds.), *Introduction to Statistical Relational Learning*. MIT Press.

Swales, J. (1990). *Genre analysis: English in academic and research settings*. Cambridge: Cambridge University Press.

Swanson, D., & Smalheiser, N. (1994). Assessing a gap in the biomedical literature: magnesium deficiency and neurologic disease. *Neuro-science Research Communications, 15*, 1-9.

Syswerda, G. (1989). Uniform crossover in Genetic Algorithms. In J. D. Schaffer (Ed.), *The Third International Conference on Genetic Algorithms* (pp. 2-9). San Mateo, California, USA: Morgan Kaufmann.

Tablan, V., Bontcheva, K., Maynard, D., & Cunningham, H. (2003). OLLIE: On-Line Learning for Information Extraction. *HLT-NAACL 2003 Workshop: Software Engineering and Architecture of Language Technology Systems (SEALTS)*. Edmonton, Canada.

Taira, R. K., & Soderland, S. G. (1999). A statistical natural language processor for medical reports. *Proc AMIA Symp.*, (pp. 970–4).

Taira, R. K., Soderland, S. G., & Jakobovits, R. M. (2001). Automatic structuring of radiology free-text reports. *RadioGraphics, 21*, 237–245.

Taira, R. K., Soderland, S. G., & Jakobovits, R. M. (2001). Automatic structuring of radiology free-text reports. *Radiographics, 21*, 237–45.

Tamames, J. & Valencia, A. (2006). The success (or not) of HUGO nomenclature. *Genome Biology, 7*(5), 402.

Tari, L., Gonzalez, G., Leaman, R., Nikkila, S., Wendt, R., & Baral, C. (2007). ASU at TREC 2006 genomics track. In *Proceedings of the Text Retrieval Conference (TREC)*.

Taskar, B., Lacoste-Julien, S., & Klein, D. (2005). A discriminative matching approach to word alignment. In J. Chai (Ed.), *Human Language Technology Conference and Conference on Empirical Methods in Natural Language Processing* (pp. 73–80). Vancouver, USA: Association for Computational Linguistics.

Teufel, S. (1999). *Argumentative zoning*. Doctoral dissertation, University of Edinburgh Edinburgh. Retrieved June 2008 from http://www.cl.cam.ac.uk/~sht25/az.html

Teufel, S., & Moens, M. (2002). Summarizing scientific articles: Experiments with relevance and rhetorical status. *Computational Linguistics, 28*(4), 409-445.

Thamvijit, D., Chanlekha, H., Sirigayon, C., Permpool, P., & Kawtrakul, A. (2005). Person Information Extraction from the Web. *In proceeding of the 6th Symposium on Natural Language Processing 2005 (SNLP 2005)*, Chiang Rai, Thailand, Dec 13-15, 2005.

Thomas, B. J., Ouellette, H., Halpern, E. F., & Rosenthal, D. I. (2005). Automated Computer-Assisted Categorization of Radiology Reports. *Am. J. Roentgenol., 184*(2), 687-690.

Tiedemann, J. (2004). Word to word alignment strategies. In *Proceedings of the 20th International Conference on Computational Linguistics, COLING 04*, (pp. 212–218), Geneva, Switzerland.

Tolentino, H. D., Matters, M. D., Walop, W., Law, & Tong, W. (2007). *BMC Medical Informatics and Decision Making.*

Tran, T. D., Garcelon, N., Burgun, A., & Le Beux, P. (2004). Experiments in cross-language medical information retrieval using a mixing translation module. In *Proceeding of the World Congress on Health and Medical Informatics MEDINFO*, San Francisco, CA, United-States of America.

TREC. (2001). *Text REtrieval Conference*. http://trec.nist.gov/.

Tsuji, K., Daille, B., & Kageura, K. (2002). Extracting French-Japanese word pairs from bilingual corpora based on transliteration rules. In *Proceedings of the Third International Conference on Language Resources and Evaluation LREC'02*, (pp. 499–502), Las Palmas de Gran Canaria, Spain.

Tsujii, J., & Ananiadou, S. (2005). Thesaurus or logical ontology, which one do we need for text mining? *Language Resources and Evaluation, Springer Sci-*

ence and Business Media B.V. 39(1), 77-90. Springer Netherlands.

Tsuruoka, Y., & Tsujii, J. (2003). Probabilistic term variant generator for biomedical terms, *Proceedings of the 26th annual international ACM SIGIR conference on Research and development in informaion retrieval.* Toronto, Canada.

Tsuruoka, Y., & Tsujii, J. (2004). Improving the performance of dictionary-based approaches in protein name recognition. *Journal of Biomedical Informatics, 37,* 461-470.

Tsuruoka, Y., Tateishi, Y., Kim, J. D., Ohta, T., McNaught, J., Ananiadou, S., & Tsujii, J. (2005). Developing a robust part-of-speech tagger for biomedical text. *Advances in Informatics - 10th Panhellenic Conference on Informatics* (pp. 382-92).

Tsuruoka, Y., Tsujii, J., & Ananiadou, S. (2008). FACTA: A text search engine for finding biomedical concepts. *Bioinformatics 2008*; doi: 10.1093/bioinformatics/btn46.

Turney, P. (2002). Thumbs up or thumbs down? Semantic orientation applied to unsupervised classification of reviews. In *Proceedings of the 40th Annual Meeting of the Association for Computational Linguistics* (pp. 417–424). Stroudsburg, PA, USA: Association for Computational Linguistics.

Tuttle, M., Sherertz, D., Olson, N., Erlbaum, M., Sperzel, D., Fuller, L., & Neslon, S. (1990). Using Meta-1 – the 1st version of the UMLS metathesaurus. In *Proceedings of the 14th annual Symposium on Computer Applications in Medical Care (SCAMC)*, Washington, D.C.

UMLS (2006). The Unified Medical Language System®. Accessed March 1st, 2008, from http://0-www.nlm.nih.gov.catalog.llu.edu/pubs/factsheets/umls.html.

Valin, V., & Robert, D. (1993). A synosis of role and reference grammar. In Robert, D., & Valin, V. (Ed.), *Advances in Role and Reference Grammar* (pp. 1–166). Amsterdam: John Benjamins Publishing Company.

van Rijsbergen, C. J. (1979). *Information Retireval.* Butterworths, London, UK: Butterworths.

Vapnik, V. (1995). *The Nature of Statistical Learning Theory.* Heidelberg, DE: Springer.

Vapnik, V. (1998). *Statistical Learning Theory.* New York, USA: Wiley.

Vapnik, V. N. (1995). *The nature of statistical learning theory.* Springer.

Véronis, J. (1999). *A study of polysemy judgements and inter-annotator agreement.* Paper presented at the Advanced Papers of the SENSEVAL Workshop Sussex, UK.

Véronis, J., (Ed.) (2000). *Parallel Text Processing.* Kluwer Academic Publishers, Dordrecht.

Verspoor, K., Cohn, J., Joslyn, C., Mniszewski, S., Rechtsteiner, A., Rocha, L. M., & Simas, T. (2005). Protein Annotation as Term Categorization in the Gene Ontology using Word Proximity Networks. *BMC Bioinformatics, 6*(Suppl 1), S20.

Vintar, S., Buitelaar, P., & Volk, M. (2003). Semantic relations in concept-based cross-language medical information retrieval. *Proceedings of the Workshop on Adaptive Text Extraction and Mining.* Cavtat-Dubrovnik, Croatia.

Vold, E. T. (2006). Epistemic modality markers in research articles. A cross-linguistic and cross-disciplinary study. *International Journal of Applied Linguistics, 16*(1), 61-87.

Voorhees, E. (1994). Query expansion using lexical-semantic relations. *In Proceedings of the 17th annual international ACM SIGIR conference on Research and development in information retrieval,* (pp. 61-69). Springer-Verlag New York, Inc.

Voorhees, E. (1994). Query expansion using lexical-semantic relations. *In Proceedings of the 17th annual international ACM SIGIR conference,* (pp. 61-69).

Wagner, R. A., & Fischer, M. J. (1974). The string-to-string correction problem. *Journal of the Association for Computing Machinery, 21*(1), 168–173.

Wattarujeekrit, T., Shah, P., & Collier, N. (2004). PASBio: predicate-argument structures for event extraction in molecular biology. In *http://www.biomedcentral.com/bmcbioinformatics/, 5*, 155.

Webber, B. (1988). Tense as discourse anaphor. *Computational Linguistics, 14*(2), 61-72.

Weeber, M., Mork, J. G., & Aronson, A. R. (2001). Developing a Test Collection for Biomedical Word Sense Disambiguation. *Proc AMIA.*

Weeber, M., Mork, J., & Aronson, A. (2001). Developing a Test Collection for Biomedical Word Sense Disambiguation. *Proc. AMIA Symp.*, (pp. 746-750).

Weeber, M., Vos, R., Klein, H., De Jong-Van Den Berg, L. T., Aronson, A. R., & Molema, G. (2003). Generating hypotheses by discovering implicit associations in the literature: A case report of a search for new potential therapeutic uses for thalidomide. *J Am Med Inform Assoc, 10,* 252-259.

Wentland, W., Knopp, J., Silberer, C., & Hartung, M. (to appear in 2008). Building a Multilingual Lexical Resource for Named Entity Disambiguation, Translation and Transliteration. *In Proceedings of the 6th Language Resources and Evaluation Conference.* Marrakech, Morocco.

Wheeler, D., Church, D., Federhen, S., Lash, A., Madden, T., Pontius, J., Schuler, G., Schriml, L., Sequeira, E., Tatusova, T., & Wagner, L. (2003). Database resources of the national center for biotechnology. *Nucleic Acids Research, 31*(1), 28–33.

Whitelaw, C., Garg, N., & Argamon, S. (2005). Using appraisal groups for sentiment analysis. In *Proceedings of the 14th ACM International Conference on Information and Knowledge management* (pp. 625–631). New York, NY, USA: Association for Computing Machinery Press.

Widdows, D., Peters, S., Cederberg, S., Chan, C. K., Steffen, D., & Buitelaar, P. (2003). Unsupervised monolingual and bilingual word-sense disambiguation of medical documents using UMLS. *Proc. ACL Workshop NLP in Biomed*, 9-16.

Wilbur, J., Rzhetsky, A., & Shatkay, H. (2006). New directions in biomedical text annotation: Definitions, guidelines and corpus construction. *BMC Bioinformatics, 7(356).* doi:10.1186/1471-2105-7-356

William, H., & Greenes, R. (1990). SAPHIRE-an information retrieval system featuring concept matching, automatic indexing, probabilistic retrieval, and hierarchical relationships. *Comput. Biomed. Res, 0010-4809, 23*(5), 410-425. I Academic Press Professional, Inc

Witten, I. H., & Frank, E. (2000). *Data Mining.* Morgan Kaufmann.

Wray, A. (2002). *Formulaic language and the lexicon.* Cambridge: Cambridge University Press.

Wren, J. D. (2005). Open access and openly accessible: A study of scientific publications shared via the internet. *BMJ.* doi 10.1136/bmj.38422.611736.E0

Wren, J. D., & Garner, H. R. (2004). Shared relationships analysis: ranking set cohesion and commonalities within a literature-derived relationships network. *Bioinformatics, 20,* 191-198.

Wright, L., Grossetta, H., Aronson, A., & Rindflesch, T. (1998). Hierarchical concept indexing of full-text documents in the UMLS information sources map. *Journal of the American Society for Information Science, 50*(6), 514-23.

Wu, C. H., Apweiler, R., Bairoch, A., Natale, D. A., Barker, W. C., Boeckmann, B., Ferro, S., Gasteiger, E., Huang, H., Lopez, R. et al. (2006). The Universal Protein Resource (UniProt): an expanding universe of protein information. *Nucleic Acids Res, 34*(Database issue), D187-191.

Xu, H., Markatou, M., Dimova, R., Liu, H., & Friedman, C. (2008). Machine learning and word sense disambiguation in the biomedical domain: design and evaluation issues. *BMC Bioinformatics*, *7*(1), 334.

Xu, J., & Croft, W. (1996). Query expansion using local and global document analysis. *In Proceedings of the Nineteenth Annual International ACM SIGIR Confer-*

ence on Research and Development in Information Retrieval, (pp. 4-11).

Yamamoto, Y., & Takagi, T. A. (2005). Sentence classification system for multi biomedical literature summarization. *Proceedings of the 21st International Conference on Data Engineering.*

Yandell, M. D., & Majoros, W.H. (2002). Genomics and natural language processing. *Nature Reviews Genetics, 3*, 601-610. doi:10.1038/nrg861.

Yang, Z., Lin, H., Li, Y., Liu, B., & Lu, Y. (2006). TREC 2005 genomics track experiments at DUTAI. In *Proceedings of the Text Retrieval Conference (TREC).*

Yangarber R., Jokipii L. (2005). Redundancy-based Correction of Automatically Extracted Facts. In *Human Language Technology Conference/ Conference on Empirical Methods in Natural Language Processing HLT/EMNLP-2005* (pp. 57-64) .Morriston, N.J.: Association for Computational Linguistics. doi: http://dx.doi.org/10.3115/1220575.1220583

Yangarber, R., Jokipii, L., Rauramo, A., & Huttunen, S. (2005). Information Extraction from Epidemiological Reports. *In Proceedings of HLT/EMNLP-2005.* Canada.

Yeh, A., Hirschman, L., & Morgan, A. (2003). Evaluation of text data mining for database curation: Lessons learned from the KDD challenge cup. *Bioinformatics, 19*(1), i331–i339.

Yeh, A., Morgan, A., Colosimo, M., & Hirschman, L. (2005). BioCreative task 1a: Gene mention finding evaluation. *BMC Bioinformatics, 6*(Suppl. 1), S2.

Yeh, A., Morgan, A., Colosimo, M., & Hirschman, L. (2005). BioCreAtIvE task 1A: gene mention finding evaluation. *BMC Bioinformatics, 6*(Suppl 1), S2.

Yu, A. C. (2006). Methods in biomedical ontology. *Journal of Biomedical Informatics, 39*, 252-266.

Yu, H., & Hatzivassiloglou, V. (2003). Towards answering opinion questions: separating facts from opinions and identifying the polarity of opinion sentences. In *Proceedings of the 2003 Conference on Empirical Methods in Natural Language Processing* (pp. 129–136). Stroudsburg, PA, USA: Association for Computational Linguistics.

Yu, H., Hripcsak, G., & Friedman, C. (2002). Mapping abbreviations to full forms in biomedical articles. *J Am Med Inform Assoc 2002*; *9*(3), 262-272.

Yu, L., Ahmed, S., Gonzalez, G., Logsdon, B., Nakamura, M., Nikkila, S., Shah, K., Tari, L., Wendt, R., Ziegler, A., & Baral, C. (2006). Genomic information retrieval through selective extraction and tagging by the ASU-BoiAI group. In *Proceedings of the Text Retrieval Conference (TREC).*

Yuan, X., Hu, Z. Z., Wu, H. T., Torii, M., Narayanaswamy, M., Ravikumar, K. E., Vijay-Shanker, K., & Wu, C. H. (2006). An online literature mining tool for protein phosphorylation. *Bioinformatics, 22*(13), 1668-9.

Zavrel, J., Berck, P., & Lavrijssen, W. (2000).Information extraction by text classification: Corpus mining for features. *In proceedings of the workshop Information Extraction Meets Corpus Linguistics.* Athens, Greece.

Zerida, N., Lucas, N., & Crémilleux, B. (2006). Combining linguistic and structural descriptors for mining biomedical literature. In *ACM Symposium on Document Engineering* (pp. 62-64). New York: ACM. doi: doi.acm.org/10.1145/1284420.1284469

Zerida, N., Lucas, N., & Crémilleux, B. (2007). Exclusion-inclusion based text categorization of biomedical articles. In *ACM Symposium on Document engineering* (pp. 202-204). New York: ACM. doi: http://doi.acm.org/10.1145/1284420.1284469

Zesch, T., Gurevych, I., & Mühlhäuser, M. (2007). Analyzing and Accessing Wikipedia as a Lexical Semantic Resource. In G. Rehm, A. Witt, & L. Lemnitzer (Eds.), *Data Structures for Linguistic Resources and Applications* (pp. 197-205), Tübingen, Germany.

Zhou, G., & Su, J. (2004). Exploring deep knowledge resources in biomedical name recognition. In *Proceedings of the International Joint Workshop on Natural Language Processing in Biomedicine and its Applications (NLPBA)*, (pp. 96-99).

Zhou, G., Zhang, J., Su, J., Shen, D., & Tan, C. (2004). Recognizing names in biomedical texts: a machine learning approach. *Bioinformatics, 20*, 1178-90.

Zhou, G., Zhang, J., Su, J., Shen, D., & Tan, C. L. (2004). Recognizing names in biomedical texts: A machine learning approach. *Bioinformatics, 20*(7), 1178-1190.

Zhou, X . S., & Huang, T. S. (2001). Small Sample Learning during Multimedia Retrieval using BiasMap. *Proceedings of the IEEE Conference on Computer Vision and Pattern Recognition,* Hawaii, December 2001.

Zhou, X., Han, H., Chankai, I., Prestrud, A., & Brooks, A. (2006). Approaches to text mining for clinical medical records. In *Proc ACM Sympos Applied Computing* (SAC 2006), (pp. 235–239). April 2006. NY: ACM Press.

Zhu, X., Ghahramani, Z., & Lafferty, J. (2003). Semi-supervised learning using Gaussian fields and harmonic functions. In T. Fawcett & N. Mishra, (Eds.) *The 20th International Conference on Machine Learning* (pp. 912–919). Menlo Park, CA, USA: AAAI Press.

Zipf, G. K. (1939). *The Psycho-biology of Language*. Boston: Houghton Mifflin.

Zou, Q., Chu, W. W., Morioka, C., et al. (2003). IndexFinder: a method of extracting key concepts from clinical texts for indexing. *Proc AMIA Symp.,* (pp. 763–7).

Zou, Q., Chu, W. W., Morioka, C., Leazer, G. H., & Kangarloo, H. (2003). Indexfinder: A method of extracting key concepts from clinical texts for indexing. *AMIA Annu Symp Proc.,* (pp. 763-7).

Zou, Q., Chu, W. W., Morioka, C., Leazer, G. H., & Kangarloo, H. (2003). IndexFinder: A Method of Extracting Key Concepts from Clinical Texts for Indexing. *AMIA Annual Symposium Proceeding,* (pp. 763-767).

About the Contributors

Violaine Prince is full professor at the University Montpellier 2 (Montpellier, France). She obtained her PhD in 1986 at the University of Paris VII, and her 'habilitation' (post-PhD degree) at the University of Paris XI (Orsay). Previous head of Computer Science department at the Faculty of Sciences in Montpellier, previous head of the National University Council for Computer Science (grouping 3,000 professors and assistant professors in Computer Science in France), she now leads the NLP research team at LIRMM (Laboratoire d'Informatique, de Robotique et de Microélectronique de Montpellier, a CNRS research unit). Her research interests are in natural language processing (NLP) and cognitive science. She has published more than 70 reviewed papers in books, journals and conferences, authored 10 research and education books, founded and chaired several conferences and belonged to program committees as well as journals reading committees. She is member of the board of the IEEE Computer Society French Chapter.

Mathieu Roche is assistant professor at the University Montpellier 2, France. He received a PhD in computer science at the University Paris XI (Orsay) in 2004. With Jérôme Azé, he created in 2005 the DEFT challenge ('DEfi Francophone de Fouille de Textes' meaning 'Text Mining Challenge') which is a francophone equivalent of the TREC Conferences. His current main research interests at LIRMM (Laboratoire d'Informatique, de Robotique et de Microélectronique de Montpellier, a CNRS research unit) are text mining, information retrieval, terminology, and natural language processing for schema mapping.

* * *

Sophia Ananiadou is director of The National Centre for Text Mining (NaCTeM)providing text mining services with particular focus on biomedicine. She is also reader in text mining in the School of Computer Science University of Manchester. She has authored over 150 publications in journals and conferences including the first edited book on text mining for biomedicine. She has received twice the IBM UIMA innovation award for her work on interoperability of text mining tools and the DAIWA award for her research in biotext mining.

Frederic Andres has been an associate professor at National Institute of Informatics (NII) since 2000 and at The Graduate University for Advanced Studies since 2002. He received is his PhD from University of PARIS VI and his Doctor Habilitate (specialization: information engine) from University of Nantes, in 1993 and 2000 respectively. He was scientist at Bull (France) from 1989 to 1993, information system architect at Ifatec/Euriware (France) between 1996 and 2000. He is project leader of the Geomedia project and Myscoper project in the Digital Content and Media Sciences Research Division. Research interests include, but are not limited to, distributed semantic information management systems for Geomedia and multimedia applications. He has been serving at The World Organization for Digital Equality (WODE), as general secretary since January 2006. He is member of IEEE, ACM, and of many other societies.

Rolf Apweiler studied biology in Heidelberg and Bath. He worked three years in drug discovery in the pharmaceutical industry and is involved in bioinformatics since 1987. Apweiler started his bioinformatics career working on Swiss-Prot at EMBL in Heidelberg, moved in 1994 to the EMBL Outstation EBI in Hinxton, UK, and is now Joint Head of the Protein and Nucleotide Data (PANDA) Group at EBI (http://www.ebi.ac.uk/panda/). This group coordinates the UniProt activities, InterPro, GOA, Reactome, PRIDE, IntAct, Ensembl, EMBL nucleotide sequence database, and some other projects at the EBI.

Pooyan Asari graduated in software engineering from Tehran Azad University in 2005 and completed a Masters of Information Technology from Macquarie University in 2007. He is currently studying for a PhD at the University of Sydney in the field of natural language processing applied to clinical settings. Since 1999, he has been involved in the IT industry as a software engineer and system developer in different industrial and commercial projects in Iran and Australia. His professional experience includes working with MIS design and implementation, embedded system development and portable transaction solutions.

Evelyn Camon, PhD, studied cellular and molecular immunology at the Institute for Animal Health (Berkshire, UK) in collaboration with University College Dublin (UCD) (Ireland). In 1998 she joined the EBI as an EMBL-Bank Scientific Curator responsible for assessment and preparation of nucleotide sequence and alignment data for inclusion in EMBL-Bank and EMBL-align databases. In October 2000 she took on a more senior role as the EBIs first Gene Ontology Annotation Project Co-ordinator project, a post funded by the NIH. Essentially this role involved training a team of curators to extract biological knowledge from the scientific literature in a standardized way (using Gene Ontology) and ensuring this data was linked to the relevant UniProtKB proteins and regularly disseminated. Camon has also been involved in evaluating data submitted to text mining competitions (BioCreative) and in reviewing bioinformatic articles. Furthermore in collaboration with EBI, MGI and UCL she has been involved in a new proposal to improve the annotation and ontology content for immunology and the immune system (http://www.geneontology.org/GO.immunology.shtml). She is currently affiliated with UCD, School of Biological Sciences.

Vincent Claveau is a researcher for the French National Center for Scientific Research (CNRS). His research area includes natural language processing, machine learning and multimedia information retrieval. Vincent Claveau was first trained as an engineer. He obtained his PhD in computer science from University of Rennes 1, France, in 2003. During his doctoral thesis he developed methods of symbolic machine learning applied to lexical information extraction. After obtaining his PhD degree, he held a post-doctoral position in the Observatoire de linguistique Sens-Texte (OLST) research group of the University of Montreal, QC, Canada, where he worked in the linguistic and terminological fields.

Besides his research activities, Vincent Claveau also teaches graduate students natural language processing and machine learning.

Francisco M. Couto has a Master (2001) in informatics and computer engineering from the Instituto Superior Técnico. He obtained a PhD (2006) in Informatics, specialization Bioinformatics, from the Universidade de Lisboa. He is currently an assistant professor with the Informatics Department at Faculdade de Ciências da Universidade de Lisboa. He teaches courses in Information Systems and coordinates the Master in Biomedical Informatics. He is currently a member of the LASIGE research group, co-coordinating the Biomedical Informatics research line.

Manuel C. Díaz-Galiano is assistant professor in the Department of Computer Science at Jaén University (Spain). He received MS degree in computer science from the University of Granada. His current main research interest is intelligent search, including search engines, search assistants, natural language processing tools for text mining and retrieval and human computer interaction. Relevant topics include multilingual-multimodal information access, ontologies (wordnets, MeSH, UMLS), Web search engines. Mr. Díaz is member of the Research Group of Intelligent Systems of Information Access in the University of Jaén and member of SEPLN. He has participated in several research projects and several contracts with companies in technology transfer.

Emily Dimmer, PhD, studied plant genetics (University of Cambridge). In 2003, she joined the EBI as a scientific database curator. She is presently the coordinator of the GOA group at the EBI (http://www.ebi.ac.uk <http://www.ebi.ac.uk/>). GOA is a central member of the Gene Ontology Consortium, providing a comprehensive set of manual and electronic annotations to proteins in the UniProt KnowledgeBase for all species. GOA has a specific remit to providing high-quality manual annotation for the human proteome, recently securing grants to support focused, community-led GO annotation projects to annotate gene products implicated in heart and kidney development and disease.

Laura Dioşan currently works as PhD student in the Computer Science Department ofBabes-Bolyai University, Cluj-Napoca, Romania and in Laboratoire d'Informatique, de Traitement de l'Information et des Systèmes, Institut National des Sciences Appliquées, Rouen, France. Her main research area is in Evolutionary Computation. Laura Dioşan is authored/co-authored of several papers in peer reviewed international journals and proceedings of the international conferences. She proposed some evolutionary techniques for optimization of algorithm's architecture, a genetic programming technique for solving symbolic regression and classification problems, an evolutionary framework for evolving kernel functions for support vector machines. She is member of the IEEE (CS), IEEE (NN) and ACM.

Anastasios D. Doulamis received the Diploma degree in electrical and computer engineering from the National Technical University of Athens (NTUA) in 1995 with the highest honor. In 2000, he has received the PhD degree in electrical and computer engineering from the NTUA. From 1996-2000, he was with the Image, Video and Multimedia Lab of the NTUA as research assistant. In 2002, he join the NTUA as senior researcher. He is now assistant professor at the Technical University of Crete. His PhD thesis was supported by the Bodosakis Foundation Scholarship. Dr. Doulamis has received several awards and prizes during his studies, including the Best Greek Student in the field of engineering in national level in 1995, the Best Graduate Thesis Award in the area of electrical engineering with A.

Doulamis in 1996 and several prizes from the National Technical University of Athens, the National Scholarship Foundation and the Technical Chamber of Greece. In 1997, he was given the NTUA Medal as Best Young Engineer. In 2000, he received the best PhD thesis award by the Thomaidion Foundation in conjunction with N. Doulamis. He has also served as program committee in several international conferences and workshops, like EUSIPCO, ICPR. He is author of more than 100 papers in the above areas, in leading international journals and conferences.

Nikolaos D. Doulamis received a Diploma in Electrical and Computer Engineering from the National Technical University of Athens (NTUA) in 1995 with the highest honor and the PhD degree from the same department in 2000. His PhD thesis was supported by the Bodosakis Foundation. Since 2002, he is a senior researcher at NTUA and at the Research Academic Computer Technology Institute. Dr. Doulamis received the Best Greek Student award in the field of engineering at national level by the Technical chamber of Greece in 1995. He is a recipient of the Best Graduate Thesis Award in the area of electrical engineering, with A. Doulamis, and of NTUA‘s Best Young Engineer Medal. He has served as Chairman or member of the program committee of several international conferences. He is author of more than 30 journals papers in the field of video transmission, content-based image retrieval, and grid computing, and of more than 120 conference papers. Among them 14 journals papers have been published in the IEEE transactions.

Laura Inés Furlong received her PhD in biological sciences from the University of Buenos Aires, Argentina in 2002, and the MSc in bioinformatics for Health from the University Pompeu Fabra (UPF) and University of Barcelona, Spain in 2007. She is a post-doctoral researcher at the Research Unit on Biomedical Informatics (GRIB) of UPF and IMIM-Hospital del Mar, Spain, and assistant professor at the UPF. She has several publications in the field of molecular biology of human fertilization, and in biomedical text mining. Her current research focus is on the development of text mining applications for the study of genotype–phenotype relationships and the mechanisms of adverse drug reactions.

Jean-Gabriel Ganascia first studied mathematics and physics to be an engineer. Then he got his graduation in physics (Orsay University), a DEA in acoustics (Paris VI University). In parallel he studied philosophy and computer science. He obtained a grant to prepare a doctorate on knowledge-based system applied to geology. He got his "Doctorat d'ingénieur" in 1983. After that, he pursued his research on machine learning from both a theoretical view and a practical one until he obtained his "Thèse d'état" in 1987. Jean-Gabriel Ganascia was successively named assistant professor at Orsay University (Paris XI) (1982), "Maître de conférences" at Orsay University (1987), and professor at Paris VI University (1988). He was also program leader in the CNRS executive from November 1988 to April 1992 before moving to direct the Cognitive Science Coordinated Research Program and head the Cognition Sciences Scientific Interest Group since January 1993 until 2000. Jean-Gabriel Ganascia is presently first class professor of computer science at Paris VI University and ACASA team group leader in the LIP6 laboratory. His main scientific interests cover different areas of artificial intelligence: Knowledge acquisition, symbolic machine learning, data mining, data fusion, scientific discovery, cognitive modeling, digital humanities, and investigation of creativity.

Jörg Hakenberg received his Diploma in computer science from Ulm University, Germany. He started his Phd in 2003 at Humboldt-Universität zu Berlin in the Knowledge Management in Bioinformatics group. From 2006-2007, he worked for the Bioinformatics group at Technische UniversitŠt Dresden. He currently is a research associate with the BioAI lab at Arizona State University. Jšrg's main research interests are text mining in the life sciences and bioinformatics.

Graeme Hirst's present research includes the problem of near-synonymy in lexical choice in language generation; computer assistance for collaborative writing; and applications of lexical chaining as an indicator of semantic distance in texts. He was a member of the Waterloo-Toronto HealthDoc project, which aimed at building intelligent systems for the creation and customization of healthcare documents, and of the EpoCare project on answering clinical questions for physicians from clinical-evidence publications. Hirst is the author of two monographs: *Anaphora in Natural Language Understanding* (Springer-Verlag, 1981) and *Semantic Interpretation and the Resolution of Ambiguity* (Cambridge University Press, 1987). He was elected chair of the North American Chapter of the Association for Computational Linguistics for 2004-05 and treasurer of the Association for 2008-2012.

Zhang-Zhi Hu received his BS/MD in medicine from Wannan Medical College, China in 1984, and his MS in physiology from Beijing University Health Science Center in 1989. He received the National Institutes of Health (NIH) Intramural Research Training Award during 1993-1998 and received the NIH Fellows Award for Research Excellence in 1996. He continued his research at the NIH until 2001 and then joined the Protein Information Resource (PIR) at the Georgetown University, Washington DC. He is currently a research associate professor at the Department of Biochemistry and Molecular & Cellular Biology, Georgetown University. His primary research focuses on the understanding of biological pathways and networks from large-scale omics data. He is also interested in text mining tool development that supports the systems biology and ontology research. He is a member of ISCB, USHUPO and the Endocrine Society. He has over 45 journal publications and book chapters.

Antonio Jimeno-Yepes received a Master Degree in computer science (Universitat Jaume I, Castellon, Spain) and a Master Degree in intelligent systems (Universitat Jaume I). He worked at CERN (European Organization for Nuclear Research) on the LHC layout database and in several projects within the EDMS document management systems. In 2006 he joined the text mining group at the European Bioinformatics Institute. He is a PhD candidate at the Universitat Jaume I.

Christophe Jouis received his PhD degree in 1993. He worked at CR2A/IBM and CAMS (Centre d'Analyse et de Mathématiques Sociales, UMR CNRS, EHESS, Université Paris Sorbonne) in knowledge modeling and expertise transfert. Currently, his research interests focus on (1) contextual exploration, a new computational method to extract semantic values and information from texts in order to build ontologies and (2) the logic of relationships between concepts in thesauri and ontologies.

Asanee Kawtrakul received the Bachelor Degree (honor) and Master Degree in electrical engineering from Kasetsart University, Bangkok, Thailand, and Doctoral Degree in information engineering from Nagoya University, Japan. Currently, she is an associate professor of Computer Engineering Department at Kasetsart University and the Deputy Director of National Electronics and Computer Technology Center, the member of National Science and Technology Development Agency. Her research interests are in natural language processing, information engineering and knowledge engineering.

Harald Kirsch is a computer scientist by training. From 2000 to 2003 he developed commercial software for biomedical text mining before joining the the Rebholz Group (Text Mining) at the EMBL-EBI in 2003. EMBL-EBI is using his IT infrastructure based on Finite State Automata for information extraction. Since 2006, he is now developing information retrieval solutions as member of the Raytion GmbH, Duesseldorf.

Dimitrios Kokkinakis received his PhD in computational linguistics from the University of Gothenburg in December 2001. He is currently a postdoctoral fellow at the Department of Swedish Language, University of Gothenburg, Sweden. His research interests include computational lexical Semantics (particularly word-sense disambiguation, automatic lexical acquisition and relation extraction), Medical and clinical informatics, corpus linguistics (particularly standardization of resources and shallow syntactic/semantic analysis) and text mining (particularly information extraction, machine learning and visualization of linguistic and multidimensional data).

Dimosthenis Kyriazis received the diploma from the Dept. of Electrical and computer engineering of the National Technical University of Athens, Athens, Greece in 2001, the MS degree in techno-economic systems (MBA) co-organized by the Electrical and Computer Engineering Dept - NTUA, Economic Sciences Dept - National Kapodistrian University of Athens, Industrial Management Dept - University of Piraeus and his PhD from the Electrical and Computer Engineering Department of the National Technical University of Athens in 2007. He is currently a researcher in the Telecommunication Laboratory of the Institute of Communication and Computer Systems (ICCS). Before joining the ICCS he has worked in the private sector as Telecom Software Engineer. He has participated in numerous EU / National funded projects (such as IRMOS, NextGRID, Akogrimo, BEinGRID, HPC-Europa, GRIA, Memphis, CHALLENGERS, FIDIS, etc). His research interests include grid computing, scheduling, quality of service provision and workflow management in heterogeneous systems and service oriented architectures.

Vivian Lee works as curator in the Rebholz Group (Text Mining) at the EMBL-EBI. She received her PhD in genetics from the University of Nottingham in 2002. She then joined the EMBL-EBI as a scientific curator in the gene ontology annotation project and the protein-protein interaction database IntAct. Following this she took up a postdoc fellowship in cancer genetic research at the Sanger Institute, UK. Vivian's expertise lies in the domain of bioinformatics (ontological design, data/text mining, database curation) and laboratory investigation (cancer research, molecular biology and protein chemistry). She has publications in all these domains.

Ulf Leser holds a Diploma in computer science from the Technical University in München and a PhD in distributed query optimization from the Technical University Berlin. After spending some years as a project manager in industry, he was appointed a professor for Knowledge Management in Bioinformatis at Humboldt-Universität Berlin in 2003. His main research interests are information integration, text mining, and modelling and scalability of complex databases, all applied in a Life Science context.

Nadine Lucas is a researcher at the French National Center for Scientific Research CNRS. She works at Université de Caen Basse-Normandie in the GREYC laboratory (Groupe de Rercherche en Informatique, Image, Automatique et Electronique de Caen). Her research in text comparative linguistics and rhetoric started with academic writing. It later included NLP and encompassed news and web-based discussions. Her main interests are scale management in discourse parsing and multilingual NLP with scarce lexical resources. She currently is a member of the French Bingo2 project relating genomics and inductive data mining, where she focuses on textual data mining.

Maria Teresa Martín-Valdivia is lecturer in the Department of Computer Science at Jaén University (Spain). She received MS degree in computer science from the University of Granada, and PhD in computer science from Software Engineering Department of Málaga. Her current research interest includes natural language processing, tools for text mining, neural networks, machine learning algorithms, text categorization, multilingual and multimodal information retrieval. In addition, she is treasurer of SEPLN (Spanish Society of Natural Language Processing) Committee from 2007. She is member of Intelligent Systems of Information Access Research Group. She is author or co-author of more than 50 scientific publications, technical reviewer in several journals and in the program committee of some major conferences.

Arturo Montejo-Ráez is assistant professor in the Department of Computer Science at Jaén University (Spain). He received a MS degree in computer science at the University of Jaén in 1999, and a PhD in computer science at Software Engineering Department of Granada University in 2006. His current research includes information retrieval, text categorization and management systems of natural language processing, and spoken language dialogue systems.

Meenakshi Narayanswamy is a co-founder of Serene Innovations, a company with business focus on text analytics. She completed both her Bachelor's and Master's degree in biotechnology and is close to completing her PhD program in in computational biology. She is University Top Rank holder in her Master's degree. She is a recipient of a research fellowship from University Grants Commission, Govt. of India for her doctoral programme. Her PhD dissertation included the design of some parts of the RLIMS-P system.

Yun Niu is a post-doctoral researcher at the Ontario Cancer Institute, University Health Network since January 2007. Niu received her PhD in computer science from the University of Toronto in 2007. Her research focuses on question answering, information extraction, probabilistic classification in natural language processing and their applications in the biomedical domain. One of such applications is to extract important relations between biological entities, such as protein protein interactions. She was a member of the EPoCare project which aimed at providing accurate answers to questions posed by clinicians in patient treatment. Her role in the project was applying computational linguistics technologies to refine the results obtained by information retrieval. In her previous work, Niu investigated cause-effect relations in medical text, and developed automatic approaches to extract causal relations.

Jon Patrick graduated with his PhD in computer science from Monash University in 1978 after completing degrees at RMIT and Trinity College, Dublin. He has subsequently completed two degrees in psychology and he is a registered psychologist. He has held the chairs of Information Systems at Massey University and Sydney University. More recently he has moved to the chair of Language Technology to give more attention to his research in language processing. His early work in this field concentrated on processing systems for second language learners (English-Basque) and more recently he developed the widely reported Scamseek system for the Australian Securities and Investment Commission (ASIC) for which he was awarded the Eureka Science prize in 2005. Since then he has worked on applying language technology to medical contexts. He has built a number of technologies with his collaborators and introduced the first real-time language processing system for ward rounds with his collaborators at the Intensive Care Service of the Royal Prince Alfred Hospital, Sydney. He is also working with the Sydney West Area Health Service to introduce a range of IT research technologies into the AHS.

Chaveevan Pechsiri achieved a Bachelor's Degree in food science and technology from Kasetsart University, Thailand. She achieved both the Masters Degree in food sciences, the Masters Degree computer sciences from Mississippi State University, USA. She also achieved a Doctoral degree in computer engineering from Kasetsart University. Currently, she is an assistant professor at Dhurakij Pundij University and is currently researching on NLP.

Jean Pierre Pecuchet currently works as a full professor in Laboratoire d'Informatique, de Traitement de l'Information et des Systèmes, Institut National des Sciences Appliquées, Rouen, France, since 1988. His main research area regards the modelling and simulation of complex systems and the interactions between the users and the information systems. He is also interested in ontology modelling and multi-agent systems. His main research results are: the creation of an education simulator (projects ANTIC2 and Métascène), the modelling and the analysis of computerized medical records (project DOPAMINE), the methods and tools for evaluating the learner on the Web (project MARWAN) and contribution of ontology for finding information on the Web (projects ATONANT et VODEL).

José M. Perea-Ortega is a research member of the Intelligent Systems of Information Access Research Group in the University of Jaén (Spain). He received a MS degree in computer science at the University of Jaén and a PhD in computer science at Software Engineering Department of Granada University. His current research includes information retrieval, text categorization and management systems of natural language processing.

Piotr Pęzik received a PhD in computational linguistics from the University of Łódź, Poland. He is currently a member of the text mining group at the European Bioinformatics Institute in Cambridge, UK. He has contributed to the development of a number of Information Extraction and Information Retrieval tools and resources as part of both UK and European research projects, including the MedEvi search engine and the BioLexicon.

Sachit Rajbhandari, received a Master degree in information and communication technologies from Asian Institute of Technology (AIT), Thailand in 2006. He received his Bachelor degree in electronics engineering and Master degree in business studies from Tribhuvan University, Nepal in 2001 and 2003 respectively. He is working as an information management consultant at Food and Agriculture Organization of the United Nations (FAO). He had been involved in many software development projects since 2001 working at different software companies and institutions. His research interests are in Semantic Web, search engine, database management system, and information management.

K. E. Ravikumar is a co-founder of Serene Innovations, a company with prime focus on text analytics. As a CSIR senior research fellow in Anna University, he has completed all formalities for his PhD programme (Anna University) and is awaiting his defence. His PhD dissertation included the design of some parts of the RLIMS-P system. He received a BTech diploma in pharmaceutical technology, and a Masters in biotechnology. During his masters program, he was recipient of Junior research Fellowship from Directorate of Biotechnology, Govt. of India and received the University Gold medal award.

Dietrich Rebholz-Schuhmann, MD, PhD, studied medicine (University of Düsseldorf) and computer science (University of Passau). He worked in medical informatics research and at LION bioscience AG, Heidelberg, Germany, where he headed a research group in text mining and led the EUREKA research project „Bio-Path?. In 2003 he joined the EBI and thereafter served as area chair in text mining for the ISMB (2004, 2005 and 2007) and co-organized the Symposium for Semantic Mining in Biomedicine (2005 and 2008). He was member of the Network of Excellence "SemanticMining" (NoE 507505) and is team leader in the FP6-IST project "BOOTStrep" (contract FP-6 028099, www.bootstrep.eu). Furthermore, he has contributed major parts to the project plan of UKPMC that is currently instantiated at Manchester Information & Associated Services (MIMAS) and co-chairs the work package in biological information infrastructures of the ELIXIR project (part of the European initiative in scientific infrastructures ESFRI).

Alexandrin Rogozan currently works as associate professor in Laboratoire d'Informatique, de Traitement de l'Information et des Systèmes, Institut National des Sciences Appliquées, Rouen, France, since 2000. Her main research area regards the models for text indexation (using techniques for automatic language processing based on a controlled vocabulary and on terminologies), the models for image indexation (in order to create a digital and symbolic signature for image searching by keywords and/or content), the hybrid models for generation of kernel function for support vector machine (with applications in the problem of concept alignment based on definitions), the fusion models for ruttier obstacle classification and the models for compression for text clusterization.

Magali Roux-Rouquie (Roux-Dosseto) received a MS degree in biochemistry and cell biology and a PhD ("Doctorat de 3e cycle", 1979 and "Thèse d'état", 1984) at the University of Aix-Marseille II, France. Magali Roux-Rouquie was successively named assistant professor (Timone Hospital, Marseille, 1979-1981), research fellow CNRS (Immunology Center, Inserm-CNRS of Marseille, 1981-1983), full-time post-doc (Harvard University, Department of Molecular Biology Cambridge, USA, 1981-1983), director of research (Centre Hospitalo-Universitaire URA CNRS 1175, Marseille, 1984-1995), representative - "chargé de mission" - Ministry of Research, Paris, 1995-2000), director of research CNRS (GENATLAS Necker-University of Paris V Hospital, Paris 1998-2000), «Biosystems Engineering Modeling» team/group leader (Institut Pasteur, Paris, 2000-2004), director of research CNRS (Computer Science Laboratory of Paris VI UMR CNRS 7606, Paris, 2004). The main scientific interests of Magali Roux-Rouquie are knowledge organisation and standards in systems biology, molecular mechanisms of regulation in breast cancer, and regulation of human major histocompatibility complex class II genes and cytotoxic genes.

Ferran Sanz is professor of Biostatistics and Biomedical Informatics at the University Pompeu Fabra (UPF), Director of the IMIM-UPF joint Research Unit on Biomedical Informatics (GRIB, www.imim.es/grib), and currently vice-rector for scientific policy of the UPF. Author of about 100 articles in SCI indexed journals. Mentor of 17 PhD thesis. Coordinator of several EC-funded initiatives, as well as a STOA report for the European Parliament. President of the European Federation for Medicinal Chemistry from 2003 to 2005. Involved as invited expert in the genesis of the Innovative Medicines Initiative (www.imi-europe.org) and currently academic coordinator of the Spanish Platform Medicamentos Innovadores. Coordinator of the node of Biomedical Informatics of the Spanish Institute of Bioinformatics (INB).

Torsten Schiemann received his Diploma in computer science from Humboldt-Humboldt-Universität zu Berlin in 2006. He wrote his Master's thesis on word sense disambiguation at the Knowledge Management in Bioinformatics group. He currently works as a software engineer in industry.

Burr Settles is a graduate student in computer sciences at the University of Wisconsin, Madison. His research interests center on machine learning and its applications to text and data mining, including information extraction, information retrieval, and modeling social and biological networks. Burr is currently finishing his PhD thesis on active learning and multiple-instance learning algorithms for the rapid development of information management systems. He has released several open-source software projects related to his research, including ABNER (A Biomedical Named Entity Recognizer), which is described in this book.

Vijay Shanker is a professor in Computer Science at the University of Delaware. His primary research focus has been in the area of natural language processing and parsing. His current interests include information extraction, text mining and machine learning. He received his PhD in computer science from the University of Pennsylvania. He has served in program committees of over 40 conferences and has served a program committee co-chair of ACL and TAG+ conferences. He has served on editorial boards of computational linguistics and grammars journals. He has published close to 100 peer-reviewed papers.

Mário J. Silva received his undergraduate and Master degrees from the Instituto Superior Técnico, Lisboa, Portugal, and PhD degrees from the University of California, Berkeley, USA (1994). He joined the University of Lisbon (Faculty of Sciences) in 1996, where he is now associate professor (with Habilitation) in the Department of Informatics. He has published over 70 refereed technical papers and book chapters. He has advised 20 Master dissertations and 5 PhD theses, and leads a research team of 15 faculty, graduate students and technical staff (XLDB Group, http://xldb.fc.ul.pt). His current research interests are on information integration, information retrieval and text mining systems, with applications in biomedical informatics and geographic information systems. Prior research interests have included mobile computing systems, VLSI CAD and microelectronics.

L. Alfonso Ureña-López is senior lecturer in the Department of Computer Science at Jaén University (Spain). He received MS degree in computer science from the University of Granada, and PhD in computer science from Software Engineering Department of Granada. His PhD thesis was the winner of the 2001 Awards of the Spanish Society for Natural Language Processing. His current main research interest is intelligent search, including search engines, search assistants, natural language processing tools for text mining and retrieval and human computer interaction. Relevant topics include multilingual-multimodal information access, information synthesis and summarization, Semantic networks (wordnets, lexical acquisition, Web as corpus, word sense disambiguation), Web search engines (clustering and visualization of search results, portal search engines). Dr. Ureña was head of the Computer Science Department at University of Jaén (1997-2004). Currently he is deputy director of the Polytechnic School at Jaén. He is head and founder of Intelligent Systems of Information Access Research Group. Also, he is President of SEPLN since 2007 and editor of **Procesamiento de Lenguaje Natural Journal.** He has directed several research projects and several contracts with companies in technology transfer, as well as several Ph. D. *in Computer Science* and research works. He is author or co-author of more than 100 scientific publications, a technical reviewer in several journals and in the Program Committee of some major conferences.

Theodora A. Varvarigou received the BTech degree from the National Technical University of Athens, Athens, Greece in 1988, the MS degrees in electrical engineering (1989) and in computer science (1991) from Stanford University, Stanford, California in 1989 and the PhD degree from Stanford University as well in 1991. She worked at AT&T Bell Labs, Holmdel, New Jersey between 1991 and 1995. Between 1995 and 1997 she worked as an assistant professor at the Technical University of Crete, Chania, Greece. Since 1997 she was elected as an assistant professor while since 2007 she is a professor at the National Technical University of Athens, and Director of the Postgraduate Course "Engineering Economics Systems". Prof. Varvarigou has great experience in the area of Semantic Web technologies, scheduling over distributed platforms, embedded systems and grid computing. In this area, she has published more than 150 papers in leading journals and conferences. She has participated and coordinated several EU funded projects such as IRMOS, SCOVIS, POLYMNIA, Akogrimo, NextGRID, BEinGRID, Memphis, MKBEEM, MARIDES, CHALLENGERS, FIDIS, and other.

Cathy H. Wu is professor of Biochemistry and Molecular Biology and director of the Protein Information Resource (PIR). With background and experience in both biology and computer science, she has conducted bioinformatics and computational biology research for 20 years. Since 1999 she has led the development of PIR as a major public bioinformatics resource that supports genomic, proteomic and systems biology research. Dr. Wu has served on several advisory boards, including the HUPO Board of Directors, the PDB Scientific Advisory Board, the NIGMS Protein Structure Initiative Advisory Committee, and the NSF TeraGrid User Advisory Committee. She has also served on numerous program committees for international bioinformatics and proteomics conferences and workshops. She has published about over peer-reviewed papers and three books, and given more than 100 invited lectures. Her research interests include protein evolution-structure-function relationships, proteomics informatics and computational systems biology, biomedical text mining and ontology, and bioinformatics cyberinfrastructure.

Yitao Zhang is a PhD student in Health Information Technologies Research Laboratory (HITRL), School of Information Technologies, The University of Sydney. He holds a Bachelor degree of engineering from Tsinghua University, China, in 1998, and a Master degree of information technology from The University of Sydney, Australia, in 2004. His current research focuses on using natural language processing techniques to extract domain-specific knowledge from medical case studies which are reported in openly-available journal articles. His other research interests include textual paraphrasing and entailment, and assigning meaningful medical concepts, such as ICD-9-CM codes, to free-text clinical notes through a text categorization approach.

Index

D

E

M

N

O

P

Q

R

S

T

U